Visceral and Ectopic Fat

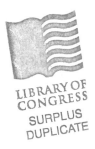

Visceral and Ectopic Fat
Risk Factors for Type 2 Diabetes, Atherosclerosis, and Cardiovascular Disease

Edited by

Hildo J. Lamb
Prof. Hildo J. Lamb, MD, PhD. Department of Radiology,
Cardio Vascular Imaging Group (CVIG), Leiden University Medical Center,
Leiden, the Netherlands

ELSEVIER

Elsevier
Radarweg 29, PO Box 211, 1000 AE Amsterdam, Netherlands
The Boulevard, Langford Lane, Kidlington, Oxford OX5 1GB, United Kingdom
50 Hampshire Street, 5th Floor, Cambridge, MA 02139, United States

Notices

Knowledge and best practice in this field are constantly changing. As new research and experience broaden our understanding, changes in research methods, professional practices, or medical treatment may become necessary.

Practitioners and researchers must always rely on their own experience and knowledge in evaluating and using any information, methods, compounds, or experiments described herein. In using such information or methods they should be mindful of their own safety and the safety of others, including parties for whom they have a professional responsibility.

To the fullest extent of the law, neither the Publisher nor the authors, contributors, or editors, assume any liability for any injury and/or damage to persons or property as a matter of products liability, negligence or otherwise, or from any use or operation of any methods, products, instructions, or ideas contained in the material herein.

ISBN: 978-0-12-822186-0

For information on all Elsevier publications visit our website at https://www.elsevier.com/books-and-journals

Publisher: Stacy Masucci
Acquisitions Editor: Patricia M. Osborn
Editorial Project Manager: Tim Eslava
Production Project Manager: Omer Mukthar
Cover Designer: Mark Rogers

Typeset by TNQ Technologies

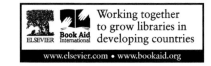

Working together
to grow libraries in
developing countries

www.elsevier.com • www.bookaid.org

Contents

List of contributors   xiii
Preface   xvii

Part I
Fat stores

1. Overall, abdominal, and visceral obesity in men and women: an introduction   3

Renée de Mutsert and Jean-Pierre Després

Overweight and obesity: definition, prevalence, and relation to disease   3
  Definition of overweight and obesity   3
  Prevalence of overweight and obesity   5
  Obesity-related mortality and diseases   6
Body fat distribution: abdominal obesity, visceral fat, and ectopic fat   8
  Body fat distribution and abdominal obesity   8
  Visceral adipose tissue and subcutaneous adipose tissue   9
  Lipid overflow hypothesis and ectopic fat accumulation   11
Sex differences in body fat distribution and health consequences   11
Summary and conclusion   14
References   14

2. Obesity and fat distribution in children and adolescents   19

Jacob C. Seidell

Childhood obesity has reached pandemic proportions   19
Abdominal obesity in children is a better indicator of health risks than BMI   19
  Visceral fat in relation to cardiomentabolic health in young people   20
Determinants of visceral fat in children and adolescents   21

Sex   21
Genetics of visceral fat accumulation   21
Ethnicity   21
Chronic stress (cortisol)   21
Behavioral determinants of visceral fat   21
Measurement of visceral fat in children   22
  Imaging techniques   22
  The waist circumference or waist/height ratio as a measure of visceral fat in clinical practice and public health   22
  Classification of abdominal obesity in children by the waist/height ratio   22
Visceral fat and metabolic risk factors in children and adolescents   23
Conclusions   23
References   24

3. Brown adipose tissue: metabolic role and non-invasive quantification in humans   25

Andreas Paulus and Matthias Bauwens

BAT physiology   25
Background on history of BAT: perceived impact on human health and scientific interest in past three decades   25
Overview of potential analysis techniques for assessing BAT activity   26
  Invasive techniques   29
  Noninvasive techniques   29
Overview of tracers with their molecular targets   31
Discussion: clinical applications?   32
References   33

4. Epicardial and pericoronary fat   39

Pál Maurovich-Horvat and György Jermendy

Introduction   39
Terminology   39
Anatomical characteristics of EAT   40
  Data based on autopsy   40
  Findings from clinical settings   41

Biochemical features and physiological
function of EAT   41
Cardiac imaging of EAT   42
EAT in the pathomechanism of atherosclerosis   44
EAT in other cardiac diseases   47
Atrial fibrillation   47
Heart failure   47
Inflammation   48
Epicardial fat necrosis   48
EAT in metabolic diseases   49
EAT in patients with COVID-19   49
Treatment options for modifying EAT volume   50
References   50

Part II
Ectopic fat stores

5. Non-invasive profiling of ectopic and adipose lipids using magnetic resonance spectroscopy and imaging   59

Radka Klepochová and Martin Krššák

Introduction   59
Lipid composition and its consequences in
magnetic resonance spectroscopy   60
In vivo magnetic resonance spectroscopy   60
Magnetic resonance spectroscopy data
acquisition   61
Analysis of the magnetic resonance
spectrscopy data   64
Magnetic resonance imaging   66
Applications   66
Adipose tissue (deep subcutaneous adipose
tissue/visceral adipose tissue/brown adipose
tissue)   66
Bone marrow fat   67
Breast   68
Liver   68
Heart   69
Skeletal muscle   70
Summary   70
References   70

6. Flexibility of ectopic lipids in skeletal/cardiac muscle and liver   75

Hannah Loher, Chris Boesch, Roland Kreis and Emanuel Christ

Measurement of the flexibility of ectopic lipids   75
Biopsy   75

Ectopic lipids in the context of negative energy
balance   75
Single bout of exercise   75
Fasting   78
Ectopic lipids in the context of positive energy
balance   78
Short-term high fat diet   78
Long-term high fat diet   78
High fructose/glucose diet   78
References   79

7. Nonalcoholic fatty liver disease: from a benign finding to a life-threatening cardiometabolic liver disease   83

Koen C. van Son, A.G. (Onno) Holleboom and Maarten E. Tushuizen

Introduction   83
Pathogenesis   84
Genetic and epigenetic determinants   84
Nutrition   85
Insulin resistance and lipotoxicity   86
Inflammation and necroapoptosis   86
Adipocytokines   86
Formation of fibrosis   86
Urea cycle dysregulation   86
Bile acids   87
Microbiome   87
Clinical consequences   87
Liver cirrhosis   87
Hepatocellular carcinoma   87
Cardiovascular disease   87
Diagnostics   88
Treatment   88
Obesity and lifestyle   88
Nutrition   89
Insulin sensitivity   89
GLP1 receptor agonists and GLP1 analogs   89
SGLT2 inhibitors   89
Lipotoxicity   89
Oxidative stress   89
Bile acids   90
Apoptosis   90
Inflammation and fibrosis   90
Combination therapy   90
Probiotics and fecal microbiome transplantation   90
Development and implementation of clinical
care paths and guidelines for NAFLD   91
Primary care   91
Secondary and tertiary care   91
Conclusion   92
References   92

8. Myocardial lipids—techniques and applications of proton magnetic resonance spectroscopy of the human heart   99

Adrianus J. Bakermans

Localized proton magnetic resonance spectroscopy of the heart	99
Quantification of myocardial metabolite content	104
Lipids in the healthy human myocardium—effects of nutrition, fasting, and exercise	106
Gender	106
Aging	106
Body mass index	106
Athletes and exercise	107
Nutrition	107
Myocardial lipids in disease	108
Insulin resistance and type 2 diabetes	108
Other diseases	109
Concluding remarks and outlook	110
References	110

9. Pancreas ectopic fat: imaging-based quantification   117

Alexandre Triay Bagur, Matthew Robson, Daniel Bulte and Michael Brady

Introduction	117
Pancreas and ectopic fat	118
Pancreas state assessment	120
Information from MRI	122
Pancreas volume	122
MRI-derived fat fraction	122
Pancreas morphology	123
Pancreas fibroinflammation	125
Big Data and AI	125
Future directions	126
References	127

10. Fat accumulation around and within the kidney   131

Ling Lin, Ilona A. Dekkers and Hildo J. Lamb

Introduction	131
Perirenal fat and renal sinus fat	131
Anatomical characteristics	131
Histological and pathophysiological characteristics	134
Imaging-based quantification	135
Renal parenchyma triglyceride	139
Histological characteristics and pathophysiological relevance	139

Imaging-based quantification	141
Clinical implications of excessive kidney fat	142
Association with chronic kidney disease and insulin resistance	142
Association with cardiovascular diseases	142
Implications for other diseases	143
Changes of excessive kidney fat after intervention	143
Summary and perspectives	143
References	144

11. Skeletal muscle fat   149

Ivica Just and Martin Krššák

Introduction	149
Skeletal muscle fat infiltration	149
Flexibility of IMAT fatty infiltration	151
Intramyocellular lipids	152
Flexibility of IMCL	154
Methods to assess lipids in the muscle	155
Computed tomography—CT	155
MRI of skeletal muscle	156
Postprocessing and assessment of fat infiltration imaging	157
MRS of skeletal muscle	158
Postprocessing and quantitation of 1H-MR spectra from skeletal muscle	159
Summary	160
References	161

12. Bone marrow adipose tissue   169

Bénédicte Gaborit, Sonia Severin and Philippe Valet

Abbreviations	169
Introduction	170
Bone marrow fat origin	170
Main characteristics in physiology	171
Main characteristics	171
Variation during growth	171
Variation with aging	172
Regional specific differences in BMAT composition	172
Effect of exercise and caloric restriction	173
Impact of unloading	173
Microscopic aspect	174
In vivo imaging	174
Computed tomography	174
Magnetic resonance imaging	176
Secretory profile and endocrine regulation of BMAT	178
BMAT and skeletal health	179
BMAT and hematopoiesis	180
BMAT in cancer	181
BMAT and metabolic diseases	181

Concluding remarks   182
References   183

Part III
Regulation of fat stores

13. Regulation of fat stores—endocrinological pathways   193

Peter Wolf, Thomas Scherer and Michael Krebs

Insulin   193
Thyroid hormone   195
Growth hormone   196
Cortisol   198
Sex hormones   198
Summary   200
Acknowledgments   201
References   201

14. Inflammation of the adipose tissue: metabolic consequences during weight (re)gain and loss   205

Mandala Ajie and Rinke Stienstra

Introduction   205
Chronic low-grade inflammation of the adipose tissue   205
Weight gain   206
Weight loss   208
Weight regain   209
Adipose tissue inflammation during obesity: how does it lead to complications?   211
Insulin resistance   211
Atherosclerosis   211
Determining adipose tissue inflammation   211
Conclusion   212
References   212

Part IV
Clinical aspects

15. Role of adipose tissue remodeling in diabetic heart disease   217

Amanda MacCannell, Sam Straw and Eylem Levelt

Adipose tissue physiology in health and the pathophysiological role of adipose tissue in transition from obesity to diabetes   217

Adipose tissue and signaling pathways in diabetes and heart disease   218
Sex differences in adipose tissue remodeling effects on cardiovascular disease   221
Adiponectin, proinflammatory adipocytokines, and cardiovascular disease in diabetes   222
Imaging ectopic adiposity in patients with type 2 diabetes mellitus   222
Conclusions   223
References   223

16. Cardiovascular disease   229

Michiel Sala, Albert de Roos and Hildo J. Lamb

Introduction   229
Obesity hypertension: role of magnetic resonance imaging   229
Fat deposits in obesity hypertension   230
Cardiovascular structure and function in obesity hypertension   232
Coronary artery disease in obesity   234
Arrhythmias   237
Heart failure   238
Conclusion   241
References   241

17. Obesity in relation to cardiorenal function   243

Isabel T.N. Nguyen, Jaap A. Joles, Marianne C. Verhaar, Hildo J. Lamb and Ilona A. Dekkers

Introduction   243
Obesity-related cardiorenal dysfunction   243
Overview of five-part classification system for cardiorenal syndrome   243
The pathophysiology of cardiorenal syndrome   244
Preclinical studies   247
Obese animal models of cardiorenal syndrome   247
The Zucker rat and substrains as proposed models of the metabolic cardiorenal syndrome   250
Abnormalities in cardiac function in obesity   250
Abnormalities in renal function in obesity   252
CKD as a risk factor for HFpEF in obese animals   252
Sex differences in the cardiorenal interaction   253
Epidemiological and translational studies in humans   253

Estimating obesity's risk for renal and cardiac dysfunction 253

Metabolic imaging studies of ectopic fat storage in heart and kidney 254

Dietary effects on ectopic fat storage in heart and kidney 255

Effects of glycemic control on ectopic fat storage in heart and kidney 258

Future outlook 258

Novel developments in preclinical studies 258

Multiorgan imaging in the management of CRS in obese individuals 258

Personalized approach in the management of obesity-related CRS 259

Conclusion 259

Funding 259

References 259

18. Obesity and asthma 265

Daisuke Murakami, Yuichi Saito and Ryota Higuchi

Physical function: lung function and genetic factors 265

Physical effects and genetic background of obesity and asthma 265

Obesity and respiratory function 265

Racial differences 266

Genetic factors in obesity and asthma 266

Epidemiology: clinical features and findings 267

Epidemiological study of obesity and asthma in children and adults 267

Epidemiological studies in children 267

Epidemiological studies in adults 269

Disease pathogenesis: immunological mechanisms 270

Pathogenesis of obesity and asthma 270

Abnormal lipid metabolism 270

Increased oxidative stress 270

Increased airway inflammation 271

Inflammation in adipose tissue 272

Abnormalities in adipokines 272

Decreased steroid responsiveness 272

Insulin resistance 272

Summary 273

Acknowledgments 273

References 273

19. Obesity and the brain: structural and functional imaging studies, and opportunities for large-scale imaging genetics 281

Ilona A. Dekkers, Janey Jiang, Hildo J. Lamb and Philip Jansen

Introduction 281

Structural brain imaging and obesity 281

Body Mass Index 282

Fat distribution 283

Diffusion tensor imaging 283

Visceral fat 283

Hypothalamic function 284

Functional brain imaging studies and obesity 285

Genetic analyses of obesity and the brain 288

Genome-wide association studies 288

Polygenic risk scores 290

Mendelian randomization 290

Future directions 290

Conclusions 291

References 291

Part V
Interventions

20. The impact of very-low-calorie diets on ectopic fat deposition 297

Jennifer J. Rayner and Ines Abdesselam

Introduction 297

Visceral adipose tissue 297

Hepatic ectopic fat 299

Very-low-calorie diet in the treatment of type II diabetes 300

Calorie restriction and cardiac lipid deposition 301

Skeletal muscle lipid metabolism and very-low-calorie diets 302

Impact of very-low-calorie diet on bone marrow fat 303

Conclusion 303

References 304

21. Intermittent fasting   307

Marjolein P. Schoonakker, Elske L. van den Burg, Petra G. van Peet, Hildo J. Lamb, Mattijs E. Numans and Hanno Pijl

Abbreviations	307
Intermittent fasting methods	307
Physiology of intermittent energy restriction	308
Effect of intermittent energy restriction on health parameters in animal models	308
Effect of intermittent energy restriction on weight and fat in animal models	308
Effect of intermittent energy restriction on metabolic parameters in animal models	310
Effect of intermittent energy restriction on other health parameters in animal models	310
Effect of intermittent energy restriction on health parameters in humans	311
Effect of intermittent energy restriction on weight and fat in humans	312
Effect of intermittent energy restriction on metabolic parameters in humans	314
Effect of intermittent energy restriction on other health parameters in humans	314
The effect of intermittent energy restriction versus continuous energy restriction on weight and fat in humans	315
Sustainability of intermittent energy restriction	316
Potential risks of intermittent energy restriction	316
Conclusion	317
References	317

22. Exercise   321

Joseph Henson, Emer M. Brady and Gaurav S. Gulsin

Introduction	321
Definition of key terms	321
Current recommendations	321
Aerobic training interventions	323
Resistance training interventions	326
Aerobic and resistance training interventions	327
The role of intensity	327
How much is enough?	327
Mechanisms underlying the effects of exercise on visceral and ectopic adipose tissue	327
The unique role of exercise in the prevention and management of chronic disease	328
Conclusion	330
References	330

23. Combined lifestyle interventions   333

Jena Shaw Tronieri, Karl Nadolsky and Monica Agarwal

Introduction	333
Medical nutrition therapy	333
Introduction	333
Dietary patterns	333
Summary	336
Physical activity	337
Introduction	337
Benefits of physical activity	337
Recommendations for physical activity	338
Adipose tissue and physical activity	339
Type and duration of physical activity	339
Recommendations	340
Sleep	340
Introduction	340
Obstructive sleep apnea	341
Recommendations	341
Behavioral interventions	341
Treatment structure	341
Behavior therapy principles	341
Goal setting	342
Self-monitoring	342
Problem-solving	343
Cognitive techniques	343
Efficacy of multicomponent behavioral interventions	343
The challenge of dissemination	344
Behavioral intervention and antiobesity medication	345
Behavioral intervention and bariatric surgery	345
Summary	345
References	346

24. Medical therapy   353

Janina Senn and Stefan Fischli

Introduction	353
Metformin	354
Mechanism of action/side effects	354
Clinical efficacy	354
Orlistat	355
Mechanism of actions/side effects	355
Clinical efficacy	356
Glucagon-like peptide 1 receptor agonists	356
Mechanisms of action/side effects	356
Clinical efficacy	357
Sodium glucose cotransporter-2 inhibitors	357
Mechanisms of action/side effects	357
Clinical efficacy	358
Conclusions	359
References	359

25. **Gastric volume reduction interventions and effects on visceral fat and metabolic biomarkers** 363

Sean M. O'Neill and Stacy A. Brethauer

Introduction 363
Endoscopic sleeve gastroplasty 364
   Meta-analyses 365
   Case series 367
   Metabolic effects 370
Primary obesity surgery endoluminal (POSE) procedure 371
   Meta-analysis 371
   Metabolic effects 371
Intragastric balloon therapy 372
   IGB types 372
   Meta-analyses and controlled trials 372
   Metabolic and visceral fat effects of intragastric balloons 373
Conclusion 373
References 374

26. **Roux-en-Y gastric bypass: influence on adipose tissue and metabolic homeostasis** 377

Christopher P. Menzel, Charles R. Flynn and Wayne J. English

Introduction 377
RYGB procedure description 377
Mechanisms of RYGB 377

RYGB—effect on weight loss and obesity-related comorbidities 380
Pathogenesis of obesity through adipose tissue 381
Molecular markers in obesity have changed quantities after RYGB 381
Changes in adipose tissue 382
Bile acids and metabolic and bariatric surgery 383
Visceral fat 383
Ectopic fat 385
Subcutaneous fat 386
Overview of metabolic benefits after RYGB 386
Class 1 obesity and metabolic and bariatric surgery 387
Conclusion 388
References 388

27. **Fecal transplant** 391

M.M. Ruissen, J.J. Keller and Maarten E. Tushuizen

The gut microbiome 391
Gut microbiome modulation 392
Fecal microbiome transplantation 393
Fecal transplantations—murine models 394
Fecal microbiome transplantation in humans 395
References 396

Index 399

List of contributors

Ines Abdesselam, Oxford Centre for Clinical Magnetic Resonance Research, Division of Cardiovascular Medicine, Radcliffe Department of Medicine, University of Oxford, Oxford, United Kingdom

Monica Agarwal, Department of Medicine, University of Alabama at Birmingham, Birmingham, AL, United States

Mandala Ajie, Department of Internal Medicine, Radboud University Medical Center, Nijmegen, the Netherlands

Adrianus J. Bakermans, Department of Radiology and Nuclear Medicine, Amsterdam University Medical Centers, University of Amsterdam, Amsterdam, the Netherlands

Matthias Bauwens, Department of Radiology and Nuclear Medicine, Maastricht University Medical Center, Maastricht, the Netherlands; School of Nutrition and Translational Research in Metabolism (NUTRIM), Maastricht University, Maastricht, the Netherlands; Department of Nuclear Medicine, University Hospital RWTH Aachen, Aachen, Germany

Chris Boesch, University of Bern, Bern, Switzerland

Emer M. Brady, University of Leicester and the NIHR Leicester Biomedical Research Centre, Leicester, United Kingdom

Michael Brady, Perspectum Ltd, Oxford, United Kingdom

Stacy A. Brethauer, Department of Surgery, Division of GI and General Surgery, The Ohio State University Wexner Medical Center, Columbus, OH, United States

Daniel Bulte, Department of Engineering Science, University of Oxford, Oxford, United Kingdom

Emanuel Christ, Division of Endocrinology, Diabetology and Metabolism, University Hospital of Basel, Basel, Switzerland

Ilona A. Dekkers, Department of Radiology, Cardio Vascular Imaging Group (CVIG), Leiden University Medical Center, Leiden, the Netherlands

Renée de Mutsert, Department of Clinical Epidemiology, Leiden University and Medical Center, Leiden, the Netherlands

Albert de Roos, Leiden University Medical Center, Radiology Department, Leiden, the Netherlands

Jean-Pierre Després, VITAM Centre de recherche en santé durable, CIUSSS Capitale-Nationale, Department of Kinesiology, Faculty of Medicine, Université Laval, Québec, Canada

Wayne J. English, Vanderbilt University Medical Center, Department of Surgery, Nashville, TN, United States

Stefan Fischli, Luzerner Kantonsspital, Division of Endocrinology, Diabetes and Clinical Nutrition, Luzern, Switzerland

Charles R. Flynn, Vanderbilt University Medical Center, Department of Surgery, Nashville, TN, United States

Bénédicte Gaborit, Aix Marseille Univ, INSERM, INRAE, C2VN, Marseille, France; Department of Endocrinology, Metabolic Diseases and Nutrition, Pôle ENDO, APHM, Marseille, France

Gaurav S. Gulsin, University of Leicester and the NIHR Leicester Biomedical Research Centre, Leicester, United Kingdom

Joseph Henson, University of Leicester and the NIHR Leicester Biomedical Research Centre, Leicester, United Kingdom

Ryota Higuchi, Department of Otorhinolaryngology, Graduate School of Medical Sciences, Kyushu University, Fukuoka, Japan

A.G. (Onno) Holleboom, Department of Internal Medicine, Amsterdam University Medical Center, Amsterdam, the Netherlands

Philip Jansen, Department of Human Genetics, Amsterdam University Medical Centers, the Netherlands; Department of Complex Trait Genetics, VU University Amsterdam, Amsterdam, the Netherlands; Netherlands Institute for Neuroscience (NIN), an Institute of the Royal Academy of Arts and Sciences, Amsterdam, the Netherlands

György Jermendy, Bajcsy-Zsilinszky Teaching Hospital, Medical Department, Budapest, Hungary

Janey Jiang, Department of Radiology, Haga Ziekenhuis, Den Haag, the Netherlands

Jaap A. Joles, Department of Nephrology and Hypertension, University Medical Center Utrecht, Utrecht, the Netherlands

Ivica Just, Division of Endocrinology and Metabolism, Department of Medicine III, Medical University of Vienna, Vienna, Austria; High-Field MR Centre, Department of Biomedical Imaging and Image-guided Therapy, Medical University of Vienna, Vienna, Austria

J.J. Keller, Department of Gastroenterology, Haaglanden Medical Center, The Hague, the Netherlands

Radka Klepochová, Division of Endocrinology and Metabolism, Department of Medicine III, Medical University of Vienna, Vienna, Austria; High-Field MR Centre, Department of Biomedical Imaging and Image-guided Therapy, Medical University of Vienna, Vienna, Austria

Michael Krebs, Division of Endocrinology and Metabolism, Department of Internal Medicine III, Medical University of Vienna, Austria

Roland Kreis, Magnetic Resonance Methodology, Institute of Diagnostic and Interventional Neuroradiology, University of Bern, Bern, Switzerland

Martin Krššák, Division of Endocrinology and Metabolism, Department of Medicine III, Medical University of Vienna, Vienna, Austria; High-Field MR Centre, Department of Biomedical Imaging and Image-guided Therapy, Medical University of Vienna, Vienna, Austria

Hildo J. Lamb, Department of Radiology, Cardio Vascular Imaging Group (CVIG), Leiden University Medical Center, Leiden, the Netherlands

Eylem Levelt, University of Leeds, Multidisciplinary Cardiovascular Research Centre and Biomedical Imaging Science Department, Leeds Institute of Cardiovascular and Metabolic Medicine, Leeds, United Kingdom; Leeds Teaching Hospitals NHS Trust, Department of Cardiology, Leeds, United Kingdom

Ling Lin, The Eighth Affiliated Hospital of Sun Yat-sen University, Shenzhen, China; Leiden University Medical Center, Leiden, the Netherlands

Hannah Loher, Division of Endocrinology and Diabetology, Kantonsspital Lucerne, Lucerne, Switzerland

Amanda MacCannell, University of Leeds, Multidisciplinary Cardiovascular Research Centre and Biomedical Imaging Science Department, Leeds Institute of Cardiovascular and Metabolic Medicine, Leeds, United Kingdom

Pál Maurovich-Horvat, Semmelweis University, Faculty of Medicine, Medical Imaging Centre, Budapest, Hungary

Christopher P. Menzel, Vanderbilt University Medical Center, Department of Surgery, Nashville, TN, United States

Daisuke Murakami, Department of Otorhinolaryngology, Graduate School of Medical Sciences, Kyushu University, Fukuoka, Japan

Karl Nadolsky, Department of Medicine, Michigan State University College of Human Medicine, Grand Rapids, MI, United States

Isabel T.N. Nguyen, Department of Nephrology and Hypertension, University Medical Center Utrecht, Utrecht, the Netherlands

Mattijs E. Numans, Public Health and Primary Care, Leiden University Medical Center, Leiden, the Netherlands

Sean M. O'Neill, Department of Surgery, Division of Minimally Invasive Surgery, University of Michigan, Ann Arbor, MI, United States

Andreas Paulus, Department of Radiology and Nuclear Medicine, Maastricht University Medical Center, Maastricht, the Netherlands

Hanno Pijl, Internal Medicine, Leiden University Medical Center, Leiden, the Netherlands

Jennifer J. Rayner, Oxford Centre for Clinical Magnetic Resonance Research, Division of Cardiovascular Medicine, Radcliffe Department of Medicine, University of Oxford, Oxford, United Kingdom

Matthew Robson, Perspectum Ltd, Oxford, United Kingdom

M.M. Ruissen, Department of Internal Medicine, Leiden University Medical Center, Leiden, the Netherlands

Yuichi Saito, Department of Otorhinolaryngology, Graduate School of Medical Sciences, Kyushu University, Fukuoka, Japan

Michiel Sala, Leiden University Medical Center, Radiology Department, Leiden, the Netherlands

Thomas Scherer, Division of Endocrinology and Metabolism, Department of Internal Medicine III, Medical University of Vienna, Austria

Marjolein P. Schoonakker, Public Health and Primary Care, Leiden University Medical Center, Leiden, the Netherlands

Jacob C. Seidell, Department of Health Sciences and Sarphati Amsterdam, Vrije Universiteit Amsterdam, Amsterdam, the Netherlands

Janina Senn, Luzerner Kantonsspital, Division of Endocrinology, Diabetes and Clinical Nutrition, Luzern, Switzerland

Sonia Severin, INSERM U1048 and Paul Sabatier University, Institute of Cardiovascular and Metabolic Diseases, Toulouse, France

Rinke Stienstra, Department of Internal Medicine, Radboud University Medical Center, Nijmegen, the Netherlands; Division of Human Nutrition and Health, Wageningen University, Wageningen, the Netherlands

Sam Straw, University of Leeds, Multidisciplinary Cardiovascular Research Centre and Biomedical Imaging Science Department, Leeds Institute of Cardiovascular and Metabolic Medicine, Leeds, United Kingdom; Leeds Teaching Hospitals NHS Trust, Department of Cardiology, Leeds, United Kingdom

Alexandre Triay Bagur, Department of Engineering Science, University of Oxford, Oxford, United Kingdom; Perspectum Ltd, Oxford, United Kingdom

Jena Shaw Tronieri, Department of Psychiatry, Perelman School of Medicine at the University of Pennsylvania, Philadelphia, PA, United States

Maarten E. Tushuizen, Department of Gastroenterology and Hepatology, Leiden University Medical Center, Leiden, the Netherlands

Philippe Valet, Restore UMR 1301 Inserm, 5070 CNRS, Université Paul Sabatier, Toulouse, France

Elske L. van den Burg, Public Health and Primary Care, Leiden University Medical Center, Leiden, the Netherlands

Petra G. van Peet, Public Health and Primary Care, Leiden University Medical Center, Leiden, the Netherlands

Koen C. van Son, Department of Gastroenterology and Hepatology, Radboud University Medical Center, Nijmegen, the Netherlands; Department of Internal Medicine, Amsterdam University Medical Center, Amsterdam, the Netherlands; Department of Gastroenterology and Hepatology, Leiden University Medical Center, Leiden, the Netherlands

Marianne C. Verhaar, Department of Nephrology and Hypertension, University Medical Center Utrecht, Utrecht, the Netherlands

Peter Wolf, Division of Endocrinology and Metabolism, Department of Internal Medicine III, Medical University of Vienna, Austria

Preface

Contemporary lifestyle is associated with a worldwide increase in obesity and poses severe challenges to sustainability of our healthcare system. Typical characteristics of obesity are accumulation of visceral and ectopic fat, which are major risk factors for development of type 2 diabetes, atherosclerosis, and cardiovascular disease. Originally I was trained as a biologist. After my PhD thesis, I developed interest in the pathophysiology and behavior of (ectopic) fat stores during and after intervention in relation to cardiovascular metabolism and function. I vividly remember that in my direct academic surrounding this topic was regarded as a dead end road, since "fat is just sitting there."

First experiments in Leiden showed intriguing unexpected changes in myocardial fat content in response to fasting and dietary interventions. For example, after three days of fasting by healthy volunteers, myocardial triglyceride content measured by ^{1}H-MR spectroscopy surprisingly increased, which is most likely an evolutionary heritage to prepare for even worse times with energy deprivation and linked to the current obesity epidemic. This finding was encouraging to try to further unravel lipid metabolism and was an inspiration for trials with medical intervention and initiated my shift to medicine and radiology. After longer-term calorie restriction, myocardial fat content decreased, which was associated with improvement of diastolic heart function. Current hypothesis we are working on is that besides visceral fat, the fatty liver plays an underestimated central role as risk factor for development of type 2 diabetes, atherosclerosis, and cardiovascular disease.

This book tries to cover a broad spectrum related to visceral and ectopic fat accumulation. In part 1 general epidemiological aspects are discussed on visceral fat, brown fat, pericardial, and peri-coronary fat. Part 2 describes ectopic fat accumulation in the liver, myocardium, pancreas, kidney, skeletal muscle, and bone marrow. Part 3 covers endocrinologic regulation of fat stores and the link between inflammation of fat tissue and obesity. Part 4 has focus on the clinical aspects relating to diabetic cardiomyopathy, cardiovascular disease, cardiorenal interaction, pulmonary function, and brain atrophy. Part 5 provides an overview of therapeutic options, ranging from very-low-calorie diet, intermittent fasting, exercise, and combined lifestyle intervention to medical therapy, gastric surgery, and fecal transplant.

I'm highly indebted to the authors from all over the world who contributed to this book during challenging times of the corona pandemic. Despite difficult personal circumstances, all authors delivered excellent quality content. Thank you very much for your commitment and continuous support! Obviously, not all topics relating to obesity and visceral fat could be covered, so I hope we have the opportunity to provide you as a reader with an update in coming years.

Prof. Hildo J. Lamb, MD, MSc, PhD, EBCR
Leiden, The Netherlands

Part I

Fat stores

Chapter 1

Overall, abdominal, and visceral obesity in men and women: an introduction

Renée de Mutsert[1] and Jean-Pierre Després[2]

[1]Department of Clinical Epidemiology, Leiden University and Medical Center, Leiden, the Netherlands; [2]VITAM Centre de recherche en santé durable, CIUSSS Capitale-Nationale, Department of Kinesiology, Faculty of Medicine, Université Laval, Québec, Canada

Overweight and obesity: definition, prevalence, and relation to disease

Definition of overweight and obesity

Overweight and obesity are defined by the World Health Organization (WHO) as abnormal or excessive body fat accumulation that presents a risk to health [1,2]. WHO defines overweight as a body mass index (BMI) equal to or more than 25, and obesity as a BMI equal to or more than 30 [1]. The BMI is a simple index of weight-for-height that is commonly used to classify overweight and obesity in adults. It is defined as a person's body weight in kilograms divided by the square of the body height in meters (kg/m^2). This weight/height^2 index was originally developed by Adolphe Quetelet (1796−874), a Belgian mathematician, astronomer, and statistician. He had observed that body weight in kilograms was proportional to the square of the height in meters and proposed the so-called Quetelet Index in 1832 [3,4]. It was not until 1970 that the Quetelet index and other indices of relative weight were compared with measures of body fatness in several studies [5−7]. Judged by the criteria of correlation with body height (lowest is best) and measures of body fatness (highest is best), the Quetelet index proved best [6,7] and was termed the body mass index in 1972 b y Ancel Keys (1904−2004) [6].

On the basis of the relation of the BMI with mortality, the WHO originally identified three grades of overweight: grade 1 overweight ($25.0−29.9\ kg/m^2$), grade 2 overweight ($30.0−39.9\ kg/m^2$), and grade 3 overweight ($\geq40.0\ kg/m^2$) [8]. In a following report of a WHO Consultation on Obesity in 1998, an additional subdivision was added because management options regarding prevention and treatment of obesity differ above a BMI of 35 [9]. The classification of overweight in adults according to BMI is shown in Table 1.1. It must be noted that this classification is the same for both men and women and that the BMI cutoff points are somewhat arbitrary along a continuum of increasing disease risk with increasing BMI. In addition, this classification is based on data from Europe and the United States. Because the health risks associated with obesity occur at a lower BMI in Asian populations than in Western populations, separate criteria to identify overweight and obesity in Asian populations were proposed by the Asia Pacific Cohort Studies Collaboration [10]. They indicated that, in Asian populations, overweight should be classified as a BMI of 23 or higher and obesity as a BMI of 25 or higher (Table 1.1) [10]. Nevertheless, because of the large variations in associations between BMI and health risks in Asian populations, in 2004 a WHO expert consultation decided not to redefine cutoff points for each population separately and agreed that the WHO BMI cutoff points should be retained as international classification [11].

In simple terms, obesity is a consequence of an energy imbalance where energy intake has exceeded energy expenditure over a considerable period [9]. Whereas unlimited access to energy-dense foods, and a lack of physical activity at work, and during leisure time, certain play a role in creating a chronic positive energy balance, obesity has a wide range of environmental and societal drivers and determinants that adversely affect food intake and physical activity patterns and thereby may overwhelm the normal regulatory processes controlling long-term energy balance in man [9,12]. Next to the availability of ultraprocessed, affordable, energy-dense palatable foods, genetics, biology, healthcare access, mental health, sociocultural factors, equity, economics, commercial determinants, and environmental determinants are all determinants of obesity [12,13]. All these complex and diverse determinants can give rise to a positive energy balance and weight gain, and it is the interaction between these determinants, rather than any single factor acting alone, which may lead to obesity [9,12]. An extensive

Visceral and Ectopic Fat. https://doi.org/10.1016/B978-0-12-822186-0.00017-1

TABLE 1.1 Classification of overall and abdominal obesity and risk of comorbidities in adults in European/United States and Asian populations according to BMI and waist circumference.

Classification	European/US	Asian	Risk of comorbidities
Overall obesity	**BMI (kg/m^2)**		
Underweight	<18.5	<18.5	Low
Normal weight	18.5−24.9	18.5−22.9	Average
Overweight	≥25.0	≥23.0	
Preobese	25.0−29.9	23.0−24.9	Increased
Obesity	≥30.0	≥25.0	
Obese class I	30.0−34.9	25.0−29.9	Moderate
Obese class II	35.0−39.9	≥30.0	Severe
Obese class III	≥40.0		Very severe
Abdominal obesity	**WC (cm)**		
Men	>94	−	Increased
Women	>80	−	Increased
Men	>102	>90	Substantially
Women	>88	>80	Increased
	WHR		
Men	≥0.90	−	Substantially
Women	≥0.85	−	Increased

BMI, body mass index; *cm*, centimeter; *kg*, kilogram; *m*, meter; *US*, United States of America; *WC*, waist circumference; *WHR*, waist-to-hip ratio. Adapted from references WHO Consultation on Obesity (1999: Geneva, Switzerland) & World Health Organization. Obesity: preventing and managing the global epidemic: report of a WHO consultation. Geneva: World Health Organization; 2000. https://apps.who.int/iris/handle/10665/63854; World Health Organization. Regional office for the western pacific. The Asia-pacific perspective: redefining obesity and its treatment. Sydney: World Health Organization; 2000. https://apps.who.int/iris/handle/10665/206936; Alberti KG, Eckel RH, Grundy SM, Zimmet PZ, Cleeman JI, Donato KA, et al. Harmonizing the metabolic syndrome: a joint interim statement of the international diabetes federation task force on epidemiology and prevention; national heart, lung, and blood institute; American heart association; world heart federation; international atherosclerosis society; and international association for the study of obesity. Circulation. 2009;120(16):1640−1645; Waist circumference and waist−hip ratio, report of a WHO expert consultation. Geneva: World Health Organization; 2008. http://apps.who.int/iris/bitstream/handle/10665/44583/9789241501491_eng.pdf; jsessionid=119F6B965A818696251E152260BE34ED?sequence=1.

discussion on the multifactorial causes of obesity and potential solutions to the obesity pandemic is outside the scope of this chapter, but it may be clear that a systemic, multistakeholder approach is needed to address the epidemic of obesity. Sustainable community-based interventions are needed that rely less on education and personal responsibility of individuals but more on changes to the current obesogenic environment and societal norms to make healthy behaviors easier [14,15].

Whereas obesity was already added to the sixth International Classification of Diseases in 1948 [12,16], and was recognized as a chronic disease by the WHO in 1997 [9], there has been a long debate on whether obesity should be considered as a disease or not [17]. Arguments against the classification of obesity as a disease included that obesity is a risk factor for other conditions rather than a disease in its own right and that declaring obesity as a disease would define a significant proportion of the population in many countries as being ill, and potentially emphasize medical approaches to treatment at the expense of behavioral and societal interventions [18−20]. Only after the American Medical Association officially recognized obesity as a disease state requiring treatment and prevention efforts in 2013, many obesity and medical societies followed. The stated purpose for this decision was to improve research into the causes of obesity, leading to improvement in methods to prevent and treat it, ultimately improving patient health and outcomes. In addition, it was expected to improve insurance coverage and reimbursement to providers for treating individuals with obesity. Finally, it would support the concept that obesity is a serious disease that requires treatment and would also remove the stigma that was associated with obesity [18−20]. In 2017, the World Obesity Federation Obesity published in a position statement that obesity should be recognized as a chronic, relapsing, multifactorial disease [20]. In March 2021, the European Commission recognized obesity as a chronic disease [12].

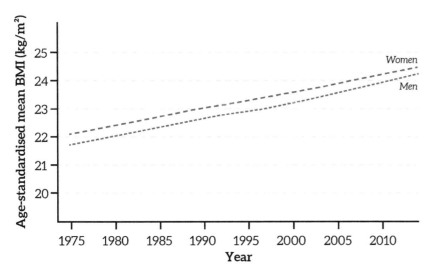

FIGURE 1.1 Worldwide trend in body index in men and women from 1975 to 2016. *Credit: identim, adapted from references NCD Risk Factor Collaboration. Trends in adult body-mass index in 200 countries from 1975 to 2014: a pooled analysis of 1698 population-based measurement studies with 19· 2 million participants. The Lancet. 2016;387(10026):1377—1396; Collaboration NCDRF. Worldwide trends in body-mass index, underweight, overweight, and obesity from 1975 to 2016: a pooled analysis of 2416 population-based measurement studies in 128.9 million children, adolescents, and adults. Lancet. 2017;390(10113):2627—2642*

Prevalence of overweight and obesity

The international WHO classification allows estimation and comparisons of the prevalence of overweight and obesity between different countries and different points in time. The prevalence of obesity has increased at an alarming rate in many parts of the world. The global age-standardized mean BMI increased from 21.7 kg/m^2 in 1975 to 24.2 kg/m^2 in 2014 in men, and from 22.1 kg/m^2 in 1975 to 24.4 kg/m^2 in 2014 in women (Fig. 1.1) [21,22]. The worldwide prevalence of obesity has nearly tripled since 1975 (Fig. 1.2) [1,23].

For example, in 1980, the global age-standardized prevalence of overweight was 25%, which increased to 34% in 2008. The age-standardized prevalence of obesity nearly doubled from 6% to 12% during the same 28-year period. These numbers have further increased to 39% for overweight and 13% for obesity in 2016 [1,24]. This corresponds to more than 1.9 billion adults of 18 years or older with overweight in 2016, of whom 650 million with obesity [1]. This exponential increase in the prevalence and incidence of obesity over the past few decades has led the WHO to declare it a global epidemic and worldwide public health crisis [25]. It must be noted that the WHO international classification of obesity of a BMI of 30 or higher was used for all countries and populations. The global prevalence of obesity may, therefore, be underestimated because many people in Asia may be inappropriately classified by their level of BMI [10,14]. While many of the same trends of an increasing obesity prevalence can be seen around the world, the global obesity landscape shows substantial variation. In some regions, such as parts of Europe and North America, the prevalence of obesity is plateauing at high levels, while in other countries, the biggest impact is yet to come. The World Obesity Atlas 2022, published by the World Obesity Federation, predicted that by 2030, 20% of women and 15% of men will be living with obesity, ranging from 9% to 5% in South East Asia, to 40% and 34% in the Americas, respectively (Fig. 1.3). In total, this equals to over 1 billion people globally [12]. Thereby, obesity is one of the 21st century's greatest public health challenges, rising fastest in low- and middle-income countries [12].

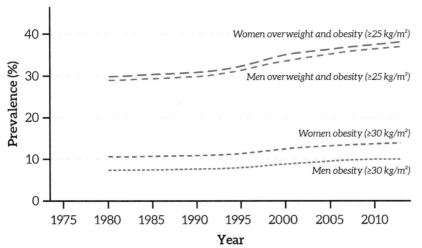

FIGURE 1.2 Worldwide prevalence of overweight and obesity in men and women during 1980—2013. *Credit: identim, adapted from reference Ng M, Fleming T, Robinson M, Thomson B, Graetz N, Margono C, et al. Global, regional, and national prevalence of overweight and obesity in children and adults during 1980-2013: a systematic analysis for the Global Burden of Disease Study 2013. Lancet. 2014;384(9945):766—781*

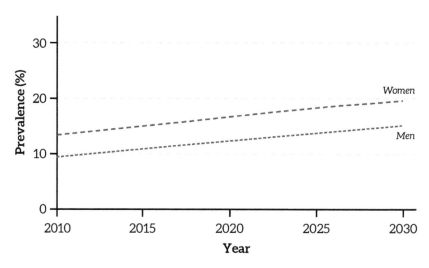

FIGURE 1.3 Estimated global prevalence of obesity among men and women in 2010–2030. *Credit: identim, adapted from references World Obesity Federation. World obesity Atlas 2022. https://data.worldobesity.org/publications/World-Obesity-Atlas-2022.pdf; Collaboration NCDRF. Worldwide trends in body-mass index, underweight, overweight, and obesity from 1975 to 2016: a pooled analysis of 2416 population-based measurement studies in 128.9 million children, adolescents, and adults. Lancet. 2017;390 (10113):2627–2642*

Obesity-related mortality and diseases

Overweight and obesity are associated with increased all-cause mortality in the general population [26–28]. In 2015, high BMI accounted for 4.0 million deaths globally, which represented 7% of the deaths from any cause; it also contributed to 120 million disability-adjusted life-years, which represented 5% of disability-adjusted life-years from any cause among adults globally. A total of 39% of the deaths and 37% of the disability-adjusted life-years that were related to high BMI occurred in persons who were not obese [28]. If the overweight and obese population had normal levels of BMI, the proportion of premature deaths that could be avoided would be about one in five in North America, one in six in Australia and New Zealand, one in seven in Europe, and one in 20 in east Asia [27].

The BMI–mortality relationship typically forms a U-shaped curve, with all-cause mortality generally being lowest with a BMI of 20.0–24.9 [26]. Whereas absolute mortality is higher in men than in women, the shape of the BMI–mortality curve is similar in men and in women (Fig. 1.4) [29]. Because underlying chronic disease and smoking may lead to unintentional weight loss and reduced BMI, the observed increased mortality risk associated with a low BMI is in part due to confounding by tobacco use or disease-related weight loss [30]. Studies limiting confounding and reverse causality by

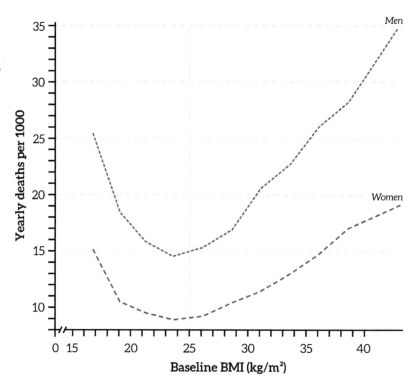

FIGURE 1.4 Body mass index and all-cause mortality in yearly deaths per 1000 for men and women. *Credit: identim, adapted from reference Prospective Studies C, Whitlock G, Lewington S, Sherliker P, Clarke R, Emberson J, et al. Body-mass index and cause-specific mortality in 900 000 adults: collaborative analyses of 57 prospective studies. Lancet. 2009;373(9669):1083–1096*

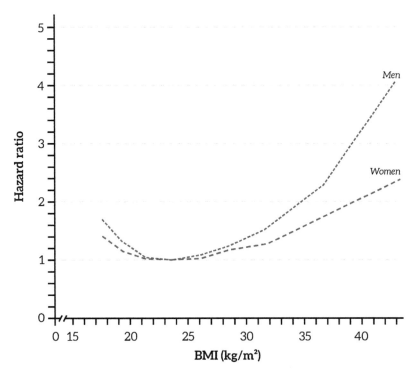

FIGURE 1.5 Relative risks of mortality in never-smokers without preexisting diseases who survived the first 5 years of follow-up. *Credit: identim, adapted from references Berrington de Gonzalez A, Hartge P, Cerhan JR, Flint AJ, Hannan L, MacInnis RJ, et al. Body-mass index and mortality among 1.46 million white adults. N Engl J Med. 2010;363(23):2211–2219; Global BMIMC, Di Angelantonio E, Bhupathiraju S.N, Wormser D, Gao P, Kaptoge S, et al. Body-mass index and all-cause mortality: individual-participant-data meta-analysis of 239 prospective studies in four continents. Lancet. 2016;388(10046):776–786*

restricting analyses to never-smokers and excluding preexisting disease and the first 5 years of follow-up have shown a more J-shaped relationship between BMI and all-cause mortality (Fig. 1.5) [26,27]. Although the prevalence of BMI differs between countries and ethnicities, the Global BMI Mortality Collaboration concluded in 2016 on the basis of 239 studies across four continents that wherever overweight and obesity are common, their associations with higher all-cause mortality are broadly similar in different populations [25].

In 2015, more than two-thirds of deaths related to high BMI were due to cardiovascular disease [28]. Diabetes was the second leading cause of BMI-related deaths in 2015, whereas chronic kidney disease and cancers each accounted for less than 10% of all BMI-related deaths in 2015. High BMI also accounted for 28.6 million years lived with disability, which represented 3.6% of years lived with disability due to any cause globally. Diabetes was the leading cause of years lived with disability related to BMI, followed by musculoskeletal disorders and cardiovascular disease [27].

The major health consequences associated with overweight and obesity are type 2 diabetes, cardiovascular diseases, gallbladder disease, gallbladder disease, osteoarthritis, certain types of cancer, sleep apnea, and psychosocial disturbances as depression [9,28,31–37]. In particular, overweight is a strong risk factor for insulin resistance and type 2 diabetes. About 90% of type 2 diabetes is attributable to excess body weight [38]. Next to type 2 diabetes, overweight and obesity are related to many cardiovascular risk factors as hypertension, hyperglycemia, and dyslipidemia, resulting in increased risks of cardiovascular disease [9,28,31,32,37]. Obesity, diabetes, and hypertension also affect the kidneys. A high BMI is a strong risk factor for chronic kidney disease and end-stage renal disease [39]. Diabetic nephropathy develops in about one-third of patients with diabetes, and its incidence is sharply increasing in the developing world [38]. A high BMI has also been associated with an increased risks of cancer of the esophagus, colon and rectum, liver, gallbladder, pancreas and kidney, and uterus, cervix, and ovary cancer in women [33,34]. It must be noted that aforementioned associations of BMI and risk of chronic diseases are based on observations in the general population and results from these observational studies may suffer from residual confounding [40,41]. Nevertheless, recent Mendelian randomization studies using genetic predisposition for high BMI have confirmed that the observed associations between BMI and type 2 diabetes, coronary artery disease, coronary heart disease, stroke, and certain types of cancer are causal [42–44].

Whereas studies in the general population have shown increased mortality risks associated with high BMI, studies in patient populations have reported inverse relations, with high BMI being associated with reduced mortality. This has also been referred to as the obesity paradox [45–48]. An extensive discussion on this topic is outside the scope of this chapter. For the interpretation of the BMI–mortality relationship in these patient populations, it is important to note that these populations often consist of patients at an older age who are followed for less than five years. It is well established that in the general population, obesity is particularly associated with an increased mortality risk after a long period of follow-up [26,27]. Whereas overweight increases mortality only after a long-term exposure, underweight is associated with short-term mortality and lower values for BMI were found to be associated with poor survival in the short term in the general population as well [49,50]. This increased short-term mortality that is associated with thinness in patient populations is most likely due to illness at baseline [49,51,52]. Therefore, for the interpretation of the BMI—mortality relationship in patient populations, differences in age at baseline and duration of follow-up should be taken into account [50].

Body fat distribution: abdominal obesity, visceral fat, and ectopic fat

Body fat distribution and abdominal obesity

The BMI provides a useful measure of obesity that can be used to estimate and monitor the prevalence of obesity at the population level. However, BMI does not account for the wide variation in body fat distribution and may not correspond to the same degree of fatness and associated health risk across different individuals and populations [9]. BMI is only dependent on body height and weight, and it does not take into consideration different levels of adiposity based on age, physical activity levels, and sex. People with a similar BMI can have substantially different health risks, and obesity is therefore a remarkably heterogenous condition when defined on the basis of BMI alone [53,54]. For example, BMI does not distinguish fat mass from lean body mass, and people with the same BMI may have a different body composition. In particular in persons with a high muscle mass, BMI may overestimate the amount of body fat. Another important drawback to use BMI as a proxy of body fatness is that BMI does not contain information on the location of the fat stored in the body. During the past decades, it has become well established that body fat distribution, in particular the regional distribution of body fat, is important for health and that abdominal obesity is a major driver of the increased disease risks associated with obesity [53—58].

Already in the 1980s, Björntorp and his group reported that body fat distribution, and mainly the regional accumulation of body fat, was closely related to metabolic diseases [59]. They showed that men with a high proportion of abdominal fat had a substantially increased risk of type 2 diabetes [60]. Many studies have shown since that measures of central obesity that more accurately describe the distribution of body fat, namely the waist circumference and the waist-to-hip ratio, are more closely associated with subsequent morbidity and mortality than BMI [61—65]. Therefore, it was proposed that measurement of waist circumference provides a simple and practical method of identifying overweight patients at increased risk of obesity-associated illness due to abdominal fat distribution [9,66,67], including cutoffs for Western and Asian populations (Table 1.1) [68,69]. Importantly, within each category of BMI, abdominal obesity assessed by waist circumference or waist-to-hip ratio is related to increased risks of morbidity and mortality [70]. Studies that reported similar associations of BMI and waist circumference with risk of cardiovascular disease [71] often did not report associations of waist circumference within categories of BMI. Because waist circumference is strongly associated with BMI and total body fat (Table 1.2), its associations also reflect associations of overall adiposity [70]. Table 1.2 further shows

TABLE 1.2 Pearson correlation coefficients of body mass index, total body fat, abdominal subcutaneous adipose tissue, visceral adipose tissue, waist circumference, waist-to-hip ratio, and liver fat content in middle-aged men and women.

M W	BMI	TBF	aSAT	VAT	WC	WHR	HTGC
BMI		0.86	0.88	0.71	0.87	0.47	0.36
TBF	0.87		0.84	0.71	0.85	0.51	0.37
aSAT	0.82	0.78		0.62	0.83	0.43	0.32
VAT	0.64	0.66	0.49		0.76	0.60	0.50
WC	0.88	0.85	0.82	0.70		0.76	0.40
WHR	0.62	0.66	0.55	0.65	0.82		0.33
HTGC	0.42	0.42	0.29	0.44	0.41	0.38	

aSAT, abdominal subcutaneous tissue; *BMI*, body mass index; *HTGC*, hepatic triglyceride content; *M*, men; *TBF*, total body fat; *VAT*, visceral adipose tissue; *W*, women; *WC*, waist circumference. Pearson correlation coefficients derived from the Netherlands Epidemiology of Obesity study (n = 1077 men, n = 985 women) [73].

that although visceral fat, as assessed with magnetic resonance imaging (MRI), is more strongly correlated with waist circumference than with the other body fat measurements, the correlations of waist circumference with total body fat and BMI are stronger than the correlation of waist circumference with visceral fat. Therefore, because abdominal fat is strongly related to total body fat, for the study of specific effects of abdominal fat, it is important to adjust the associations for total body fat [72]. The waist-to-hip ratio is a dimensionless ratio of the circumference of the waist to that of the hip circumference. As a result, the waist-to-hip ratio is a measure of body shape rather than of body fat. People with the same waist-to-hip ratio may have a completely different BMI ranging from lean to obese individuals, which is represented by the low correlation with measures of BMI and total body fat (Table 1.2).

Visceral adipose tissue and subcutaneous adipose tissue

With the development of imaging techniques such as computed tomography (CT) and MRI, it became possible to scan the body and discriminate between different types of abdominal adipose tissue [74,75]. Researchers from the University of Osaka were the first to use CT to distinguish the fat located in the abdominal cavity, the visceral fat, from the fat located subcutaneously [74]. They observed that people with excess visceral fat displayed higher fasting plasma triglycerides levels and higher plasma glucose responses following an oral glucose challenge than those with the same BMI but fat mainly stored subcutaneously [76]. In 1989, Seidell et al. showed that visceral fat area as measured with CT was also associated with serum triglycerides, plasma insulin, glucose, and diastolic and systolic blood pressure [77]. Després and colleagues have also reported early evidence that among equally obese individuals, those with high levels of visceral adipose tissue were at increased risk of developing type 2 diabetes and cardiovascular disease [78]. Many imaging studies since have revealed that there are major individual differences in the way people accumulate body adipose tissue. Factors that influence fat deposition in various depots include age, race or ethnic origin, genetics and gene expression, and lifestyle factors such as diet, exercise, and smoking [53,54]. Fig. 1.6 shows that for a given waist circumference, there is a large variation in visceral fat in both men and women. Although a marker of central body fat, waist circumference cannot distinguish visceral fat from abdominal subcutaneous adipose tissue. For example, individuals with a waist circumference of 100 cm may either suffer from abdominal subcutaneous obesity or from visceral obesity (Fig. 1.6).

The imaging studies also consistently showed that at any given BMI, individuals with visceral obesity are at much higher risk of adverse clinical outcomes, such as type 2 diabetes and cardiovascular disease, than people with subcutaneous obesity [53,54,79,80]. Visceral adipose tissue appeared more strongly associated with metabolic risk factors than subcutaneous adipose tissue and therefore the major contributor to cardiovascular risk above body mass [53,79,80]. It is now well established that

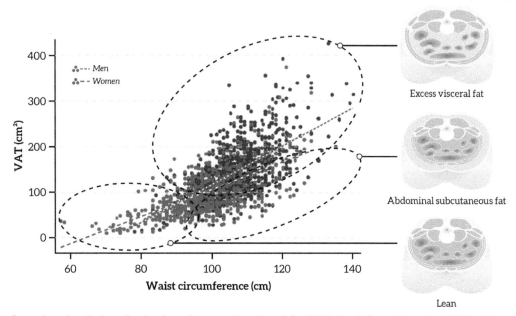

FIGURE 1.6 Scatterplot of crude data of waist circumference against visceral fat (VAT) in middle-aged men (n = 1190) and women (n = 1063) participating in the Netherlands Epidemiology of Obesity study. *Credit: identim/Shutterstock, adapted from references de Mutsert R, den Heijer M, Rabelink TJ, Smit JW, Romijn JA, Jukema JW, et al. The Netherlands Epidemiology of Obesity (NEO) study: study design and data collection. Eur J Epidemiol. 2013;28(6):513−523.*

visceral adipose tissue drives the increased risks of type 2 diabetes, atherosclerosis, and cardiovascular disease that are associated with obesity [53,81]. Mendelian randomization studies have proved that visceral adipose tissue is causally associated with cardiovascular risk factors, coronary heart disease, and type 2 diabetes [42,82]. In addition to cardiometabolic diseases, visceral fat has also been associated with increased risks of respiratory diseases such as sleep apnea and chronic obstructive pulmonary disease, dementia, reduced bone density, polycystic ovary syndrome, and different types of cancer [54].

Although subcutaneous fat seems to be related to a more beneficial metabolic profile than visceral fat, some studies showed that abdominal subcutaneous adipose tissue is important also in the pathogenesis of insulin resistance [83,84]. Whereas peripheral gluteofemoral subcutaneous adipose tissue, located at the hips and thighs, has been shown to be inversely related to the risk of diabetes and cardiovascular disease [85–87], several studies have shown relations between abdominal subcutaneous adipose tissue insulin resistance as well [83,84,88]. This supports that subcutaneous adipose tissue is not an inert depot but is also an active endocrine organ that may contribute to the circulating pool of cytokines and free fatty acids [89]. In particular, abdominal subcutaneous adipose tissue may have different properties and exert different effects than peripheral subcutaneous adipose tissue [88]. The abdominal subcutaneous adipose tissue can be further divided by the fascia superficialis into superficial and deep subcutaneous adipose tissue [90]. It has been suggested that the adipocytes from deep subcutaneous adipose tissue have higher lipolytic activity than superficial subcutaneous adipose tissue adipocytes [91] and that abdominal deep subcutaneous adipose tissue thereby exhibits an intermediate phenotype between visceral adipose tissue and abdominal superficial subcutaneous adipose tissue [92,93], but more research is needed to confirm this.

Three not mutually exclusive hypotheses as to why visceral obesity is deleterious to cardiometabolic health have been proposed, including the seminal "lipid overflow hypothesis" [53,94,95]. First, visceral adipose tissue has a high rate of lipolysis exposing the liver to high concentrations of nonesterified fatty acids that contribute to impaired hepatic metabolic functions, a chronic, low-grade inflammatory state, and reduced insulin sensitivity (Fig. 1.7) [96,97]. Second, visceral adipose tissue becomes infiltrated with inflammatory macrophages and is a source of low-grade chronic inflammation through a high secretion rate of cytokines such as interleukin-6 and tumor necrosis factor-alpha (Fig. 1.7) [96]. Thereby,

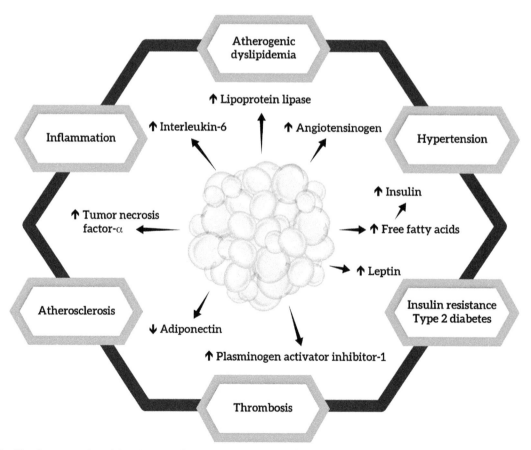

FIGURE 1.7 Visual representation of the adverse cardiometabolic effects of intraabdominal visceral adipocytes. *Credit: identim, adapted from references Wajchenberg BL, Giannella-Neto D, da Silva ME, Santos RF. Depot-specific hormonal characteristics of subcutaneous and visceral adipose tissue and their relation to the metabolic syndrome. Horm Metab Res. 2002;34(11−12):616−621; Lyon CJ, Law RE, Hsueh WA. Minireview: adiposity, inflammation, and atherogenesis. Endocrinology. 2003;144(6):2195−2200; Trayhurn P, Wood IS. Adipokines: inflammation and the pleiotropic role of white adipose tissue. Br J Nutr. 2004;92(3):347−355; Eckel RH, Grundy SM, Zimmet PZ. The metabolic syndrome. Lancet. 2005;365(9468):1415−1428*

visceral adipose tissue is an active endocrine organ. Compared with subcutaneous adipose tissue, the effect of insulin is lower and that of catecholamine is higher in visceral adipose tissue, with its metabolites and its secretions draining through the portal system, partially at least, to the liver [98,99]. Visceral adipocytes transfer and release fatty acids more extensively have increased glucocorticoid and reduced thiazolidinedione responses, produce more angiotensinogen, interleukin-6, and plasminogen activator inhibitor-1, and secrete less leptin and adiponectin than subcutaneous adipose tissue [98,100–102]. Fig. 1.7 illustrates the adverse cardiometabolic effects of intraabdominal visceral adipocytes.

The third hypothesis proposes that excess visceral fat is a marker of the relative inability of subcutaneous adipose tissue to act as a metabolic buffer, which would normally store excess fatty acids, thereby protecting normally lean tissues such as the liver, heart, kidney, and skeletal muscle against toxic ectopic fat deposition [53,54,94,95]. This third scenario is also referred to as the so-called "lipid overflow hypothesis" (Fig. 1.8) [53].

Lipid overflow hypothesis and ectopic fat accumulation

When the body is in a positive energy disbalance, lipids accumulate primarily in subcutaneous adipose tissue, which is located just beneath the skin and amounts to 82%–97% of total body fat [53,103]. Lipids can also accumulate in the visceral adipose tissue, which is located deeper in the abdomen and situated around the organs, and amounts to 5%–10% of all adipose tissue [103]. Subcutaneous adipose tissue has the capability to expand when there is a positive energy balance. However, the response to excess caloric intake might vary, and there is considerable variation between individuals where the fat is stored [104]. The propensity to preferentially accumulate visceral fat in conditions of excess energy intake varies between individuals, and the ability of subcutaneous adipose tissue to store excess fat is a major determinant of metabolic health. According to the "lipid overflow hypothesis" [53,94,95], the subcutaneous adipose tissue compartment has a maximum capacity to store excess fat, which may differ for each individual. When the caloric surplus is led into the subcutaneous adipose tissue, which is sensitive to insulin, the individual is unlikely to develop the metabolic syndrome as the subcutaneous fat can expand. When, however, the subcutaneous adipose tissue becomes dysfunctional, for example, under the influence of age, sex, genetic factors, hormones, or lifestyle factors, it may reach its maximum capacity. When the subcutaneous adipose tissue compartment is unable to expand further to store the energy surplus, the fatty acids will "overflow" to the visceral adipose tissue compartment, leading to visceral fat accumulation and ectopic fat deposition in normally lean tissues as the heart, the liver, the pancreas, and the kidneys (Fig. 1.8) [53,54,103,105]. Ectopic fat is thereby defined by the deposition of triglycerides within cells of nonadipose tissue [53,54,103,105].

Adipose tissue dysfunction and ectopic fat deposition are characterized by adipocyte hypertrophy, impaired adipogenesis, low free fatty acid uptake, reduced triglyceride synthesis, resistance to the inhibitory effect of insulin on lipolysis, immune cell infiltration, and inflammatory cytokine secretion [53,98,106]. Compared with other organs, ectopic fat in the liver is well studied. Excess visceral fat may lead to nonalcoholic fatty liver disease, due to its high lipolytic rate, and a continuous excess of free fatty acids, which are released into the portal circulation and transported to the liver, leading to hepatic steatosis and gluconeogenesis [99,105]. Nonalcoholic fatty liver disease is defined as a hepatic fat content of more than 5%, not due to excessive alcohol consumption [107,108]. Nonalcoholic fatty liver disease covers a broad clinical spectrum, ranging from simple hepatic steatosis to nonalcoholic steatohepatitis, and cirrhosis. Nonalcoholic fatty liver disease is a leading cause of chronic liver diseases worldwide [109] and is also strongly associated with the metabolic syndrome, insulin resistance, type 2 diabetes, and cardiovascular disease [109–111]. With the increase in obesity over the past decades, the prevalence of nonalcoholic fatty liver disease increased as well and is now present in 25% of the general adult population, and 65%–85% in adults with obesity [112,113].

Although individuals with nonalcoholic steatohepatitis are at increased risk of cardiometabolic diseases, the specific contribution of excess liver fat to clinical outcomes remains uncertain. For instance, although nonalcoholic steatohepatitis is clearly associated with an increased risk of type 2 diabetes, recent studies have suggested that excess visceral adipose tissue was responsible for the link between excess liver fat and cardiovascular diseases [54,114]. Further studies are underway to quantify the respective contributions of specific ectopic fat depots to various clinical outcomes.

Sex differences in body fat distribution and health consequences

The French physician Jean Vague (1911–2003) was the first physician who proposed, in 1947, that body fat topography was the key factor involved in explaining the health hazards of obesity [115]. He identified two body shapes and proposed the terms gynoid obesity and android obesity. He coined the term android obesity to refer to adipose tissue accumulated preferentially in the trunk/upper body area and suggested that this was a form of obesity closely associated with diabetes

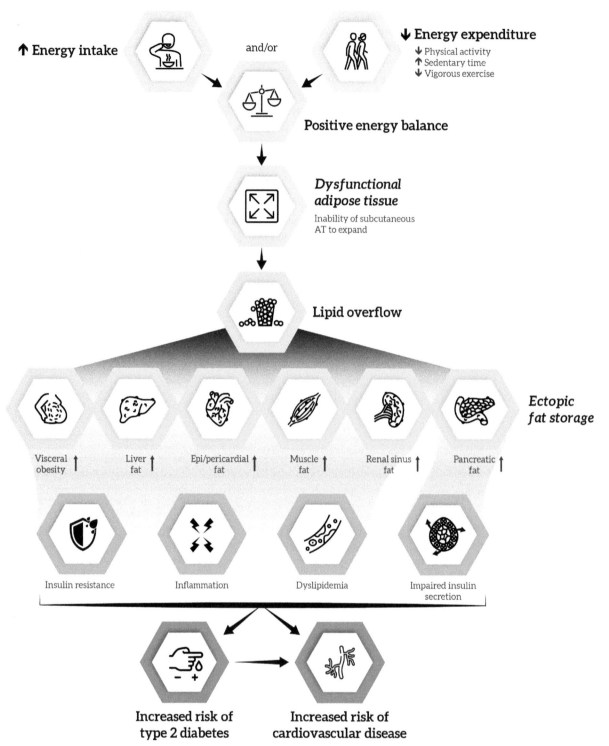

FIGURE 1.8 Visual interpretation of the lipid overflow hypothesis. *Credit: identim, adapted from references Tchernof A, Despres JP. Pathophysiology of human visceral obesity: an update. Physiol Rev. 2013;93(1):359-404; Despres JP, Lemieux I. Abdominal obesity and metabolic syndrome. Nature. 2006;444(7121):881−887.*

and heart disease. He also proposed the term gynoid obesity to refer to preferential adipose tissue accumulation in the hips and thighs, typically described as female obesity, a form much less associated with complications [53,115]. At present, it is well established that body fat distribution is sexually dimorphic and sex hormones play a major role in the regulation of adipose tissue distribution, function, and stores [116−120]. Factors that contribute to the sex difference in body fat distribution are differences between men and women in basal fatty acid oxidation, postprandial fatty acid storage, and regional differences in the regulation of lipolysis [121].

For the same BMI, women have a higher percentage of body fat than men and are more likely to store fat subcutaneously in the gluteal—femoral region [117,122,123]. Men, however, store more fat in the visceral area [117,121]. Although women have on average 10% more total body fat [120,124], they have a lower risk of type 2 diabetes and cardiovascular diseases than men [125—127]. Differences in both gluteofemoral subcutaneous adipose tissue [85—87] and visceral fat may explain these differences in cardiometabolic risk between men and women [128,129]. Estrogens are thought to underly the gluteal—femoral fat distribution that seems to protect women from cardiometabolic disease [116,117,130]. The role of male sex hormones (androgens) in body fat distribution and cardiovascular risk is less clear and appears to be opposite in women to that in men. In a large study, opposite relations were observed in 1835 men and women between bioavailable testosterone and visceral fat [131]. Whereas in men, androgen deficiency contributes to the development of metabolic syndrome and type 2 diabetes [132], excess androgens in postmenopausal women and in women with polycystic ovary syndrome have been associated with abdominal fat and cardiovascular disease [133]. While women have less visceral fat than men, this typically increases after menopause, with a shift toward a more abdominal fat distribution [131,134,135]. Some studies have suggested that women are particularly susceptible to the detrimental metabolic effects of excess visceral fat [83,136]. In this light, it is important to note that although women are more likely to store fat in the gluteal—femoral region, around 40% of women between 30 and 79 years store fat predominantly in the abdominal area [117]. Future studies should continue to unravel the underlying mechanisms of the detrimental metabolic effects of visceral adipose tissue in men and women. As an illustration and to conclude, Fig. 1.9 shows an example of body fat distribution in a male and a female body, with both excess visceral fat and ectopic fat accumulation.

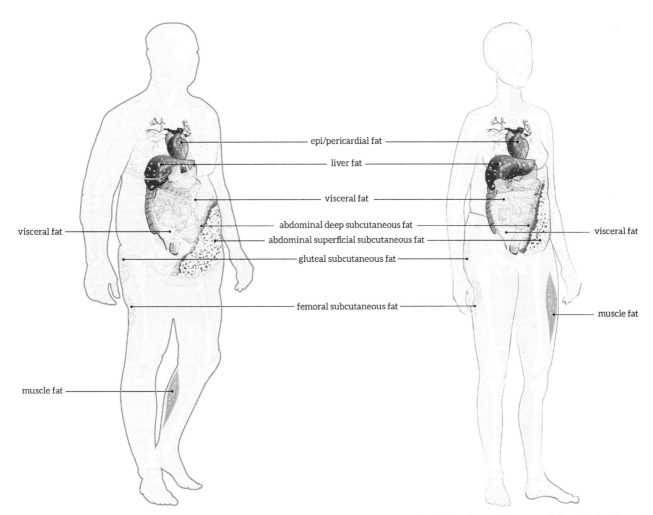

FIGURE 1.9   Illustration of body fat distribution in a male and a female body, with both excess visceral fat and ectopic fat accumulation. *Credit: identim/ Shutterstock*

Summary and conclusion

Overweight and obesity are defined as excessive fat accumulation that may impair health. In addition to overall obesity, body fat distribution is relevant for cardiometabolic health. In particular, abdominal obesity is driving the increased disease risks associated with obesity. The intraabdominal visceral adipose tissue is an active endocrine organ, and excess visceral fat increases risks of type 2 diabetes and cardiovascular disease. Ectopic fat accumulation is defined as storage of excess fat in normally lean tissues as the liver, the heart, the kidney, and the pancreas and contributes to impaired cardiometabolic health. Differences in body fat distribution between men and women in part explain the observed sex differences in cardiometabolic disease risk. Because of the established health risks and substantial increases in prevalence, obesity has become a major global health challenge. There is an urgent need for therapeutic strategies to target visceral and ectopic fat and for public health action to manage and prevent obesity. The amount of visceral adipose tissue is an important target to measure for cardiometabolic risk stratification. However, imaging techniques such as magnetic resonance imaging or computed tomography to directly assess visceral adipose tissue are expensive and time-consuming and therefore not well suited for clinical practice. Several studies have developed noninvasive alternatives to direct measurements of visceral adipose tissue, including the hypertriglyceridemic waist phenotype [137], the visceral adiposity index [138], and the lipid accumulation product [139]. Although most of these indices include waist circumference, it is not measured routinely in clinical settings [66]. Because imaging is unfeasible in clinical practice, the International Atherosclerosis Society and the International Chair on Cardiometabolic Risk Working Group on Visceral Obesity emphasized the need for more research into simple, clinically applicable tools to identify individuals with excess visceral fat [54]. Because waist circumference is such important predictor of visceral fat, this strengthens the call to measure waist circumference routinely in clinical practice [66].

References

[1] World Health Organization. Fact Sheet Obesity and overweight. www.who.int/news-room/fact-sheets/detail/obesity-and-overweight. [Accessed 01 April 2022].

[2] Garrow JS. Health implications of obesity. Obesity and related diseases. London: Churchill Livingstone; 1988. p. 1−16.

[3] Quetelet A. Recherces sur le poids de l'homme aux differents ages. Nouveaux Memoires de l'Academie Royale des Sciences et Belles-Lettres de Bruxelles. 1832.

[4] Eknoyan G. Adolphe Quetelet (1796−1874)–the average man and indices of obesity. Nephrol Dial Transplant 2008;23(1):47−51.

[5] Florey CV. The use and interpretation of ponderal index and other weight-height ratios in epidemiological studies. J Chron Dis 1970;23(2):93−103.

[6] Keys A, Fidanza F, Karvonen MJ, Kimura N, Taylor HL. Indices of relative weight and obesity. J Chron Dis 1972;25(6):329−43.

[7] Garrow JS, Webster J. Quetelet's index (W/H2) as a measure of fatness. Int J Obes 1985;9(2):147−53.

[8] WHO Expert Committee on Physical Status : the Use and Interpretation of Anthropometry (1993 : Geneva, Switzerland) & World Health Organization. Physical status: the use of and interpretation of anthropometry, report of a WHO expert committee. World Health Organization; 1995. https://apps.who.int/iris/handle/10665/37003.

[9] WHO Consultation on Obesity (1999: Geneva, Switzerland) & World Health Organization. Obesity: preventing and managing the global epidemic: report of a WHO consultation. Geneva: World Health Organization; 2000. https://apps.who.int/iris/handle/10665/63854.

[10] World Health Organization. Regional office for the western pacific. The Asia-pacific perspective : redefining obesity and its treatment. Sydney: World Health Organization; 2000. https://apps.who.int/iris/handle/10665/206936.

[11] WHO Expert Consultation. Appropriate body-mass index for Asian populations and its implications for policy and intervention strategies. Lancet 2004;363(9403):157−63.

[12] World Obesity Federation. World obesity Atlas. 2022. https://data.worldobesity.org/publications/World-Obesity-Atlas-2022.pdf.

[13] Swinburn BA, Sacks G, Hall KD, McPherson K, Finegood DT, Moodie ML, et al. The global obesity pandemic: shaped by global drivers and local environments. Lancet 2011;378(9793):804−14.

[14] Seidell JC, Halberstadt J. The global burden of obesity and the challenges of prevention. Ann Nutr Metab 2015;66(Suppl. 2):7−12.

[15] Huang TT, Drewnowski A, Kumanyika SK, Glass TA. A systems-oriented multilevel framework for addressing obesity in the 21st century. Prev Chronic Dis 2009;6(3).

[16] World Health Organization. International statistical classification of diseases and related health problems (ICD). 2019. www.who.int/standards/classifications/classification-of-diseases. [Accessed 1 April 2022].

[17] Bray GA. Obesity is a chronic, relapsing neurochemical disease. Int J Obes Relat Metab Disord 2004;28(1):34−8.

[18] Rosen H. Is obesity A disease or A behavior abnormality? Did the AMA get it right? Mo Med 2014;111(2):104−8.

[19] Kyle TK, Dhurandhar EJ, Allison DB. Regarding obesity as a disease: evolving policies and their implications. Endocrinol Metab Clin North Am 2016;45(3):511−20.

[20] Bray GA, Kim KK, Wilding JPH, World Obesity F. Obesity: a chronic relapsing progressive disease process. A position statement of the World Obesity Federation. Obes Rev 2017;18(7):715−23.

[21] NCD Risk Factor Collaboration. Trends in adult body-mass index in 200 countries from 1975 to 2014: a pooled analysis of 1698 population-based measurement studies with 19.2 million participants. The lancet 2016;387(10026):1377−96.

[22] Collaboration NCDRF. Worldwide trends in body-mass index, underweight, overweight, and obesity from 1975 to 2016: a pooled analysis of 2416 population-based measurement studies in 128.9 million children, adolescents, and adults. Lancet 2017;390(10113):2627−42.

[23] Ng M, Fleming T, Robinson M, Thomson B, Graetz N, Margono C, et al. Global, regional, and national prevalence of overweight and obesity in children and adults during 1980-2013: a systematic analysis for the Global Burden of Disease Study 2013. Lancet 2014;384(9945):766−81.

[24] Stevens GA, Singh GM, Lu Y, Danaei G, Lin JK, Finucane MM, et al. National, regional, and global trends in adult overweight and obesity prevalences. Popul Health Metr 2012;10(1):22.

[25] World Health Organization. Preventing chronic diseases: a vital investment: WHO global report. World Health Organization; 2005. https://apps.who.int/iris/handle/10665/43314.

[26] Berrington de Gonzalez A, Hartge P, Cerhan JR, Flint AJ, Hannan L, MacInnis RJ, et al. Body-mass index and mortality among 1.46 million white adults. N Engl J Med 2010;363(23):2211−9.

[27] Global BMIMC, Di Angelantonio E, Bhupathiraju SN, Wormser D, Gao P, Kaptoge S, et al. Body-mass index and all-cause mortality: individual-participant-data meta-analysis of 239 prospective studies in four continents. Lancet 2016;388(10046):776−86.

[28] Collaborators GBDO, Afshin A, Forouzanfar MH, Reitsma MB, Sur P, Estep K, et al. Health effects of overweight and obesity in 195 countries over 25 years. N Engl J Med 2017;377(1):13−27.

[29] Prospective Studies C, Whitlock G, Lewington S, Sherliker P, Clarke R, Emberson J, et al. Body-mass index and cause-specific mortality in 900 000 adults: collaborative analyses of 57 prospective studies. Lancet 2009;373(9669):1083−96.

[30] Manson JE, Bassuk SS, Hu FB, Stampfer MJ, Colditz GA, Willett WC. Estimating the number of deaths due to obesity: can the divergent findings be reconciled? J Womens Health (Larchmt) 2007;16(2):168−76.

[31] Singh GM, Danaei G, Farzadfar F, Stevens GA, Woodward M, Wormser D, et al. The age-specific quantitative effects of metabolic risk factors on cardiovascular diseases and diabetes: a pooled analysis. PLoS One 2013;8(7):e65174.

[32] Emerging Risk Factors C, Wormser D, Kaptoge S, Di Angelantonio E, Wood AM, Pennells L, et al. Separate and combined associations of body-mass index and abdominal adiposity with cardiovascular disease: collaborative analysis of 58 prospective studies. Lancet 2011;377(9771):1085−95.

[33] Lauby-Secretan B, Scoccianti C, Loomis D, Grosse Y, Bianchini F, Straif K, et al. Body fatness and cancer−viewpoint of the IARC working group. N Engl J Med 2016;375(8):794−8.

[34] World Cancer Research Fund/American Institute for Cancer Research. Food, nutrition, physical activity, and the prevention of cancer: a global perspective. Washington, DC: American Institute for Cancer Research; 2007.

[35] Jiang L, Rong J, Wang Y, Hu F, Bao C, Li X, et al. The relationship between body mass index and hip osteoarthritis: a systematic review and meta-analysis. Joint Bone Spine 2011;78(2):150−5.

[36] Jiang L, Tian W, Wang Y, Rong J, Bao C, Liu Y, et al. Body mass index and susceptibility to knee osteoarthritis: a systematic review and meta-analysis. Joint Bone Spine 2012;79(3):291−7.

[37] Bluher M. Obesity: global epidemiology and pathogenesis. Nat Rev Endocrinol 2019;15(5):288−98.

[38] Hossain P, Kawar B, El Nahas M. Obesity and diabetes in the developing world−a growing challenge. N Engl J Med 2007;356(3):213−5.

[39] Hsu CY, McCulloch CE, Iribarren C, Darbinian J, Go AS. Body mass index and risk for end-stage renal disease. Ann Intern Med 2006;144(1):21−8.

[40] Vandenbroucke JP. When are observational studies as credible as randomised trials? Lancet 2004;363(9422):1728−31.

[41] Pearce N, Lawlor DA. Causal inference-so much more than statistics. Int J Epidemiol 2016;45(6):1895−903.

[42] Dale CE, Fatemifar G, Palmer TM, White J, Prieto-Merino D, Zabaneh D, et al. Causal associations of adiposity and body fat distribution with coronary heart disease, stroke subtypes, and type 2 diabetes mellitus: a mendelian randomization analysis. Circulation 2017;135(24):2373−88.

[43] Richardson TG, Sanderson E, Elsworth B, Tilling K, Davey Smith G. Use of genetic variation to separate the effects of early and later life adiposity on disease risk: mendelian randomisation study. BMJ 2020;369:m1203.

[44] Fang Z, Song M, Lee DH, Giovannucci EL. The role of mendelian randomization studies in deciphering the effect of obesity on cancer. J Natl Cancer Inst 2022;114(3):361−71.

[45] Romero-Corral A, Montori VM, Somers VK, Korinek J, Thomas RJ, Allison TG, et al. Association of bodyweight with total mortality and with cardiovascular events in coronary artery disease: a systematic review of cohort studies. Lancet 2006;368(9536):666−78.

[46] Kalantar-Zadeh K, Abbott KC, Salahudeen AK, Kilpatrick RD, Horwich TB. Survival advantages of obesity in dialysis patients. Am J Clin Nutr 2005;81(3):543−54.

[47] Curtis JP, Selter JG, Wang Y, Rathore SS, Jovin IS, Jadbabaie F, et al. The obesity paradox: body mass index and outcomes in patients with heart failure. Arch Intern Med 2005;165(1):55−61.

[48] Niedziela J, Hudzik B, Niedziela N, Gasior M, Gierlotka M, Wasilewski J, et al. The obesity paradox in acute coronary syndrome: a meta-analysis. Eur J Epidemiol 2014;29(11):801−12.

[49] Manson JE, Stampfer MJ, Hennekens CH, Willett WC. Body weight and longevity. A reassessment. JAMA 1987;257(3):353−8.

[50] de Mutsert R, Snijder MB, van der Sman-de Beer F, Seidell JC, Boeschoten EW, Krediet RT, et al. Association between body mass index and mortality is similar in the hemodialysis population and the general population at high age and equal duration of follow-up. J Am Soc Nephrol 2007;18(3):967−74.

[51] Stevens J, Cai J, Pamuk ER, Williamson DF, Thun MJ, Wood JL. The effect of age on the association between body-mass index and mortality. N Engl J Med 1998;338(1):1—7.

[52] Stevens J, Juhaeri, Cai J. Changes in body mass index prior to baseline among participants who are ill or who die during the early years of follow-up. Am J Epidemiol 2001;153(10):946—53.

[53] Tchernof A, Despres JP. Pathophysiology of human visceral obesity: an update. Physiol Rev 2013;93(1):359—404.

[54] Neeland IJ, Ross R, Despres JP, Matsuzawa Y, Yamashita S, Shai I, et al. Visceral and ectopic fat, atherosclerosis, and cardiometabolic disease: a position statement. Lancet Diabetes Endocrinol 2019;7(9):715—25.

[55] Katzmarzyk PT, Janssen I, Ross R, Church TS, Blair SN. The importance of waist circumference in the definition of metabolic syndrome: prospective analyses of mortality in men. Diabetes Care 2006;29(2):404—9.

[56] Katzmarzyk PT, Malina RM, Song TM, Bouchard C. Physique, subcutaneous fat, adipose tissue distribution, and risk factors in the Quebec Family Study. Int J Obes Relat Metab Disord 1999;23(5):476—84.

[57] Larsson B, Seidell J, Svardsudd K, Welin L, Tibblin G, Wilhelmsen L, et al. Obesity, adipose tissue distribution and health in men–the study of men born in 1913. Appetite 1989;13(1):37—44.

[58] Bjorntorp P. Metabolic implications of body fat distribution. Diabetes Care 1991;14(12):1132—43.

[59] Krotkiewski M, Bjorntorp P, Sjostrom L, Smith U. Impact of obesity on metabolism in men and women. Importance of regional adipose tissue distribution. J Clin Invest 1983;72(3):1150—62.

[60] Ohlson LO, Larsson B, Svardsudd K, Welin L, Eriksson H, Wilhelmsen L, et al. The influence of body fat distribution on the incidence of diabetes mellitus. 13.5 years of follow-up of the participants in the study of men born in 1913. Diabetes 1985;34(10):1055—8.

[61] Wang Y, Rimm EB, Stampfer MJ, Willett WC, Hu FB. Comparison of abdominal adiposity and overall obesity in predicting risk of type 2 diabetes among men. Am J Clin Nutr 2005;81(3):555—63.

[62] Huxley R, Mendis S, Zheleznyakov E, Reddy S, Chan J. Body mass index, waist circumference and waist:hip ratio as predictors of cardiovascular risk–a review of the literature. Eur J Clin Nutr 2010;64(1):16—22.

[63] InterAct C, Langenberg C, Sharp SJ, Schulze MB, Rolandsson O, Overvad K, et al. Long-term risk of incident type 2 diabetes and measures of overall and regional obesity: the EPIC-InterAct case-cohort study. PLoS Med 2012;9(6):e1001230.

[64] Pischon T, Boeing H, Hoffmann K, Bergmann M, Schulze MB, Overvad K, et al. General and abdominal adiposity and risk of death in Europe. N Engl J Med 2008;359(20):2105—20.

[65] Sluik D, Boeing H, Montonen J, Pischon T, Kaaks R, Teucher B, et al. Associations between general and abdominal adiposity and mortality in individuals with diabetes mellitus. Am J Epidemiol 2011;174(1):22—34.

[66] Ross R, Neeland IJ, Yamashita S, Shai I, Seidell J, Magni P, et al. Waist circumference as a vital sign in clinical practice: a consensus statement from the IAS and ICCR working group on visceral obesity. Nat Rev Endocrinol 2020;16(3):177—89.

[67] Pouliot MC, Despres JP, Lemieux S, Moorjani S, Bouchard C, Tremblay A, et al. Waist circumference and abdominal sagittal diameter: best simple anthropometric indexes of abdominal visceral adipose tissue accumulation and related cardiovascular risk in men and women. Am J Cardiol 1994;73(7):460—8.

[68] Alberti KG, Eckel RH, Grundy SM, Zimmet PZ, Cleeman JI, Donato KA, et al. Harmonizing the metabolic syndrome: a joint interim statement of the international diabetes federation task force on epidemiology and prevention; national heart, lung, and blood institute; American heart association; world heart federation; international atherosclerosis society; and international association for the study of obesity. Circulation 2009;120(16):1640—5.

[69] Waist circumference and waist—hip ratio, report of a WHO expert consultation. Geneva: World Health Organization; 2008. http://apps.who.int/iris/bitstream/handle/10665/44583/9789241501491_eng.pdf;jsessionid=119F6B965A818696251E152260BE34ED?sequence=1.

[70] Seidell JC. Waist circumference and waist/hip ratio in relation to all-cause mortality, cancer and sleep apnea. Eur J Clin Nutr 2010;64(1):35—41.

[71] van Dis I, Kromhout D, Geleijnse JM, Boer JM, Verschuren WM. Body mass index and waist circumference predict both 10-year nonfatal and fatal cardiovascular disease risk: study conducted in 20,000 Dutch men and women aged 20-65 years. Eur J Cardiovasc Prev Rehabil 2009;16(6):729—34.

[72] Seidell JC, Bouchard C. Visceral fat in relation to health: is it a major culprit or simply an innocent bystander? Int J Obes Relat Metab Disord 1997;21(8):626—31.

[73] de Mutsert R, den Heijer M, Rabelink TJ, Smit JW, Romijn JA, Jukema JW, et al. The Netherlands Epidemiology of Obesity (NEO) study: study design and data collection. Eur J Epidemiol 2013;28(6):513—23.

[74] Tokunaga K, Matsuzawa Y, Ishikawa K, Tarui S. A novel technique for the determination of body fat by computed tomography. Int J Obes 1983;7(5):437—45.

[75] van der Kooy K, Seidell JC. Techniques for the measurement of visceral fat: a practical guide. Int J Obes Relat Metab Disord 1993;17(4):187—96.

[76] Fujioka S, Matsuzawa Y, Tokunaga K, Tarui S. Contribution of intra-abdominal fat accumulation to the impairment of glucose and lipid metabolism in human obesity. Metabolism 1987;36(1):54—9.

[77] Seidell JC, Bjorntorp P, Sjostrom L, Sannerstedt R, Krotkiewski M, Kvist H. Regional distribution of muscle and fat mass in men–new insight into the risk of abdominal obesity using computed tomography. Int J Obes 1989;13(3):289—303.

[78] Despres J-P, Moorjani S, Lupien PJ, Tremblay A, Nadeau A, Bouchard C. Regional distribution of body fat, plasma lipoproteins, and cardiovascular disease. Arteriosc Off J Am Heart Assoc Inc 1990;10(4):497—511.

[79] Neeland IJ, Ayers CR, Rohatgi AK, Turer AT, Berry JD, Das SR, et al. Associations of visceral and abdominal subcutaneous adipose tissue with markers of cardiac and metabolic risk in obese adults. Obesity 2013;21(9):E439—47.

[80] Fox CS, Massaro JM, Hoffmann U, Pou KM, Maurovich-Horvat P, Liu CY, et al. Abdominal visceral and subcutaneous adipose tissue compartments: association with metabolic risk factors in the Framingham Heart Study. Circulation 2007;116(1):39—48.

[81] Despres JP. Body fat distribution and risk of cardiovascular disease: an update. Circulation 2012;126(10):1301—13.

[82] Karlsson T, Rask-Andersen M, Pan G, Hoglund J, Wadelius C, Ek WE, et al. Contribution of genetics to visceral adiposity and its relation to cardiovascular and metabolic disease. Nat Med 2019;25(9):1390—5.

[83] de Mutsert R, Gast K, Widya R, de Koning E, Jazet I, Lamb H, et al. Associations of abdominal subcutaneous and visceral fat with insulin resistance and secretion differ between men and women: The Netherlands epidemiology of obesity study. Metab Syndr Relat Disord 2018;16(1):54—63.

[84] Goodpaster BH, Thaete FL, Simoneau JA, Kelley DE. Subcutaneous abdominal fat and thigh muscle composition predict insulin sensitivity independently of visceral fat. Diabetes 1997;46(10):1579—85.

[85] Amati F, Pennant M, Azuma K, Dube JJ, Toledo FG, Rossi AP, et al. Lower thigh subcutaneous and higher visceral abdominal adipose tissue content both contribute to insulin resistance. Obesity 2012;20(5):1115—7.

[86] Snijder MB, Dekker JM, Visser M, Bouter LM, Stehouwer CD, Kostense PJ, et al. Associations of hip and thigh circumferences independent of waist circumference with the incidence of type 2 diabetes: the Hoorn Study. Am J Clin Nutr 2003;77(5):1192—7.

[87] Neeland IJ, Turer AT, Ayers CR, Berry JD, Rohatgi A, Das SR, et al. Body fat distribution and incident cardiovascular disease in obese adults. J Am Coll Cardiol 2015;65(19):2150—1.

[88] Patel P, Abate N. Role of subcutaneous adipose tissue in the pathogenesis of insulin resistance. J Obes 2013;2013:489187.

[89] Tordjman J, Divoux A, Prifti E, Poitou C, Pelloux V, Hugol D, et al. Structural and inflammatory heterogeneity in subcutaneous adipose tissue: relation with liver histopathology in morbid obesity. J Hepatol 2012;56(5):1152—8.

[90] Deschenes D, Couture P, Dupont P, Tchernof A. Subdivision of the subcutaneous adipose tissue compartment and lipid-lipoprotein levels in women. Obes Res 2003;11(3):469—76.

[91] Monzon JR, Basile R, Heneghan S, Udupi V, Green A. Lipolysis in adipocytes isolated from deep and superficial subcutaneous adipose tissue. Obes Res 2002;10(4):266—9.

[92] Golan R, Shelef I, Rudich A, Gepner Y, Shemesh E, Chassidim Y, et al. Abdominal superficial subcutaneous fat: a putative distinct protective fat subdepot in type 2 diabetes. Diabetes Care 2012;35(3):640—7.

[93] Brand T, van den Munckhof ICL, van der Graaf M, Schraa K, Dekker HM, Joosten LAB, et al. Superficial vs deep subcutaneous adipose tissue: sex-specific associations with hepatic steatosis and metabolic traits. J Clin Endocrinol Metab 2021;106(10):e3881—9.

[94] Despres JP, Lemieux I. Abdominal obesity and metabolic syndrome. Nature 2006;444(7121):881—7.

[95] Chartrand DJ, Murphy-Despres A, Almeras N, Lemieux I, Larose E, Despres JP. Overweight, obesity, and CVD risk: a focus on visceral/ectopic fat. Curr Atheroscler Rep 2022;24(4):185—95.

[96] Mauer J, Chaurasia B, Goldau J, Vogt MC, Ruud J, Nguyen KD, et al. Signaling by IL-6 promotes alternative activation of macrophages to limit endotoxemia and obesity-associated resistance to insulin. Nat Immunol 2014;15(5):423—30.

[97] Nielsen S, Guo Z, Johnson CM, Hensrud DD, Jensen MD. Splanchnic lipolysis in human obesity. J Clin Invest 2004;113(11):1582—8.

[98] Wajchenberg BL, Giannella-Neto D, da Silva ME, Santos RF. Depot-specific hormonal characteristics of subcutaneous and visceral adipose tissue and their relation to the metabolic syndrome. Horm Metab Res 2002;34(11—12):616—21.

[99] Bjorntorp P. "Portal" adipose tissue as a generator of risk factors for cardiovascular disease and diabetes. Arteriosclerosis 1990;10(4):493—6.

[100] Lyon CJ, Law RE, Hsueh WA. Minireview: adiposity, inflammation, and atherogenesis. Endocrinology 2003;144(6):2195—200.

[101] Trayhurn P, Wood IS. Adipokines: inflammation and the pleiotropic role of white adipose tissue. Br J Nutr 2004;92(3):347—55.

[102] Eckel RH, Grundy SM, Zimmet PZ. The metabolic syndrome. Lancet 2005;365(9468):1415—28.

[103] Gastaldelli A, Basta G. Ectopic fat and cardiovascular disease: what is the link? Nutr Metab Cardiovasc Dis 2010;20(7):481—90.

[104] Neeland IJ, Poirier P, Despres JP. Cardiovascular and metabolic heterogeneity of obesity: clinical challenges and implications for management. Circulation 2018;137(13):1391—406.

[105] Gastaldelli A, Cusi K, Pettiti M, Hardies J, Miyazaki Y, Berria R, et al. Relationship between hepatic/visceral fat and hepatic insulin resistance in nondiabetic and type 2 diabetic subjects. Gastroenterology 2007;133(2):496—506.

[106] Shulman GI. Ectopic fat in insulin resistance, dyslipidemia, and cardiometabolic disease. N Engl J Med 2014;371(12):1131—41.

[107] Chalasani N, Younossi Z, Lavine JE, Charlton M, Cusi K, Rinella M, et al. The diagnosis and management of nonalcoholic fatty liver disease: practice guidance from the American Association for the Study of Liver Diseases. Hepatology 2018;67(1):328—57.

[108] Szczepaniak LS, Nurenberg P, Leonard D, Browning JD, Reingold JS, Grundy S, et al. Magnetic resonance spectroscopy to measure hepatic triglyceride content: prevalence of hepatic steatosis in the general population. Am J Physiol Endocrinol Metab 2005;288(2):E462—8.

[109] Armstrong MJ, Adams LA, Canbay A, Syn WK. Extrahepatic complications of nonalcoholic fatty liver disease. Hepatology 2014;59(3):1174—97.

[110] Targher G, Day CP, Bonora E. Risk of cardiovascular disease in patients with nonalcoholic fatty liver disease. N Engl J Med 2010;363(14):1341—50.

[111] Ortiz-Lopez C, Lomonaco R, Orsak B, Finch J, Chang Z, Kochunov VG, et al. Prevalence of prediabetes and diabetes and metabolic profile of patients with nonalcoholic fatty liver disease (NAFLD). Diabetes Care 2012;35(4):873—8.

[112] Fabbrini E, Sullivan S, Klein S. Obesity and nonalcoholic fatty liver disease: biochemical, metabolic, and clinical implications. Hepatology 2010;51(2):679—89.

[113] Younossi ZM, Koenig AB, Abdelatif D, Fazel Y, Henry L, Wymer M. Global epidemiology of nonalcoholic fatty liver disease-Meta-analytic assessment of prevalence, incidence, and outcomes. Hepatology 2016;64(1):73—84.

[114] Tejani S, McCoy C, Ayers CR, Powell-Wiley TM, Després J-P, Linge J, et al. Cardiometabolic health outcomes associated with discordant visceral and liver fat phenotypes: insights from the Dallas Heart Study and UK Biobank. Mayo Clin Proc 2022;97(2):225−37.

[115] Vague J. The degree of masculine differentiation of obesities: a factor determining predisposition to diabetes, atherosclerosis, gout, and uric calculus disease. Am J Clin Nutr 1956;4:20−34. 1956.

[116] Geer EB, Shen W. Gender differences in insulin resistance, body composition, and energy balance. Gend Med 2009;6(Suppl. 1):60−75.

[117] Karastergiou K, Smith SR, Greenberg AS, Fried SK. Sex differences in human adipose tissues - the biology of pear shape. Biol Sex Differ 2012;3(1):13.

[118] Mayes JS, Watson GH. Direct effects of sex steroid hormones on adipose tissues and obesity. Obes Rev 2004;5(4):197−216.

[119] Federman DD. The biology of human sex differences. N Engl J Med 2006;354(14):1507−14.

[120] Wells JC. Sexual dimorphism of body composition. Best Pract Res Clin Endocrinol Metab 2007;21(3):415−30.

[121] Blaak E. Gender differences in fat metabolism. Curr Opin Clin Nutr Metab Care 2001;4(6):499−502.

[122] Camhi SM, Bray GA, Bouchard C, Greenway FL, Johnson WD, Newton RL, et al. The relationship of waist circumference and BMI to visceral, subcutaneous, and total body fat: sex and race differences. Obesity 2011;19(2):402−8.

[123] Schreiner PJ, Terry JG, Evans GW, Hinson WH, Crouse 3rd JR, Heiss G. Sex-specific associations of magnetic resonance imaging-derived intra-abdominal and subcutaneous fat areas with conventional anthropometric indices. The Atherosclerosis Risk in Communities Study. Am J Epidemiol 1996;144(4):335−45.

[124] Jackson AS, Stanforth PR, Gagnon J, Rankinen T, Leon AS, Rao DC, et al. The effect of sex, age and race on estimating percentage body fat from body mass index: the Heritage Family Study. Int J Obes Relat Metab Disord 2002;26(6):789−96.

[125] Manolopoulos KN, Karpe F, Frayn KN. Gluteofemoral body fat as a determinant of metabolic health. Int J Obes 2010;34(6):949−59.

[126] Kautzky-Willer A, Harreiter J. Sex and gender differences in therapy of type 2 diabetes. Diabetes Res Clin Pract 2017;131:230−41.

[127] Leening MJ, Ferket BS, Steyerberg EW, Kavousi M, Deckers JW, Nieboer D, et al. Sex differences in lifetime risk and first manifestation of cardiovascular disease: prospective population based cohort study. BMJ 2014;349:g5992.

[128] Lemieux S, Despres JP, Moorjani S, Nadeau A, Theriault G, Prud'homme D, et al. Are gender differences in cardiovascular disease risk factors explained by the level of visceral adipose tissue? Diabetologia 1994;37(8):757−64.

[129] Nordstrom A, Hadrevi J, Olsson T, Franks PW, Nordstrom P. Higher prevalence of type 2 diabetes in men than in women is associated with differences in visceral fat mass. J Clin Endocrinol Metab 2016;101(10):3740−6.

[130] Karpe F, Pinnick KE. Biology of upper-body and lower-body adipose tissue–link to whole-body phenotypes. Nat Rev Endocrinol 2015;11(2):90−100.

[131] Mongraw-Chaffin ML, Anderson CA, Allison MA, Ouyang P, Szklo M, Vaidya D, et al. Association between sex hormones and adiposity: qualitative differences in women and men in the multi-ethnic study of atherosclerosis. J Clin Endocrinol Metab 2015;100(4):E596−600.

[132] Gibb FW, Strachan MW. Androgen deficiency and type 2 diabetes mellitus. Clin Biochem 2014;47(10−11):940−9.

[133] Nandi A, Chen Z, Patel R, Poretsky L. Polycystic ovary syndrome. Endocrinol Metab Clin North Am 2014;43(1):123−47.

[134] Lovejoy JC, Champagne CM, de Jonge L, Xie H, Smith SR. Increased visceral fat and decreased energy expenditure during the menopausal transition. Int J Obes 2008;32(6):949−58.

[135] Janssen I, Powell LH, Kazlauskaite R, Dugan SA. Testosterone and visceral fat in midlife women: the Study of Women's Health across the Nation (SWAN) fat patterning study. Obesity 2010;18(3):604−10.

[136] Hanley AJ, Wagenknecht LE, Norris JM, Bryer-Ash M, Chen YI, Anderson AM, et al. Insulin resistance, beta cell dysfunction and visceral adiposity as predictors of incident diabetes: the Insulin Resistance Atherosclerosis Study (IRAS) Family study. Diabetologia 2009;52(10):2079−86.

[137] Lemieux I, Poirier P, Bergeron J, Almeras N, Lamarche B, Cantin B, et al. Hypertriglyceridemic waist: a useful screening phenotype in preventive cardiology? Can J Cardiol 2007;23(Suppl. B):23B−31B.

[138] Amato MC, Giordano C, Galia M, Criscimanna A, Vitabile S, Midiri M, et al. Visceral Adiposity Index: a reliable indicator of visceral fat function associated with cardiometabolic risk. Diabetes Care 2010;33(4):920−2.

[139] Kahn HS. The "lipid accumulation product" performs better than the body mass index for recognizing cardiovascular risk: a population-based comparison. BMC Cardiovasc Disord 2005;5:26.

Chapter 2

Obesity and fat distribution in children and adolescents

Jacob C. Seidell

Department of Health Sciences and Sarphati Amsterdam, Vrije Universiteit Amsterdam, Amsterdam, the Netherlands

Childhood obesity has reached pandemic proportions

Worldwide, the proportion of children and adolescents in developed countries is high. In 2013, 24% of boys and 23% of girls were overweight or obese [1]. The prevalence of overweight and obesity has also increased in children and adolescents in developing countries, from 8% to 13% in 2013 for boys and from 8% to 13% in girls [1]. The rising trends in children's and adolescents' BMI have plateaued in many high-income countries, albeit at high levels, but have accelerated in parts of Asia [2]. Fig. 2.1 shows the dramatic increase in overweight in children around the world. At the same time, many children are still underweight although there is a gradual decline.

Overweight and obesity are usually determined on the basis of height and weight in the form of BMI or standard deviations from BMI distributions in reference populations. This has important implications. The use of BMI to define obesity (the degree of excess body fat) is highly specific, but has low to moderate sensitivity. As a result, BMI-based estimates of obesity prevalence are highly conservative for all ages and both sexes. At least 25%−50% of children and adolescents defined as having a healthy BMI for age will also have excess body fat [3]. In addition, BMI says nothing about the distribution of fat over the body. BMI in childhood is not a consistent marker of body fatness across different ethnic groups. For instance, BMI has been shown to overestimate body fatness in black African children and underestimate body fatness in children of Asian origin.

Three critical periods in childhood have been identified in the development and persistence of obesity. The first period is the first 1000 days after conception (pregnancy and the first twoyears of life). Birthweight (both low and high birthweight), especially if combined with excessive weight gain, is associated with a higher risk of later overweight and obesity. A second period is the period of "adiposity rebound" (the age at which body fatness increases following a period of decrease between the ages of 5 and 8 years). Early adiposity rebound is associated with a higher risk of subsequent obesity. The third risk period is adolescence. In this period, hormonal changes do not only affect body fatness but also body fat distribution. Differences between genders and ethnic groups then also become more pronounced.

Abdominal obesity in children is a better indicator of health risks than BMI

BMI (and also sds-BMI) is commonly used in clinical practice, but it is a relatively poor measure of body fatness especially in adolescence. In addition, overall body fatness does not reflect differences in body fat distribution. Especially fat accumulation in the abdominal region is related to health outcomes. As in adults, abdominal obesity is related to cardiometabolic risk factors in children and adolescence. Abdominal obesity is determined by the accumulation of both subcutaneous adipose tissue (SAT) and visceral adipose tissue (VAT). VAT depots, located in the body cavity beneath the abdominal muscles, are composed of the greater and lesser omentum (peritoneum that is attached to the stomach and links it with other abdominal organs) and mesenteric fat. In addition, there is a compartment called retroperitoneal fat which surrounds the kidneys. But it is particularly the omental and mesenteric fat that are related to cardiometabolic problems, partially because they are drained by the portal vein which implies that fatty acids and other bioactive compounds released by these depots are transported directly to the liver [4,5].

Visceral and Ectopic Fat. https://doi.org/10.1016/B978-0-12-822186-0.00013-4

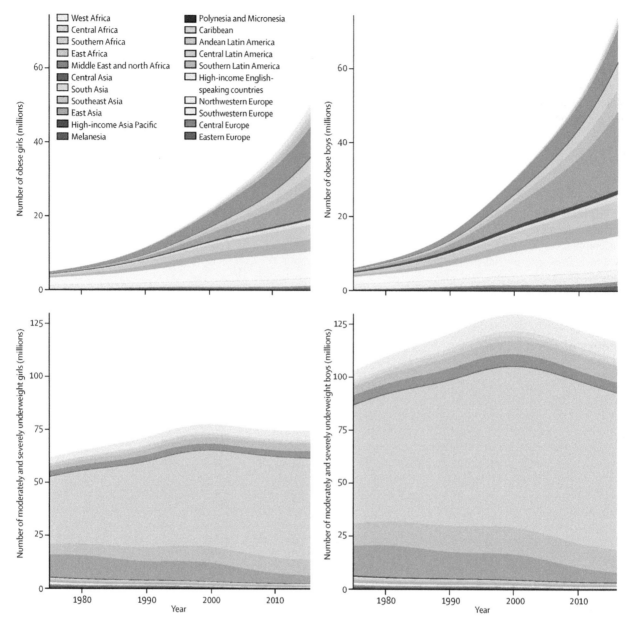

FIGURE 2.1 Worldwide trends in body mass index, underweight, overweight, and obesity from 1975 to 2016: a pooled analysis of 2416 population-based measurement studies in 128·9 million children, adolescents, and adults. *Reproduced from NCD Risk Factor Collaboration (NCD-RisC). Worldwide trends in body-mass index, underweight, overweight, and obesity from 1975 to 2016: a pooled analysis of 2416 population-based measurement studies in 128·9 million children, adolescents, and adults. Lancet 2017;390:2627—42.*

Visceral fat in relation to cardiomentabolic health in young people

Cardiometabolic risk factors are more prevalent in children and adolescents with visceral obesity than those with overweight or general obesity [4]. Visceral fat, or intra-abdominal adipose tissue, lies deep within the abdominal cavity and can only be directly quantified with imaging techniques. Visceral fat has been detected in children as young as 5 years of age. Visceral fat generally increases in proportion with general fatness, but the relationship between visceral and total body fat is complex; in children, a major portion of the variance in visceral fat is independent of total body fat. The majority of fat in children is, however, subcutaneous fat. Visceral adipose tissue accumulation becomes notable in puberty (especially in boys). Preliminary evidence in children also suggests that acquisition of visceral fat during growth is a linear process that occurs in proportion to general increases in body fat.

Determinants of visceral fat in children and adolescents

Sex

In many studies no or only small significant sex differences in visceral fat were seen in prepubertal children. The gender differences in fat distribution are influenced by sex differences in hormone concentrations, anatomical differences in the number and density of specific hormone receptors, capillary blood flow, and the activity of enzymes promoting lipid synthesis or degradation. Hormones influencing the amount and regional distribution of adipose tissue during puberty include cortisol, insulin, growth hormone, and the sex steroids. Cortisol and insulin promote fat deposition while the sex steroids and GH stimulate lipolysis. An overly sensitive hypothalamic−pituitary−adrenal axis may exist in obesity and disrupt the balance between the lipogenic effects of cortisol and insulin and the lipolytic effects of sex steroids and growth hormone. Leptin is released from the adipocytes and may act as a metabolic signal to the hypothalamic areas controlling satiety, energy expenditure, and the regulation of cortisol, insulin, sex steroid, and growth hormone release.

The gender difference in visceral fat particularly becomes apparent during puberty. In boys there is an increase in muscle mass and a decrease in subcutaneous adipose tissue due to increases in testosterone. In girls, female sex steroids stimulate the accumulation of subcutaneous fat compartments (breasts, hips, thighs). But in addition to sex steroids, also leptin may play a role. Pubertal girls have two- to threefold greater serum leptin concentrations than pubertal boys after correction for adiposity. The lower serum leptin concentrations in males may be due to androgen-induced reduction in leptin production. However, the gender difference in serum leptin concentration is also present prepubertally, suggesting that factors other than sex steroids (e.g., body fat patterning, energy expenditure, aerobic fitness) influence serum leptin concentrations [5,6].

Genetics of visceral fat accumulation

It has been estimated that between 50% and 55% of the variance in visceral fat levels, adjusted for total fatness, is attributable to genetic factors [7]. It appears that phenotypes reflecting body fat distribution (abdominal, visceral, and subcutaneous fat; waist:hip ratio; waist circumference; sagittal diameter) were associated with: ACE, ADIPOQ, ADRB2, APOAQ, FABP2, LTA, MTTP, PLIN, PPARG, and UCP1 (angiotensin-converting enzyme, adiponectin, β-2-adrenergic receptor, apoAQ, fatty acid-binding protein 2, lymphotoxin-α, microsomal TAG transfer protein, perilipin, PPAR-γ and uncoupling protein 1 genes) [7].

Ethnicity

In adults, Caucasian men have (after adjustment for overall body fatness) relatively less visceral fat than South Asian men and also less than Hispanics in the United States, but they have more visceral adipose tissue than African American men. These ethnic differences are less pronounced in women.

In children these ethnic differences are also seen, especially during and after puberty. The predominance of visceral adipose tissue accumulation in South Asian children may relate to intrauterine growth retardation. The thin-fat phenotype in South Asian children is present at birth. Indian babies are centrally adipose but thin in muscle and viscera (protein-rich tissues) [8]. These differences early in life suggest that ethnic differences in fat distribution are genetic and/or determined through exposure to maternal physiology, rather than a consequence of behaviors or diet in childhood or at older ages [8].

Chronic stress (cortisol)

Some studies suggest that visceral adiposity could represent a nonoptimal physiological adaptation to chronic stress. Stress-induced activation of the HPA axis may contribute to the antecedents of the metabolic syndrome by promoting central adiposity and inducing an inflammatory response and insulin resistance. The increase in cortisol levels during puberty or an oversensitive HPA axis in an adolescent may influence body fat distribution. Adipose tissue-specific regulation of glucocorticoid metabolism is primarily determined by the enzyme 11β-hydroxysteroid dehydrogenase type 1 (11β-HSD1), which catalyzes the conversion of cortisone to hormonally active cortisol. 11β-HSD1 is highly expressed in VAT [9,10].

Behavioral determinants of visceral fat

Several studies have confirmed that increased levels of physical activity and higher levels of fitness are associated with less visceral adipose tissue [11]. Studies among adults showed that acute energy restriction, using very-low-energy diets, produces early preferential loss of visceral fat. Results of some studies suggest that in reducing deposits of visceral tissue, the glycemic index and glycemic load of consumed products (i.e., refined carbohydrates and sugary drinks) may be very important [11]. Glucose raises insulin concentration, which can stimulate 11β-HSD1, increase active cortisol in visceral fat, and enhance visceral fat accumulation. Cigarette smoking and excessive alcohol consumption seem to be associated with a preferential accumulation of visceral fat [11].

Also in children and adolescents combined lifestyle interventions that have focused on improving dietary habits and increasing physical activity lead to improvements in cardiometabolic risk factors [12].

Measurement of visceral fat in children

Imaging techniques

Visceral fat can be directly measured by imaging techniques. MRI does not require exposure to ionizing radiation, making it advantageous over CT, particularly for multiple measurements. However, MRI is also expensive and not widely available for research. An alternative method of assessing visceral adiposity may be ultrasonography. Indirect measurements of visceral fat include dual-energy X-ray absorptiometry (DXA) to measure fat mass in the trunk region and anthropometry. The main limitation of DXA assessment of body composition is the inability to distinguish subcutaneous from intraabdominal fat mass [13].

The waist circumference or waist/height ratio as a measure of visceral fat in clinical practice and public health

Imaging techniques such as MRI, CT, or DEXA are usually not available in population studies or in clinical practice. But there is a variety of easily measured anthropometric indices that reflect abdominal obesity and visceral fat. In several studies it was found that the waist circumference and sagittal diameter were highly correlated with visceral fat. The waist circumference, however, changes rapidly during maturation and lateral growth and therefore requires age- and gender-specific reference curves. The waist-over-height ratio (WHtR) is not dependent on age and height. This ratio was devised to correct for the over- and underestimation of risk among tall and short individuals with similar waist circumference. This index is strongly correlated with abdominal fat measures which are obtained using advanced imaging techniques [14,15].

In a systematic review conducted in children and adolescents, WHtR was associated with systolic and diastolic blood pressure (BP), high levels of insulin, HDL-cholesterol (HDL-C), and serum triglycerides. WHtR has also been associated with resistin levels in children and adolescents, with plasminogen activator inhibitor-1 (PAI-1) levels in obese adolescents and with CRP levels in children and adolescents [16].

Classification of abdominal obesity in children by the waist/height ratio

In the adult population, the WHtR is related to cardiovascular risk and the recommendation for keeping it ≥ 0.5 has been used as a mass prevention measure. Although the suggested cutoff point for children is equal to that of adults in some studies, evidence suggests that this value may not be adequate, and there is the need to increase its sensitivity to become a good screening tool for childhood obesity. Mehta suggested that a WHtR between ≥ 0.5 and < 0.55 identified children at risk for central obesity and WC/HT ≥ 0.55 identified central obesity with a high probability (Table 2.1) [15].

TABLE 2.1 Tentative classification of abdominal obesity by waist/height ratio.

Children (≤15 years)	Boys (>15 years)	Girls (>15 years)	Categorization	Clinical management
≤0.34	≤0.34	≤0.34	Very lean	—
0.35−0.45	0.35−0.52	0.35−0.42	Lean	—
0.46−0.51	0.43−0.52	0.42−0.48	Healthy	—
0.52−0.63	0.53−0.62	0.49−0.57	Overweight	Refer to combined lifestyle intervention
≥0.64	≥0.63	≥0.58	Obesity	Assess cardiometabolic profile and refer to combined lifestyle intervention

Visceral fat and metabolic risk factors in children and adolescents

The correlations between visceral fat and cardiometabolic risk factors in adolescents are similar to those observed in adults [16]. In most studies the association between visceral fat and these risk factors were stronger than other measures of adiposity.

Associations between visceral fat and cardiometabolic risk factors (positive unless indicated):

- Serum triglycerides.
- HDL-cholesterol (negative association).
- Basal and stimulated insulin responses. Homeostasis model assessment of insulin resistance (HOMA) score.
- M/I index of insulin sensitivity (inverse association; the ratio between glucose infusion rate and plasma insulin levels during the hyperglycaemic clamp)
- Systolic and diastolic blood pressure.
- Early macrophage-rich coronary lesions were associated with increased amounts of visceral fat in adolescent male individuals.

Conclusions

The global prevalence of obesity is increasing rapidly. Unhealthy lifestyles in combination with genetic susceptibility are the main cause for this global epidemic. Particularly the accumulation of visceral fat poses a great risk for cardiometabolic diseases and other chronic noncommunicable diseases.

Fig. 2.2 summarizes the main learnings in this chapter.

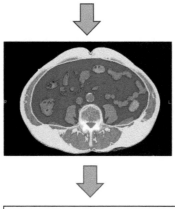

FIGURE 2.2 Relationships between determinants of visceral fat (red area in the abdominal scan) and cardiometabolic risk factors.

References

[1] Ng M, Fleming T, Robinson M, et al. Global, regional, and national prevalence of overweight and obesity in children and adults during 1980—2013: a systematic analysis for the Global Burden of Disease Study 2013. Lancet 2014;384:766—81.

[2] NCD Risk Factor Collaboration (NCD-RisC). Worldwide trends in body-mass index, underweight, overweight, and obesity from 1975 to 2016: a pooled analysis of 2416 population-based measurement studies in 128·9 million children, adolescents, and adults. Lancet 2017;390:2627—42.

[3] Reilly JJ, El-Hamdouchi A, Diouf A, Monyeki A, Somda SA. Determining the worldwide prevalence of obesity. Lancet 2018;391:1773—4.

[4] Forkert ECO, Rendo-Urteaga T, Nascimento-Ferreira MV, et al. Abdominal obesity and cardiometabolic risk in children and adolescents, are we aware of their relevance? Nutrire 2016;41:15.

[5] Goran MI. Visceral fat in prepubertal children: influence of obesity, anthropometry, ethnicity, gender, diet, and growth. Am J Hum Biol 1999;11:201—7.

[6] Roemmich JN, Rogol AD. Hormonal changes during puberty and their relationship to fat distribution. Am J Hum Biol 1999;11:209—24.

[7] Sung YJ, Pérusse L, Sarzynski MA, et al. Genome-wide association studies suggest sex-specific loci associated with abdominal and visceral fat. Int J Obes 2016;40:662—74.

[8] Stanfield KM, Wells JC, Fewtrell MS, Frost C, Leon DA. Differences in body composition between infants of South Asian and European ancestry: the London mother and baby study. Int J Epidemiol 2012;41:1409—18.

[9] Drapeau V, Therrien F, Richard D, et al. Is visceral obesity a physiological adaptation to stress? Panminerva Med 2003;45:189—95.

[10] Goldbacher EM, Matthews KA, Salomon K. Central adiposity and hemodynamic functioning at rest and during stress in adolescents. Health Psychol 2005;24:375—84.

[11] Vissers D, Hens W, Hansen D, Taeymans J. The effect of diet or exercise on visceral adipose tissue in overweight youth. Med Sci Sports Exerc 2016;48:1415—24.

[12] Bondyra-Wiśniewska B, Myszkowska-Ryciak J, Harton A. Impact of lifestyle intervention programs for children and adolescents with overweight or obesity on body weight and selected cardiometabolic factors-A systematic review. Int J Environ Res Publ Health 2021;18:2061.

[13] Olza J, Aguilera C, Gil-Campos M, et al. Waist-to-height ratio, inflammation and CVD risk in obese children. Publ Health Nutr 2014;17:2378—85.

[14] Lobor Cancelier AC, Trevisol D, Schuelter-Trevisol F. Waist-to-height ratio as a screening tool for childhood obesity: a systematic literature review. Ann Pediatr Child Health 2018;6:1141.

[15] Mehta SK. Waist circumference to height ratio in children and adolescents. Clin Pediatr 2015;54:652—8.

[16] Suliga E. Visceral adipose tissue in children and adolescents: a review. Nutr Res Rev 2009;22:137—47.

Chapter 3

Brown adipose tissue: metabolic role and non-invasive quantification in humans

Andreas Paulus[1] and Matthias Bauwens[1,2,3]

[1]Department of Radiology and Nuclear Medicine, Maastricht University Medical Center, Maastricht, the Netherlands; [2]School of Nutrition and Translational Research in Metabolism (NUTRIM), Maastricht University, Maastricht, the Netherlands; [3]Department of Nuclear Medicine, University Hospital RWTH Aachen, Aachen, Germany

BAT physiology

Brown adipose tissue (BAT), or brown fat, is a type of tissue with characteristics similar to both muscle tissue and white adipose tissue [1]. On the one hand, both brown adipocytes and muscle cells have the intrinsic capacity to activate the myogenic factor 5 promoter that can induce differentiation of fibroblasts to myoblasts. In in vitro conditions, muscle cells cocultured with the transcription factor PRDM16, a regulator for BAT-cell differentiation, were converted into brown fat cells, and brown fat cells without PRDM16 were converted into muscle cells. On the other hand, brown adipocytes share with white adipocytes their capacity to store lipids, although the lipid droplets in white adipocytes are much larger compared to those in brown adipocytes. BAT is also more highly vascularized compared to white adipose tissue (WAT). This higher vascularization, together with the high density of iron-rich mitochondria in BAT, causes its brownish color.

BAT is not restricted to a single location in the body (see Fig. 3.1). Each location contains brown adipocytes as well as preadipocytes, embedded interstitial cells, and endothelial cells of the capillaries. The activity of each location is determined further by the presence and signaling of nerve terminals.

The physiological role of BAT is to generate heat: thermogenesis. This is achieved by uncoupling the mitochondrial oxidative phosphorylation from ATP production and instead using a specific protein (UnCoupling Protein 1, or UCP-1). In this way, energy generated by lipolysis is wasted resulting in "only" generation of heat. This heat production can be intensified by stimulation of lipolysis (by signaling by norepinephrine from the nerve endings). There are a number of reviews on the exact mechanism, which we gladly refer to Refs. [2–4]. This thermogenic effect is a defining effect in warm-blooded animals, and especially abundant in newborns and hibernating animals [5]. Of the endothermic animals, mammals are the only ones with a functional brown adipose tissue, as birds only have an expression of (avian) UCP in muscular tissue and use muscular shivering to maintain body heat.

There is more to adipose tissue than just brown and white; however, as over the past decade also beige adipocytes have been discovered [6]. Beige adipocytes are aroused in white fat depots and respond to stimuli like brown adipocytes (mainly cold-induced hormones). As beige adipocytes contain abundant mitochondria and are active in dissipating energy, they have drawn much attention as a therapeutic target for obesity. It is currently not entirely clear how the amount and metabolic activity of beige tissue could be altered in humans, but the mere possibility of adjusting this "new" type of cell does draw a lot of researchers into this field so we can expect more information in the coming decade [7–10] (Table 3.1).

Background on history of BAT: perceived impact on human health and scientific interest in past three decades

Brown adipose tissue was thought to have limited effect in adult humans and was therefore for a long time an underestimated research field. Already in the 1920s BAT was described and studies were performed to investigate BAT's function in newborns [11–14]. It could be observed that BAT's size decreased with aging and therefore the general belief

Visceral and Ectopic Fat. https://doi.org/10.1016/B978-0-12-822186-0.00016-X

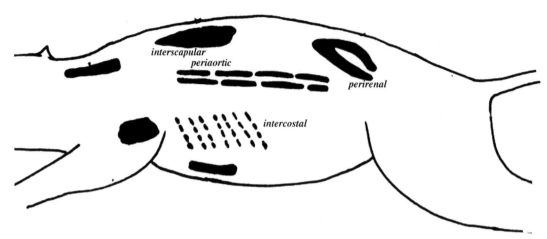

FIGURE 3.1 Locations of BAT in a rodent. *From Cannon B, Nedergaard J. Brown adipose tissue: function and physiological significance. Physiol Rev 2004;8(1):277—359. https://doi.org/10.1152/physrev.00015.2003 with permission.*

was that it is irrelevant for human adults [15—17]. This view changed when significant amounts of BAT were found in Finnish outdoor workers in the 1980s. [18] (See Fig. 3.2 for a schematic overview of the current understanding of BAT distribution in humans.) Active BAT in adult humans was reported for the first time in the beginning of this century by retrospective Positron Emission Tomography/Computed Tomography (PET/CT) scans with the glucose analog [18F]fluoro-2-deoxy-2-D-glucose ([18F]FDG) and consecutive biopsies [19—22]. Since then BAT research gained more and more interest and many studies were conducted to unravel BAT's functions. Dedicated cold exposure studies showed increased [18F]FDG uptake and concluded therefore an increase in BAT activity [22—24]. Also short-term cold exposure in obese patients showed BAT recruitment which might give an option to increase whole body energy expenditure by BAT activation to decrease body weight in those subjects [25]. BAT's research is ranging nowadays from development of new techniques to visualize and quantify BAT's activity over activation of BAT by pharmacological or external factors up to recruitment of BAT in obese individuals. Until now BAT's role in whole body metabolism as well as in certain metabolic conditions and diseases is not completely understood and therefore needs more investigation.

The primary focus of this multidisciplinary interest regarding BAT research focuses on a worldwide pandemic: obesity. Obesity is the result of a positive energy balance and could theoretically be easily addressed by lowering the energy intake and increasing energy expenditure by physical activity. It was shown however that subjects have serious problems to follow their diet plans and keep themselves active [26,27]. An alternative strategy would be to increase energy expenditure by mitochondrial activation. The concept of applying mitochondrial uncoupling as a means for weight loss has been proven with the pharmaceutical dinitrophenol—even though this compound was quickly outbanned in the 1940s as overdosing led to heat death [28]. A more specific approach, targeting BAT, is often seen as a potential solution. Closely related to obesity is diabetes type II. Here, BAT was found to increase insulin sensitivity in those patients after BAT activation by cold exposure for several days [25]. Much work remains to be done however, as until now BAT's contribution to energy expenditure in humans was estimated by different research groups to be 2%—30% with a large interpatient deviation rendering any studies investigating a potential effect of an increase in BAT energy expenditure difficult.

On the other side of the spectrum, BAT research can also help cancer patients' cachexia [29]. Kir et al. showed in 2014 that by neutralization of PTHrP (a known promoter of browning in adipose tissue) in tumor-bearing mice cachexia could be significantly reduced [30]. Parathyroid hormone appears to also be a potent regulator of BAT activity and may be an important mediator of elevated expenditure during cancer cachexia, although this is disputed by observations that cachexia wasting is not blunted in UCP1 KO mice [31]. In patients with catecholamine secreting tumors this may be clinically relevant, as catecholamines were found to activate BAT and therefore lead to increased metabolic activity and weight loss [32—34]. Controlling BATs activity in these patients would counteract weight loss and lead to a better quality of life.

Overview of potential analysis techniques for assessing BAT activity

During the past decades multiple BAT analysis methods have been developed or adapted from other fields. Especially the field of nuclear medicine allowed visualization but also quantification of BAT's metabolism. Invasive and noninvasive techniques are discussed in this chapter and pros and cons of different methods are explained.

TABLE 3.1 Characteristics of myocyte (muscle cell), brown, beige and white adipocytes.

Myocyte	Brown adipocyte	Beige adipocyte	White adipocyte
Properties			
Many mitochondria	Many small lipid droplets	Moderate mitochondria	Few mitochondria
Few small lipid droplets			One large lipid droplet
Highly vascularized tissue		Embedded in white adipose tissue, increasing vascularization	Adequate vascularization (compromised in obesity)
No UCP1 expression	High UCP1 expression	Medium UCP1 expression	No or very limited UCP1 expression
Shared Myf5-expressing progenitors from mesenchymal stem cell		Myf5-negative progenitors from mesenchymal stem cell	
Converts to brown adipocyte in presence of PRDM16	Converts to muscle cell in absence of PRDM16	Converts back to white adipocytes in absence of stimuli	Can convert to beige adipocyte by PPARγ or cold (for tissue)
Function			
Muscle movement	Heat generation (lipid clearance?)	Heat generation (lipid clearance?)	Lipid storage

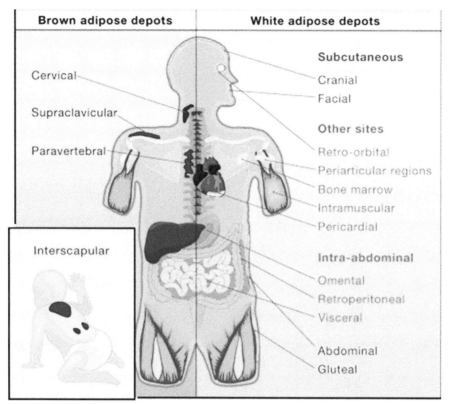

FIGURE 3.2   Locations of brown and white adipose tissue in humans. *From Gesta S, Tseng YH, Kahn CR. Developmental origin of fat: tracking obesity to its source. Cell 2007;131(2):242–256. https://doi.org/10.1016/j.cell.2007.10.004 with permission.*

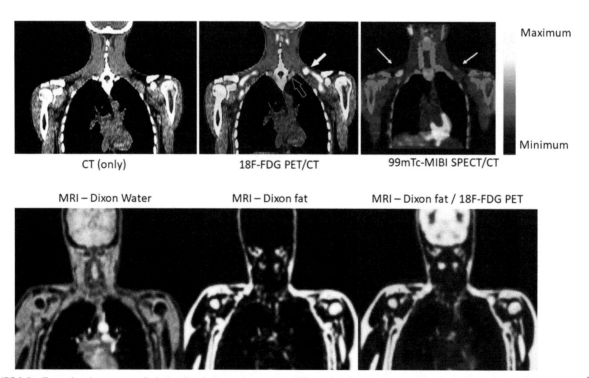

FIGURE 3.3   Exemplary images compiled, showing the human torso using different imaging equipment: CT-only; PET combined with CT (using [^{18}F]-FDG as a tracer), SPECT combined with CT (using [^{99m}Tc]-MIBI as a tracer) and MRI (either fat only, water only, or fat signal fraction). Filled arrows indicate examples of brown adipose tissue; open arrows indicate examples of white adipose tissue. *From Gariani K, Gariani J, Amzalag G, Delattre BM, Ratib O, Garibotto V. Hybrid PET/MRI as a tool to detect brown adipose tissue: proof of principle. Obes Res Clin Pract 2015;9(6):613–617. https://doi. org/10.1016/j.orcp.2015.05.004; Belhocine T, Shastry A, Driedger A, Urbain J.-L. Detection of 99mTc-sestamibi uptake in brown adipose tissue with SPECT-CT. Eur J Nucl Med Mol Imag 2006;34(1):149. https://doi.org/10.1007/s00259-006-0244-x; Hu HH, Tovar JP, Pavlova Z, Smith ML, Gilsanz V. Unequivocal identification of brown adipose tissue in a human infant. J Magn Reson Imaging. 2012;35(4):938–942. doi: 10.1002/jmri.23531. Epub 2011 Dec 16. PMID: 22180228; PMCID: PMC3310283.*

Invasive techniques

Invasive techniques for BAT assessment play a significant role in preclinical BAT studies, but less so in clinical studies simply due to their invasive nature. Biopsies can either be used for direct staining or for additional in vitro experiments, and it is even possible to culture biopsy-derived adipocytes, allowing for a multitude of subsequent in vitro experiments, as recently demonstrated by Nascimento et al. [35]. Biopsies are powerful in exploring highly localized tissues or analyzing the expression of cells embedded in a larger tissue, as is the case in beige adipocytes (embedded in white adipose tissue) [36,37]. Staining of different constituents of BAT metabolism also helped to understand processes involved in energy homeostasis. One prominent example is ADIFAB (Acrylodan labeled Intestinal Fatty Acid Binding Protein) staining for unbound fatty acids. Different mechanisms related to fatty acid uptake by BAT have been investigated with this stain in vitro [38,39] but also others are available for fatty acid/triglyceride staining and quantification [40−42].

An important example of BAT metabolism quantification is triolein radiolabeled with tritium. The radiolabeled triglyceride is applied in small animals and after certain times animals are euthanized, organs can be harvested and counted for their radioactivity uptake. By incorporation of tritium labeled triolein into lipoproteins, it was, for example, found that the majority of fatty acids internalized into BAT after lipoprotein lipase liberation [43,44]. Dual labeled particles were utilized to follow-up lipoproteins after triglyceride depletion by additional incorporation of cholesteryl oleate labeled by carbon-14. A more indirect method would be blood sampling after certain timepoints and cold exposure. Increased triolein labeled triglyceride uptake from the blood could be measured due to cold exposure and therefore increased metabolic activity, but this elevated clearance can not only be attributed to BAT as also other tissues will experience an higher energy demand [45,46].

Autoradiography with tritium-labeled triglycerides can be conducted as well. This method does not reflect in vivo surrounding for BAT cells as also endothelial cells are important for triglyceride uptake in BAT. Anyhow important information was found using this method, i.e., lipids are stored first in intracellular lipid droplets before they are metabolized in the mitochondria [47].

Noninvasive techniques

For in vivo studies, either preclinically or clinically, noninvasive techniques are often necessary to visualize and quantify BAT activity. Here different BAT visualization techniques are summarized.

Computed Tomography (CT) relies on an X-ray source that is rotated around an object and differences in beam attenuation by different types of tissue are detected by multiple detectors which are located in the gantry. As CT measures differences in attenuation, expressed as Hounsfield Units, it is challenging to identify BAT with a standalone CT especially when white adipose tissue (WAT) is located next to it.

There are also differences in interpreting Hounsfield units by different research groups, e.g., Gortel et al. used a threshold of −200 to −30, Maurovic-Horvat et al. used a threshold from −149 to −30, and Mahabadi et al. a threshold of −195 to −45 [48−51]. As this is not a direct measure for BAT an over or underestimation of BAT's tissue amount is easily possible and therefore results in inconsistent quantification.

Nonetheless, CT can be a good addition to other imaging approaches to give excellent anatomical information and therefore make BAT identification more intuitive. In addition, the density as measured by CT can be translated into a fat/water ratio, rendering medium-term changes in BAT composition possible. Taken together, this implies that although CT has some difficulty in locating and quantifying BAT, once found, it is able to quantify changes in BAT density, which is directly linked to water and lipid content. A true determination of the amount of lipids that are being metabolized in BAT is not an easy feature however, as it requires information on the influx of new lipids (to be assessed using molecular imaging, but which tracer mimics this best?) and the local depletion of lipids (but does a single CT density measurement correlate 1:1 with BAT's preferred lipids?).

As the determination of the composition of a tissue becomes easier when using multiple energies in CT, more advanced CT techniques such as dual-energy CT can be helpful (see Ref. [52] for an excellent overview on dual-energy CT techniques). There are a number of different technical approaches to dual-energy CT, but they all rely on the principle that different energies have different attenuations in tissue; and this attenuation is dependent on the elemental composition of the tissue. Instead of the usual single quantity "density" that is obtained from a normal CT, dual-energy CT allows to decompose the tissue into two or three main components (i.e., "water" and "lipid"). Dual energy CT is widely used in the clinic, and although not being routinely used to investigate BAT it is being routinely used to assess (muscle) cachexia, liver fattiness, and diabetes—all applications where it is required to measure lipid content in a tissue [53−56]. Dual-energy CT, regardless of the technical approach (dual sources, slow kV switching, fast kV switching, dual layer energy counting, or even photon counting detectors), do have their limits: they cannot distinguish short-chained fatty acids (from lipids) from longer-chained fatty acids (from lipids), but BAT only uses mediate to long-chain fatty acids, so more information is needed to fully quantify BAT's use of lipids.

In Single Photon Emission Computed Tomography (SPECT) a radioactive substance, called radiotracer or tracer, is injected into a test subject and emission of single gamma rays can be measured and localized from outside the subject by a detector. After tomographic reconstruction, the detected signals can be transformed into a 3D image of the activity distribution within the entire subject.

Any substance class, important for BAT metabolism or directed toward specific BAT proteins, can be potentially radiolabeled by SPECT-emitting radioisotopes and therefore different aspects of BAT and its metabolism can be investigated. Although it is possible to simultaneously use different tracers (each labeled with a different isotope suitable for SPECT), these combinations are complex and rarely applied outside of the preclinical level—so in daily practice SPECT allows for the visualization of a single metabolic feature in humans per imaging session and often per study (for examples see Refs. [57−60]).

In Positron Emission Tomography (PET) a radiotracer labeled with a positron emitting radioisotope is injected into a subject and annihilation rays are measured in coincidence under 180 degrees with a detector ring. Like in SPECT, a 3D image of a specific tracer distribution is created which allows BAT visualization but additionally allows quantification of radiotracer uptake. Dependent on the substance class used as radiotracer, quantification of BAT's metabolic activity is possible with PET. Nonetheless, similar to SPECT but even more strict due to physical properties of the radionuclides, only a single metabolic feature can be quantified per imaging session, restricting research to one or a few features per study and prohibiting array-type studies (for examples, see Refs. [61,62]).

MRI is a nonradioactive measurement technique. A subject is measured within a magnetic field where the protons of the subject are all aligned. The direction of the magnetization is flipped toward the transversal direction which induces the protons to spin and emit a radiofrequency (RF) which is dependent on the chemical surrounding. This RF can be measured from outside the subject and a 3D image can be computed, allowing T1 and/or T2 weighted images of the anatomical structure. To enhance contrast or follow-up metabolic activities, functional MRI (fMRI) can be used. Here superparamagnetic particles are injected in the subject and followed by MRI. It is also possible to use Magnetic Resonance Spectroscopy to determine the fat/water ratio of a tissue (with strong differences between WAT, BAT, and muscle), or even quantify the temperature of a (piece of) tissue in vivo, a useful feature when assessing BAT activity [63]. BOLD MRI allows the quantification of blood flow and oxygenation. Combining all of these techniques would provide excellent information, but as MRI is a time-consuming technique choices have be made in order to facilitate patient comfort. As MRI is a technique with many interesting and different aspects, we gladly refer to the following recent reviews for further information [64,65].

Near-infrared spectroscopy (NIRS) has been used for measuring changes in O_2-dependent light absorption in the tissue in a noninvasive manner. Among NIRS, time-resolved NIRS (NIRTRS) can quantify the concentrations of oxygenated and deoxygenated hemoglobin ([oxy-Hb] and [deoxy-Hb], respectively) by emitting ultrashort light pulses and counts photons, which are scattered and absorbed in the tissue [66]. This allows the quantification of certain aspects of BAT activity, as BAT is highly vascularized in comparison to WAT. Research so far has shown that [oxy-Hb] and [deoxy-Hb] concentrations are correlated to typical 18F-FDG PET data in BAT, although future research is required to investigate its potential as the relatively low-cost continuous wavelength NIRS (NIRCWS) (used for measuring relative changes in oxygenation in tissues) does not show this correlation.

Infrared thermography (IRT) is being increasingly recognized as a valid and complementary method to standard imaging modalities. It is noninvasive, cheap, and quick and does not use any radiation, allowing the possibility of large studies of BAT on healthy populations and children [67]. IRT following BAT stimulation consistently shows a change in supraclavicular skin temperature and a close association with results from BAT measurements from other methods. The current variations in study protocols prevent a direct comparison to clinical study protocols with 18F-FDG, so some optimization is required to allow true large-scale studies.

As should now be clear: different techniques each have their advantages and disadvantages. Therefore, combinations of different techniques have been developed to increase image quality, resolution, and to gain additional information from one single scan. Most important here is the combination of PET/CT. By PET/CT and the glucose analog [18F]FDG, BAT has been visualized for the first time in humans [19−22]. CT provides important anatomical information and helps to identify adipose tissue. [18F]FDG PET shows regions with high glucose uptake. Combining these information BAT can be identified and glucose uptake can be quantified. Recently PET/MRI has been brought to clinical applications. First retrospective [68] and later dedicated studies [69−71] have been published for preclinical as well as clinical applications, most often with [18F]FDG as the radiotracer.

Overview of tracers with their molecular targets

Historically, [18F]FDG was the first radiotracer used to visualize BAT in humans [19−21]. For a long time, symmetrical accumulations found during [18F]FDG-scans in the supraclavicular area were thought to originate from muscle tissue but multimodal scans with PET/CT revealed that those signals show Hounsfield units in the range of adipose tissue. This led to a high number of retrospective studies all conducted with [18F]FDG as the radiotracer, as [18F]FDG is also most often used in cancer scans.

The prevalence to visualize BAT during a [18F]FDG PET/CT is strongly dependent on external factors such as age, BMI, outdoor temperature [72]. [18F]FDG is still the gold standard for BAT visualization and quantification approaches, with good efforts being made to standardize this technique [73,74].

As [18F]FDG is a glucose analog, its main uptake mechanism is through the GLUT family protein transporters, mainly the fat muscle specific isoform GLUT4 [75]. Once it has been taken up by BAT, glucose can be processed in different pathways, e.g., in citric acid cycle or it is converted to FA [76]. [18F]FDG is "trapped" intracellularly as the tracer, after uptake in the cell through GLUT, is phosphorylated once (preventing any exit through GLUT) but can then no longer be metabolized due to the presence of 18F [77]. This property is one of the key advantages of [18F]FDG as a tracer and perhaps the main reason for its clinical success: more than 90% of PET scans in cancer patients worldwide are performed with this specific tracer [78].

Although [18F]FDG is used frequently for BAT scans it is suffering from a severe problem:

Fatty acids have been identified as the main metabolized substance class in BAT [79−81]. Therefore one can largely underestimate BATs activity just by [18F]FDG scans. Additionally [18F]FDG is dependent on the insulin sensitivity of the specific subject, which might prevent BAT from taking up any kind of glucose. This does not necessarily mean that BAT does not show any metabolic activity, but instead fatty acids are preferably metabolized—rendering the diagnostic capacity of [18F]FDG as a passe-partout tool questionable [61].

In tracer development for assessing BATs contribution to whole body energy expenditure, fatty acid (FA)−based radiotracers have gained more and more interest as they reflect BATs primary substance class for energy turnover. Multiple FA-based tracers have been proposed lately or have been adapted from other approaches, mainly myocardial imaging.

One prominent example is [18F]FTHA. Originating from cardiac research it can also be used to visualize BAT. Most important, neither the sulfur atom at the sixth position nor the introduction of fluorine-18 has influence on the uptake kinetics [82]. During oxidation processes in the mitochondria it is irreversibly bound to mitochondria proteins, which make it an ideal candidate to investigate FA consumption during BAT activation [83].

[11C]palmitate is a radiolabeled FA where the radioisotope has no influence on the pharmacokinetics of the FA as it is a radioactive carbon in the backbone of the FA. Like [18F]FTHA it has evolved from a myocardial imaging agent toward application in BAT clinical imaging [84−87].

Other prominent examples of FAs used for myocardial imaging with a potential for BAT imaging are [123I]BMIPP [88,89] Syamsunarno, [123I]IHXA and [123I]IHDA [90], and [123I]IPPA [91].

BAT imaging with FA-based tracers is already an improvement to imaging with [18F]FDG when it comes to quantification of BAT's contribution to whole body energy expenditure. Nevertheless, it was found that FAs are predominantly taken up as triglyceride-derived FAs originating from triglyceride-rich lipoproteins (TRL) and therefore FA tracers injected as such rely on multiple uptake mechanisms before they can be incorporated into BAT [92,93]. This, in fact, might reduce the uptake probability and therefore might not reflect the real FA consumption. Triglyceride-derived FA internalization was shown to be dependent on the presence of several proteins, namely: lipoprotein lipase (LPL), cluster of differentiation 36 (CD36), and fatty acid transport proteins (FATP) [93−96].

To overcome the limitation of not mimicking the uptake mechanism in vivo, in first attempts tri[3H]oleate and [14C] cholesteryl oleate double-labeled TRL-like particles were developed. Those particles proved that they could reach BAT and that FAs are taken up. As tritium and carbon-14 are not suitable for noninvasive applications, our group recently developed TRLs with a Bodipy-triglyceride suitable for radiolabeling with fluorine-18. With this multimodal approach, where in vitro behavior can also be observed by fluorescence microscopy, our group was able to visualize and quantify BAT's incorporation of TRL-derived FAs and investigate the effect of cold activation and metabolic syndromes [97,98].

BAT is activated by norepinephrine which is secreted by sympathetic nerve endings and imaging agents like [123I] MIBG, 6-[18F]fluorodopamine and (S,S)-[11C]-O-methylreboxetine are targeting the sympathetic nervous system [99−101]. Therefore, those imaging agents are good indicators for BAT to get activated.

BAT cells have a high number of mitochondria which gives the possibility to image with [99mTc]Tc-MIBI. [99mTc]Tc-MIBI binds to mitochondria rich cells and BAT has been visualized with it previously under basal conditions [59,102].

Other types of perfusion and tracers that rely on oxygen consumption are $[^{15}O]H_2O$, $[^{15}O]O_2$, and $[^{11}C]$acetate [103,104]. Although these last tracers may represent the true perfusion and oxidative metabolism of BAT, the short physical half-life of the radionuclides (2 min for ^{15}O, 20 min for ^{11}C) prohibits any large-scale studies.

Except for FA-based tracers and to some extent to $[^{18}F]FDG$, a quantification of BATs metabolic state is currently not possible. Anyhow, those tracers are a good addition to gain more information about BAT's condition and likelihood to get activated.

Discussion: clinical applications?

Noninvasive imaging of BAT certainly has a future, although the jury is still out on which imaging technique (combination) is best to go forward. While anatomical imaging (CT, classical MRI) is useful, it lacks the necessary metabolic information to determine the real activity of any given tissue. Near-infrared imaging and thermal imaging provide blood flow or temperature-specific information but currently lack sufficient spatial resolution, and PET/SPECT imaging using specific tracers, informative as they are, may be too specific to acquire all the desired knowledge (Fig. 3.3). The choice of technique will therefore depend on the question that has to be answered, and in BAT the main question (beyond the existing very interesting fundamental research) is centered on lipid metabolism in the body.

The ongoing obesity pandemic, accompanied by a large increase in diabetes prevalence, is a large motivator for evaluating BAT, and thus requires the quantification of BAT activity with respect to the metabolic syndrome [107]. As shown above, BAT can already be visualized and quantified in nondisease conditions. In certain cases, activation is necessary, especially when it comes to clinical imaging. Currently most BAT scans are performed with $[^{18}F]FDG$, even though this method has several drawbacks such as problems to quantify BAT's activity, as glucose is not the primary substance class to be taken up by BAT and that during diabetes the insulin sensitivity is reduced, which makes it more unlikely to visualize BAT with a glucose tracer. $[^{18}F]FDG$ provided the first information on the difference of BAT activity in humans in a nonclinical setting, with obese persons having less active BAT compared to lean persons. In addition to BAT's clear (reverse) correlation to obesity, it has also been shown via noninvasive imaging to be involved in other diseases as well, such as cancer. A recent clinical case illustrates this nicely: $[^{18}F]FDG$ PET/CT demonstrated that the increased metabolic BAT activity as observed in a paraganglioma cancer patient disappeared after the tumor was surgically removed (Fig. 3.4) [108]. Blood analysis before and after surgery explained the phenomenon: the tumor was inducing high

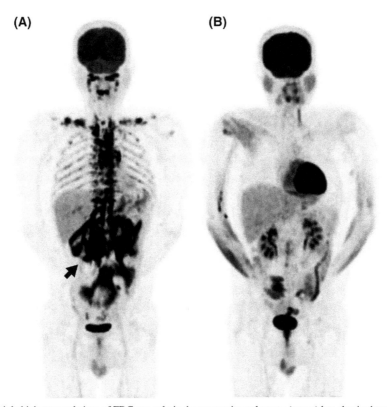

FIGURE 3.4   (left, A) Multiple high accumulations of FDG not only in the retroperitoneal tumor (arrow) but also in the peritracheal, upper mediastinal, supraclavicular, perispinal, periaortic, and perirenal spaces (corresponding to known locations of BAT); (right, B) Disappearance of multiple FDG accumulations 1 month after the resection of the right retroperitoneal paraganglioma. *Image reproduced according to creative commons license Terada E, Ashida K, Ohe K, Sakamoto S, Hasuzawa N, Nomura M. Brown adipose activation and reversible beige coloration in adipose tissue with multiple accumulations of 18 F-fluorodeoxyglucose in sporadic paraganglioma: a case report. Clin Case Rep 2019;7(7):1399−1403. https://doi.org/10.1002/CCR3.2259.*

levels of circulating catecholamines, a hormone known to activate BAT. While this may seem harmless, the danger for a misdiagnosis was clear (single primary tumor with surgical approach vs. metastasized tumor needing chemotherapy).

By cold exposure it was found that not only BAT got more active in diabetic patients but also their insulin sensitivity increased, making BAT an important organ to modulate blood glucose levels in diabetic patients. Important to mention here is that even though [^{18}F]FDG uptake in BAT was impaired in diabetic patients, uptake of the FA-based tracer [^{18}F] FTHA was not altered when compared to nondiabetic controls. Therefore BAT might be active in diabetic conditions even though it was not possible to visualize it with the most prominent imaging method via [^{18}F]FDG. More studies with FA-based tracers should be conducted to investigate BAT's role during diabetes.

The metabolic uncertainties about specific tracers, combined with the use of radiation, are significant inhibitors of large-scale studies on BAT clinically. At this moment, obese people are generally not considered as sufficiently ill in order to justify the use of performing studies with ionizing radiation and its inherent (small) risk of developing cancer. This is less of a problem in preclinical experiments with mice or rats, but the essential role of BAT in small rodents is not easily translated to the human setting where BAT is merely facultative.

The current list of possible techniques to visualize and quantify BAT does yield a large amount of new knowledge about BAT. Up to date (January 2022), there are over 13.000 publications on BAT listed in PubMed, out of which roughly 1000 are imaging-related. Armed with this knowledge, and counting on the foreseeable technical improvements, we expect BAT imaging to play an increasing role in the clinical setting. This may be in the form of support in clinical trials as companion-diagnostics during diabetes or even obesity treatment, or even in the form of a subsection of large-scale population studies investigating lipid metabolism. By 2030, we should know if BAT is merely a facultative evolutionary remnant or one of the key-players in human metabolism.

References

[1] Enerbäck S. The origins of Brown adipose tissue. N Engl J Med May 2009;360(19):2021–3. https://doi.org/10.1056/nejmcibr0809610.

[2] Cannon B, Nedergaard J. Brown adipose tissue: function and physiological significance. Physiol Rev 2004;84(1):277–359. https://doi.org/10.1152/physrev.00015.2003.

[3] Argentato PP, De Cássia César H, Estadella D, Pisani LP. Programming mediated by fatty acids affects uncoupling protein 1 (UCP-1) in brown adipose tissue. Br J Nutr 2018;120(6):619–27. https://doi.org/10.1017/S0007114518001629.

[4] Bargut TCL, Aguila MB, Mandarim-de-Lacerda CA. Brown adipose tissue: updates in cellular and molecular biology. Tissue Cell Oct. 01, 2016;48(5):452–60. https://doi.org/10.1016/j.tice.2016.08.001. Churchill Livingstone.

[5] Gesta S, Tseng YH, Kahn CR. Developmental origin of fat: tracking obesity to its source. Cell Oct. 19, 2007;131(2):242–56. https://doi.org/10.1016/j.cell.2007.10.004. Elsevier B.V.

[6] Qian S, Tang Y, Tang Q. Adipose tissue plasticity and the pleiotropic roles of BMP signaling. J Biol Chem Apr. 2021:100678. https://doi.org/10.1016/j.jbc.2021.100678.

[7] McNeill BT, Suchacki KJ, Stimson RH. Human Brown adipose tissue as a therapeutic target - warming up or cooling down? Eur J Endocrinol Mar. 2021. https://doi.org/10.1530/EJE-20-1439.

[8] Lizcano F, Arroyave F. Control of adipose cell browning and its therapeutic potential. Metabolites Nov. 01, 2020;10(11):1–27. https://doi.org/10.3390/metabo10110471. MDPI AG.

[9] Lizcano F. The beige adipocyte as a therapy for metabolic diseases. Int J Mol Sci Oct. 02, 2019;20(20). https://doi.org/10.3390/ijms20205058. MDPI AG.

[10] Rui L. Brown and beige adipose tissues in health and disease. Compr Physiol Oct. 2017;7(4):1281–306. https://doi.org/10.1002/cphy.c170001.

[11] Cramer W. On glandular adipose tissue, and its relation to other endocrine organs and to the vitamine problem. Br J Exp Pathol 1920;1(4):184–96.

[12] Aherne W, Hull D. Brown adipose tissue and heat production in the newborn infant. J Pathol Bacteriol 1966;91(1):223–34. https://doi.org/10.1002/path.1700910126.

[13] Ito S, Kuroshima A. Distribution of brown adipose tissue in Japanese new-born infants. Nihon Seirigaku Zasshi 1967;29(11):660–1.

[14] Heim T, Kellermayer M, Dani M. Thermal conditions and the mobilization of lipids from brown and white adipose tissue in the human neonate. Acta Paediatr Acad Sci Hung 1968;9(2):109–20.

[15] Heaton JM. The distribution of brown adipose tissue in the human. J Anat 1972;112(Pt 1):35–9.

[16] Tanuma Y, Tamamoto M, Ito T, Yokochi C. The occurrence of brown adipose tissue in perirenal fat in Japanese. Arch Histol Jpn 1975;38(1):43–70.

[17] Astrup A, Bulow J, Madsen J, Christensen NJ. Contribution of BAT and skeletal muscle to thermogenesis induced by ephedrine in man. Am J Physiol 1985;248(5 Pt 1):E507–15. https://doi.org/10.1152/ajpendo.1985.248.5.E507.

[18] Huttunen P, Hirvonen J, Kinnula V. The occurrence of brown adipose tissue in outdoor workers. Eur J Appl Physiol Occup Physiol 1981;46(4):339–45.

[19] Hany TF, Gharehpapagh E, Kamel EM, Buck A, Himms-Hagen J, von Schulthess GK. Brown adipose tissue: a factor to consider in symmetrical tracer uptake in the neck and upper chest region. Eur J Nucl Med Mol Imag 2002;29(10):1393–8. https://doi.org/10.1007/s00259-002-0902-6.

[20] Cohade C, Mourtzikos KA, Wahl RL. 'USA-Fat': prevalence is related to ambient outdoor temperature-evaluation with 18F-FDG PET/CT. J Nucl Med 2003;44(8):1267−70.

[21] Lee P, Greenfield JR, Ho KKY, Fulham MJ. A critical appraisal of the prevalence and metabolic significance of brown adipose tissue in adult humans. Am J Physiol Endocrinol Metab 2010;299(4):E601−6. https://doi.org/10.1152/ajpendo.00298.2010.

[22] van Marken Lichtenbelt WD, et al. Cold-activated brown adipose tissue in healthy men. N Engl J Med 2009;360(15):1500−8. https://doi.org/10.1056/NEJMoa0808718.

[23] Virtanen KA, et al. Functional brown adipose tissue in healthy adults. N Engl J Med 2009;360(15):1518−25. https://doi.org/10.1056/NEJMoa0808949.

[24] Saito M, et al. High incidence of metabolically active brown adipose tissue in healthy adult humans: effects of cold exposure and adiposity. Diabetes 2009;58(7):1526−31. https://doi.org/10.2337/db09-0530.

[25] Hanssen MJ, et al. Short-term cold acclimation improves insulin sensitivity in patients with type 2 diabetes mellitus. Nat Med 2015;21(8):863−5. https://doi.org/10.1038/nm.3891.

[26] Mann T, Tomiyama AJ, Westling E, Lew AM, Samuels B, Chatman J. Medicare's search for effective obesity treatments: diets are not the answer. Am Psychol 2007;62(3):220−33. https://doi.org/10.1037/0003-066x.62.3.220.

[27] Ge L, et al. Comparison of dietary macronutrient patterns of 14 popular named dietary programmes for weight and cardiovascular risk factor reduction in adults: systematic review and network meta-analysis of randomised trials. BMJ 2020;369. https://doi.org/10.1136/bmj.m696. m696.

[28] Goldgof M, Xiao C, Chanturiya T, Jou W, Gavrilova O, Reitman ML. The chemical uncoupler 2,4-dinitrophenol (DNP) protects against diet-induced obesity and improves energy homeostasis in mice at thermoneutrality. J Biol Chem Jul. 2014;289(28):19341−50. https://doi.org/10.1074/jbc.M114.568204.

[29] Sun X, Feng X, Wu X, Lu Y, Chen K, Ye Y. Fat wasting is damaging: role of adipose tissue in cancer-associated cachexia. Front Cell Dev Biol Feb. 12, 2020;8. https://doi.org/10.3389/fcell.2020.00033. Frontiers Media S.A.

[30] Kir S, et al. Tumour-derived PTH-related protein triggers adipose tissue browning and cancer cachexia. Nature 2014;513(7516):100−4. https://doi.org/10.1038/nature13528.

[31] Li L, Li B, Li M, Speakman JR. Switching on the furnace: regulation of heat production in brown adipose tissue. Mol Aspect Med Aug. 2019;68:60−73. https://doi.org/10.1016/j.mam.2019.07.005.

[32] Puar T, et al. Genotype-dependent Brown adipose tissue activation in patients with pheochromocytoma and paraganglioma. J Clin Endocrinol Metab 2016;101(1):224−32. https://doi.org/10.1210/jc.2015-3205.

[33] V Joshi P, Lele VR. Unexpected visitor on FDG PET/CT–brown adipose tissue (BAT) in mesentery in a case of retroperitoneal extra-adrenal pheochromocytoma: is the BAT activation secondary to catecholamine-secreting pheochromocytoma? Clin Nucl Med 2012;37(5):e119−20. https://doi.org/10.1097/RLU.0b013e31824437e7.

[34] Wang Q, et al. Brown adipose tissue in humans is activated by elevated plasma catecholamines levels and is inversely related to central obesity. PLoS One 2011;6(6). https://doi.org/10.1371/journal.pone.0021006. e21006.

[35] Nascimento EBM, et al. Nicotinamide riboside enhances in vitro beta-adrenergic Brown adipose tissue activity in humans. J Clin Endocrinol Metab Apr. 2021;106(5). https://doi.org/10.1210/clinem/dgaa960.

[36] Finlin BS, et al. Adipose tissue mast cells promote human adipose beiging in response to cold. Sci Rep Dec. 2019;9(1). https://doi.org/10.1038/s41598-019-45136-9.

[37] Finlin BS, et al. Mast cells promote seasonal white adipose beiging in humans. Diabetes May 2017;66(5):1237−46. https://doi.org/10.2337/db16-1057.

[38] Kampf JP, Parmley D, Kleinfeld AM. Free fatty acid transport across adipocytes is mediated by an unknown membrane protein pump. Am J Physiol Endocrinol Metab 2007;293(5):E1207−14. https://doi.org/10.1152/ajpendo.00259.2007.

[39] Cupp D, Kampf JP, Kleinfeld AM. Fatty acid-albumin complexes and the determination of the transport of long chain free fatty acids across membranes. Biochemistry 2004;43(15):4473−81. https://doi.org/10.1021/bi036335l.

[40] Thumser AE, Storch J. Characterization of a BODIPY-labeled fluorescent fatty acid analogue. Binding to fatty acid-binding proteins, intracellular localization, and metabolism. Mol Cell Biochem 2007;299(1−2):67−73. https://doi.org/10.1007/s11010-005-9041-2.

[41] Paulus A, et al. Synthesis, radiosynthesis and in vitro evaluation of 18F-Bodipy-C16/triglyceride as a dual modal imaging agent for brown adipose tissue. PLoS One 2017;12(8). https://doi.org/10.1371/journal.pone.0182297. e0182297.

[42] Henkin AH, et al. Real-time noninvasive imaging of fatty acid uptake in vivo. ACS Chem Biol 2012;7(11):1884−91. https://doi.org/10.1021/cb300194b.

[43] Berbee JF, et al. Brown fat activation reduces hypercholesterolaemia and protects from atherosclerosis development. Nat Commun 2015;6:6356. https://doi.org/10.1038/ncomms7356.

[44] Khedoe PPSJ, et al. Brown adipose tissue takes up plasma triglycerides mostly after lipolysis. J Lipid Res 2015;56(1):51−9. https://doi.org/10.1194/jlr.M052746.

[45] Bartelt A, et al. Brown adipose tissue activity controls triglyceride clearance. Nat Med 2011;17(2):200−5. https://doi.org/10.1038/nm.2297.

[46] Labbé SM, et al. Organ-specific dietary fatty acid uptake in humans using positron emission tomography coupled to computed tomography. Am J Physiol Endocrinol Metab 2011;300(3):E445−53. https://doi.org/10.1152/ajpendo.00579.2010.

[47] Stein O, Scow RO, Stein Y. FFA-3H uptake by perfused adipose tissue: electron microscopic autoradiographic study. Am J Physiol 1970;219(2):510−8.

[48] Gorter PM, et al. Quantification of epicardial and peri-coronary fat using cardiac computed tomography; reproducibility and relation with obesity and metabolic syndrome in patients suspected of coronary artery disease. Atherosclerosis 2008;197(2):896−903. https://doi.org/10.1016/j.atherosclerosis.2007.08.016.

[49] Gorter PM, et al. Relation of epicardial and pericoronary fat to coronary atherosclerosis and coronary artery calcium in patients undergoing coronary angiography. Am J Cardiol 2008;102(4):380−5. https://doi.org/10.1016/j.amjcard.2008.04.002.

[50] Maurovich-Horvat P, et al. Influence of pericoronary adipose tissue on local coronary atherosclerosis as assessed by a novel MDCT volumetric method. Atherosclerosis Nov. 2011;219(1):151−7. https://doi.org/10.1016/j.atherosclerosis.2011.06.049.

[51] Mahabadi AA, et al. Association of pericoronary fat volume with atherosclerotic plaque burden in the underlying coronary artery: a segment analysis. Atherosclerosis 2010;211(1):195−9. https://doi.org/10.1016/j.atherosclerosis.2010.02.013.

[52] McCollough CH, Leng S, Yu L, Fletcher JG. Dual- and multi-energy CT: principles, technical approaches, and clinical applications. Radiology Sep. 2015;276(3):637−53. https://doi.org/10.1148/radiol.2015142631.

[53] Sneed NM, Morrison SA. Body composition methods in adults with type 2 diabetes or at risk for T2D: a clinical review. Curr Diabetes Rep May 2021;21(5). https://doi.org/10.1007/s11892-021-01381-9.

[54] Han J, et al. Imaging modalities for diagnosis and monitoring of cancer cachexia. EJNMMI Res Sep. 2021;11(1):94. https://doi.org/10.1186/s13550-021-00834-2.

[55] Heymsfield SB, Gonzalez MC, Lu J, Jia G, Zheng J. Skeletal muscle mass and quality: evolution of modern measurement concepts in the context of sarcopenia. Proc Nutr Soc Nov. 2015;74(4):355−66. https://doi.org/10.1017/S0029665115000129.

[56] Yamada A, Yoshizawa E. Quantitative assessment of liver steatosis using ultrasound: dual-energy CT. J Med Ultrason Oct. 2021;48(4):507−14. https://doi.org/10.1007/s10396-021-01136-9.

[57] Zhang F, et al. An adipose tissue atlas: an image-guided identification of human-like BAT and beige depots in rodents. Cell Metabol Jan. 2018;27(1):252−62. https://doi.org/10.1016/j.cmet.2017.12.004. e3.

[58] Goetze S, Lavely WC, Ziessman HA, Wahl RL. Visualization of brown adipose tissue with 99mTc- methoxyisobutylisonitrile on SPECT/CT. J Nucl Med May 2008;49(5):752−6. https://doi.org/10.2967/jnumed.107.048074.

[59] Baba S, Engles JM, Huso DL, Ishimori T, Wahl RL. Comparison of uptake of multiple clinical radiotracers into brown adipose tissue under cold-stimulated and nonstimulated conditions. J Nucl Med Oct. 2007;48(10):1715−23. doi: jnumed.107.041715 [pii]10.2967/jnumed.107.041715 [doi].

[60] Haghighatafshar M, Farhoudi F. Is brown adipose tissue visualization reliable on 99mTc-methoxyisobutylisonitrile diagnostic SPECT scintigraphy? Medicine (United States) Jan. 2016;95(2). https://doi.org/10.1097/MD.0000000000002498.

[61] Blondin DP, et al. Selective impairment of glucose but not fatty acid or oxidative metabolism in Brown adipose tissue of subjects with type 2 diabetes. Diabetes Jul. 2015;64(7):2388−97. https://doi.org/10.2337/db14-1651.

[62] Cypess AM, et al. Quantification of human and rodent brown adipose tissue function using 99mTc-Methoxyisobutylisonitrile SPECT/CT and 18F-FDG PET/CT. J Nucl Med Nov. 2013;54(11):1896−901. https://doi.org/10.2967/jnumed.113.121012.

[63] Paulus A, et al. Characterization of BAT activity in rats using invasive and non-invasive techniques. PLoS One May 2019;14(5). https://doi.org/10.1371/journal.pone.0215852. pp. e0215852−e0215852.

[64] Hu HH. Magnetic resonance of Brown adipose tissue: a review of current techniques. Crit Rev Biomed Eng 2015;43(2−3):161−81. https://doi.org/10.1615/critrevbiomedeng.2015014377.

[65] Chondronikola M, Beeman SC, Wahl RL. Non-invasive methods for the assessment of brown adipose tissue in humans. J Physiol Feb. 2018;596(3):363−78. https://doi.org/10.1113/JP274255.

[66] Hamaoka T, et al. Near-infrared time-resolved spectroscopy for assessing Brown adipose tissue density in humans: a review. Front Endocrinol May 2020;11:261. https://doi.org/10.3389/fendo.2020.00261.

[67] Law J, Chalmers J, Morris DE, Robinson L, Budge H, Symonds ME. The use of infrared thermography in the measurement and characterization of brown adipose tissue activation. Temperature (Austin, Tex.) Apr. 2018;5(2):147−61. https://doi.org/10.1080/23328940.2017.1397085.

[68] Gariani K, Gariani J, Amzalag G, Delattre BM, Ratib O, Garibotto V. Hybrid PET/MRI as a tool to detect brown adipose tissue: proof of principle. Obes Res Clin Pract 2015;9(6):613−7. https://doi.org/10.1016/j.orcp.2015.05.004.

[69] Fischer JGW, et al. Comparison of [18F]FDG PET/CT with magnetic resonance imaging for the assessment of human brown adipose tissue activity. EJNMMI Res 2020;10(1):85. https://doi.org/10.1186/s13550-020-00665-7.

[70] Loeliger RC, et al. Relation of diet-induced thermogenesis to brown adipose tissue activity in healthy men. Am J Physiol Endocrinol Metab 2021;320(1):E93−e101. https://doi.org/10.1152/ajpendo.00237.2020.

[71] Weiner J, et al. Thyroid hormone status defines brown adipose tissue activity and browning of white adipose tissues in mice. Sci Rep 2016;6:38124. https://doi.org/10.1038/srep38124.

[72] Pace L, et al. Determinants of physiologic 18F-FDG uptake in Brown adipose tissue in sequential PET/CT examinations. Mol Imag Biol 2010;13(5):1029−35. https://doi.org/10.1007/s11307-010-0431-9.

[73] Cypess AM, Haft CR, Laughlin MR, Hu HH. Brown fat in humans: consensus points and experimental guidelines. Cell Metabol 2014;20(3):408−15. https://doi.org/10.1016/j.cmet.2014.07.025.

[74] Chen KY, et al. Brown adipose reporting criteria in imaging STudies (BARCIST 1.0): recommendations for standardized FDG-PET/CT experiments in humans. Cell Metabol Aug. 09, 2016;24(2):210−22. https://doi.org/10.1016/j.cmet.2016.07.014. Cell Press.

[75] Santalucía T, et al. Developmental regulation of GLUT-1 (erythroid/Hep G2) and GLUT-4 (muscle/fat) glucose transporter expression in rat heart, skeletal muscle, and brown adipose tissue. Endocrinology 1992;130(2):837−46. https://doi.org/10.1210/endo.130.2.1370797.

[76] Cannon B, Nedergaard J. Cultures of adipose precursor cells from brown adipose tissue and of clonal brown-adipocyte-like cell lines. Methods Mol Biol 2001;155:213−24. https://doi.org/10.1385/1-59259-231-7:213.

[77] Lim MMD, Gnerre J, Gerard P. Mechanisms of uptake of common radiopharmaceuticals. Radiographics Sep. 01, 2018;38(5):1550−1. https://doi.org/10.1148/rg.2018180072. Radiological Society of North America Inc.

[78] Petersen H, et al. FDG PET/CT in cancer: comparison of actual use with literature-based recommendations. Eur J Nucl Med Mol Imag Apr. 2016;43(4):695−706. https://doi.org/10.1007/s00259-015-3217-0.

[79] Ouellet V, et al. Brown adipose tissue oxidative metabolism contributes to energy expenditure during acute cold exposure in humans. J Clin Invest 2012;122(2):545−52. https://doi.org/10.1172/JCI60433.

[80] Yu XX, Lewin DA, Forrest W, Adams SH. Cold elicits the simultaneous induction of fatty acid synthesis and β-oxidation in murine brown adipose tissue: prediction from differential gene expression and confirmation in vivo. Faseb J 2002;16(2):155−68. https://doi.org/10.1096/fj.01-0568com.

[81] Townsend KL, Tseng Y-H. Brown fat fuel utilization and thermogenesis. Trends Endocrinol Metabol Apr. 2014;25(4):168−77. https://doi.org/10.1016/j.tem.2013.12.004.

[82] Degrado TR. Synthesis of 14 (R,S)-[18F]fluoro-6-thia-heptadecanoic acid (FTHA). J Label Compd Radiopharm 1991;29(9):989−95. https://doi.org/10.1002/jlcr.2580290903.

[83] Bauwens M, et al. Molecular imaging of brown adipose tissue in health and disease. Eur J Nucl Med Mol Imag 2014;41(4):776−91. https://doi.org/10.1007/s00259-013-2611-8.

[84] Tamaki N, et al. Assessment of myocardial fatty acid metabolism with positron emission tomography at rest and during dobutamine infusion in patients with coronary artery disease. Am Heart J 1993;125(3):702−10. https://doi.org/10.1016/0002-8703(93)90161-2.

[85] Schelbert HR, et al. Effects of substrate availability on myocardial C-11 palmitate kinetics by positron emission tomography in normal subjects and patients with ventricular dysfunction. Am Heart J 1986;111(6):1055−64. https://doi.org/10.1016/0002-8703(86)90006-2.

[86] Schelbert HR. Myocardial ischemia and clinical applications of positron emission tomography. Am J Cardiol 1989;64(9):E46−53. https://doi.org/10.1016/0002-9149(89)90734-0.

[87] Bucci M, et al. Enhanced fatty acid uptake in visceral adipose tissue is not reversed by weight loss in obese individuals with the metabolic syndrome. Diabetologia 2014;58(1):158−64. https://doi.org/10.1007/s00125-014-3402-x.

[88] Syamsunarno MRAA, et al. Fatty acid binding protein 4 and 5 play a crucial role in thermogenesis under the conditions of fasting and cold stress. PLoS One Mar. 2014;9(6). https://doi.org/10.1371/journal.pone.0090825. pp. e90825−e90825.

[89] Putri M, et al. CD36 is indispensable for thermogenesis under conditions of fasting and cold stress. Biochem Biophys Res Commun Feb. 2015;457(4):520−5. https://doi.org/10.1016/j.bbrc.2014.12.124.

[90] Poe ND, Robinson GD, MacDonald NS. Myocardial extraction of labeled long-chain fatty acid analogs. Exp Biol Med 1975;148(1):215−8. https://doi.org/10.3181/00379727-148-38509.

[91] Corbett JR. Fatty acids for myocardial imaging. Semin Nucl Med 1999;29(3):237−58. https://doi.org/10.1016/s0001-2998(99)80013-0.

[92] Festuccia WT, Blanchard P-GG, Deshaies Y. Control of Brown adipose tissue glucose and lipid metabolism by PPARγ. Front Endocrinol 2011;2:84. https://doi.org/10.3389/fendo.2011.00084.

[93] Hoeke G, Kooijman S, Boon MR, Rensen PC, Berbee JF. Role of Brown fat in lipoprotein metabolism and atherosclerosis. Circ Res 2016;118(1):173−82. https://doi.org/10.1161/circresaha.115.306647.

[94] Labbé SM, et al. In vivo measurement of energy substrate contribution to cold-induced brown adipose tissue thermogenesis. Faseb J 2015;29(5):2046−58. https://doi.org/10.1096/fj.14-266247.

[95] Coburn CT, Hajri T, Ibrahimi A, Abumrad NA. Role of CD36 in membrane transport and utilization of long-chain fatty acids by different tissues. J Mol Neurosci 2001;16(2−3):117. https://doi.org/10.1385/jmn:16:2-3:117.

[96] Stahl A. A current review of fatty acid transport proteins (SLC27). Pflügers Archiv 2004;447(5):722−7. https://doi.org/10.1007/s00424-003-1106-z.

[97] Paulus A, et al. [18F]BODIPY-triglyceride-containing chylomicron-like particles as an imaging agent for brown adipose tissue in vivo. Sci Rep 2019;9(1). https://doi.org/10.1038/s41598-019-39561-z.

[98] Paulus A, Drude N, Van Marken Lichtenbelt W, Mottaghy FM, Bauwens M. Brown adipose tissue uptake of triglyceride-rich lipoprotein-derived fatty acids in diabetic or obese mice under different temperature conditions. EJNMMI Res 2020;10(1). https://doi.org/10.1186/s13550-020-00701-6.

[99] Bachman ES, et al. Beta AR signaling required for diet-induced thermogenesis and obesity resistance. Science 2002;297(5582):843−5. https://doi.org/10.1126/science.1073160.

[100] Hadi M, Chen CC, Whatley M, Pacak K, Carrasquillo JA. Brown fat imaging with 18F-6-Fluorodopamine PET/CT, 18F-FDG PET/CT, and 123I-MIBG SPECT: a study of patients being evaluated for pheochromocytoma. J Nucl Med 2007;48(7):1077−83. https://doi.org/10.2967/jnumed.106.035915.

[101] Lin S-F, et al. Ex vivo and in vivo evaluation of the norepinephrine transporter ligand [11C]MRB for Brown adipose tissue imaging. Nucl Med Biol 2012;39(7):1081−6. https://doi.org/10.1016/j.nucmedbio.2012.04.005.

[102] Kyparos D, et al. Effect of aerobic training on99mTc-methoxy isobutyl isonitrile (99mTc-sestamibi) uptake by myocardium and skeletal muscle: implication for noninvasive assessment of muscle metabolic profile. Acta Physiol 2008;193(2):175−80. https://doi.org/10.1111/j.1748-1716.2007.01825.x.

[103] Muzik O, Mangner TJ, Granneman JG. Assessment of oxidative metabolism in brown fat using PET imaging. Front Endocrinol Feb. 2012;3:15. https://doi.org/10.3389/fendo.2012.00015.

[104] Muzik O, Mangner TJ, Leonard WR, Kumar A, Janisse J, Granneman JG. 15O PET measurement of blood flow and oxygen consumption in cold-activated human brown fat. J Nucl Med Apr. 2013;54(4):523−31. https://doi.org/10.2967/jnumed.112.111336.

[105] Belhocine T, Shastry A, Driedger A, Urbain J-L. Detection of 99mTc-sestamibi uptake in brown adipose tissue with SPECT-CT. Eur J Nucl Med Mol Imag 2006;34(1):149. https://doi.org/10.1007/s00259-006-0244-x.

[106] Yu Q, Huang S, Xu T, Wang Y, Ju S. Measuring Brown fat Using MRI and implications in the metabolic syndrome. J Magn Reson Imag 2020. https://doi.org/10.1002/jmri.27340.

[107] Reguero M, de Cedrón MG, Wagner S, Reglero G, Quintela JC, de Molina AR. Precision nutrition to activate thermogenesis as a complementary approach to target obesity and associated-metabolic-disorders. Cancers Feb. 01, 2021;13(4):1−36. https://doi.org/10.3390/cancers13040866. MDPI AG.

[108] Terada E, Ashida K, Ohe K, Sakamoto S, Hasuzawa N, Nomura M. Brown adipose activation and reversible beige coloration in adipose tissue with multiple accumulations of 18 F-fluorodeoxyglucose in sporadic paraganglioma: a case report. Clin Case Rep Jul. 2019;7(7):1399−403. https://doi.org/10.1002/CCR3.2259.

Chapter 4

Epicardial and pericoronary fat

Pál Maurovich-Horvat[1] and György Jermendy[2]

[1]*Semmelweis University, Faculty of Medicine, Medical Imaging Centre, Budapest, Hungary;* [2]*Bajcsy-Zsilinszky Teaching Hospital, Medical Department, Budapest, Hungary*

Introduction

In the 19th century it was believed that fatty degeneration of the heart is the main cause of every heart disease [1]. *Richard Quain* was the most well-known person of this theory recognizing the relationship of increased fat volume on the epicardial surface with coronary artery obstruction. The diagnosis of fatty heart was very popular in the Victorian era but was later changed to the fibrosous heart disease and chronic myocarditis. All these diagnoses were replaced by the ischemia theory in the middle of the 20th century. Interestingly, it was recognized at that time that 70% of the fatty heart diagnosis in Quain's pathological records corresponded with the ischemic heart disease. Although the relationship between the increased epicardial fat and cardiac diseases was described nearly 150 years ago, medicine did not dedicate much attention to this field. However, cardiovascular research has begun to explore the role of different fat compartments in line with the pandemic spread of obesity and the dynamic development of radiological imaging techniques [2]. In this regard, special attention was paid to the epicardial fat due to its anatomical proximity to the coronary arteries [3]. While anatomical and biochemical characteristics of the epicardial fat compartment were described in early studies, its potential role in the pathophysiological mechanism of coronary artery disease (CAD) and other cardiac dysfunction has only been investigated in the last couple of years. Beyond latest results of original investigations regarding clinical significance of EAT, several review papers [4—11] and a monography [12] were published recently.

Terminology

The terminology of fat compartments around the heart is not standardized; imprecise uses of the definitions may occur in the literature, even in recent years. Nevertheless, the most widely used and accepted terms are summarized in Table 4.1.

The epicardial fat as a part of the visceral fat is localized between the myocardial surface and the visceral layer of the pericardium. Importantly, there is no separating fascia between the myocardium and the epicardial fat. Pericardial fat

TABLE 4.1 Terminology of fat compartments around the heart.

Visceral fat	Adipose tissue around the visceral organs
Epicardial fat	Visceral fat between the myocardial surface and the visceral layer of the pericardium
Pericardial fat	Adipose tissue outside the visceral pericardium, between the visceral and parietal layears of the serous pericardium
Perivascular fat	Adipose tissue around the vessels irrespective of location
Pericoronary fat	Adipose tissue around the coronary artery adventitia
Intrathoracic fat	Entire fat within the thorax including the areas of fat within the pericardium and external to the pericardium

Visceral and Ectopic Fat. https://doi.org/10.1016/B978-0-12-822186-0.00015-8

involves adipose tissues externally to the visceral layer of the pericardium, located between the two (visceral and parietal) pericardial serous (Fig. 4.1) [13]. Unfortunately, there is often some confusion in the use of the term pericardial instead of epicardial fat or conversely, however, these terms are not interchangeable. Perivascular fat is adipose tissue around the arteries irrespective of location while pericoronary fat is the surrounding adipose tissue around the coronary artery adventitia [14]. In other words, pericoronary fat is a part of EAT that directly surrounds the coronary arteries [15]. Paracardial fat is located externally to the parietal layer of the pericardium; this term is inconsistently used in the literature leading to confusion [6,16], therefore, we have avoided using it. In practice, EAT is the fat compartment with immediate proximity to the heart while pericardial adipose tissue is the outer fat compartment of the heart [13]. Intrathoracic fat is the entire fat within the thorax including fat areas within the pericardium and external to the pericardium.

The clear distinction of epicardial fat from pericardial fat is of great clinical importance [17]. From embryological aspect they differ from each other. While the epicardial fat is similar to the visceral fat and originates from mesodermal cells, the pericardial fat has an ectodermal origin, similar to subcutaneous fat. Moreover, there is also a difference in the blood supply between these two fat compartments; the epicardial fat is supplied by the small myocardial coronary arteries but the circulation of pericardial fat is provided from the thoracic vessels (Table 4.2).

Anatomical characteristics of EAT

Interestingly, EAT can be present in humans and large mammals but is lacking or minimal in laboratory animals such as mice or rats [18]. Early findings about anatomical characteristics of EAT were based mainly on human autopsy studies while more recent data became available form clinical settings, measuring EAT by different imaging techniques.

Data based on autopsy

The epicardial fat covers nearly 80% of the heart surface but the range of covered regions may vary from 56% to 100%, depending on the absence or presence of fat accumulation [19]. In normal circumstances, EAT covers the atrioventricular and the interventricular sulci and the main coronary arteries, therefore, coronary arteries and their main epicardial branches are surrounded by adipose tissue. In line with increasing lipid accumulation, the EAT-covered heart region includes the heart basis and the apex, the entire surface of the right ventricle. The distribution of EAT is mostly inhomogeneous, the biggest mass is localized on the lateral and anterior walls of the right ventricle. In case of extremely enlarged EAT, it can accumulate also on the surface of atria and along the vessel's adventitia with spreading into the myocardium [20].

According to autopsy studies, EAT may in average contribute 20% to the whole heart weight [19,21,22]. EAT was nearly 20% of ventricular weight in another pathological investigation [23]. Nevertheless, the amount of EAT may vary widely in humans with a range from 4% to 52% and "floating heart" should not be considered a rare pathological finding [24].

Slightly greater amount of EAT was observed in women than men [21,23], although others found no gender-difference in EAT amount by autopsy [19].

The age-dependency of EAT volume is controversial. No relationship between age and EAT was found at autopsy [21,25]. However, others found an association between age and EAT in subjects with younger ages (<20 years) [26]. Another study documented with measurements of histologic sections that EAT over right ventricle was not affected in subjects aged over 40 years [27]. Taken together, EAT is probably expanding with increasing age until 20−40 years but thereafter its amount is independent on age [20].

The fat-muscle ratio was also investigated in autopsy study. Using a total of 117 autoptic human hearts Corradi et al. found a constant fat-muscle ratio in each ventricle, indicating that epicardial fat and the underlying myocardium exhibit a parallel increase during hypertrophic process [23].

In histological investigations it has been earlier established that adipocytes in the EAT are smaller than those in the abdominal or the subcutaneous fat compartments [28]. Beyond adipocytes, EAT includes nerves, ganglions, vessels, inflammatory cells, and fibrocytes as well (Fig. 4.2). The lack of separating fascia layer between the epicardial fat and the myocardium provides a close proximity of these two different tissues [18].

Although early autopsy studies provided basic information about epicardial fat in human hearts, the methodology for measuring EAT in these studies often had technical difficulties [20].

Findings from clinical settings

Age, gender, body weight, and ethnicity should be taken into consideration among physiological determinants of EAT [29−32]. EAT seems to increase with age [16]. The quantity of EAT depends on gender and body mass index. For example, pericardial fat was reported to be $137 \pm 54\ cm^3$ among men and $108 \pm 41\ cm^3$ among women of the Framingham offspring cohort [33]. In patients with high BMI ($>27\ kg/m^2$) EAT volume was more than two times higher compared to those with a BMI $<27\ kg/m^2$ ($155 \pm 15\ cm^3$ vs. $67 \pm 12\ cm^3$) [34]. Some ethnic differences in epicardial and pericardial fat thickness may also occur; non-Hispanic white men have more epicardial and pericardial fat than African Americans [35].

Both genetic and environmental factors may contribute to the quantity of EAT. According to the results of a recent, classical twin study (BUDAPEST-GLOBAL) [36], genetic effects predominated over environmental influences (80% vs. 20%) in contributing to the phenotype of EAT quantity, similar to quantities of abdominal subcutaneous and visceral adipose tissues (SAT and VAT) [37].

Biochemical features and physiological function of EAT

EAT is a white adipose tissue; however, some characteristics of EAT resemble brown or beige fat. It has been suggested that some functions of EAT might diminish during aging and this downregulation might be due to aging or advancing stages of coronary artery disease or both [38].

The biochemical features of small adipocytes in EAT may also differ from those of other fat compartments. In experimental studies EAT had higher rate of free fatty acid (FFA) release than adipose tissue elsewhere in the body suggesting that EAT might play a role in local energy supply of the myocardium. In addition, a lower oxidative capacity and a lower rate of glucose utilization were also documented [39]. On the other hand, a fivefold higher expression of uncoupled protein-1 (UCP-1) was found in EAT compared to other fat depots [40]. The UCP-1 is a specific protein in brown fat, which is necessary to its energy production and does not appear in other type of fat tissues. This latter feature is in line with the fact that epicardial fat evolves from the brown adipose tissue during embryogenesis.

Several physiological functions of EAT were described by previous investigations and derived from its biochemical or anatomical features. Unfortunately, experimental evidence supporting these observations are limited due to the very small amount of EAT in experimental animals (rodents).

It is suggested that functions of EAT may include protection of the myocardium against hypothermia [40]. In addition, EAT can provide a mechanical protective role for coronary circulation. It can attenuate the torsion developed by the myocardium contraction or the arterial pulse wave, but it has a permissive role as well in positive remodeling of coronary arteries [41].

Besides this, EAT has a substantial role in energy supply to the myocardium and should be considered as a provider of energy source during period of high energy demand [18]. On the other hand, EAT may protect the myocardium from cardiotoxic effect of large amount of FFA due to its capacity of fast FFA utilization [42]. Taken together EAT may serve as a unique energy buffering pool in the homeostasis of the myocardium.

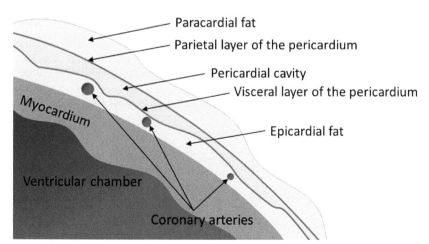

FIGURE 4.1 Adipose tissue compartments around the heart. Epicardial fat is located between the myocardium and the visceral layer of the pericardium, that directly surrounds the coronary arteries. Pericardial fat may occur between the visceral and parietal layers of the serous pericardium (in the pericardial cavity) while paracardial fat may appear externally to the parietal layer.

TABLE 4.2 Differences between epicardial and pericardial fat compartments.

	Epicardial fat	Pericardial fat
Location	Between the myocardial surface and the visceral pericardium	Outside the visceral pericardium
Embryologic origin	Splanchopleuric mesoderm	Primitive thoracic mesenchyme
Blood supply	Branches form the coronary arteries	Noncoronary sources (branches from the internal mammary artery)

In addition, adiponectin secretion from epicardial adipocytes may improve the coronary circulation. Adiponectin improves the endothelial function through stimulation of the nitrogen monoxide synthase, reduces the oxidative stress, and indirectly decreases the level of interleukin-6 (IL-6) and C-reactive protein (CRP) by reducing tumor necrosis factor-α (TNFα) production [43,44]. Adiponectin also has some extracardiac effect such as increased glucose utilization in the hepatocytes and muscle cells which may result in improving insulin sensitivity [45].

Although EAT may secrete cardioprotective adipokines in physiological condition, this beneficial function is lost under pathological circumstances and proinflammatory characteristics may become more prominent. The exact mechanism of this alteration is not fully understood in humans [38].

Cardiac imaging of EAT

The most commonly used noninvasive modalities for the visualization and quantification of EAT are echocardiography, magnetic resonance imaging (MRI), and cardiac computed tomography (CT).

Echocardiography provides a simple, cheap, and readily available assessment which pictures directly the EAT thickness on the free wall of the right ventricle. Imaging by echocardiography requires parasternal short- and long-axis view in three following end-systolic phases (Fig. 4.3). EAT can be identified as the echo-free space between the myocardial surface and the visceral layer of pericardium. Thickness of EAT may vary from 1 mm to 20–25 mm. Several studies have established the general EAT thickness under 7 mm in asymptomatic population [46]. Nevertheless, this method has several disadvantages including the poor reproducibility and the high dependence on observer's experience. In addition, it may not reflect accurately the whole quantity of the epicardial fat due to the two-dimensional nature of the measurement. In other words, the thickness rather than the entire quantity of the pericardial fat compartment can be assessed by echocardiography. Moreover, the method has poor intra- and interobserver variability, and its results may differ significantly from the measurements with CT [47,48].

The MRI technique—in contrast to echocardiography—provides accurate area measurements and, in this way, EAT volume can be calculated (Fig. 4.4). Area measurements with MRI correspond well with fat thickness determination with echocardiography, although a systemic bias through overestimation of EAT with echocardiography might occur [49,50]. Although the lack of ionizing radiation is preferable, there are disadvantages of this modality; it is less available in routine clinical practice, is more expensive, and has worse spatial resolution comparing to CT.

The multidetector-row CT (MDCT) provides a true volume assessment of EAT; this technique has superior spatial resolution among the imaging modalities (Fig. 4.5). This imaging technique should be considered the gold standard, especially in cardiovascular research. It is of note that the specificity and sensitivity of measurements with MDCT are the best comparing to alternative imaging methods. Epicardial fat quantification is performed in a standardized fashion on prospectively ECG triggered noncontrast enhanced CT scans which extend from the pulmonary artery bifurcation to the diaphragm. The identification of the EAT is based on thresholds of fat attenuation. Typically, lower thresholds of attenuation range from −250 to −190 Hounsfield Unit (HU) and upper thresholds are set between −50 and −30 HU. In contrast to area and thickness measurements, volume quantification provides the most accurate way for assessing the true epicardial fat quantity which can be performed on volume rendered image reconstruction [34]. In addition, noncontrast enhanced cardiac CT scans can be used for the quantification of coronary artery calcification resulting in more reliable cardiovascular risk assessment [51–53]. CT imaging provides reliable evaluation of both EAT volume and attenuation; the latter is reflecting inflammatory activity of EAT [54–56]. Importantly, native CT results in a very small (1 mSv) radiation dose. Maurovich-Horvat et al. found in a collaborative work that the measurement of pericoronary adipose tissue proved to

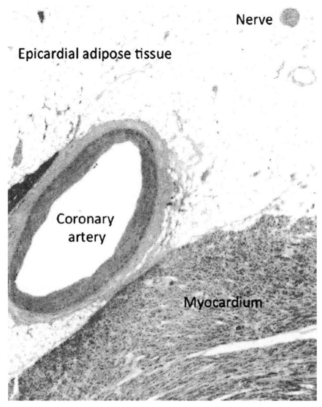

FIGURE 4.2 Microscopic view of the epicardial adipose tissue. It is of note that there is no separating fascia layer between the epicardial fat and the myocardium. *From Nagy E, et al. Arch Med Sci 2017;13:864−874, with permission.*

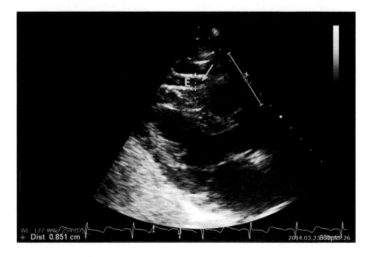

Figure 4.3   Quantification of epicardial adipose tissue by echocardiography (parasternal view). The thickness of the area between the myocardium and the visceral layer of the pericardium is 8.5 mm indicating epicardial adipose tissue. *From Nagy E, et al. Arch Med Sci 2017;13:864−874, with permission.*

be highly reproducible by using MDCT (intra-observer intraclass correlation (ICC): 0.997, inter-observer ICC:0.951) [57]. Additionally, similar reliability of measurements was found for assessing EAT in twin studies (intra-reader ICC: 0.99; inter-reader ICC: 0.98) [37].

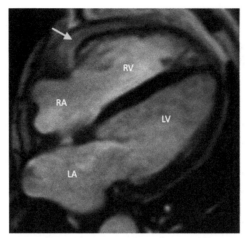

FIGURE 4.4 Epicardial adipose tissue (*green arrow*) demonstrated using magnetic resonance imaging (MRI) technique. *LA*, left atrium; *LV*, left ventricle; *RA*, right atrium; *RV*, right ventricle.

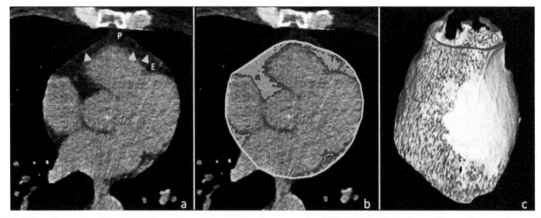

FIGURE 4.5 Measuring epicardial adipose tissue by cardiac computed tomography (CT). (A) Axial section at the aortic root. *Arrows* indicate the visceral layer of the pericardium. Epicardial fat (E) is located inside while pericardial fat (P) outside of the visceral layer. (B) Epicardial adipose tissue (yellow) at the corresponding section. (C) Three-dimension reconstruction of the total epicardial fat compartment (yellow). The volume of epicardial adipose tissue was 112 cm^3. *From Nagy E, et al. Arch Med Sci 2017;13:864–874, with permission.*

EAT in the pathomechanism of atherosclerosis

Recently, a hypothesis regarding the direct role of EAT in the development and progression of coronary atherosclerosis has been raised and paracrine and vasocrine effects of EAT due to close proximity of epicardial fat to coronary arteries has been suggested [58]. The hypothesis was indirectly supported by a pathological study in subjects with myocardial bridge. Namely, no atherosclerosis was observed in coronary segments beneath myocardial bridge where surrounding fat on the coronary arteries was lacking [59].

In a landmark study, Mazurek et al. analyzed epicardial and subcutaneous fat from the lower extremity in obese patients referred for coronary artery bypass grafting. They found increased level of inflammatory mediators (interleukin-6 (IL-6), tumor necrosis factor-α (TNF-α), interleukin-1β (IL-1β), monocyte chemoattractant protein-1 (MCP-1)), macrophages, lymphocytes, and basophils in epicardial fat as compared to subcutaneous fat compartments [60]. Others found that epicardial and omental fat exhibited a broadly comparable pathogenic messenger ribonucleotide acid (mRNA) profile indicating macrophage infiltration into epicardial fat [61]. In another study, mediators of the nuclear factor-kappaB (NFkappaB) and c-Jun N-terminal kinase (JNK) pathways were suggested to involve in the inflammatory profile of EAT highlighting the role of the macrophages in the inflammation within this tissue [62]. These studies indicate that chronic inflammation occurs locally as well as systemically potentially contributing further to the pathogenesis of CAD.

It was documented that the epicardial adipocytes had impaired adiponectin secretion and increased leptin production in obese patients with hypertension, metabolic syndrome and CAD [63,64]. This shift in the adiponectin/leptin ratio enhances the development of atherosclerosis. Namely, the decreased adiponectin expression attenuates endothelial function and leads to increased TNF-α production triggering systematic inflammation and oxidative stress. The altered leptin level promotes atherogenic changes in endothelial cells such as increased adhesion of monocytes, higher level of macrophage-to-foam cell transformation, unfavorable changes in lipid levels, and elevation of C-reactive-protein (CRP) and inflammatory cytokine levels. All these alterations may lead to development and destabilization of atherosclerotic plaques in coronary arteries [65].

Based on several studies, it became widely accepted that EAT should be considered as a source of inflammatory mediators that might directly influence the myocardium and coronary arteries (Fig. 4.6) [66,67]. Two mechanisms of influence (paracrine and vasocrine) were suggested [58]. Paracrine way of influence means that adipokines released from pericoronary fat may diffuse across the arterial wall (adventitia, media, and intima) and finally can interact with endothelial cells in the intima and with vascular smooth cells in the media. The alternative vasocrine effect can be realized by release of adipocytokines and FFAs from EAT directly into vasa vasorum of the coronary arterial wall [68]. It was suggested that vasocrine influence may be predominant over paracrine effect in case of more advanced atherosclerotic lesions where inflammatory mediators may diffuse only with difficulties [61].

The relationship between EAT and CAD was analyzed in several clinical studies and meta-analyses [69−74]. In the Framingham and the MESA (Multiethnic Study of Atherosclerosis) epidemiological studies a significant association of epicardial fat with coronary artery calcification was found which remained significant after adjustment for traditional cardiovascular risk factors [52,75]. The increased epicardial fat proved to be associated with more advanced atherosclerosis [76] and other investigations have demonstrated an association between epicardial fat and noncalcified coronary plaques [77,78]. A significant relationship of increased epicardial fat volume ($>130.7 \text{ cm}^3$) with vulnerable plaques was also documented [79]. The relationship of morphological features of vulnerable plaques (positive remodeling, spotty calcifications, and low CT attenuation in necrotic core) with the pericardial fat was also studied and the volume of pericardial fat proved to be nearly twice as high in patients with vulnerable plaques as compared to those without CAD [80,81]. Pericardial fat was associated with myocardial ischemia detected by single photon emission computed tomography (SPECT) in patients without known CAD [82]. EAT correlated with the severity of coronary atherosclerosis suggesting that its excessive accumulation might contribute to the development of acute coronary syndrome and coronary total occlusions [83,84]. In another study, EAT thickness was independently associated with the thrombolysis in myocardial infarction (TIMI) risk score in patients with non-ST-elevation myocardial infarction (NSTEMI) and unstable angina pectoris [85]. In patients with the metabolic syndrome, increased EAT was associated with impaired coronary flow reserve [86]. In women with chest pain and angiographically normal coronary arteries EAT thickness was correlated with reduced coronary flow reserve [87]. Different surrogate parameters of atherosclerosis were also investigated by others and an association between EAT thickness and carotis intima-media thickness in type 2 diabetic patients as well as in children and adolescents with

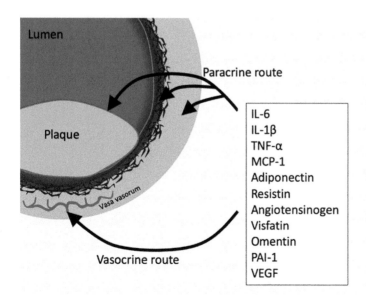

FIGURE 4.6 Routes for paracrine and vasocrine effects of epicardial adipose tissue on coronary arteries and plaque formation. IL: interleukin, TNF-α: tumor necrosis factor-α, MCP-1: monocyte chemoattractant protein-1, PAI-1: plasminogen activator inhibitor-1, VEGF: vascular endothelial growth factor. *From Nagy E, et al. Arch Med Sci 2017;13:864−874, with permission.*

obesity was found [88,89]. Moreover, EAT showed an independent association with arterial stiffness in an asymptomatic Korean cohort [90].

Maurovich-Horvat et al. investigated the relationship of different thoracic fat depots (pericoronary, epicardial, peri-aortic, extracardiac-intrathoracic) with coronary atherosclerosis (assessed by coronary CT angiography) in 342 patients (age: 52 ± 11 years, 61% male, BMI 29.1 ± 5.9 kg/m^2) and found an independent association between pericoronary fat and CAD. Interestingly, all four thoracic fat depots were higher in patients with coronary plaque compared to those without despite no difference in BMI. Correlation of the fat depots to BMI was moderate for epicardial, periaortic, and extracardiac-intrathoracic fat depots, and it was modest for the pericoronary fat compartment (Table 4.3).

The smallest fat depots yet closest in proximity to the coronary vasculature (pericoronary fat) were most consistently associated with CAD (Table 4.4). The association between pericoronary fat and inflammatory biomarkers suggests that while systemic inflammation plays a role in the pathogenesis of CAD, there are additional local effects that may exist [91].

A systematic review and meta-analysis demonstrated an association between obstructive CAD and elevated EAT thickness in the left atrioventricular groove [74]. Multiple investigations have shown an association between increased EAT volume and obstructive coronary artery disease [92,93]. A recent, much larger study (5743 consecutive patients investigated by coronary CT angiography) was published from China documenting that epicardial fat volume improved prediction above conventional risk factors and coronary calcium score (area under the receiver operating characteristic curve increased from 0.856 to 0.874, integrated discrimination improvement 0.0487, net reclassification improvement 0.1181, $P < .0001$ for all). This new method provided a more accurate and effective estimation for pretest probability of obstructive coronary artery disease [94]. As these studies were cross-sectional in nature, it is uncertain whether EAT plays a causal role in the development of atherosclerosis. Nevertheless, longitudinal, prospective studies reported supportive data for the "outside to inside signaling" hypothesis as a causal mechanism in the process of atherosclerotic plaque development [75,95]. In these studies, intrathoracic fat and EAT volume were measured and an increase of their quantity was associated with incident coronary heart disease and with major adverse cardiac events. Associations were independent from BMI and other risk factors, suggesting that EAT is one of the factors contributing to CAD. Importantly, a systematic review from 2015 evaluated the prognostic value of EAT; analyzing the results of one prospective investigation, three case-control studies, and five retrospective reanalyses of previously published prospective studies on calcium scoring the authors concluded that epicardial fat volume has prognostic value for adverse cardiac events and, in addition, its quantification can improve risk assessment with calcium scoring [96]. Recently, results of a prospective clinical study were published from Denmark. Patients with type 2 diabetes were recruited (n = 1030) and followed for 4.7 years, EAT was measured by echocardiography and the endpoint was the composite of incident cardiovascular disease and all-cause mortality. High (>median) EAT levels were associated with the composite endpoint, particularly in men, after adjusting for cardiovascular risk factors [97]. Similar results were observed by the authors in a former clinical study, investigating patients with type 2 diabetes and microalbuminuria: high-levels of cardiac fat were associated with increased risk of incident cardiovascular disease or total mortality in a five-year follow-up study [98].

The predictive value of EAT in the cardiovascular risk assessment was extensively investigated in prospective studies. In the Heinz Nixdorf Recall Study (3630 subjects, 9.9 ± 2.6 years of follow-up) EAT volume had a predictive value on major adverse cardiovascular events (HR: 1.15 [95% CI: 1.01−1.30]) and improved the combined predictive value of Framingham risk score and Ca-scoring (area under curve: AUC = 0.749 vs. 0.764; $P = .011$) [99]. In addition, Cheng et al. found that adding pericardial fat volume (≥ 125 cm^3) to Framingham risk score and calcium score (≥ 400 Agatston score) resulted in a trend toward improved prediction compared to the latter two only (ROC analysis, AUC 0.73 vs. 0.68;

TABLE 4.3 Correlation between fat measures and body mass index (BMI).

	BMI	Pericoronary	Epicardial	Periaortic	Extracardiac-intrathoracic
BMI	–	0.21	0.44	0.44	0.45
Pericoronary	0.21	–	0.70	0.54	0.49
Epicardial	0.44	0.67	–	0.69	0.70
Periaortic	0.44	0.54	0.69	–	0.75
Extracardiac-intrathoracic	0.45	0.49	0.70	0.75	–

All $P < .001$.
From: Maurovich-Horvat, et al. Obesity 2015;23:1278−1284.

TABLE 4.4 Unadjusted and adjusted analysis of pericoronary fat volume to presence of any plaque on a per patient basis per 10 cm³ increase in fat volume.

	Unadjusted OR (95% CI)	P value	Adjusted[a] OR (95% CI)	P value
Pericoronary	1.66 (1.41–1.97)	<0.0001	1.31 (1.08–1.59	0.006
Epicardial	1.21 (1.12–1.29)	<0.0001	1.09 (0.99–1.19)	0.08
Periaortic	2.74 (1.98–3.78)	<0.0001	1.40 (0.87–2.23)	0.16
Extracardiac-intrathoracic	1.10 (1.06.1.15)	<0.0001	1.04 (0.99–1.10)	0.13

CI, confidence interval; *OR*, odds ratio.
[a]*Adjusted for age, gender, diabetes, hypertension, dyslipidemia, smoking, BMI, aspirin use, statin use.*
From: Maurovich-Horvat, et al. Obesity 2015;23:1278–1284.

$P = .058$) [95]. In the study from Denmark, EAT modestly improved risk prediction over cardiovascular risk factors [97]. Despite the results gained, further studies are needed to assess whether adding EAT quantity to other risk factors may really improve the accuracy of CAD prediction in clinical practice.

EAT in other cardiac diseases

It was reasonable to assume that EAT may have a potential role in the pathomechanism of atrial fibrillation and heart failure.

Atrial fibrillation

The relationship of EAT with atrial fibrillation was analyzed in several clinical studies [100–106] and the potential role of EAT in the pathomechanism of atrial fibrillation was discussed in review articles [107–110].

It is widely accepted that there is a relationship between EAT and the occurrence of atrial fibrillation. In the Framingham Heart Study, higher pericardial fat volume was associated with higher prevalence of atrial fibrillation, even after adjustment of several risk factors [100]. A strong association between EAT and atrial fibrillation (both paroxysmal and persistent) was documented by Al Chekakie et al.; the relationship proved to independent of traditional risk factors and atrial enlargement [101]. In addition, patients with extensive EAT increase had a higher risk of atrial fibrillation recurrence after ablation intervention. Taken together, EAT proved to be an independent predictor of the presence, severity, and recurrence of atrial fibrillation [101]. In another study, left atrial epicardial fat thickness was measured using cardiac CT in patients with no (n = 73), paroxysmal (n = 60), or persistent (n = 36) atrial fibrillation; patients with persistent atrial fibrillation had significantly thicker EAT as compared to patients with paroxysmal or without atrial fibrillation [102]. In patients (n = 110) with first-time ablation for atrial fibrillation, pericardial fat volumes (assessed by MRI) were significantly associated with the presence of atrial fibrillation and its chronicity as well as with clinical symptom burden. Pericardial fat depots were predictive of long-term atrial fibrillation recurrence after ablation. Pericardial fat depots were associated with left atrial volume. Importantly, systemic measures of adiposity (BMI) were not associated with these outcomes in multivariate-adjusted models [103]. EAT thickness (measured by echocardiography) was an independent predictor for postablation recurrence of atrial fibrillation in a study of 283 patients [104]. In a small cross-sectional study of 84 consecutive patients investigated by echocardiography, higher EAT thickness was observed in permanent vs. paroxysmal atrial fibrillation (4.8 ± 2.5 vs. 3.5 ± 2.4 mm, $P < .05$) [105]. In a study of 105 patients, EAT was measured using MRI, and patients with atrial fibrillation had higher EAT than those without [106].

Several potential factors and mechanisms (inflammation, adipocyte infiltration, electrical remodeling, fibrosis and structure remodeling, autonomic nervous system dysfunction, oxidative stress, gene expression, local aromatase effect, ventricular diastolic dysfunction) were considered to explain the relationship between EAT and atrial fibrillation [109].

Heart failure

Although the close proximity of EAT to myocardium substantiates metabolic and functional interaction between the two different tissues, it remained questionable for a long time, whether EAT has any influence on systolic (HFrEF: heart failure with reduced ejection fraction) or diastolic (HFpEF: heart failure with preserved ejection fraction) heart failure in the clinical practice. Now we have data that support the role of EAT in HFpEF, however, data with HFrEF are controversial.

In a retrospective single center study, EAT thickness (measured by echocardiography) increased in patients with HFpEF compared to controls [111]. In a cross-sectional MRI study with a total of 64 heart failure patients (left ventricular ejection fraction >40%) 20 control subjects were investigated. Heart failure patients had more epicardial fat volume compared to controls, despite similar BMI. Epicardial fat volume was associated with the presence of atrial fibrillation and type 2 diabetes mellitus and with biomarkers related to myocardial injury [112]. In another study, patients with heart failure and a left ventricular ejection fraction >45% underwent right and left heart catheterization with simultaneous echocardiography; obesity and increased EAT were associated with higher right-sided filling pressures and with reduced exercise capacity [113]. In a recent study, the contributing role of EAT to the pathophysiology of obesity-related HFpEF was documented as subjects with HFpEF and obesity who have excess epicardial fat deposition demonstrated significantly greater impairments in rest and exercise hemodynamics and reduced exercise capacity compared with patients with obesity and HFpEF but without excess EAT [114].

In patients with HFrEF the results are inconsistent as both increased and decreased EAT volumes (vs. controls) were observed in different investigations [115–117].

Regarding the underlying pathomechanism of increased EAT and heart failure relationship, several factors should be considered. Obesity, type 2 diabetes, HFpEF, and atrial fibrillation often coexist. This is due to the very similar effects of obesity and type 2 diabetes on left ventricle and atrium, namely, both cause expansion and inflammation of EAT leading to microvascular dysfunction and fibrosis of the myocardium. On the other hand, the same process may also lead to atrial myopathy, manifesting as atrial fibrillation. In this way, EAT expansion and inflammation could be contributing factors to heart failure development [67,118]. In an MRI study, patients with HFpEF had significantly more intramyocardial fat than HFrEF patients or controls. Intramyocardial fat correlated with left ventricular diastolic dysfunction parameters in HFpEF patients. These data emphasize the role of myocardial lipid accumulation in the pathomechanism [119,120].

Concerning the pathomechanism of decreased EAT and heart failure relationship it was suggested that this alteration might result in a decreased buffering capacity for excess fatty free acids as well as a diminished responsiveness to adjust to special energy demands of the heart. Furthermore, a reduced adiponectin production might be suggested leading to diminished protective effects under ischemic conditions [115].

In a recent study, EAT thickness (assessed by echocardiography) and EAT volume (evaluated by MRI) were measured in patients with HFpEF or HFrEF. EAT volume increased but EAT/LVM (epicardial adipose tissue/left ventricular mass ratio) and EAT thickness reduced in HFrEF and HFpEF. Greater total EAT was more closely associated with worse functional parameters in HFpEF than in HFrEF suggesting a divergent role of EAT in the pathophysiology of HFrEF and HFpEF [121].

Although data are accumulating about the role of EAT in the pathomechanism of heart failure, long-term observations in this regard are still lacking.

Inflammation

Infections, most commonly viral infections, may cause myocarditis and/or pericarditis leading to alterations in both EAT volume and EAT density (attenuation). In a retrospective cohort study with 614 patients (mean age 61 years) with a high cardiovascular risk, EAT volume and attenuation significantly correlated but this relationship gradually diminished with increasing calcium scores. It was suggested that EAT attenuation might reflect fibrotic and inflammatory changes within the EAT, providing additional information to EAT volume alone [122]. In the editorial to this publication, it was postulated that fat density (attenuation) reflects higher inflammatory status rather than an inactive tissue fibrosis [123].

Epicardial fat necrosis

The epicardial fat necrosis is a rare clinical condition, 26 cases were reported till 2011 [124], additional case reports were published thereafter [125–128]. This clinical entity should be considered among differential diagnosis of chest pain. The etiology is obscure, the prognosis is good. In general, the presenting symptom is left-sided chest pain in a previously healthy individual with an associated juxtacardiac mass seen in chest radiography. CT or MRI may confirm the correct diagnosis resulting in the avoidance of surgical intervention. It should be considered as an overlooked and underdiagnosed condition; reviewing 3604 chest scans referred by an emergency department, 11 cases were retrospectively confirmed but only 27% of the cases were correctly diagnosed at the time of presentation [129].

EAT in metabolic diseases

Typically, type 2 diabetes is preceded by prediabetes but insulin resistance syndrome due to obesity may be the first pathological stage in the long-lasting asymptomatic period of diabetes. The insulin resistance syndrome (called also as the metabolic syndrome) includes insulin resistance and different metabolic abnormalities (elevated serum triglycerides, lower HDL-cholesterol, hyperglycemia) as well as elevated blood pressure. Obesity, especially abdominal visceral fat accumulation plays a central role in this syndrome. Although the use of term and the suggested pathomechanism of the metabolic syndrome became debatable some years ago, the association between the enlarged abdominal visceral fat compartment and the increased cardiovascular risk remained unquestionable [130]. The enlarged visceral fat depot is characterized primarily with increased lipolysis leading to hepatic steatosis.

Generally, EAT volumes are increased in obesity showing a stronger correlation with visceral (abdominal) lipid accumulation [3,7,131].

Several clinical investigations were dedicated to assess the characteristics of EAT in the metabolic syndrome, prediabetes, and type 2 diabetes. In a metaanalysis, EAT was 7.5 ± 0.1 mm in thickness in the metabolic syndrome (n = 427) compared to 4.0 ± 0.1 mm in controls (n = 301) and EAT correlated significantly with the components of the metabolic syndrome [132]. EAT volume was significantly higher in patients with type 2 diabetes than in nondiabetic subjects and EAT volume was significantly associated with components of the metabolic syndrome [133]. In asymptomatic type 2 diabetic patients the thickness of EAT proved to be an independent risk factor for significant coronary artery stenosis but not for silent myocardial ischemia [134]. A strong correlation was found between fasting plasma glucose and EAT measured with CT or echocardiography [135]. EAT quantity was higher in patients with type 2 diabetes mellitus compared to lean subjects or obese patients without diabetes. In addition, the difference in EAT volume between men and women was more pronounced in subjects with impaired fasting glucose or diabetes mellitus [136]. A clear relationship of epicardial fat and serum alanine aminotransferase (ALT) and aspartate aminotransferase (AST) activity, surrogate markers of fatty liver, were documented in a cross-sectional, observational study [137].

Interestingly, higher epicardial fat volume and serum leptin levels were found in subjects with type 1 diabetes than in nondiabetic controls. The epicardial fat thickness and serum leptin levels proved to be the best independent correlates of each other in patients with type 1 diabetes independently of BMI, glycemic control and daily insulin requirement [138]. Patients with type 1 diabetes (n = 100) from the Diabetes Control and Complications Trial/Epidemiology of Diabetes Interventions and Complications (DCCT/EDIC) study were also investigated. In this pilot study, the accumulation of adipose tissue in epicardial and intrathoracic spaces were highly associated with greater BMI, bigger waist-to-hip ratio, greater weighted glycated hemoglobin values, elevated triglycerides, and a history of elevated albumin excretion rate, or end-stage renal disease [139].

Taken together, obesity, the insulin resistance syndrome (the metabolic syndrome), type 2 diabetes, prediabetes, and nonalcoholic fatty liver disease are associated with increased amount of EAT [13]. Accumulation of EAT may occur even in patients with type 1 diabetes [138].

EAT in patients with COVID-19

EAT volume is associated with cardiometabolic disturbances, is a source of proinflammatory cytokines, and a marker of visceral obesity. In addition, EAT attenuation (assessed in HU) reflects inflammatory changes within the adipose tissue. Moreover, it has been postulated that EAT may transduce inflammation to the heart [140−145]. Therefore, it is worth investigating the potential role of EAT in the outcomes of patients with COVID-19 (coronavirus disease 2019).

In a post-hoc analysis of a prospective international registry (109 consecutive patients; age 64 ± 16 years) with laboratory-confirmed COVID-19 and noncontrast chest CT imaging, EAT volume (mL) and attenuation (HU) were measured and a composite endpoint of clinical deterioration (intensive care unit admission, invasive mechanical ventilation, or vasopressor therapy) or in-hospital death was assessed. In multivariable logistic regression analysis, EAT volume per doubling (OR 5.1; 95% CI 1.8−14.1; $P = 0.011$] and EAT attenuation per 5 Hounsfield unit increase (OR 3.4; 95% CI 1.5−7.5; $P = .003$) were independent predictors of clinical deterioration or death, as was total pneumonia burden, chronic lung disease, and history of heart failure [146].

In another retrospective analysis of 41 patients with confirmed COVID-19, EAT thickness (mm) and attenuation (HU) were evaluated. EAT attenuation significantly increased with increasing COVID-19 severity, patients with severe and critical COVID-19 had significantly greater EAT attenuation than those presenting with mild and moderate COVID-19. CT-measured EAT attenuation could have diagnostic and prognostic value in patients with COVID-19 [147].

In a study from Italy, clinical outcomes were investigated in adult patients with confirmed SARS-CoV-2 (severe acute respiratory syndrome coronavirus 2) infection admitted to San Raffaele University Hospital in Milan from February 25 to April 19, 2020. Chest CT scan for pneumonia were performed in each patient (n = 192, median age 60 years). EAT volume and attenuation, a marker of EAT inflammation were measured. Primary outcome was critical illness (admission to intensive care unit, invasive ventilation or death). In this study, EAT attenuation but not EAT volume or obesity independently predicted critical illness (HR 1.12; 95% CI: 1.04−1.21). The results should be considered hypothesis-generating due to the study design (post-hoc analysis) and several limitations [148].

Further clinical studies are needed to better understand the potential role of EAT in the clinical course of patients with COVID-19.

Treatment options for modifying EAT volume

Lifestyle changes, bariatric surgery, and pharmacological intervention with different drugs may be considered.

Reduction in weight (BMI) by using very-low calorie diet resulted in a decrease of EAT volume in severely obese subjects (n = 20; echocardiographic EAT thickness at baseline: 12.3 ± 1.8 mm, at 6 months follow-up: 8.3 ± 1.0 mm; $P = .001$) [149]. Similarly, beneficial effect was observed as a result of regular exercise training in a small group of patients (n = 24; echocardiographic EAT volume at baseline: 8.11 ± 1.64 mm, at 12 weeks follow-up: 7.39 ± 1.54; $P < .001$) [150].

EAT volume decreased after bariatric surgery as well, however one study found that myocardial triglyceride content did not change significantly [151,152]. In a meta-analysis, diet or bariatric surgery proved to be more beneficial than exercise training in reducing EAT volume [153].

Pharmacological intervention may imply statins and/or antihyperglycemic agents [154,155]. Generally, these clinical studies were small with a relatively short follow-up. Atorvastatin resulted in a more pronounced decrease of EAT than simvastatin/ezetimibe [156]. Metformin monotherapy significantly decreased EAT and BMI in patients with newly diagnosed diabetes [157]. Pioglitazone compared with metformin increased pericardial fat volume in patients with type 2 diabetes [158]. Short-term (3 months) use of glucagon-like peptide-1 (GLP1) receptor agonists (exenatide, liraglutide) decreased the volume of EAT in patients with type 2 diabetes [159]. In a longer (26 weeks) randomized controlled trial exenatide twice daily (vs. standard antidiabetic treatment) proved to be effective in reducing both epicardial and liver fat content in obese patients with type 2 diabetes; the beneficial effect was mainly weight loss dependent [160]. Liraglutide added on metformin (vs. metformin alone) caused large and rapid epicardial fat reduction [161]. In a recent study, new GLP1-receptor agonists (weekly administration of semaglutide or dulaglutide) caused rapid, substantial, and dose-dependent reduction in EAT thickness [162]. In a pilot study, sitagliptin, a dipeptidyl-peptidase-4 (DPP4)-inhibitor, decreased the volume of EAT in a 24-week long study with obese type 2 diabetic patients [163]. Sodium-glucose co-transporter (SGLT2) inhibitors such as dapagliflozin, canagliflozin or empagliflozin proved to be effective in reducing EAT volume in patients with type 2 diabetes [164−167]. However, in the EMPACEF trial, empagliflozin had no effect on myocardial or epicardial fat in patients with type 2 diabetes [168]. Interestingly, metformin treatment had no effect on EAT compared with placebo in patients with CAD but without type 2 diabetes [169].

A recent systematic review and meta-analysis provided evidence that exercise, diet, bariatric surgery, and pharmaceutical interventions could reduce EAT volume [170].

In summary, EAT was considered as a novel therapeutic target in the last couple of years, and statins as well as antihyperglycemic agents proved to be the best candidates [171,172]. Among antihyperglycemic agents, SLGT2-inhibitors and GLP1-receptor agonists should be preferable as they have cardiac benefits beyond appropriate glucose lowering effect [173].

References

[1] Bedford E. The story of fatty heart. A disease of Victorian times. Br Heart J 1972;34:23−8.

[2] Despres JP, Cartier A, Cote M, Arsenault BJ. The concept of cardiometabolic risk: bridging the fields of diabetology and cardiology. Ann Med 2008;40:514−23.

[3] Iacobellis G, Ribaudo MC, Assael F, Vecci E, Tiberti C, Zappaterreno A, Di Mario U, Leonetti F. Echocardiographic epicardial adipose tissue is related to anthropometric and clinical parameters of metabolic syndrome: a new indicator of cardiovascular risk. J Clin Endocrinol Metab 2003;88:5163−8.

[4] Nagy E, Jermendy AL, Merkely B, Maurovich-Horvat P. Clinical importance of epicardial adipose tissue. Arch Med Sci 2017;13:864−74.

[5] Douglass E, Greif S, Frishman WH. Epicardial fat: pathophysiology and clinical significance. Cardiol Rev 2017;25:230−5.

[6] Gaborit B, Sengenes C, Ancel P, Jacquier A, Dutour A. Role of epicardial adipose tissue in health and disease: a matter of fat? Compr Physiol 2017;7:1051−82.

[7] Guglielmi V, Sbraccia P. Epicardial adipose tissue: at the heart of the obesity complications. Acta Diabetol 2017;54:805−12.

[8] Ansaldo AM, Montecucco F, Sahebkar A, Dallegri F, Carbone F. Epicardial adipose tissue and cardiovascular diseases. Int J Cardiol 2019;278:254−60.

[9] Iacobellis G, Barbaro G. Epicardial adipose tissue feeding and overfeeding the heart. Nutrition 2019;59:1−6.

[10] Guglielmo M, Lin A, Dey D, Baggiano A, Fusini L, Muscogiuri G, Pontone G. Epicardial fat and coronary artery disease: role of cardiac imaging. Atherosclerosis 2021;321:30−8.

[11] Ayton SL, Gulsin GS, McCann GP, Moss AJ. Epicardial adipose tissue in obesity-related cardiac dysfunction. Heart May 2021;13. https://doi.org/10.1136/heartjnl-2020-318242. heartjnl-2020-318242. [Epub ahead of print].

[12] Iacobellis G, editor. Epicardial adipose tissue from cell to clinic. Springer; 2020.

[13] Iacobellis G. Local and systemic effects of the multifaceted epicardial adipose tissue depot. Nat Rev Endocrinol 2015:363−71.

[14] Iacobellis G, Bianco AC. Epicardial adipose tissue: emerging physiological, pathophysiological and clinical features. Trends Endocrinol Metabol 2011;22:450−7.

[15] Hirata Y, Yamada H, Sata M. Epicardial fat and pericardial fat surrounding the heart have different characteristics. Circ J 2018;82:2475−6.

[16] Bertaso AG, Bertol D, Duncan BB, Foppa M. Epicardial fat: definition, measurements and systematic review of main outcomes. Arq Bras Cardiol 2013;101:E18−28.

[17] Iacobellis G. Epicardial and pericardial fat: close, but very different. Obesity 2009;17. 625-625.

[18] Iacobellis G, Corradi D, Sharma AM. Epicardial adipose tissue: anatomic, biomolecular, and clinical relationships with the heart. Nat Clin Pract Cardiovasc Med 2005;2:536−43.

[19] Shirani J, Berezowski K, Roberts WC. Quantitative measurement of normal and excessive (cor adiposum) subepicardial adipose tissue, its clinical significance, and its effect on electrocardiographic QRS voltage. Am J Cardiol 1995;76:414−8.

[20] Rabkin SW. Epicardial fat: properties, function and relationship to obesity. Obes Rev 2007;8:253−61.

[21] Reiner L, Mazzoleni A, Rodriguez FL. Statistical analysis of the epicardial fat weight in human hearts. AMA Arch Pathol 1955;60:369−73.

[22] Sons HU, Hoffmann V. Epicardial fat cell size, fat distribution and fat infiltration of the right and left ventricle of the heart. Anat Anzeiger 1986;161:355−73.

[23] Corradi D. The ventricular epicardial fat is related to the myocardial mass in normal, ischemic and hypertrophic hearts. Cardiovasc Pathol 2004;13:313−6.

[24] Roberts WC, Roberts JD. The floating heart or the heart too fat to sink: analysis of 55 necropsy patients. Am J Cardiol 1983;52:1286−9.

[25] Smith HL, Willius FA. Adiposity of the heart. A clinical and pathologic study of one hundred and thirty size obese patients. Arch Intern Med 1933;52:911−31.

[26] Tansey DK, Aly Z, Sheppard MN. Fat in the right ventricle of the normal heart. Histopathology 2005;46:98−104.

[27] Schejbal V. Epicardial fatty tissue of the right ventricle − morphology, morphometry and functional significance. Pneumologie 1989;43:490−9.

[28] Bambace C, Telesca M, Zoico E, Sepe A, Olioso D, Rossi A, Corzato F, Di Francesco V, Mazzucco A, Santini F, Zamboni M. Adiponectin gene expression and adipocyte diameter: a comparison between epicardial and subcutaneous adipose tissue in men. Cardiovasc Pathol 2011;20:e153−6.

[29] Adams DB, Narayan O, Munnur RK, Cameron JD, Wong DT, Talman AH, Harper RW, Seneviratne SK, Meredith IT, Ko BS. Ethnic differences in coronary plaque and epicardial fat volume quantified using computed tomography. Int J Cardiovasc Imag 2017;33:241−9.

[30] Hanley C, Matthews KA, Brooks MM, Janssen I, Budoff MJ, Sekikawa A, Mulukutla S, El Khoudary SR. Cardiovascular fat in women at midlife: effects of race, overall adiposity, and central adiposity. The SWAN cardiovascular fat study. Menopause 2018;25:38−45.

[31] Kim SA, Kim MN, Shim WJ, Park SM. Epicardial adipose tissue is related to cardiac function in elderly women, but not in men. Nutr Metab Cardiovasc Dis 2017;27:41−7.

[32] Mancio J, Pinheiro M, Ferreira W, Carvalho M, Barros A, Ferreira N, Vouga L, Ribeiro VG, Leite-Moreira A, Falcao-Pires I, Bettencourt N. Gender differences in the association of epicardial adipose tissue and coronary artery calcification: EPICHEART study: EAT and coronary calcification by gender. Int J Cardiol 2017;249:419−25.

[33] Fox CS, Gona P, Hoffmann U, Porter SA, Salton CJ, Massaro JM, Levy D, Larson MG, D'Agostino RB, O'Donnell CJ, Manning WJ. Pericardial fat, intrathoracic fat, and measures of left ventricular structure and function the Framingham heart study. Circulation 2009;119:1586−91.

[34] Gorter PM, van Lindert ASR, de Vos AM, Meijs MSFL, van der Graaf Y, Doevendans PA, Prokop M, Visseren FLJ. Quantification of epicardial and peri-coronary fat using cardiac computed tomography; reproducibility and relation with obesity and metabolic syndrome in patients suspected of coronary artery disease. Atherosclerosis 2008;197:896−903.

[35] Willens HJ, Gomez-Marin O, Chirinos JA, Goldberg R, Lowery MH, Iacobellis G. Comparison of epicardial and pericardial fat thickness assessed by echocardiography in African American and non-Hispanic white men: a pilot study. Ethnic Dis 2008;18:311−6.

[36] Maurovich-Horvat P, Tárnoki DL, Tárnoki ÁD, Horváth T, Jermendy ÁL, Kolossváry M, Szilveszter B, Vörös V, Kovács A, Molnár AÁ, Littvay L, Lamb HJ, Vörös S, Jermendy G, Merkely B. Rationale, design and methodological aspects of the BUDAPEST-GLOBAL study (burden of atherosclerotic plaques study in twins - genetic loci and the burden of atherosclerotic lesions). Clin Cardiol 2015;38:699−707.

[37] Jermendy AL, Kolossvary M, Drobni ZD, Tarnoki AD, Tarnoki DL, Karady J, Voros S, Lamb HJ, Merkely B, Jermendy G, Maurovich-Horvat P. Assessing genetic and environmental influences on epicardial and abdominal adipose tissue quantities: a classical twin study. Int J Obes 2018;42:163−8.

[38] Iacobellis G. Aging effects on epicardial adipose tissue. Front Aging May 13, 2021. https://doi.org/10.3389/fragi.2021.666260.

[39] Marchington JM, Mattacks CA, Pond CM. Adipose tissue in the mammalian heart and pericardium: structure, foetal development and biochemical properties. Comp Biochem Physiol B 1989;94:225–32.

[40] Sacks HS, Fain JN, Holman B, Cheema P, Chary A, Parks F, Karas J, Optican R, Bahouth SW, Garrett E, Wolf RY, Carter RA, Robbins T, Wolford D, Samaha J. Uncoupling protein-1 and related messenger ribonucleic acids in human epicardial and other adipose tissues: epicardial fat functioning as brown fat. J Clin Endocrinol Metab 2009;94:3611–5.

[41] Prati F, Arbustini E, Labellarte A, Sommariva L, Pawlowski T, Manzoli A, Pagano A, Motolese M, Boccanelli A. Eccentric atherosclerotic plaques with positive remodelling have a pericardial distribution: a permissive role of epicardial fat? A three-dimensional intravascular ultrasound study of left anterior descending artery lesions. Eur Heart J 2003;24:329–36.

[42] Iozzo P. Metabolic toxicity of the heart: insights from molecular imaging. Nutr Metab Cardiovas 2010;20:147–56.

[43] Deng G, Long Y, Yu YR, Li MR. Adiponectin directly improves endothelial dysfunction in obese rats through the AMPK-eNOS Pathway. Int J Obes 2010;34:165–71.

[44] Li R, Wang WQ, Zhang H, Yang X, Fan Q, Christopher TA, Lopez BL, Tao L, Goldstein BJ, Gao F, Ma XL. Adiponectin improves endothelial function in hyperlipidemic rats by reducing oxidative/nitrative stress and differential regulation of eNOS/iNOS activity. Am J Physiol-Endoc M 2007;293:E1703–8.

[45] Payne GA, Kohr MC, Tune JD. Epicardial perivascular adipose tissue as a therapeutic target in obesity-related coronary artery disease. Br J Pharmacol 2012;165:659–69.

[46] Iacobellis G, Willens HJ. Echocardiographic epicardial fat: a review of research and clinical applications. J Am Soc Echocardiogr 2009;22:1311–9.

[47] Saura D, Oliva MJ, Rodriguez D, Pascual-Figal DA, Hurtado JA, Pinar E, de la Morena G, Valdes M. Reproducibility of echocardiographic measurements of epicardial fat thickness. Int J Cardiol 2010;141:311–3.

[48] Kim BJ, Kang JG, Lee SH, Lee JY, Sung KC, Kim BS, Kang JH. Relationship of echocardiographic epicardial fat thickness and epicardial fat volume by computed tomography with coronary artery calcification: data from the CAESAR study. Arch Med Res 2017;48:352–9.

[49] Flüchter S, Haghi D, Dinter D, Heberlein W, Kühl HP, Neff W, Sueselbeck T, Borggrefe M, Papavassiliu T. Volumetric assessment of epicardial adipose tissue with cardiovascular magnetic resonance imaging. Obesity (Silver Spring) 2007;15:870–8.

[50] Sicari R, Sironi AM, Petz R, Frassi F, Chubuchny V, De Marchi D, Positano V, Lombardi M, Picano E, Gastaldelli A. Pericardial rather than epicardial fat is a cardiometabolic risk marker: an MRI vs echo study. J Am Soc Echocardiogr 2011;24:1156–62.

[51] Agatston AS, Janowitz WR, Hildner FJ, Zusmer NR, Viamonte Jr M, Detrano R. Quantification of coronary artery calcium using ultrafast computed tomography. J Am Coll Cardiol 1990;15:827–32.

[52] Rosito GA, Massaro JM, Hoffmann U, Ruberg FL, Mahabadi AA, Vasan RS, et al. Pericardial fat, visceral abdominal fat, cardiovascular disease risk factors, and vascular calcification in a community-based sample: the Framingham Heart Study. Circulation 2008;117:605–13.

[53] Madaj P, Budoff MJ. Risk stratification of non-contrast CT beyond the coronary calcium scan. J Cardiovasc Comput 2012;6:301–7.

[54] Hell MM, Achenbach S, Schuhbaeck A, Klinghammer L, May MS, Marwan M. CT-based analysis of pericoronary adipose tissue density: relation to cardiovascular risk factors and epicardial adipose tissue volume. J Cardiovasc Comput Tomogr 2016;10:52–60.

[55] Oikonomou EK, Marwan M, Desai MY, Mancio J, Alashi A, Hutt Centeno E, Thomas S, Herdman L, Kotanidis CP, Thomas KE, Griffin BP, Flamm SD, Antonopoulos AS, Shirodaria C, Sabharwal N, Deanfield J, Neubauer S, Hopewell JC, Channon KM, Achenbach S, Antoniades C. Non-invasive detection of coronary inflammation using computed tomography and prediction of residual cardiovascular risk (the CRISP CT study): a post-hoc analysis of prospective outcome data. Lancet 2018;392:929–39.

[56] Mahabadi AA, Rassaf T. Imaging of coronary inflammation for cardiovascular risk prediction. Lancet 2018;392:894–6.

[57] Maurovich-Horvat P, Kallianos K, Engel LC, Szymonifka J, Fox CS, Hoffmann U, Truong QA. Influence of pericoronary adipose tissue on local coronary atherosclerosis as assessed by a novel MDCT volumetric method. Atherosclerosis 2011;219:151–7.

[58] Sacks HS, Fain JN. Human epicardial adipose tissue: a review. Am Heart J 2007;153:907–17.

[59] Ishii T, Asuwa N, Masuda S, Ishikawa Y. The effects of a myocardial bridge on coronary atherosclerosis and ischaemia. J Pathol 1998;185:4–9.

[60] Mazurek T, Zhang LF, Zalewski A, Mannion JD, Diehl JT, Arafat H, Sarov-Blat L, O'Brien S, Keiper EA, Johnson AG, Martin J, Goldstein BJ, Shi Y. Human epicardial adipose tissue is a source of inflammatory mediators. Circulation 2003;108:2460–6.

[61] Baker AR, da Silva NF, Quinn DW, Harte AL, Pagano D, Bonser RS, Kumar S, McTernan PG. Human epicardial adipose tissue expresses a pathogenic profile of adipocytokines in patients with cardiovascular disease. Cardiovasc Diabetol 2006;5:1.

[62] Baker AR, Harte AL, Howell N, Pritlove DC, Ranasinghe AM, da Silva NF, Youssef EM, Khunti K, Davies MJ, Bonser RS, Kumar S, Pagano D, McTernan PG. Epicardial adipose tissue as a source of nuclear factor-kappa B and c-Jun N-terminal kinase mediated inflammation in patients with coronary artery disease. J Clin Endocrinol Metab 2009;94:261–7.

[63] Eiras S, Teijeira-Fernandez E, Shamagian LG, Fernandez AL, Vazquez-Boquete A, Gonzalez-Juanatey JR. Extension of coronary artery disease is associated with increased IL-6 and decreased adiponectin gene expression in epicardial adipose tissue. Cytokine 2008;43:174–80.

[64] Iacobellis G, Pistilli D, Gucciardo M, Leonetti F, Miraldi F, Brancaccio G, Gallo P, di Gioia CRT. Adiponectin expression in human epicardial adipose tissue in vivo is lower in patients with coronary artery disease. Cytokine 2005;9:251–5.

[65] Iacobellis G, Malazavos AE, Corsi MM. Epicardial fat: from the biomolecular aspects to the clinical practice. Int J Biochem Cell Biol 2011;43:1651–4.

[66] Matloch Z, Cinkajzlova A, Mraz M, Haluzik M. The role of inflammation in epicardial adipose tissue in heart diseases. Curr Pharmaceut Des 2018;24:297–309.

[67] Packer M. Epicardial adipose tissue may mediate deleterious effects of obesity and inflammation on the myocardium. J Am Coll Cardiol 2018;71:2360–72.

[68] Yudkin JS, Eringa E, Stehouwer CDA. "Vasocrine" signalling from perivascular fat: a mechanism linking insulin resistance to vascular disease. Lancet 2005;365:1817—20.

[69] Wang TD, Lee WJ, Shih FY, Huang CH, Chen WJ, Lee YT, Shih TTF, Chen MF. Association of epicardial adipose tissue with coronary atherosclerosis is region-specific and independent of conventional risk factors and intra-abdominal adiposity. Atherosclerosis 2010;213:279—87.

[70] Yerramasu A, Dey D, Venuraju S, Anand DV, Atwal S, Corder R, Berman DS, Lahiri A. Increased volume of epicardial fat is an independent risk factor for accelerated progression of sub-clinical coronary atherosclerosis. Atherosclerosis 2012;220:223—30.

[71] Acele A, Baykan AO, Yuksel Kalkan G, Celiker E, Gur M. Epicardial fat thickness is associated with aortic intima-media thickness in patients without clinical manifestation of atherosclerotic cardiovascular disease. Echocardiography 2017;34:1146—51.

[72] Mancio J, Azevedo D, Saraiva F, Azevedo AI, Pires-Morais G, Leite-Moreira A, Falcao-Pires I, Lunet N, Bettencourt N. Epicardial adipose tissue volume assessed by computed tomography and coronary artery disease: a systematic review and meta-analysis. Eur Heart J Cardiovasc Imaging 2018;19:490—7.

[73] Patel VB, Shah S, Verma S, Oudit GY. Epicardial adipose tissue as a metabolic transducer: role in heart failure and coronary artery disease. Heart Fail Rev 2017;22:889—902.

[74] Wu FZ, Chou KJ, Huang YL, Wu MT. The relation of location-specific epicardial adipose tissue thickness and obstructive coronary artery disease: systemic review and meta-analysis of observational studies. BMC Cardiovasc Disord 2014;14:62.

[75] Ding JZ, Hsu FC, Harris TB, Liu YM, Kritchevsky SB, Szklo M, Ouyang P, Espeland MA, Lohman KK, Criqui MH, Allison M, Bluemke DA, Carr JJ. The association of pericardial fat with incident coronary heart disease: the multi-ethnic study of atherosclerosis (MESA). Am J Clin Nutr 2009;90:499—504.

[76] Wang CP, Hsu HL, Hung WC, Yu TH, Chen YH, Chiu CA, Lu LF, Chung FM, Shin SJ, Lee YJ. Increased epicardial adipose tissue (EAT) volume in type 2 diabetes mellitus and association with metabolic syndrome and severity of coronary atherosclerosis. Clin Endocrinol 2009;70:876—82.

[77] Alexopoulos N, McLean DS, Janik M, Arepalli CD, Stillman AE, Raggi P. Epicardial adipose tissue and coronary artery plaque characteristics. Atherosclerosis 2010;210:150—4.

[78] Konishi M, Sugiyama S, Sugamura K, Nozaki T, Ohba K, Matsubara J, Matsuzawa Y, Sumida H, Nagayoshi Y, Nakaura T, Awai K, Yamashita Y, Jinnouchi H, Matsui K, Kimura K, Umemura S, Ogawa H. Association of pericardial fat accumulation rather than abdominal obesity with coronary atherosclerotic plaque formation in patients with suspected coronary artery disease. Atherosclerosis 2010;209:573—8.

[79] Ito T, Nasu K, Terashima M, Ehara M, Kinoshita Y, Ito T, Kimura M, Tanaka N, Habara M, Tsuchikane E, Suzuki T. The impact of epicardial fat volume on coronary plaque vulnerability: insight from optical coherence tomography analysis. Eur Heart J-Card Img 2012;13:408—15.

[80] Schlett CL, Ferencik M, Kriegel MF, Bamberg F, Ghoshhajra BB, Joshi SB, Nagurney JT, Fox CS, Truong QA, Hoffmann U. Association of pericardial fat and coronary high-risk lesions as determined by cardiac CT. Atherosclerosis 2012;222:129—34.

[81] Nerlekar N, Brown AJ, Muthalaly RG, Talman A, Hettige T, Cameron JD, Wong DTL. Association of epicardial adipose tissue and high-risk plaque characteristics: a systematic review and meta-analysis. J Am Heart Assoc 2017;6:e006379.

[82] Tamarappoo B, Dey D, Shmilovich H, Nakazato R, Gransar H, Cheng VY, Friedman JD, Hayes SW, Thomson LEJ, Slomka PJ, Rozanski A, Berman DS. Increased pericardial fat volume measured from noncontrast CT predicts myocardial ischemia by SPECT. JACC Cardiovasc Imaging 2010;3:1104—12.

[83] Ueno K, Anzai T, Jinzaki M, Yamada M, Jo Y, Maekawa Y, Kawamura A, Yoshikawa T, Tanami Y, Sato K, Kuribayashi S, Ogawa S. Increased epicardial fat volume quantified by 64-multidetector computed tomography is associated with coronary atherosclerosis and totally occlusive lesions. Circ J 2009;73:1927—33.

[84] Nasri A, Najafian J, Derakhshandeh SM, Madjlesi F. Epicardial fat thickness and severity of coronary heart disease in patients with diabetes mellitus type II. ARYA Atheroscler 2018;14:32—7.

[85] Ozcan F, Turak O, Canpolat U, Kanat S, Kadife I, Avci S, Isleyen A, Cebeci M, Tok D, Basar FN, Aras D, Topaloglu S, Aydogdu S. Association of epicardial fat thickness with TIMI risk score in NSTEMI/USAP patients. Herz 2014;39:755—60.

[86] Tok D, Cagli K, Kadife I, Turak O, Ozcan F, Basar FN, Golbasi Z, Aydogdu S. Impaired coronary flow reserve is associated with increased echocardiographic epicardial fat thickness in metabolic syndrome patients. Coron Artery Dis 2013;24:191—5.

[87] Sade LE, Eroglu S, Bozbas H, Ozbicer S, Hayran M, Haberal A, Muderrisoglu H. Relation between epicardial fat thickness and coronary flow reserve in women with chest pain and angiographically normal coronary arteries. Atherosclerosis 2009;204:580—5.

[88] Cabrera-Rego JO, Iacobellis G, Castillo-Herrera JA, Valiente-Mustelier J, Gandarilla-Sarmientos JC, Marin-Julia SM, Navarrete-Cabrera J. Epicardial fat thickness correlates with carotid intima-media thickness, arterial stiffness, and cardiac geometry in children and adolescents. Pediatr Cardiol 2014;35:450—6.

[89] Cetin M, Cakici M, Polat M, Suner A, Zencir C, Ardic I. Relation of epicardial fat thickness with carotid intima-media thickness in patients with type 2 diabetes mellitus. Internet J Endocrinol 2013:769175.

[90] Park HE, Choi SY, Kim HS, Kim MK, Cho SH, Oh BH. Epicardial fat reflects arterial stiffness: assessment using 256-slice multidetector coronary computed tomography and cardio-ankle vascular index. J Atherosclerosis Thromb 2012;9:570—6.

[91] Maurovich-Horvat P, Kallianos K, Engel LC, Szymonifka J, Schlett CL, Koenig W, Hoffmann U, Truong QA. Relationship of thoracic fat depots with coronary atherosclerosis and circulating inflammatory biomarkers. Obesity 2015;23:1178—84.

[92] Picard FA, Gueret P, Laissy JP, Champagne S, Leclercq F, Carrie D, Juliard JM, Henry P, Niarra R, Chatellier G, Steg PG. Epicardial adipose tissue thickness correlates with the presence and severity of angiographic coronary artery disease in stable patients with chest pain. PLoS One 2014;9:e110005.

[93] Sinha SK, Thakur R, Jha MJ, Goel A, Kumar V, Kumar A, Mishra V, Varma CM, Krishna V, Singh AK, Sachan M. Epicardial adipose tissue thickness and its association with the presence and severity of coronary artery disease in clinical setting: a cross-sectional observational study. J Clin Med Res 2016;8:410—9.

[94] Zhou J, Chen Y, Zhang Y, Wang H, Tan Y, Liu Y, Huang L, Zhang H, Ma Y, Cong H. Epicardial fat volume improves the prediction of obstructive coronary artery disease above traditional risk factors and coronary calcium score. Circ Cardiovasc Imaging 2019;12(1):e008002.

[95] Cheng VY, Dey D, Tamarappoo B, Nakazato R, Gransar H, Miranda-Peats R, Ramesh A, Wong ND, Shaw LJ, Slomka PJ, Berman DS. Pericardial fat burden on ECG-gated noncontrast CT in asymptomatic patients who subsequently experience adverse cardiovascular events. JACC Cardiovasc Imaging 2010;3:352—60.

[96] Spearman JV, Renker M, Schoepf UJ, Krazinski AW, Herbert TL, De Cecco CN, Nietert PJ, Meinel FG. Prognostic value of epicardial fat volume measurements by computed tomography: a systematic review of the literature. Eur Radiol 2015;25:3372—81.

[97] Christensen RH, von Scholten BJ, Hansen CS, Jensen MT, Vilsbøll T, Rossing P, Jørgensen PG. Epicardial adipose tissue predicts incident cardiovascular disease and mortality in patients with type 2 diabetes. Cardiovasc Diabetol 2019;18(1):114.

[98] Christensen RH, von Scholten BJ, Hansen CS, Heywood SE, Rosenmeier JB, Andersen UB, Hovind P, Reinhard H, Parving HH, Pedersen BK, Jørgensen ME, Jacobsen PK, Rossing P. Epicardial, pericardial and total cardiac fat and cardiovascular disease in type 2 diabetic patients with elevated urinary albumin excretion rate. Eur J Prev Cardiol 2017;24:1517—24.

[99] Mahabadi AA, Lehmann N, Mohlenkamp S, Pundt N, Dykun I, Roggenbuck U, Moebus S, Jockel KH, Erbel R, Kalsch H, Groups HNI. Non-coronary measures enhance the predictive value of cardiac CT above traditional risk factors and CAC score in the general population. JACC Cardiovasc Imaging 2016;9:1177—85.

[100] Thanassoulis G, Massaro JM, O'Donnell CJ, Hoffmann U, Levy D, Ellinor PT, Wang TJ, Schnabel RB, Vasan RS, Fox CS, Benjamin EJ. Pericardial fat is associated with prevalent atrial fibrillation: the Framingham Heart Study. Circ Arrhythm Electrophysiol 2010;3:345—50.

[101] Al Chekakie MO, Welles CC, Metoyer R, Ibrahim A, Shapira AR, Cytron J, Santucci P, Wilber DJ, Akar JG. Pericardial fat is independently associated with human atrial fibrillation. J Am Coll Cardiol 2010;56:784—8.

[102] Batal O, Schoenhagen P, Shao M, Ayyad AE, Van Wagoner DR, Halliburton SS, Tchou PJ, Chung MK. Left atrial epicardial adiposity and atrial fibrillation. Circ Arrhythm Electrophysiol 2010;3:230—6.

[103] Wong CX, Abed HS, Molaee P, Nelson AJ, Brooks AG, Sharma G, Leong DP, Lau DH, Middeldorp ME, Roberts-Thomson KC, Wittert GA, Abhayaratna WP, Worthley SG, Sanders P. Pericardial fat is associated with atrial fibrillation severity and ablation outcome. J Am Coll Cardiol 2011;57:1745—51.

[104] Chao TF, Hung CL, Tsao HM, Lin YJ, Yun CH, Lai YH, Chang SL, Lo LW, Hu YF, Tuan TC, Chang HY, Kuo JY, Yeh HI, Wu TJ, Hsieh MH, Yu WC, Chen SA. Epicardial adipose tissue thickness and ablation outcome of atrial fibrillation. PLoS One 2013;8:e74926.

[105] Iacobellis G, Zaki MC, Garcia D, Willens HJ. Epicardial fat in atrial fibrillation and heart failure. Horm Metab Res 2014;46:587—90.

[106] Nakamori S, Nezafat M, Ngo LH, Manning WJ, Nezafat R. Left atrial epicardial fat volume is associated with atrial fibrillation: a prospective cardiovascular magnetic resonance 3D Dixon study. J Am Heart Assoc 2018;7:e008232.

[107] Zhu W, Zhang H, Guo L, Hong K. Relationship between epicardial adipose tissue volume and atrial fibrillation: a systematic review and meta-analysis. Herz 2016;41:421—7.

[108] Gaeta M, Bandera F, Tassinari F, Capasso L, Cargnelutti M, Pelissero G, Malavazos AE, Ricci C. Is epicardial fat depot associated with atrial fibrillation? A systematic review and meta-analysis. Europace 2017;19:747—52.

[109] Zhou M, Wang H, Chen J, Zhao L. Epicardial adipose tissue and atrial fibrillation: possible mechanisms, potential therapies, and future directions. Pacing Clin Electrophysiol 2020;43:133—45.

[110] Couselo-Seijas M, Rodríguez-Mañero M, González-Juanatey JR, Eiras S. Updates on epicardial adipose tissue mechanisms on atrial fibrillation. Obes Rev May 2021;17:e13277. https://doi.org/10.1111/obr.13277 [Online ahead of print].

[111] Obokata M, Reddy YNV, Pislaru SV, Melenovsky V, Borlaug BA. Evidence supporting the existence of a distinct obese phenotype of heart failure with preserved ejection fraction. Circulation 2017;136:6—19.

[112] van Woerden G, Gorter TM, Westenbrink BD, Willems TP, van Veldhuisen DJ, Rienstra M. Epicardial fat in heart failure patients with mid-range and preserved ejection fraction. Eur J Heart Fail 2018;20:1559—66.

[113] Gorter TM, van Woerden G, Rienstra M, Dickinson MG, Hummel YM, Voors AA, Hoendermis ES, van Veldhuisen DJ. Epicardial adipose tissue and invasive hemodynamics in heart failure with preserved ejection fraction. JACC Heart Fail 2020;8:667—76.

[114] Koepp KE, Obokata M, Reddy YNV, Olson TP, Borlaug BA. Hemodynamic and functional impact of epicardial adipose tissue in heart failure with preserved ejection fraction. JACC Heart Fail 2020;8:657—66.

[115] Doesch C, Haghi D, Fluchter S, Suselbeck T, Schoenberg SO, Michaely H, Borggrefe M, Papavassiliu T. Epicardial adipose tissue in patients with heart failure. J Cardiovasc Magn Reson 2010;12:40.

[116] Khawaja T, Greer C, Chokshi A, Chavarria N, Thadani S, Jones M, et al. Epicardial fat volume in patients with left ventricular systolic dysfunction. Am J Cardiol 2011;108:397—401.

[117] Tabakci MM, Durmuş Hİ, Avci A, Toprak C, Demir S, Arslantaş U, Cerşit S, Fidan S, **Kulahçioğlu Ş**, Batgerel U, Kargin R. Relation of epicardial fat thickness to the severity of heart failure in patients with nonischemic dilated cardiomyopathy. Echocardiography 2015;32:740—8.

[118] Packer M. Do most patients with obesity or type 2 diabetes, and atrial fibrillation, also have undiagnosed heart failure? A critical conceptual framework for understanding mechanisms and improving diagnosis and treatment. Eur J Heart Fail 2020;22:214—27.

[119] Wu CK, Lee JK, Hsu JC, Su MM, Wu YF, Lin TT, Lan CW, Hwang JJ, Lin LY. Myocardial adipose deposition and the development of heart failure with preserved ejection fraction. Eur J Heart Fail 2020;22:445—54.

[120] Van Woerden G, van Veldhuisen DJ, Rienstra M, Westenbrink BD. Myocardial adiposity in heart failure with preserved ejection fraction: the plot thickens. Eur J Heart Fail 2020;22:455−7.

[121] Tromp J, Bryant JA, Jin X, van Woerden G, Asali S, Yiying H, Liew OW, Ching JCP, Jaufeerally F, Loh SY, Sim D, Lee S, Soon D, Tay WT, Packer M, van Veldhuisen DJ, Chin C, Richards AM, Lam CSP. Epicardial fat in heart failure with reduced versus preserved ejection fraction. Eur J Heart Fail March 2021;16. https://doi.org/10.1002/ejhf.2156 [Epub ahead of print].

[122] Liu Z, Wang S, Wang Y, Zhou N, Shu J, Stamm C, Jiang M, Luo F. Association of epicardial adipose tissue attenuation with coronary atherosclerosis in patients with a high risk of coronary artery disease. Atherosclerosis 2019;284:230−6.

[123] Iacobellis G, Mahabadi AA. Is epicardial fat attenuation a novel marker of coronary inflammation? Atherosclerosis 2019;284:212−3.

[124] Baig A, Campbell B, Russell M, Singh J, Borra S. Epicardial fat necrosis: an uncommon etiology of chest pain. Cardiol J 2012;19:424−8.

[125] Ferretti GR, Rigaud D. Acute chest pain related to pericardial fat necrosis. Can Respir J 2016;2016:1948325.

[126] Nguyen DN, Tran CD, Rudkin SM, Mueller JS, Hartman MS. Epipericardial fat necrosis: uncommon cause of acute pleuritic chest pain. Radiol Case Rep 2018;13:1276−8.

[127] Friedman YE, Gayer G, Livne Margolin M, Kneller A, Mouallem M. Epipericardial fat necrosis. Isr Med Assoc J 2018;20:327−8.

[128] Couto J, Pontes Dos Santos L, Marques Mendes E, Brito A, López R, Santos C. Epicardial fat necrosis: a rare and benign cause of chest pain. Rev Port Cardiol 2020;39:113−4.

[129] Giassi K de S, Costa AN, Bachion GH, Apanavicius A, Filho JR, Kairalla RA, Lynch DA. Epipericardial fat necrosis: an underdiagnosed condition. Br J Radiol 2014;87(1038):20140118.

[130] Borch-Johnsen K, Wareham N. The rise and fall of the metabolic syndrome. Diabetologia 2010;53:597−9.

[131] Cikim AS, Topal E, Harputluoglu M, Keskin L, Zengin Z, Cikim K, Ozdemir R, Aladag M, Yologlu S. Epicardial adipose tissue, hepatic steatosis and obesity. J Endocrinol Invest 2007;30:459−64.

[132] Rabkin SW. The relationship between epicardial fat and indices of obesity and the metabolic syndrome: a systematic review and meta-analysis. Metab Syndr Relat Disord 2014;12:31−42.

[133] Wang TD, Lee WJ, Shih FY, Huang CH, Chang YC, Chen WJ, Lee YT, Chen MF. Relations of epicardial adipose tissue measured by multi-detector computed tomography to components of the metabolic syndrome are region-specific and independent of anthropometric indexes and intraabdominal visceral fat. J Clin Endocrinol Metab 2009;94:662−9.

[134] Kim HM, Kim KJ, Lee HJ, Yu HT, Moon JH, Kang ES, Cha BS, Lee HC, Lee BW, Kim YJ. Epicardial adipose tissue thickness is an indicator for coronary artery stenosis in asymptomatic type 2 diabetic patients: its assessment by cardiac magnetic resonance. Cardiovasc Diabetol 2012;11:83.

[135] Iacobellis G, Barbaro G, Gerstein HC. Relationship of epicardial fat thickness and fasting glucose. Int J Cardiol 2008;128:424−6.

[136] Iozzo P, Lautamaki R, Borra R, Lehto HR, Bucci M, Viljanen A, Parkka J, Lepomaki V, Maggio R, Parkkola R, Knuuti J, Nuutila P. Contribution of glucose tolerance and gender to cardiac adiposity. J Clin Endocrinol Metab 2009;94:4472−82.

[137] Iacobellis G, Pellicelli AM, Grisorio B, Barbarini G, Leonetti F, Sharma AM, Barbaro G. Relation of epicardial fat and alanine aminotransferase in subjects with increased visceral fat. Obesity (Silver Spring) 2008;16:179−83.

[138] Iacobellis G, Diaz S, Mendez A, Goldberg R. Increased epicardial fat and plasma leptin in type 1 diabetes independently of obesity. Nutr Metab Cardiovasc Dis 2014;24:725−9.

[139] Darabian S, Backlund JY, Cleary PA, Sheidaee N, Bebu I, Lachin JM, Budoff MJ, Group DER. Significance of epicardial and intrathoracic adipose tissue volume among type 1 diabetes patients in the DCCT/EDIC: a pilot study. PLoS One 2016;11:e0159958.

[140] Franssens BT, Nathoe HM, Leiner T, van der Graaf Y, Visseren FL, SMART study group. Relation between cardiovascular disease risk factors and epicardial adipose tissue density on cardiac computed tomography in patients at high risk of cardiovascular events. Eur J Prev Cardiol 2017;24:660−70.

[141] Goeller M, Achenbach S, Marwan M, Doris MK, Cadet S, Commandeur F, Chen X, Slomka PJ, Gransar H, Cao JJ, Wong ND, Albrecht MH, Rozanski A, Tamarappoo BK, Berman DS, Dey D. Epicardial adipose tissue density and volume are related to subclinical atherosclerosis, inflammation and major adverse cardiac events in asymptomatic subjects. J Cardiovasc Comput Tomogr 2018;12:67−73.

[142] Malavazos AE, Goldberger JJ, Iacobellis G. Does epicardial fat contribute to COVID-19 myocardial inflammation? Eur Heart J 2020;41:2333.

[143] Kim IC, Han S. Epicardial adipose tissue: fuel for COVID-19-induced cardiac injury? Eur Heart J 2020;41:2334−5.

[144] Zhao Y, Chen M, Yang X, Zhao L. COVID-19 letter to the editor: epicardial fat inflammation as possible enhancer in COVID-19? Metabolism 2021;117:154722.

[145] Abrishami A, Eslami V, Baharvand Z, Khalili N, Saghamanesh S, Zarei E, Sanei-Taheri M. Epicardial adipose tissue, inflammatory biomarkers and COVID-19: is there a possible relationship? Int Immunopharm 2021;90:107174.

[146] Grodecki K, Lin A, Razipour A, Cadet S, McElhinney PA, Chan C, et al. Epicardial adipose tissue is associated with extent of pneumonia and adverse outcomes in patients with COVID-19. Metabolism 2020;115:154436.

[147] Iacobellis G, Secchi F, Capitanio G, Basilico S, Schiaffino S, Boveri S, Sardanelli F, Corsi Romanelli MM, Malavazos AE. Epicardial fat inflammation in severe COVID-19. Obesity (Silver Spring) 2020;28:2260−2.

[148] Conte C, Esposito A, De Lorenzo R, Di Filippo L, Palmisano A, Vignale D, Leone R, Nicoletti V, Ruggeri A, Gallone G, Secchi A, Bosi E, Tresoldi M, Castagna A, Landoni G, Zangrillo A, De Cobelli F, Ciceri F, Camici P, Rovere-Querini P. Epicardial adipose tissue characteristics, obesity and clinical outcomes in COVID-19: a post-hoc analysis of a prospective cohort study. Nutr Metab Cardiovasc Dis 2021. https://doi.org/10.1016/j.numecd.2021.04.020 [online ahead of print].

[149] Iacobellis G, Singh N, Wharton S, Sharma AM. Substantial changes in epicardial fat thickness after weight loss in severely obese subjects. Obesity (Silver Spring) 2008;16:1693−7.

[150] Kim MK, Tomita T, Kim MJ, Sasai H, Maeda S, Tanaka K. Aerobic exercise training reduces epicardial fat in obese men. J Appl Physiol 1985;106:5–11. 2009.

[151] Gaborit B, Jacquier A, Kober F, Abdesselam I, Cuisset T, Boullu-Ciocca S, Emungania O, Alessi MC, Clement K, Bernard M, Dutour A. Effects of bariatric surgery on cardiac ectopic fat: lesser decrease in epicardial fat compared to visceral fat loss and no change in myocardial triglyceride content. J Am Coll Cardiol 2012;60:1381–9.

[152] Altin C, Erol V, Aydin E, Yilmaz M, Tekindal MA, Sade LE, Gulay H, Muderrisoglu H. Impact of weight loss on epicardial fat and carotid intima media thickness after laparoscopic sleeve gastrectomy: a prospective study. Nutr Metab Cardiovasc Dis 2018;28:501–9.

[153] Rabkin SW, Campbell H. Comparison of reducing epicardial fat by exercise, diet or bariatric surgery weight loss strategies: a systematic review and meta-analysis. Obes Rev 2015;16:406–15.

[154] Raggi P, Gadiyaram V, Zhang C, Chen Z, Lopaschuk G, Stillman AE. Statins reduce epicardial adipose tissue attenuation independent of lipid lowering: a potential pleiotropic effect. J Am Heart Assoc 2019;8:e013104.

[155] Xourgia E, Papazafiropoulou A, Melidonis A. Effects of antidiabetic drugs on epicardial fat. World J Diabetes 2018;9:141–8.

[156] Park JH, Park YS, Kim YJ, Lee IS, Kim JH, Lee JH, Choi SW, Jeong JO, Seong IW. Effects of statins on the epicardial fat thickness in patients with coronary artery stenosis underwent percutaneous coronary intervention: comparison of atorvastatin with simvastatin/ezetimibe. J Cardiovasc Ultrasound 2010;18:121–6.

[157] Ziyrek M, Kahraman S, Ozdemir E, Dogan A. Metformin monotherapy significantly decreases epicardial adipose tissue thickness in newly diagnosed type 2 diabetes patients. Rev Port Cardiol 2019;38:419–23.

[158] Jonker JT, Lamb HJ, van der Meer RW, Rijzewijk LJ, Menting LJ, Diamant M, Bax JJ, de Roos A, Romijn JA, Smit JW. Pioglitazone compared with metformin increases pericardial fat volume in patients with type 2 diabetes mellitus. J Clin Endocrinol Metab 2010;95:456–60.

[159] Morano S, Romagnoli E, Filardi T, Nieddu L, Mandosi E, Fallarino M, Turinese I, Dagostino MP, Lenzi A, Carnevale V. Short-term effects of glucagon-like peptide 1 (GLP-1) receptor agonists on fat distribution in patients with type 2 diabetes mellitus: an ultrasonography study. Acta Diabetol 2015;52:727–32.

[160] Dutour A, Abdesselam I, Ancel P, Kober F, Mrad G, Darmon P, Ronsin O, Pradel V, Lesavre N, Martin JC, Jacquier A, Lefur Y, Bernard M, Gaborit B. Exenatide decreases liver fat content and epicardial adipose tissue in patients with obesity and type 2 diabetes: a prospective randomized clinical trial using magnetic resonance imaging and spectroscopy. Diabetes Obes Metabol 2016;18:882–91.

[161] Iacobellis G, Mohseni M, Bianco SD, Banga PK. Liraglutide causes large and rapid epicardial fat reduction. Obesity (Silver Spring) 2017;25:311–6.

[162] Iacobellis G, Villasante Fricke AC. Effects of semaglutide versus dulaglutide on epicardial fat thickness in subjects with type 2 diabetes and obesity. J Endocr Soc 2020;4(4):bvz042.

[163] Lima-Martinez MM, Paoli M, Rodney M, Balladares N, Contreras M, D'Marco L, Iacobellis G. Effect of sitagliptin on epicardial fat thickness in subjects with type 2 diabetes and obesity: a pilot study. Endocrine 2016;51:448–55.

[164] Diaz-Rodriguez E, Agra RM, Fernandez AL, Adrio B, Garcia-Caballero T, Gonzalez-Juanatey JR, Eiras S. Effects of dapagliflozin on human epicardial adipose tissue: modulation of insulin resistance, inflammatory chemokine production, and differentiation ability. Cardiovasc Res 2018;114:336–46.

[165] Sato T, Aizawa Y, Yuasa S, Kishi S, Fuse K, Fujita S, Ikeda Y, Kitazawa H, Takahashi M, Sato M, Okabe M. The effect of dapagliflozin treatment on epicardial adipose tissue volume. Cardiovasc Diabetol 2018;17:6.

[166] Yagi S, Hirata Y, Ise T, Kusunose K, Yamada H, Fukuda D, Salim HM, Maimaituxun G, Nishio S, Takagawa Y, Hama S, Matsuura T, Yamaguchi K, Tobiume T, Soeki T, Wakatsuki T, Aihara KI, Akaike M, Shimabukuro M, Sata M. Canagliflozin reduces epicardial fat in patients with type 2 diabetes mellitus. Diabetol Metab Syndrome 2017;9:78.

[167] Iacobellis G, Gra-Menendez S. Effects of dapagliflozin on epicardial fat thickness in patients with type 2 diabetes and obesity. Obes (Silver Spring) 2020;28:1068–74.

[168] Gaborit B, Ancel P, Abdullah AE, Maurice F, Abdesselam I, Calen A, Soghomonian A, Houssays M, Varlet I, Eisinger M, Lasbleiz A, Peiretti F, Bornet CE, Lefur Y, Pini L, Rapacchi S, Bernard M, Resseguier N, Darmon P, Kober F, Dutour A. Effect of empagliflozin on ectopic fat stores and myocardial energetics in type 2 diabetes: the EMPACEF study. Cardiovasc Diabetol 2021;20(1):57.

[169] Al-Talabany S, Mohan M, Weir-McCall J, Gandy S, Singh JSS, Mordi IR, Baig F, Choy AMJ, Geroge J, Houston JG, Struthers AD, Khan S, Lang CC. Effect of metformin on epicardial adipose tissue in patients with coronary artery disease without diabetes: a cardiac MRI substudy of the MET-remodel trial. Obes Med 2021;24:100349.

[170] Launbo N, Zobel EH, von Scholten BJ, Faerch K, Jørgensen PG, Christensen RH. Targeting epicardial adipose tissue with exercise, diet, bariatric surgery or pharmaceutical interventions: a systematic review and meta-analysis. Obes Rev 2021;22(1):e13136.

[171] Mazurek T, Opolski G. Pericoronary adipose tissue: a novel therapeutic target in obesity-related coronary atherosclerosis. J Am Coll Nutr 2015;34:244–54.

[172] Iacobellis G. Epicardial fat: a new cardiovascular therapeutic target. Curr Opin Pharmacol 2016;27:13–8.

[173] Packer M. Disease-treatment interactions in the management of patients with obesity and diabetes who have atrial fibrillation: the potential mediating influence of epicardial adipose tissue. Cardiovasc Diabetol 2019;18(1):121.

Part II

Ectopic fat stores

Chapter 5

Non-invasive profiling of ectopic and adipose lipids using magnetic resonance spectroscopy and imaging

Radka Klepochová[1,2] and Martin Kriššák[1,2]

[1]Division of Endocrinology and Metabolism, Department of Medicine III, Medical University of Vienna, Vienna, Austria; [2]High-Field MR Centre, Department of Biomedical Imaging and Image-guided Therapy, Medical University of Vienna, Vienna, Austria

Introduction

The number of people with obesity has increased dramatically over the past decades to an estimated 650 million adults worldwide in 2016 [1]. Obesity predisposes a person to the development of insulin resistance, type 2 diabetes mellitus, and cardiovascular disease.

Obesity is due to a chronic positive energy balance, which increases the amount of triglycerides in adipose tissue. Adipose tissue consists of adipocytes, which have the unique capacity to store large amounts of energy in the form of triglycerides. In addition to this, adipose tissue acts as an endocrine organ by secreting various hormones and cytokines with subsequent effects on glucose and lipid metabolism and energy homeostasis. However, the triglycerides can also be stored in nonadipose tissue, such as muscle, liver, pancreas, and heart. Indeed, obesity has been shown to lead to excessive deposition of triglycerides in these organs, which is termed ectopic fat deposition [2,3]. Ectopic fat is defined as storage of triglycerides in tissues other than adipose tissue, which normally contain only small amounts of fat, such as in hepatocytes (intrahepatocellular lipids; IHCL), skeletal (intramyocellular lipids; IMCL), or cardiac muscle cells (myocardial lipids; MYCL), and pancreatic beta cells (intrapancreatic lipids; IPCL) [4,5]. Most importantly, the amount of visceral fat mass (visceral adipose tissue; VAT) has been related to ectopic fat deposits [2,6,7].

The problem with the accumulation of ectopic lipids and their association with insulin resistance and type 2 diabetes mellitus is not only their presence alone, but also the functionality of their metabolism, the accumulation of metabolic intermediates, and their quality, expressed as a saturation profile [2,8], or fatty acid composition. Profiling offers additional information, such as lipid saturation and (poly)-unsaturation status. It is already well documented that levels of fat unsaturation in various adipose tissue compartments vary with diseases, such as osteoporosis [9], type 2 diabetes [10], or cardiovascular disease [11]. The information about the composition of ectopic lipids yields new insights on their possible role in pathology and their value as potential biomarkers. This may, in turn, influence our understanding of organ biochemistry in health and various diseases.

Gas chromatography analysis of biopsy samples is the gold standard for lipid profiling. A noninvasive alternative would simplify and improve the accessibility of future clinical research studies. Magnetic resonance spectroscopy (MRS) and, to some extent, magnetic resonance imaging (MRI) enable the assessment of quantitative fractions of the degree of various bulk saturation that is fully comparable with independent analytical measures, and thus, have the potential to replace invasive biopsy exams. Measures provided by both magnetic resonance imaging (MRI) [12−14], and MRS [13,15,16], have been shown to correlate with the results of with gas chromatography. In addition to eliminating the need for tissue biopsy, MR does not expose subjects to ionizing radiation. Furthermore, for this purpose, MR does not require injection with a contrast agent, which otherwise can be limiting in patients with renal disease [17].

Compared to MRI, MRS may be able to provide more detail on the in vivo lipid composition at higher field strengths and can, therefore, contribute to our understanding of metabolism in humans [17]. Moreover, it can be used to gain

Visceral and Ectopic Fat. https://doi.org/10.1016/B978-0-12-822186-0.00003-1

dynamic information and, therefore, can determine the response to physiological challenges. The MR signal of various nuclei can be detected, and, in metabolic research, proton (^{1}H) and carbon (^{13}C) MRS can unravel different aspects of lipid storage and fatty acid metabolism.

This chapter will describe the basics of lipid composition and its appearance in in vivo ^{1}H MR spectra, ^{1}H MRS data acquisition, and processing. In the applications of noninvasive ^{1}H MRS for lipid profiling, we will mention not only the studies on ectopic lipid compartments (liver, skeletal muscle, pancreas), but also the studies on subcutaneous and visceral adipose tissue, bone marrow fat, and breast tissue as these share the same methodology. Thus, the technical know-how gained in these studies can often be transformed to measurements of inner organs. Furthermore, the physiology and pathologic consequences of increased fat accumulation and derailed fat metabolism in adipose and ectopic compartments are often interrelated.

Lipid composition and its consequences in magnetic resonance spectroscopy

Triglycerides contribute to the carbon and proton MR signal [18]. Triglycerides consist of a glycerol backbone with three fatty acid chains each of which is characterized by the number of carbon atoms that make up the chain, and the number of double bonds between them. Fatty acids may be categorized in terms of their degree of saturation, as saturated (no double bonds, saturation index SI), unsaturated (at least one double bond, unsaturation index [UI]), monounsaturated (one double bond, monounsaturation index [MUI]), or polyunsaturated (at least two double bonds, polyunsaturated index [PUI]) fatty acids [19]. From the protons in a triglyceride molecule, up to 10 different ^{1}H MRS signals can be resolved, as shown in Fig. 5.1.

In vivo magnetic resonance spectroscopy

Research on ectopic fat accumulation took a major leap forward when it became possible to study lipid content in non-adipose tissue with volume-selected ^{1}H magnetic resonance spectroscopy (^{1}H MRS). In the 1980 and 1990s, a noninvasive method was introduced to measure IMCL [20−22] and IHCL [23−25] accumulation using localized ^{1}H MRS. The method is noninvasive, and the voxel (volume-pixel) covers, typically, 1−27 cm^3, which enables the study of the same area repeatedly. With the advent of higher field strengths ($\geq$3T), the focus was also directed at localized spectroscopy of adipose tissue [26] and bone marrow [27]. Improved spectral resolution and a less prominent water signal allowed

FIGURE 5.1 Schematic illustration of a fatty acid chains (top) and the corresponding MR spectrum (bottom). Numerical values of chemical shifts are given in Table 5.1.

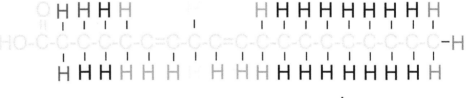

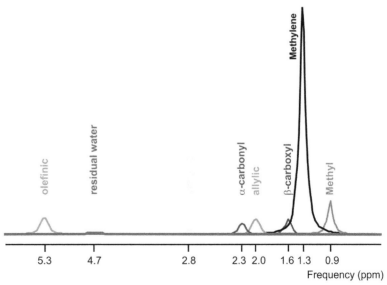

identification of up to nine spectral lines from fatty acids (see below) and endorsed noninvasive lipid profiling in different adipose tissue compartments [28]. Prior knowledge on in vivo fatty acid spectral line position and appearance was then brought back into MRS of liver, pancreas, and skeletal muscle and permitted the profiling of ectopic lipids [29].

Magnetic resonance spectroscopy data acquisition

The MR spectra needed for fatty acid composition assessment may be acquired by localized single-voxel techniques with either Point REsolved SpectroScopy (PRESS) or STimulated Echo Acquisition Mode (STEAM) sequences, depending on whether a $90°-180°-180°$ or a $90°-90°-90°$ RF excitation and refocusing scheme is used (Fig. 5.2). The choice between STEAM and PRESS has an impact on lipid composition estimation accuracy [30]. PRESS and STEAM differ in their sensitivity to J-coupling, causing these sequences to yield different peak amplitudes for resonances that exhibit J-coupling and provide different estimates of the peak T_2 relaxation time values [30]. Although the STEAM technique yields only half signal of that from the PRESS sequence, it is preferred for an accurate quantification of the peak areas of a lipid spectrum because it is less affected by the J-couplings of the lipid protons, and allows for shorter echo time (TE) of the sequence, which makes it less prone to T_2 underestimation and fat peak area overestimation [30,31]. It is, however, possible to design the PRESS sequence in such a way that minimizes the effects of J-couplings [31,32] and use it for quantitative MRS of lipid composition, but the choice of the volume in the PRESS sequence may be more affected by the chemical shift displacement, causing an underestimation of off-resonance frequency components that are not subjected to all three localization pulses. On the other hand, moderately longer TE inherently applied in PRESS sequences may be favorable to suppress the signal from flowing blood when spectra are acquired from beating heart. Examples of 1H MR spectra obtained from adipose tissue, bone marrow, liver, and skeletal muscle are given in Fig. 5.3.

Differences in the molecular environment of specific chemical groups in the fatty acid molecule yield different T_1 and T_2 relaxation times of distinct spectral lines. For lipid composition measurements, the different T_1 relaxation times do not represent a problem because the TR of an MRS experiment is typically much longer than the longest T_1 of fat, allowing for full relaxation of magnetization between repeated excitation of the volume-of-interest. However, different T_2 relaxation times may pose a quantitation problem. It is known from the MR literature that J-coupling accelerates signal decay and reduces the apparent T_2 value of fat [33–35]. Therefore, a further advantage of STEAM is the possibility to set the minimum echo time (TE) to typically 20 ms or even less, whereas, in PRESS, the minimal possible TE is 30 ms. For example, the UI of hepatic lipids in the work of Ye et al. [36] was found to be underestimated by 20% with a TE of 30 ms if a T_2 correction is not performed, but only by 7% if TE was set to 10 ms. Gajdosik et al. [37] were able reduce the TE of a STEAM sequence to 6 ms, by optimizing both the radiofrequency pulse shapes and the spoiler gradients (Fig. 5.4). With this, it is possible to minimize the underestimation of T_2 effect. Definitely, accurate fat quantification requires correction for T_2.

On the other hand, long TEs are favorable for the improvement of spectral resolution of longer T_2 signals and for the suppression of overwhelming signals with shorter T_2 relaxation times. Setting the TE to 200 ms allowed for the clear distinction of the olefinic (5.3 ppm; CH=CH) signal from the dominant water signal in the liver even at the lower field strength of 1.5T [26]. A similar approach enabled resolution of the signal that arose from terminal protons of an n-3 methyl group in the fatty acid chain at 0.98 ppm T_2 relaxation times of terminal methyl lipid peaks are normally in a range between 50 and 80 ms. Nevertheless, the T_2 of an n-3 fatty acid terminal methyl group in an oil phantom was found to be much longer (623 ± 34 ms) [39]. Using this knowledge and setting the TE of the PRESS sequence to 1000 ms enabled the detection and quantification of an n-3 methyl group in vivo (Fig. 5.5). Alternatively, using the J-coupling between the

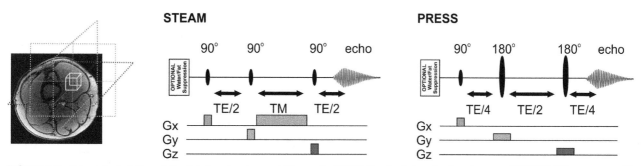

FIGURE 5.2 Schematic depiction of stimulated mode echo acquisition mode (STEAM) and point-resolved spectroscopy (PRESS) MRS sequences with RF pulse, gradient, and acquisition timing (*TE*, echo time; *TM*, mixing time). Cross section of gradient selected planes (red, blue, green) results in the excitation of signal from selected volume of interest (VOI; *yellow box*). Depiction is underlined with T1-weighted MRI image of skeletal muscle.

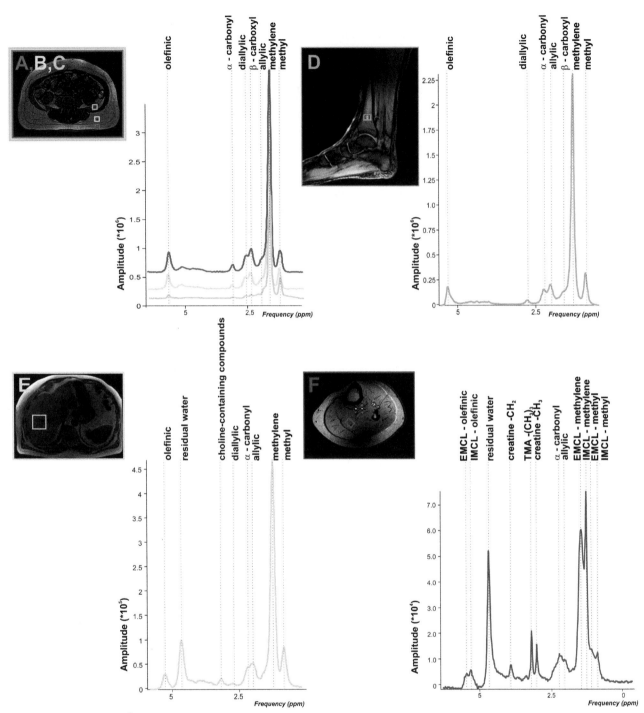

FIGURE 5.3 Examples of ¹H MR spectra obtained at 3T with short TE from (A) superficial subcutaneous adipose tissue, (B) deep subcutaneous adipose tissue, (C) visceral adipose tissue, (D) tibialis bone marrow, (E) liver, and (F) soleus. All spectra are acquired with STEAM sequence, and different number of acquisition (SAT; VAT; bone marrow, liver: NA = 4, soleus muscle: NA = 16) in (E) liver and (F) soleus water suppression was used. Note higher amplitudes and SNR in adipose tissue and bone marrow spectra and specific spectral pattern due to the EMCL/IMCL splitting in skeletal muscle spectra.

chemical groups within the fatty acid chain called spectral editing, Skoch et al. [40] were able to assess the n-3 fraction of triglycerides in deep subcutaneous tissue.

While in vivo data acquisition by localized, single ¹H MRS of superficial/deep adipose tissue and subcutaneous fat is relatively easy and straightforward, detection of IMCL, IHCL, MYCL, and IPCL needs water signal suppression. In

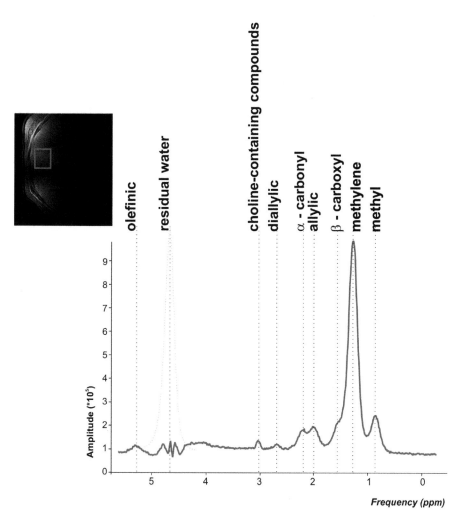

FIGURE 5.4 Example of ^{1}H MR spectrum from liver measured with surface coil at 7T with GUSTEAU sequence [37]. with TE of 6 ms and eight acquisitions during free shallow breathing. To detect olefinic lipid signal (5.3 ppm), water signal was suppressed in the postprocessing.

TABLE 5.1 Peak assignments, subcutaneous white subcutaneous adipose tissue (wSAT) relaxation times at 3T [38], human tibial bone marrow (tBM), and calf subcutaneous fat (cSAT) relaxation times at 7T [27].

	Type	wSAT		tBM		cSAT	
Chemical shift (ppm)	Chemical group	T_1 (ms)	T_2 (ms)	T_1 (ms)	T_2 (ms)	T_1 (ms)	T_2 (ms)
		3T		7T		7T	
0.90	Methyl	610	58	1160	74	1080	67
1.30	Methylene	370	83	550	69	530	63
1.59	β-Carboxyl	500	88	390	33	320	30
2.03	Allylic	370	34	420	42	390	39
2.25	α-Carbonyl	360	89	440	60	400	55
2.77	Diallylic	430	64	600	59	580	58
5.31	Olefinic	440	87	—	—	—	—

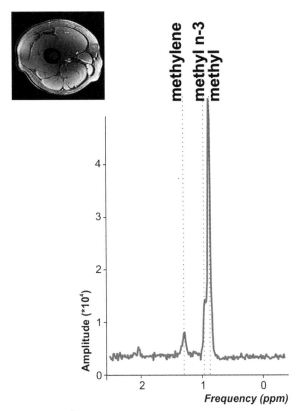

FIGURE 5.5 Detection of n-3 fatty acids. Example of ^{1}H MR spectrum acquired with multichannel volume coil at 7T from subcutaneous fat in thigh with ultralong TE (1000 ms) PRESS sequence [39].

addition, ectopic lipid data acquisition of the liver, pancreas, and heart requires cancellation of movement artifacts. The effects of breathing can be reduced by signal acquisition during expiratory or inspiratory breath-holding, by signal acquisition triggered to the diaphragm or belly movement, or by postprocessing elimination of corrupt transients. The effects of heartbeat can usually be avoided by prospective triggering of signal acquisition to the ECG signal. Breath movement and cardiac cycle triggering can be combined in one signal acquisition scheme. For the signal acquisition in skeletal muscle, voxel placement must be chosen carefully with respect to the anatomical borders of a single muscle group and also to avoid subcutaneous fat.

The number of acquisitions (NA) required for MRS-based fatty acid composition assessment is provided by the resulting signal-to-noise of the lowest assessable fatty acid signal (olefinic 5.3, or diallylic 2.77 ppm) and varies with the overall tissue TG accumulation and magnetic field strength used for measurement. The number of acquisitions starts by 4−8 in subcutaneous adipose tissue at any field strength and goes up to 64−128 transients for liver, skeletal muscle, or heart measurement at 1.5 or 3 T. Typical measurement may take few minutes per voxel [19], including localized shimming and frequency adjustment.

Specific situation is encountered in the data acquisition of breast tissue. The distribution of breast adipose tissue and mammary glands is nonuniform, and positioning of single voxel for STEAM or PRESS sequence into homogenous compartment can be very challenging [41]. To overcome this problem, three-dimensional chemical shift imaging (CSI) can be applied, and MRS signal of voxel containing fat or metabolite information only can be extracted in the postprocessing [42]. Further on, rather small size of the organ and custom RF coils adapted to the breast anatomy provided by system manufacturers favor 3D CSI acquisitions, which can cover whole breast [43,44].

Analysis of the magnetic resonance spectrscopy data

To compute the various measures of unsaturation, the amplitudes of the individual resonances are calculated by fitting line shape functions to the data. Commonly used algorithms are AMARES time domain [45] and LCModel in the frequency domain [46] (Fig. 5.6).

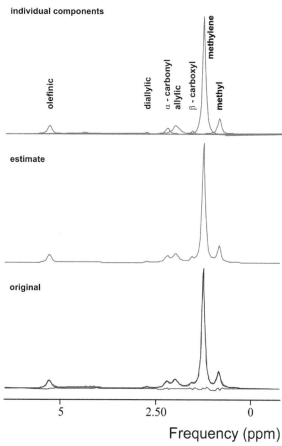

FIGURE 5.6 MRS data processing and spectral line quantification by AMARES algorithm in jMRUI package. Acquired spectrum (bottom panel, cyan), summed estimate (middle panel, red), and individual components (upper panel, red). Measured signal is deconvoluted in the time domain into the sum of individual harmonic functions yielding minimized residuum (bottom trace in the bottom panel).

Many methods to define and calculate the MRS-derived degree of saturation and unsaturation have been proposed [9,19,26,28,47−50].

Every fatty acid chain, whether saturated or unsaturated, contains large amount of methylene protons at 1.3 ppm, two α-carbonyl protons at 2.25 ppm, two β-carboxyl protons at 1.59 ppm, and three methyl protons at 0.9 ppm, terminating the fatty acid chain. The β-carboxyl peak is visible only in spectra with excellent quality, and α-carbonyl protons, in some cases, are not well separated from allylic protons and may be contaminated.

Furthermore, every unsaturated fatty acid chain contains two allylic protons at 2.03 ppm and two olefinic protons in double bonds at 5.3 ppm, and in polyunsaturated fatty acid chains with two or more double bonds, there are two diallylic protons at 2.77 ppm attached to carbon between double bonds. But, again, diallylic protons often cannot be resolved in the spectrum, and moreover, in tissues with a strong water signal, the estimation of the olefinic peak is very challenging.

Based on all those facts, the UI can be calculated as

$$UI(allylic) = \frac{3}{4} * \frac{S(allylic)}{S(methyl)}$$

where S is the signal intensity of the mentioned peak.

Alternatively, when the resolution of the allylic peak is problematic and ^{1}H MRS acquisition can enable the resolution of the olefinic signal at 5.3 ppm, then the olefinic signal may be used to calculate fatty acid UI as

$$UI(olefinic) = \frac{S(olefinic)}{S(methyl)}$$

Saturation index (SI) can be calculated as

$$SI = 1 - UI$$

and, under the assumption that the fraction of fatty acids with three or more double bonds can be ignored because fatty acids with zero, one, and two double bonds constitute $\sim 97\%-98\%$ of the total fat in humans on ordinary Western diets [27]. We can, therefore, calculate the polyunsaturated index as

$$PUFA = \frac{3}{2} * \frac{S(diallylic)}{S(methyl)}$$

Similar expressions have been derived by other authors [9,19,26−28,47−51].

Magnetic resonance imaging

Using Dixon's chemical shift−encoded (CSE) MRI-based techniques, the signals from fat and water may be sorted into separate images based on their different phase evolution during echo time-dependent signal acquisition.

The original implementation by Dixon used so-called double-echo "in-phase" and "opposed-phase" images. After selecting a specific area in the organ, using regions of interest (ROIs), and the numerical values of the signal intensity on the generated fat and water, images can be obtained. Based on the acquired signal intensity values, the content of fat fractions in individual organs can be calculated.

Quantitative assessment of the fat accumulation is achieved by computing the percentage value of the fat fraction, which is the fat signal intensity divided by the sum of the fat and water signals and then multiplied by 100. In other words, fat fraction (FF) is computed as follows:

$$FF = \frac{S(F)}{S(W + F)} * 100\%$$

where S is the signal intensity contribution from water (W) and fat (F). ROIs are placed manually within the target organs and then copied to ensure that the size and location are the same on both fat-only (F) and water-only (W) images [52].

The development of the Dixon technique includes improved description of signal evolution by multiecho acquisition, preventing the T_1 effects by low flip-angle excitation and better definition of fat signal by a complex spectral model. These refinements allow for robust and accurate estimation of the proton density fat fraction [53] in a large range of values. Although attempts to apply the CSE-MRI methods to describe the number of double bonds, the number of methylene-interrupted double bonds, and the chain length in adipose tissue, bone marrow, and liver have been undertaken [14,54], these methods are not yet sensitive enough to characterize and detect subtle intraindividual or interindividual variations in lipid composition, but they are attractive for their future potential to provide a spatial map of lipid composition distributions [19].

Applications

As the applications of the measurement of fat fraction or fat accumulations in different organs and adipose tissue compartments are mentioned in other chapters ("Part I Fat Stores" "Part II Ectopic Fat Stores"), here, we would like to review the studies of noninvasive profiling of lipid compartments and point out the links to human pathophysiology. We will also mention technical details that are specific for data acquisition, processing, and interpretation in the respective measurement positions.

Adipose tissue (deep subcutaneous adipose tissue/visceral adipose tissue/brown adipose tissue)

First attempt to characterize the lipid composition of adipose tissue has been undertaken using natural abundance ^{13}C-MRS [55−57]. However, they pointed toward clinical potential in detection of compositional changes due to the malnourishment [55] or diet intervention [57], or worldwide availability of multinuclear RF components at clinical systems did not foster these applications. T_1-weighted ^{1}H MRI provides a reliable basis for interindividual comparison of body fat distribution and allows a fast and reliable quantification of total body adipose tissue, and subcutaneous and visceral fat compartments in different body regions [8]. It has been reported that the relative volume of visceral adipose tissue, assessed with MRI and

MRS, seems to be a predictive factor for an improvement of insulin sensitivity in lifestyle interventions Subsequently, Machann et al. found that the fraction of unsaturated fatty acids in visceral adipose tissue was lower in subjects with high total visceral adipose tissue volume [58]. The characterization of the lipid composition in adipose tissue is performed, in general, using a single-voxel ^{1}H MRS STEAM technique with a short TE to minimize relaxation effects and signal dephasing due to dipolar coupling, and a long TR, allowing for full magnetization recovery [59]. Examples of proton MR spectra of adipose tissue are given in Fig. 5.3A−C. As we have already mentioned, ^{1}H MRS data acquisition from adipose tissue is easier than, for instance, from the liver, because there is no strong water signal interfering with the olefinic peak (5.3 ppm), which can be resolved in MR spectra without water suppression. Good resolution of the olefinic peak in these spectra suggests that the olefinic peak could be used as a direct measure of bulk lipid unsaturation.

Several studies were able to show that the amount of subcutaneous and visceral adipose tissue correlated with metabolic disorders and obesity [60−66]. In a study targeting the volume and composition of visceral fat in healthy volunteers, Machann et al. found that the fraction of unsaturated fatty acids in visceral adipose tissue (VAT) were lower in subjects with a high total visceral adipose tissue volume [58]. It was also found that the visceral lipids were more saturated than both deep and superficial subcutaneous fat and that deep, subcutaneous fat was more saturated than superficial fat in patients with nonalcoholic fatty liver disease [67,68]. These results that reported different lipid profiles of SAT and VAT complement volumetric studies, which found a strong correlation between the marker of whole-body glucose homeostatis, HOMA-IR, and visceral fat mass, as well as total fat mass [69]. In another review of the effects of diet- and exercise-induced weight loss on visceral adipose tissue distribution in both men and women, Ross mentioned that a diet-induced loss of approximately 12 kg corresponded to a 30%−35% reduction in visceral fat mass [70], pointing again to a specific role for VAT in whole-body metabolism. Visceral adipose tissue remains more strongly associated with an adverse metabolic risk profile [71] and contributes significantly to the levels of free fatty acids [72], which interfere with the glucose homeostasis and leads to insulin resistance [61]. Moreover, VAT seems to be a predictive factor for an improvement of insulin sensitivity in lifestyle interventions [59].

Positron emission tomography has traditionally been used for the detection of brown adipose tissue. Brown and white adipose tissue could be differentiated by their signal fat fraction values due to their different water content [73]. Nevertheless, ^{1}H MRS, applied in several acquisitions with a range of echo times, showed shorter T_2 and lower unsaturated fatty acids in brown adipose tissue than that in white adipose tissue in healthy humans. This study allowed for identification and characterization of brown adipose tissue with MRS without the use of positron emission tomography or cold stimulation [38].

Bone marrow fat

The association of bone marrow adiposity and bone health has become of increasing interest recently. Both MRI and MRS have been used to investigate an association between the amount of bone marrow lipid, composition, and bone quality. Example of proton MR spectra of tibial bone marrow is given in Fig. 5.3D.

Vertebral marrow fat was studied by Yeung et al. in a group of postmenopausal women, and these authors found that the unsaturation index was lower in osteoporotic and osteopenic subjects, compared with normal subjects and young controls [9]. Patsch et al. showed that altered bone marrow fat composition is linked with fragility fractures and diabetes, since diabetic patients with fragility fractures had a significantly lower unsaturation index in vertebral bone marrow than controls [49]. MRS of spinal bone marrow fat may, therefore, serve as a novel tool for the independent fracture risk assessment of bone mineral density and the unsaturation index in bone marrow was suggested as a biomarker of skeletal integrity. The link between the unsaturation index of vertebral bone marrow, based on the olefinic peak (5.3 ppm), and measures of metabolic risk, was also suggested in a study of postmenopausal women with or without type 2 diabetes [10] and in a study of morbidly obese patients. The unsaturation index of the femur was significantly lower in subjects with type 2 diabetes compared with nondiabetic subjects [74]. The effect of gender was detected in a study investigating an elderly population (age >80 years) [75], which reported a lower unsaturation index of vertebral bone marrow in women than in men.

From technical point of view, the MRS data acquisition in vertebral bone marrow applies the same principle and parameters as in other adipose tissue compartments, but special care should be given to localized shimming in preparation for the measurement. The details and heterogeneity of the vertebral anatomy (vertebra, spine cord, cerebrospinal liquid, and muscles) increase the effects of magnetic susceptibility jumps on the tissue border and can deteriorate the MRS data quality. Increased line width often does not allow for individual detection of allylic, diallylic, and α-carbonyl (2.0−2.7 ppm) resonance lines. In this case, again, the olefinic line is taken as a measure of unsaturation.

Nevertheless, good accessibility and easy motion restriction during the measurement favor the studies in different populations and clinical settings. MRS of bone marrow was also applied in a study that compared women with anorexia nervosa to normal-weight controls [76]. The degree of fat saturation in the femur was inversely related to the bone mineral density, suggesting that saturated fat may have a more negative effect on bone [76], but another study did not find a statistically significant association between bone mineral density and unsaturation index [77].

Breast

Applications of single voxel ^{1}H MRS of breast were driven by the goal of mammary cancer diagnosis and grading [41]. Total choline signal was taken as a measure of malignancy, and the presence of strong lipid resonance lines and inhomogenous morphology of breast tissue hampered reliable applications [78,79]. Advance of 3D MRS imaging (MRSI) allowed for selecting metabolite information in the postprocessing [42] and combination with fat-selective Dixon MRI-enabled partial volume correction [80]. With the improvement in hardware and acquisition performance and enhanced spectral resolution, lipid resonances and their respective ratio came into the focus of investigations also in the breast MRS. Single-voxel MRS studies did characterize the bulk saturation profile [81,82] and relaxation behavior of lipid resonances at 3 and 7T. Saturation indices were found to be similar to those in other adipose tissue compartments in healthy tissue [81,82]. In later reports focused on cancer diagnosis and treatment response, increased measures of saturated fatty acids and decreased measures of monounsaturated and/or polyunsaturated fatty acid in malignant breast tissue with invasive ductal carcinoma when compared with benign tissue were found [44,83–85]. Recent methodological improvements show the possibility of two-dimensional double-quantum filtered correlation spectroscopy for sensitive acquisition of olefinic lipid signal at clinical field strength [86].

Liver

^{1}H MRS measurements of the hepatic fatty acid composition are more difficult due to liver motion caused by breathing and a prominent water signal. Nevertheless, this technique is considered the gold standard for the noninvasive determination of liver fat accumulation, and the example of proton MR spectrum with typical spectral resolution achieved with short TE acquisition at 3T is given in Fig. 5.3E.

The hepatic ^{1}H MR spectrum consists of dominant resonances from water and lipids (CH$_2$ and CH$_3$ groups). Lipid resonances are normalized to the water resonance and corrected for relaxation effects, allowing for quantification of IHCL. Results from this technique show good agreement with measurements from tissue biopsies in the liver [87], and were used to validate a quantitative MRI-derived proton density fat fraction (Fig. 5.7) [88].

As in Fig. 5.1, each of the resonance lines present in the fat ^{1}H MRS corresponds to a structurally different proton group. However, because of significant spectral line overlap at clinical field strengths ($\leq$3T), resolution of the individual components of the allylic and α-carbonyl lines at 2.03 and 2.25 ppm is often not possible and the 4.2 and 5.3 ppm fat peaks are often not clearly distinguishable from the 4.7 ppm water signal. This can lead to fat quantification error [89] and hamper the possibility of lipid profiling. Nevertheless, Hamilton et al. showed that, with a short TE STEAM sequence, careful individual shimming, and prior knowledge-based postprocessing in the time domain, it is possible to use detectable ^{1}H MRS fat resonance lines to characterize bulk liver triglyceride composition. This molecular structure-based method for fat spectral characterization allowed a more accurate quantification of liver fat using MRS and MRI methods that incorporate spectral correction [89]. This was an improvement to the previous suggestions to use the usually well-resolved, but rather small, diallylic resonance line (2.77 ppm) as the main surrogate for the saturation profile [48]. Further improvements in MR hardware, data acquisition, and processing strategy allowed for direct detection of the olefinic resonance (5.3 ppm) at a higher field strength ($\geq$3T) [39,47]. Acquisition triggered to breath movement, a high number of acquisitions, single transient data storage, and advanced postprocessing—including elimination of corrupted transients, individual phase correction, and frequency alignment—were used on a clinical MR system [47] with an ultrashort TE (6 ms). Similarly, advanced postprocessing was used in another approach [37]. The olefinic peak could also be detected in long echo time ^{1}H MRS (TE = 200 ms) of the liver at a rather low magnetic field strength (1.5 T) [51]. All three methods were validated with measurements in oil samples and in adipose tissue and provide a robust basis for an accurate assessment of the hepatocellular content of lipids and fatty acid chain composition.

When considering the physiological meaning of hepatic lipid profiling, it should be pointed out that initial studies that used liver biopsy showed a higher monounsaturated fatty acid fraction at the expense of the polyunsaturated fatty acid fraction in people with nonalcoholic fatty liver disease, compared with people without nonalcoholic fatty liver disease [90,91]. In this respect, pivotal MR-based studies investigated spectral parameters that are linked to the degree of

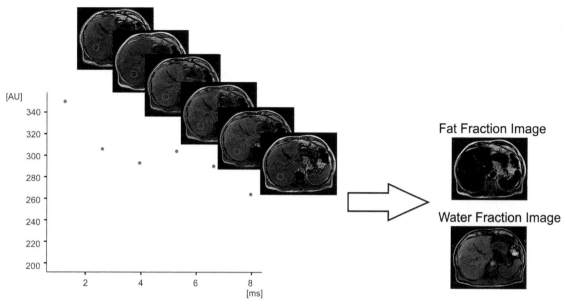

FIGURE 5.7   Multiecho chemical shift—encoded MRI (Dixon) for tissue fat fraction acquisition. Echo images (n = 6) and echo time signal evolution are shown in the left part of the figure. Numeric signal values are derived from the circular region of interest placed in the homogenous liver region in postprocessing. Pixel-by-pixel echo time signal evolution is used to calculate proton density fat fraction (PDFF) and water fraction images, which are depicted on the right. Measurement yielded hepatic PDFF of ca. 11%.

unsaturation [37,48,51,92]. Even though these studies did not specifically and robustly quantify hepatic saturated, monounsaturated, and poly-unsaturated fatty acid fraction separately, they did show a higher fraction of saturated lipids and a lower fraction of (poly-)unsaturated lipids in individuals with hepatic steatosis [37,48]. A comparison of fatty acid saturation indices from the liver, subcutaneous, and visceral adipose tissue yielded a linear correlation of UI between the sites, with the highest saturated fatty acid fraction in the liver followed by subcutaneous and visceral adipose sites [51].

Using the latest improvements in ^{1}H MRS by Roumans et al. [47], and combining the ^{1}H MRS measurement into a comprehensive metabolic study protocol, it could be shown that saturated fatty acid fraction was elevated in patients with nonalcoholic fatty liver and type 2 diabetes and that it is positively associated with de novo lipogenesis [47]. Furthermore, saturated fatty acid fraction shows a strong, negative correlation with hepatic insulin sensitivity, which was previously also linked to total hepatic fat accumulation in the same negative way [93]. This is also in line with previous studies that have linked high rates of de novo lipogenesis to increased metabolic risk [94−96].

Heart

The acquisition of ^{1}H MRS for the assessment MYCL is more challenging when compared with the liver or muscle. The anatomy of the heart does not offer large volumes of homogenous tissue, which challenges signal-to-noise ratio in the cardiac spectra. Also, the heart is a continuously moving organ, making cardiac MRS more sensitive to phase distortions and signal losses. Moreover, shimming, frequency adjustment, and necessary water signal suppression are challenging as well. The combination of ECG triggering and respiratory gating and/or breath-hold during acquisition of the spectra is essential. Nevertheless, the method was pioneered in the 1990s [97,98] and validated in volunteers and against biopsies taken during heart transplantation [99−101]. This robust assessment of total MYCL content has been applied in studies designed to detect the links between MYCL accumulation and cardiovascular or metabolic disease [102−105].

Recently, a non−water-suppressed metabolite-cycling ^{1}H MRS method [106] has been used to improve the spectral resolution of myocardial spectroscopy, but the rather low overall fat fraction (<1%), the higher creatine signal, and possible extracellular lipid contribution do not allow robust assessment of lipid resonances in the region of 2.0−2.8 ppm. This leaves myocardial spectroscopy with the possibility to roughly estimate the saturation surrogate from the ratio of methylene (CH_2, 1.3 ppm) to methyl (CH_3, 0.9 ppm) resonance lines, but its potential has not yet been studied.

Skeletal muscle

The measurement of intramyocellular lipids (IMCLs) by volume-selective ^{1}H MRS was introduced by Schick et al. [20] and employs the effect of the orientation dependence of susceptibility changes. Differences in magnetic properties of a bulk cylinder, such as extramyocellular lipids (EMCLs) and spherical vesicle-accumulated IMCLs, give the potential to separate these two compartments. Example of proton MR spectra from soleus muscle is given in Fig. 5.3F. Macro- and microscopic susceptibility differences cause local magnetic fields to vary strongly, such that lipid peaks of different compartments can be shifted in resonance frequency by up to ~ 0.2 ppm [21,107]. Methods for ^{1}H MRS of skeletal muscle have recently been reviewed, and recommendations for data acquisition, processing, and interpretation have been given [108]. Some details can also be found in the following chapter of this book ("Part II Ectopic Fat Stores/Skeletal muscle").

When considering the potential of ^{1}H MRS for the noninvasive lipid profiling of skeletal muscle, we need to consider the specific characteristics of the skeletal muscle spectra. The inhomogenous distribution of EMCL, the rather low IMCL content, and the partially overlapping EMCL and IMCL resonances in all chemical shift positions do not allow for robust detection and quantification of allylic, α-carbonyl, diallylic (2.0—2.7 ppm), and olefinic (5.3 ppm) peaks. Thus, similar to the situation in myocardial spectroscopy, in the one-dimensional MRS, only the potential of a saturation fraction surrogate formed by the ratio of methylene (CH_2, 1.3—IMCL, 1.5 ppm—EMCL) to methyl (CH_3, 0.9 ppm—IMCL, 1.1 ppm—EMCL) for noninvasive lipid profiling can be explored. This approach has been employed in pilot validation and cross-sectional studies, and different ratios of the CH_2 to CH_3 signal have been found in lipodystrophic, trained, and untrained populations [109]. Similar variations of the CH_2/CH_3 ratio, which can also mark the fatty acid chain length, have been reported for IMCL during a fasting protocol [110], resembling lipids in other adipose tissue compartments where diet affects the fatty acid saturation and chain length as well [28].

Two-dimensional correlation spectroscopy (2D COSY) technique, well established in high-resolution NMRS, can help to resolve the overlapping resonances by depicting the cross-correlation signals between neighboring chemical groups in second spectral dimension. This was first implemented in in vivo muscle investigation on clinical scanner in single-voxel manner [111], and the feasibility of detecting 2D cross-peaks between different groups of IMCL and EMCL, including the unsaturated protons within these two lipids pools, was demonstrated. Later, it was combined with multiecho planar spectroscopic imaging [112], and decrease in UI of IMCL and EMCL was observed in the soleus and tibialis anterior muscle regions of subjects with type 2 diabetes mellitus compared with healthy controls. Similar differences were observed in EMCL lipid profile of obese but otherwise healthy volunteers [113].

Summary

Proton MRS allows for the noninvasive lipid profiling of subcutaneous and bone marrow adipose tissue, and the prior knowledge gained from these measurements has successfully been introduced in studies of the liver and skeletal muscle. From a methodological point of view, the comparison between published studies and the interpretation of the results is hampered by different acquisition (STEAM vs. PRESS, water suppression or not, etc.) and postprocessing approaches to spectrum analysis (time domain vs. frequency domain, line shape). There is also no consensus about the issue of calculating universal indices for fatty acid saturation, unsaturation, and polyunsaturation from the results of ^{1}H MRS. The lack of consensus in methodology is also true for the MRI techniques, and further method development and validation studies are needed before such a consensus can be reached. In addition to the presence of a strong water signal, which also proves problematic for the MRI-based methods, an artifactual spatial gradient in the readout direction of the resulting FAC maps is an important challenge to overcome.

Nevertheless, MRS-based noninvasive lipid profiling has been applied in several metabolic studies, and the relation of fatty acid (un)saturation indices to different pathologies and diet interventions has been suggested. In the breast tissue, the links between the lipid profile and the malignancy of mammary carcinoma have been suggested, and its clinical value for lesion grading is currently under investigation.

References

[1] Obesity [Internet].

[2] Snel M, Jonker JT, Schoones J, Lamb H, De Roos A, Pijl H, et al. Ectopic fat and insulin resistance: pathophysiology and effect of diet and lifestyle interventions. Internet J Endocrinol 2012;2012.

[3] Coen PM, Goodpaster BH. Role of intramyocelluar lipids in human health. Trends Endocrinol Metab 2012;23(8):391—8.

[4] McQuaid SE, Hodson L, Neville MJ, Dennis AL, Cheeseman J, Humphreys SM, et al. Downregulation of adipose tissue fatty acid trafficking in obesity. Diabetes 2011;60(1):47—55.

[5] Szendroedi R. Ectopic lipids and organ function. Curr Opin Lipidol 2009;20(1):50−6.

[6] Kotronen W, Bergholm P, Yki-Järvinen. Liver fat in the metabolic syndrome. J Clin Endocrinol Metab 2007;92(9):3490−7.

[7] Taira S, Higa Y, Kozuka U, et al. Lipid deposition in various sites of the skeletal muscles and liver exhibits a positive correlation with visceral fat accumulation in middle-aged Japanese men with metabolic syndrome. Intern Med 2013;52(14):1561−71.

[8] Machann J, Thamer C, Schnoedt B, Haap M, Haring H-U, Claussen CD, et al. Standardized assessment of whole body adipose tissue topography by MRI. J Magn Reson Imag 2005;21(4):455−62.

[9] Yeung G, Lee A, Woo L. Osteoporosis is associated with increased marrow fat content and decreased marrow fat unsaturation: a proton MR spectroscopy study. J Magn Reson Imag 2005;22(2):279−85.

[10] Baum T, Yap SP, Karampinos DC, Nardo L, Kuo D, Burghardt AJ, et al. Does vertebral bone marrow fat content correlate with abdominal adipose tissue, lumbar spine bone mineral density, and blood biomarkers in women with type 2 diabetes mellitus? J Magn Reson Imag 2012;35(1):117−24.

[11] Souza RJ de, Mente A, Maroleanu A, Cozma AI, Ha V, Kishibe T, et al. Intake of saturated and trans unsaturated fatty acids and risk of all cause mortality, cardiovascular disease, and type 2 diabetes: systematic review and meta-analysis of observational studies. BMJ 2015;351.

[12] Martel D, Leporq B, Bruno M, Regatte R, Honig S, Chang G. Chemical shift-encoded MRI for assessment of bone marrow adipose tissue fat composition: pilot study in premenopausal versus postmenopausal women. Magn Reson Imaging 2018;53:148−55.

[13] Nemeth S, Leporq S, Faraz S, et al. 3D chemical shift-encoded MRI for volume and composition quantification of abdominal adipose tissue during an overfeeding protocol in healthy volunteers. J Magn Reson Imag 2019;49(6):1587−99.

[14] Martel L, Saxena B, Turyan H, et al. 3T chemical shift-encoded MRI: detection of altered proximal femur marrow adipose tissue composition in glucocorticoid users and validation with magnetic resonance spectroscopy. J Magn Reson Imag 2019;50(2):490−6.

[15] Lundbom H, Fielding H, Taskinen L. PRESS echo time behavior of triglyceride resonances at 1.5T: detecting omega-3 fatty acids in adipose tissue in vivo. J Magn Reson 2009;201(1):39−47.

[16] Ruschke K, Baum K, Settles H, et al. Diffusion-weighted stimulated echo acquisition mode (DW-STEAM) MR spectroscopy to measure fat unsaturation in regions with low proton-density fat fraction. Magn Reson Med 2016;75(1):32−41.

[17] Van de Weijer T, Schrauwen-Hinderling VB. Application of magnetic resonance spectroscopy in metabolic research. Biochim Biophys Acta - Mol Basis Dis. 2019;1865(4):741−8.

[18] Hakumäki J, Kauppinen R. 1H NMR visible lipids in the life and death of cells. Trends Biochem Sci 2000;25(8):357−62.

[19] Peterson P, Trinh L, Månsson S. Quantitative 1H MRI and MRS of fatty acid composition. Magn Reson Med 2021;85(1):49−67.

[20] Schick E, Jung B, Bunse L. Comparison of localized proton NMR signals of skeletal muscle and fat tissue in vivo: two lipid compartments in muscle tissue. Magn Reson Med 1993;29(2):158−67.

[21] Boesch C, Slotboom J, Hoppeler H, Kreis R. In vivo determination of intra-myocellular lipids in human muscle by means of localized 1H-MR-spectroscopy. Magn Reson Med 1997;37(4):484−93.

[22] Boesch C, Kreis R. Observation of intramyocellular lipids by1H-magnetic resonance spectroscopy. Ann N Y Acad Sci 2006;904(1):25−31.

[23] Szczepaniak B, Schick D, Garg B, et al. Measurement of intracellular triglyceride stores by H spectroscopy: validation in vivo. Am J Physiol 1999;276(5).

[24] Longo R, Masutti V, Crocé B, et al. Fatty infiltration of the liver. Quantification by 1H localized magnetic resonance spectroscopy and comparison with computed tomography. Invest Radiol 1993;28(4):297−302.

[25] Thomsen B, Winkler C, Jensen H. Quantification of liver fat using magnetic resonance spectroscopy. Magn Reson Imaging 1994;12(3):487−95.

[26] Lundbom J, Hakkarainen A, Fielding B, Söderlund S, Westerbacka J, Taskinen MR, et al. Characterizing human adipose tissue lipids by long echo time 1H-MRS in vivo at 1.5 Tesla: validation by gas chromatography. NMR Biomed 2010;23(5):466−72.

[27] Ren J, Dimitrov I, Sherry AD, Malloy CR. Composition of adipose tissue and marrow fat in humans by 1H NMR at 7 Tesla. J Lipid Res 2008;49(9):2055−62.

[28] Machann J, Stefan N, Wagner R, Bongers M, Schleicher E, Fritsche A, et al. Intra- and interindividual variability of fatty acid unsaturation in six different human adipose tissue compartments assessed by 1H-MRS in vivo at 3 T. NMR Biomed 2017;30(9):1−10.

[29] Loher H, Kreis R, Boesch C, Christ E. The flexibility of ectopic lipids. Int J Mol Sci 2016;17(9):1−32.

[30] Hamilton G, Middleton MS, Bydder M, Yokoo T, Schwimmer JB, Kono Y, et al. Effect of PRESS and STEAM sequences on magnetic resonance spectroscopic liver fat quantification. J Magn Reson Imag 2009;30(1):145−52.

[31] Yahya, Tessier, Fallone. Effect of J-coupling on lipid composition determination with localized proton magnetic resonance spectroscopy at 9.4 T. J Magn Reson Imag 2011;34(6):1388−96.

[32] Yablonskiy DA, Neil JJ, Raichle ME, Ackerman JJH. Homonuclear J coupling effects in volume localized NMR spectroscopy: pitfalls and solutions. Magn Reson Med 1998;39(2):169−78.

[33] Stables K, Anderson G. Density matrix simulations of the effects of J coupling in spin echo and fast spin echo imaging. J Magn Reson 1999;140(2):305−14.

[34] Stables K, Anderson C, Gore. Analysis of J coupling-induced fat suppression in DIET imaging. J Magn Reson 1999;136(2):143−51.

[35] Henkelman H, Bishop P, Plewes. Why fat is bright in RARE and fast spin-echo imaging. J Magn Reson Imag 1992;2(5):533−40.

[36] Ye D, Fuchs W, Rudin. Hepatic lipid composition differs between ob/ob and ob/+ control mice as determined by using in vivo localized proton magnetic resonance spectroscopy. MAGMA 2012;25(5):381−9.

[37] Gajdošík C, Hangel M, Chmelík V, et al. Ultrashort-TE stimulated echo acquisition mode (STEAM) improves the quantification of lipids and fatty acid chain unsaturation in the human liver at 7 T. NMR Biomed 2015;28(10):1283−93.

[38] Ouwerkerk R, Hamimi A, Matta J, Abd-Elmoniem KZ, Eary JF, Sater ZA, et al. Proton MR spectroscopy measurements of white and Brown adipose tissue in healthy humans: relaxation parameters and unsaturated fatty acids. Radiology 2021;299(2):396–406. https://doi.org/10.1148/radiol2021202676.

[39] Gajdošík M, Hingerl L, Škoch A, Freudenthaler A, Krumpolec P, Ukropec J, et al. Ultralong TE in vivo 1H MR spectroscopy of omega-3 fatty acids in subcutaneous adipose tissue at 7 T. J Magn Reson Imag 2019;50(1):71–82.

[40] Škoch A, Tošner Z, Hájek M. The in vivo J-difference editing MEGA-PRESS technique for the detection of n-3 fatty acids. NMR Biomed 2014;27(11):1293–9.

[41] Haddadin IS, McIntosh A, Meisamy S, Corum C, Snyder ALS, Powell NJ, et al. Metabolite quantification and high-field MRS in breast cancer. NMR Biomed 2009;22(1):65–76.

[42] Gruber S, Debski B-K, Pinker K, Chmelik M, Grabner G, Helbich T, et al. Three-dimensional proton MR spectroscopic imaging at 3 T for the differentiation of benign and malignant breast lesions. Radiology 2011;261(3). https://doi.org/10.1148/radiol11102096. 752–61.

[43] He S, Hooley L, Weinreb B. In vivo MR spectroscopic imaging of polyunsaturated fatty acids (PUFA) in healthy and cancerous breast tissues by selective multiple-quantum coherence transfer (Sel-MQC): a preliminary study. Magn Reson Med 2007;58(6):1079–85.

[44] Lewin S, Moccaldi M, Kim G. Fatty acid composition in mammary adipose tissue measured by Gradient-echo Spectroscopic MRI and its association with breast cancers. Eur J Radiol 2019;116:205–11.

[45] Vanhamme L, van den Boogaart A, Van Huffel S, van den Boogaart A, Van Huffel S, van den Boogaart A, et al. Improved method for accurate and efficient quantification of MRS data with use of prior knowledge. J Magn Reson 1997;129(1):35–43.

[46] Provencher SW. Automatic quantitation of localized in vivo 1H spectra with LCModel. NMR Biomed 2001;14(4):260–4.

[47] Roumans KHM, Lindeboom L, Veeraiah P, Remie CME, Phielix E, Havekes B, et al. Hepatic saturated fatty acid fraction is associated with de novo lipogenesis and hepatic insulin resistance. Nat Commun 2020;11(1):1–11.

[48] Johnson NA, Walton DW, Sachinwalla T, Thompson CH, Smith K, Ruell PA, et al. Noninvasive assessment of hepatic lipid composition: advancing understanding and management of fatty liver disorders. Hepatology 2008;47(5):1513–23.

[49] Patsch JM, Li X, Baum T, Yap SP, Karampinos DC, Schwartz AV, et al. Bone marrow fat composition as a novel imaging biomarker in postmenopausal women with prevalent fragility fractures. J Bone Miner Res 2013;28(8):1721–8.

[50] Corbin IR, Furth EE, Pickup S, Siegelman ES, Delikatny EJ. In vivo assessment of hepatic triglycerides in murine non-alcoholic fatty liver disease using magnetic resonance spectroscopy. Biochim Biophys Acta - Mol Cell Biol Lipids 2009;1791(8):757–63.

[51] Lundbom J, Hakkarainen A, Söderlund S, Westerbacka J, Lundbom N, Taskinen MR. Long-TE 1H MRS suggests that liver fat is more saturated than subcutaneous and visceral fat. NMR Biomed 2011;24(3):238–45.

[52] Pieńkowska J, Brzeska B, Kaszubowski M, Kozak O, Jankowska A, Szurowska E. The correlation between the MRI-evaluated ectopic fat accumulation and the incidence of diabetes mellitus and hypertension depends on body mass index and waist circumference ratio. PLoS One 2020;15(1):e0226889.

[53] Reeder W, Yu P, Gold M, et al. Multicoil Dixon chemical species separation with an iterative least-squares estimation method. Magn Reson Med 2004;51(1):35–45.

[54] Nemeth S, Leporq C, Gambarota S, et al. Comparison of MRI-derived vs. traditional estimations of fatty acid composition from MR spectroscopy signals. NMR Biomed 2018;31(9).

[55] Thomas T-R, Barnard F, Sargentoni D, et al. Changes in adipose tissue composition in malnourished patients before and after liver transplantation: a carbon-13 magnetic resonance spectroscopy and gas-liquid chromatography study. Hepatology 1997;25(1):178–83.

[56] Thomas H, Ala-Korpela J, Azzopardi I, et al. Noninvasive characterization of neonatal adipose tissue by 13C magnetic resonance spectroscopy. Lipids 1997;32(6):645–51.

[57] Hwang B, Leaf R. In vivo characterization of fatty acids in human adipose tissue using natural abundance 1H decoupled 13C MRS at 1.5 T: clinical applications to dietary therapy. NMR Biomed 2003;16(3):160–7.

[58] Machann J, Stefan N, Schabel C, Schleicher E, Fritsche A, Würslin C, et al. Fraction of unsaturated fatty acids in visceral adipose tissue (VAT) is lower in subjects with high total VAT volume - a combined 1H MRS and volumetric MRI study in male subjects. NMR Biomed 2013;26(2):232–6.

[59] Machann T, Stefan S, Kantartzis H, et al. Follow-up whole-body assessment of adipose tissue compartments during a lifestyle intervention in a large cohort at increased risk for type 2 diabetes. Radiology 2010;257(2):353–63.

[60] Fox M, Hoffmann P, Maurovich-Horvat L, et al. Abdominal visceral and subcutaneous adipose tissue compartments: association with metabolic risk factors in the Framingham Heart Study. Circulation 2007;116(1):39–48.

[61] Wajchenberg B. Subcutaneous and visceral adipose tissue: their relation to the metabolic syndrome. Endocr Rev 2000;21(6):697–738.

[62] von Eyben F, Mouritsen, Holm M, Dimcevski S, et al. Intra-abdominal obesity and metabolic risk factors: a study of young adults. Int J Obes Relat Metab Disord 2003;27(8):941–9.

[63] Goodpaster BH, Krishnaswami S, Harris TB, Katsiaras A, Kritchevsky BS, Simonsick ME, et al. Obesity, regional body fat distribution, and the metabolic syndrome in older men and women. Arch Intern Med 2005;165(7):777–83.

[64] Imbeault P, Lemieux S, Prud'homme D, Tremblay A, Nadeau A, Després JP, et al. Relationship of visceral adipose tissue to metabolic risk factors for coronary heart disease: is there a contribution of subcutaneous fat cell hypertrophy? Metabolism 1999;48(3):355–62.

[65] Després JP. Health consequences of visceral obesity. Ann Med 2001;33(8):534–41.

[66] Pascot LS, Lemieux I, Prud'homme, Tremblay, Bouchard, et al. Age-related increase in visceral adipose tissue and body fat and the metabolic risk profile of premenopausal women. Diabetes Care 1999;22(9):1471–8.

[67] Hamilton G, Schlein AN, Middleton MS, Hooker CA, Wolfson T, Gamst AC, et al. In vivo triglyceride composition of abdominal adipose tissue measured by 1H MRS at 3T. J Magn Reson Imag 2017;45(5):1455.

[68] Lundbom J, Hakkarainen A, Lundbom N, Taskinen MR. Deep subcutaneous adipose tissue is more saturated than superficial subcutaneous adipose tissue. Int J Obes 2013;37(4):620−2.

[69] Zhang M, Hu, Zhang S, Zhou. Associations of different adipose tissue depots with insulin resistance: a systematic review and meta-analysis of observational studies. Sci Rep 2015;5.

[70] Ross R. Effects of diet- and exercise-induced weight loss on visceral adipose tissue in men and women. Sport Med 1997;24(1):55−64.

[71] Fontana L, Eagon JC, Trujillo ME, Scherer PE, Klein S. Visceral fat adipokine secretion is associated with systemic inflammation in obese humans. Diabetes 2007;56(4):1010−3.

[72] Björntorp P. Metabolic implications of body fat distribution. Diabetes Care 1991;14(12):1132−43.

[73] Baum T, Cordes C, Dieckmeyer M, Ruschke S, Franz D, Hauner H, et al. MR-based assessment of body fat distribution and characteristics. Eur J Radiol 2016;85(8):1512−8.

[74] Yu G, Eajazi T, Bredella. Marrow adipose tissue composition in adults with morbid obesity. Bone 2017;97:38−42.

[75] Xu K, Sigurdsson S, Gudnason V, Hue T, Schwartz A, Li X. Reliable quantification of marrow fat content and unsaturation level using in vivo MR spectroscopy. Magn Reson Med 2018;79(3):1722.

[76] Bredella F, Daley M, Rosen K, et al. Marrow fat composition in anorexia nervosa. Bone 2014;66:199−204.

[77] Ecklund K, Vajapeyam S, Mulkern RV, Feldman HA, O'Donnell JM, DiVasta AD, et al. Bone marrow fat content in 70 adolescent girls with anorexia nervosa: magnetic resonance imaging and magnetic resonance spectroscopy assessment. Pediatr Radiol 2017;47(8):952.

[78] Bolan M, Baker L, Emory N, et al. In vivo quantification of choline compounds in the breast with 1H MR spectroscopy. Magn Reson Med 2003;50(6):1134−43.

[79] Bolan PJ, DelaBarre L, Baker EH, Merkle H, Everson LI, Yee D, et al. Eliminating spurious lipid sidebands in 1H MRS of breast lesions. Magn Reson Med 2002;48(2):215−22.

[80] Minarikova, Gruber, Bogner P-D, Baltzer H, et al. Dixon imaging-based partial volume correction improves quantification of choline detected by breast 3D-MRSI. Eur Radiol 2015;25(3):830−6.

[81] Coum O, Noury B, Saint-Hilaire V, et al. In vivo MR spectroscopy of human breast tissue: quantification of fatty acid composition at a clinical field strength (3 T). MAGMA 2016;29(1):1−4.

[82] Dimitrov IE, Douglas D, Ren J, Smith NB, Webb AG, Sherry AD, et al. In vivo determination of human breast fat composition by 1H MRS at 7T. Magn Reson Med 2012;67(1):20.

[83] Freed M, Storey P, Lewin AA, Babb J, Moccaldi M, Moy L, et al. Evaluation of breast lipid composition in patients with benign tissue and cancer by using multiple gradient-echo MR imaging. Radiology 2016;281(1):43−53. https://doi.org/10.1148/radiol2016151959.

[84] Bitencourt S, Morris P, Thakur. Fat composition measured by proton spectroscopy: a breast cancer tumor marker? Diagnostics (Basel, Switzerland) 2021;11(3).

[85] Cheung H, Mallikourti M, Heys H. Intra-tumoural lipid composition and lymphovascular invasion in breast cancer via non-invasive magnetic resonance spectroscopy. Eur Radiol 2021;31(6):3703−11.

[86] Mallikourti V, Cheung SM, Gagliardi T, Masannat Y, Heys SD, He J. Optimal phased-array signal combination for polyunsaturated fatty acids measurement in breast cancer using multiple quantum coherence MR spectroscopy at 3T. Sci Rep 2019;9(1):1−9.

[87] Szczepaniak LS, Babcock EE, Schick F, Dobbins RL, Garg A, Burns DK, et al. Measurement of intracellular triglyceride stores by 1H spectroscopy: validation in vivo. Am J Physiol 1999;276(5). https://doi.org/10.1152/ajpendo19992765E977. 39−5.

[88] Bohte WV, Bipat S. The diagnostic accuracy of US, CT, MRI and 1H-MRS for the evaluation of hepatic steatosis compared with liver biopsy: a meta-analysis. Eur Radiol 2011;21(1):87−97.

[89] Hamilton G, Yokoo T, Bydder M, Cruite I, Schroeder ME, Sirlin CB, et al. In vivo characterization of the liver fat 1H MR spectrum. NMR Biomed 2011;24(7):784−90.

[90] Araya R, Videla T, Orellana P, et al. Increase in long-chain polyunsaturated fatty acid n - 6/n - 3 ratio in relation to hepatic steatosis in patients with non-alcoholic fatty liver disease. Clin Sci (Lond). 2004;106(6):635−43.

[91] Puri B, Wiest M, Choudhury OC, et al. A lipidomic analysis of nonalcoholic fatty liver disease. Hepatology 2007;46(4):1081−90.

[92] Hamilton G, Smith DL, Bydder M, Nayak KS, Hu HH. MR properties of brown and white adipose tissues. J Magn Reson Imag 2011;34:468−73.

[93] Krssak M, Brehm A, Bernroider E, Anderwald C, Nowotny P, Man CD, et al. Alterations in postprandial hepatic glycogen metabolism in type 2 diabetes. Diabetes 2004;53(12):3048−56.

[94] Gluchowski G, Chitraju B, Mejhert B, et al. Hepatocyte deletion of triglyceride-synthesis enzyme acyl CoA: diacylglycerol acyltransferase 2 reduces steatosis without increasing inflammation or fibrosis in mice. Hepatology 2019;70(6):1972−85.

[95] Lambert R-R, Browning P. Increased de novo lipogenesis is a distinct characteristic of individuals with nonalcoholic fatty liver disease. Gastroenterology 2014;146(3):726−35.

[96] Matikainen A, Söderlund S, Ahola H, et al. Hepatic lipogenesis and a marker of hepatic lipid oxidation, predict postprandial responses of triglyceride-rich lipoproteins. Obesity 2014;22(8):1854−9.

[97] Felblinger J, Jung B, Slotboom J, C Boesch RK. Methods and reproducibility of cardiac/respiratory double-triggered (1)H-MR spectroscopy of the human heart - PubMed [Internet]. Magn Reson Med 1999:903−10.

[98] Hollander D, Evanochko P. Observation of cardiac lipids in humans by localized 1H magnetic resonance spectroscopic imaging. Magn Reson Med 1994;32(2):175−80.

[99] O'Connor RD, Xu J, Ewald GA, Ackerman JJH, Peterson LR, Gropler RJ, et al. Intramyocardial triglyceride quantification by magnetic resonance spectroscopy: in vivo and ex vivo correlation in human subjects. Magn Reson Med 2011;65(5):1234−8.

[100] Meer van der D, Kozerke S, Bax H, et al. Metabolic imaging of myocardial triglyceride content: reproducibility of 1H MR spectroscopy with respiratory navigator gating in volunteers. Radiology 2007;245(1):251−7.

[101] Reingold JS, McGavock JM, Kaka S, Tillery T, Victor RG, Szczepaniak LS. Determination of triglyceride in the human myocardium by magnetic resonance spectroscopy: reproducibility and sensitivity of the method. Am J Physiol Endocrinol Metab 2005;289(5):935−9. https://doi.org/10.1152/ajpendo000952005. 52−5.

[102] McGavock L, Zib T, Salas U, et al. Cardiac steatosis in diabetes mellitus: a 1H-magnetic resonance spectroscopy study. Circulation 2007;116(10):1170−5.

[103] Meer van der RW, Hammer S, Smit F, Bax D, et al. Short-term caloric restriction induces accumulation of myocardial triglycerides and decreases left ventricular diastolic function in healthy subjects. Diabetes 2007;56(12):2849−53.

[104] Szczepaniak D, Metzger S-D'Ambrosia, Arbique V, et al. Myocardial triglycerides and systolic function in humans: in vivo evaluation by localized proton spectroscopy and cardiac imaging. Magn Reson Med 2003;49(3):417−23.

[105] Krššák, Winhofer, Göbl B, Reiter, Kautzky-Willer, et al. Insulin resistance is not associated with myocardial steatosis in women. Diabetologia 2011;54(7):1871−8.

[106] Fillmer A, Hock A, Cameron D, Henning A. Non-water-suppressed 1H MR spectroscopy with orientational prior knowledge shows potential for separating intra- and extramyocellular lipid signals in human myocardium. Sci Rep 2017;7(1):1−14.

[107] Szczepaniak LS, Dobbins RL, Stein DT, Denis McGarry J. Bulk magnetic susceptibility effects on the assessment of intra- and extramyocellular lipids in vivo. Magn Reson Med 2002;47(3):607−10.

[108] Krššák M, Lindeboom L, Schrauwen-Hinderling V, Szczepaniak LS, Derave W, Lundbom J, et al. Proton magnetic resonance spectroscopy in skeletal muscle : experts' consensus recommendations. NMR Biomed January 2020:1−20.

[109] Savage DB, Watson L, Carr K, Adams C, Brage S, Chatterjee KK, et al. Accumulation of saturated intramyocellular lipid is associated with insulin resistance. J Lipid Res 2019;60(7):1323−32.

[110] Thankamony A, Kemp GJ, Koulman A, Bokii V, Savage DB, Boesch C, et al. Compositional marker in vivo reveals intramyocellular lipid turnover during fasting-induced lipolysis. Sci Rep 2018;8(1):1−8.

[111] Velan D, Lemieux R, Sridhar S, et al. Investigation of muscle lipid metabolism by localized one- and two-dimensional MRS techniques using a clinical 3T MRI/MRS scanner. J Magn Reson Imag 2007;25(1):192−9.

[112] Furuyama, Nagarajan, Roberts L, Hahn T. A pilot validation of multi-echo based echo-planar correlated spectroscopic imaging in human calf muscles. NMR Biomed 2014;27(10):1176−83.

[113] Nagarajan R, Carpenter CL, Lee CC, Michael N, Sarma MK, Souza R, et al. Assessment of lipid and metabolite changes in obese calf muscle using multi-echo echo-planar correlated spectroscopic imaging. Sci Rep 2017;7(1):1−10.

Chapter 6

Flexibility of ectopic lipids in skeletal/cardiac muscle and liver

Hannah Loher[1], Chris Boesch[2], Roland Kreis[3] and Emanuel Christ[4]

[1]Division of Endocrinology and Diabetology, Kantonsspital Lucerne, Lucerne, Switzerland; [2]University of Bern, Bern, Switzerland; [3]Magnetic Resonance Methodology, Institute of Diagnostic and Interventional Neuroradiology, University of Bern, Bern, Switzerland; [4]Division of Endocrinology, Diabetology and Metabolism, University Hospital of Basel, Basel, Switzerland

Measurement of the flexibility of ectopic lipids

Biopsy

In the first studies that investigated ectopic lipids, they were quantified with biopsies [1]. In general, the ectopic lipids can be quantified in the tissue biopsies by biochemical, electron microscopic, or histochemical methods [2,3].

Biopsies were mainly used for the quantification of intramyocellular lipids but also for intrahepatocellular lipids. The latter has been used primarily for the diagnosis of nonalcoholic fatty liver disease (NAFLD) and nonalcoholic steatohepatitis (NASH) [4]. Since liver biopsy carries an increased risk for complications, its use for study purposes is limited. Other organs such as the heart can only be examined with biopsies in very selected cases, and due to the potential complications, it is difficult to examine intramyocardial lipids in the context of research.

Especially when repeated measurements are necessary, as is the case when examining the influence of interventions such as diet or physical exercise on ectopic lipids, biopsies are invasive procedures and, therefore, not ideal.

Consequently, noninvasive examination methods are warranted. Various methods are available for the noninvasive quantification of ectopic lipids, in particular CT, MRI, and MR-spectroscopy. For the assessment of the flexibility of ectopic lipids, in particular MR-spectroscopy has proven to be a reliable and helpful tool.

^{1}H-magnetic resonance spectroscopy (MRS)

MR-spectroscopy can be used for the quantification of numerous metabolites, including energy stores such as glycogen (using ^{13}C-MRS), high-energy phosphates (^{31}P-MRS), and intramyocellular lipids (IMCL, ^{1}H-MRS) [5]. Following the observation [6] and identification [7] of IMCL-resonances in the ^{1}H-MR spectrum, an in-vivo validation study in humans showed an excellent correlation between ^{1}H-MRS IMCL results and electron microscopy of biopsies [3].

While ^{1}H-MRS is generally accepted in clinical trials as gold standard for the quantification of intrahepatic lipids (IHCL) [8,9], various specialized MR imaging sequences are also established meanwhile [10]. ^{1}H-MRI/MRS proved to be particularly credible tools for quantification of NAFLD, an important complication in patients with the metabolic syndrome.

Quantification of ectopic lipid depots in the myocardium using ^{1}H-MRS required additional methodological steps to overcome the motion of the heart ([11,12] and references therein). Examples of ^{1}H-MR spectra in skeletal muscle and liver before and after exercise are shown in Figs. 6.1 and 6.2, respectively [13].

Ectopic lipids in the context of negative energy balance

Single bout of exercise

During exercise there is an increased demand for energy which can be met by carbohydrate (short-term) or fatty acid (longer duration of exercise) oxidation in the mitochondria of the skeletal muscles [14]. Fatty acids originate on one hand

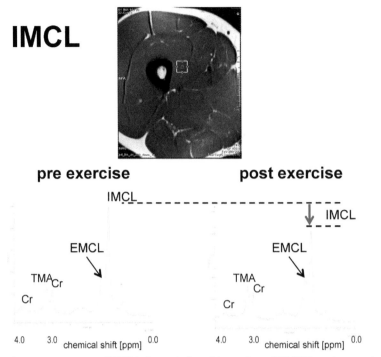

FIGURE 6.1 Typical 1H magnetic resonance spectrum (MRS) before and after a 2-h exercise at 50% VO2max in a voxel of the tibialis anterior muscle. A significant decrease in IMCL is documented (red arrow). *IMCL*, intramyocellular lipids; *EMCL*, extramyocellular lipids; *Cr*, Creatinine; *TMA*, trimethyl-ammonium. *From Loher H, Kreis R, Boesch C, Christ E. The Flexibility of Ectopic Lipids. International Journal of Molecular Sciences 2016;17(9). https://doi.org/10.3390/ijms17091554.*

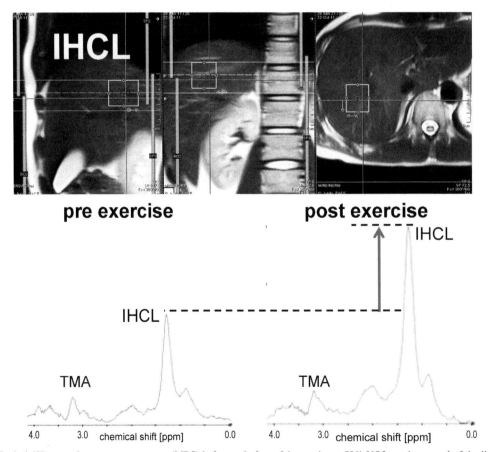

FIGURE 6.2 Typical 1H magnetic resonance spectrum (MRS) before and after a 2-h exercise at 50% VO2max in a voxel of the liver. A significant increase in IHCL is documented (red arrow). IHCL, intrahepatocellular lipids; TMA, trimethyl-ammonium. *From Loher H, Kreis R, Boesch C, Christ E. The Flexibility of Ectopic Lipids. International Journal of Molecular Sciences 2016;17(9). https://doi.org/10.3390/ijms17091554.*

from the fat tissue and can be delivered within lipoproteins to the muscle tissue via the blood stream. The endothelial-bound lipoprotein lipase of the skeletal muscle catalyzes the hydrolysis of triglycerides. The free fatty acids can then be taken up into the muscle tissue through CD36. Skeletal muscle-lipoprotein lipase as well as CD36 is influenced among others by muscle contraction and fasting [15]. This pathway with multiple steps implies that there is a certain delay until the fuel is available for energy generation in the target tissue (Fig. 6.3).

On the other hand, fatty acids can also originate from lipolysis of IMCL [16], i.e., from lipid droplets located next to the skeletal muscle mitochondria. This implies that energy availability is much faster since there is no need for transport of FFA from fat tissue to the exercising muscle. In this context it has been shown that during moderate-intensity exercise about 30%−50% of total lipid oxidation derive from intramyocellular lipids [17,18]. In skeletal muscle, lipolysis is mainly regulated by adipose triglyceride lipase and hormone sensitive lipase [19]. As suggested by its name, the hormone sensitive lipase and the adipose tissue lipase are regulated by hormones such as insulin, growth hormone, or catecholamines [20]; [21]; [22].

During a two-to-three-hour workout (at 50% VO$_2$max), lipids in the muscle are reduced by 25%−59% (among others [7,23−34]). So far, it has been shown that gender has an influence on flexibility of intramyocellular lipid breakdown: the reduction is less pronounced in women compared to men [35].

Patients with growth hormone deficiency have also been studied, and this group of patients is known to have impaired lipid metabolism/reduced lipolysis [20−22]. Importantly, growth hormone replacement therapy does not lead to a significant increase in flexibility of ectopic lipids [36,37]. However, it may have an effect on recovery of intramyocellular lipids 24 h after the physical exercise [38].

In contrast to IMCL, the ectopic lipid depots in the liver (IHCL) behave differently during exercise: after 90−120 min of exercise, the lipid content of the liver is increased in healthy subjects [39,40]. This phenomenon is called spillover effect [41]: it probably occurs due to increased systemic lipolysis during exercise with increased levels of free fatty acids. The available fatty acids are not fully used by the working tissue and thus, the excess fatty acids are stored in the liver and interestingly, also in nonexercising muscle [42]. Again, growth hormone deficiency or growth hormone replacement therapy does not significantly impact on the flexibility of IHCL [36].

Lipids in cardiac muscle (intramyocardial lipids = ICCL) appear to behave similarly to those in skeletal muscle during exercise, i.e., are decreased in intramyocardial lipids. This was observed during a 2-h bout of exercise [24] as well as during a marathon [43].

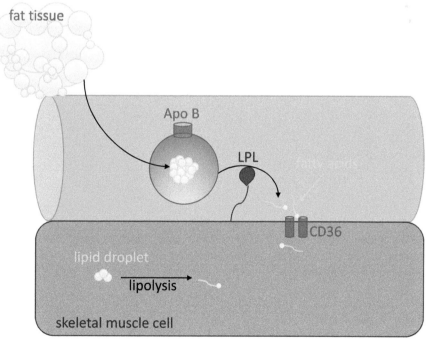

FIGURE 6.3 Lipids as an energy source are stored in fat tissue and, if neede,d transported in apolipoprotein B (apoB) containg lipoproteines to the exercising skeletal muslce skeletal muscle. Upon lipolysis by the lipoprotein lipase (LPL) the free fatty acids are transported via CD36 into the skeletal muscle where they are oxidised. Alternatively, lipid droplets (intramyocellular lipids, IMCL) are located in the skeletal muscle and can be used as fuel, if needed.

Fasting

During fasting, the energy needs of the working tissue must be met by consuming energy reserves, similar to exercise. During fasting, insulin levels are low due to low blood glucose levels. Low insulin levels disinhibit lipolysis and hepatic gluconeogenesis and glycogenolysis, thereby increasing the availability of fuel.

Almost all studies that have investigated the effect of fasting on intramyocellular lipids have shown a significant increase of intramyocellular lipid content after 48—120 h of fasting [44—46].

An increase in lipids was also observed in the hepatocytes of men during short-term fasting, but not in women. In women, serum triglycerides are lower than in men [44]. It is, therefore, conceivable that men may have elevated IHCL after fasting due to the spillover effect, similar to the effect of exercise.

Ectopic lipids in the context of positive energy balance

Short-term high fat diet

An isocaloric moderate—high fat diet for 2—3 days resulted in an increase in IMCL [47—49]. This effect has also been observed with a hypercaloric diet [50]. Training status had no relevant influence on flexibility: an increase in IMCL was observed in sedentary subjects [48,50] as well as in endurance-trained cyclists/runners [47,49]. One possible explanation is an increase in muscle lipoprotein lipase activity after a high fat meal [16,51]. In these studies, IMCL was analyzed with ^{1}H-MRS except for the last two studies [47,49] where it was quantified with muscle biopsies.

However, no increase in IMCL was observed after a single high fat meal. Nevertheless, an increase in IHCL was measured. The cause of this discrepancy is not clear [52]. An increase in IHCL could also be measured during a prolonged high fat diet during 3—4 days [53,54].

Bachmann et al. [50] have also investigated the effect of intravenous intralipid infusion on IMCL levels by repetitive ^{1}H-MRS measurements. The maximum IMCL content was determined 2 h after the infusion.

Long-term high fat diet

Even during a longer intervention period lasting 1—4 weeks, an increase in IMCL was observed after a high fat diet [55—57]. There is evidence that in this context this increase is due to an increased storage of fatty acids in the myocytes [56].

A single study [58] did not show a significant increase in IMCL after a high fat diet for 3 weeks. One possible cause is that in this study the participants were overweight, which is associated with an increased free fatty acid availability already at baseline, i.e., before high fat diet thereby disguising a possible increase, in contrast to the other studies where subjects were normal weight [55—57].

High fructose/glucose diet

High fructose as well as high glucose diet increased IHCL [59—61]. Since plasma free fatty acids decrease during the high fructose diet, it is assumed that the increase in IHCL occurs through de novo lipogenesis in the liver and not through re-esterification of fatty acids [59]. Consistently, a low fructose diet during 6 weeks led to a lower intrahepatocellular lipid content [62].

A high fructose diet also induced an increase in IMCL, although the mechanism is not completely elucidated as there are conflicting data [63].

In summary (Table 6.1), ectopic lipids, especially IMCL and IHCL, can be significantly altered by simple interventions in different energetic situations (positive/negative energy balance). This must be kept in mind especially when planning studies that investigate ectopic lipids: standardization with regard to diet and exercise/sport is critical.

Although multiple hormones influence lipid metabolism, the available data suggest that the lack of a hormone, such as growth hormone for instance, does not significantly impact on the short-term flexibility of ectopic lipids. This is most likely because there are redundant hormonal systems such as catecholamines, cortisol, and growth hormone, which are capable of promoting lipolysis thereby providing energy resources in the form of FFA in the situation of negative energy balance. All of them increase in the context of negative energy balance. The redundant hormonal systems, which promote lipolysis, may have been important in guaranteeing enough energy resources in case of a negative energy balance (i.e., fasting or exercise). On the other hand, in a situation of increased fuel availability (positive energy balance, obesity) there are no redundant hormonal systems but only insulin as a regulator. It is conceivable that the lack of redundant hormonal systems in this situation results in the epidemic of the metabolic syndrome and type 2 diabetes.

TABLE 6.1 Changes of ectopic lipids in relation to energy status and diet. *IMCL,* intramyocellular lipids; *IHCL,* intrahepatocellular lipids; *ICCL,* intramyocardiallipids.

Positive energy balance			
Short-term high fat diet	IMCL ↑	ICCL ?	IHCL ↑
High fructose/glucose diet	IMCL ↑	ICCL ?	IHCL ↑
Negative energy balance			
Acute bout of exercise	IMCL ↓	ICCL ↓	IHCL ↑
Fasting	IMCL ↑	ICCL ?	IHCL ↑

References

[1] Folch J, Lees M, Sloane Stanley GH. A simple method for the isolation and purification of total lipides from animal tissues. J Biol Chem 1957;226(1):497−509.

[2] De Bock K, Dresselaers T, Kiens B, Richter EA, Van Hecke P, Hespel P. Evaluation of intramyocellular lipid breakdown during exercise by biochemical assay, NMR spectroscopy, and Oil Red O staining. Am J Physiol Endocrinol Metab 2007;293(1):E428−34.

[3] Howald H, Boesch C, Kreis R, Matter S, Billeter R, Essen-Gustavsson B, Hoppeler H. Content of intramyocellular lipids derived by electron microscopy, biochemical assays, and (1)H-MR spectroscopy. J Appl Physiol 2002;92(6):2264−72.

[4] Chalasani N, Younossi Z, Lavine JE, Diehl AM, Brunt EM, Cusi K, Charlton M, Sanyal AJ. The diagnosis and management of non-alcoholic fatty liver disease: practice guideline by the American association for the study of liver diseases, American college of gastroenterology, and the American gastroenterological association. Am J Gastroenterol 2012;107(6):811−26. https://doi.org/10.1038/ajg.2012.128.

[5] Krššák M, Lindeboom L, Schrauwen-Hinderling V, Szczepaniak LS, Derave W, Lundbom J, Befroy D, Schick F, Machann J, Kreis R, Boesch C. Proton magnetic resonance spectroscopy in skeletal muscle: experts' consensus recommendations. NMR Biomed 2021;34(5):e4266. https://doi.org/10.1002/nbm.4266.

[6] Schick F, Eismann B, Jung WI, Bongers H, Bunse M, Lutz O. Comparison of localized proton NMR signals of skeletal muscle and fat tissue in vivo: two lipid compartments in muscle tissue. Magn Reson Med 1993;29(2):158−67.

[7] Boesch C, Slotboom J, Hoppeler H, Kreis R. In vivo determination of intra-myocellular lipids in human muscle by means of localized 1H-MR-spectroscopy. Magn Reson Med 1997;37(4):484−93.

[8] EASL-EASD-EASO Clinical Practice Guidelines for the management of non-alcoholic fatty liver disease. Diabetologia 2016;59(6):1121−40. https://doi.org/10.1007/s00125-016-3902-y.

[9] Schaapman JJ, Tushuizen ME, Coenraad MJ, Lamb HJ. Multiparametric MRI in patients with nonalcoholic fatty liver disease. J Magn Reson Imag : JMRI 2021;53(6):1623−31. https://doi.org/10.1002/jmri.27292.

[10] Yokoo T, Serai SD, Pirasteh A, Bashir MR, Hamilton G, Hernando D, Hu HH, Hetterich H, Kühn J-P, Kukuk GM, Loomba R, Middleton MS, Obuchowski NA, Song JS, Tang A, Wu X, Reeder SB, Sirlin CB. Linearity, bias, and precision of hepatic proton density fat fraction measurements by using MR imaging: a meta-analysis. Radiology 2018;286(2):486−98. https://doi.org/10.1148/radiol.2017170550.

[11] Fillmer A, Hock A, Cameron D, Henning A. Non-water-suppressed ¹H MR spectroscopy with orientational prior knowledge shows potential for separating intra- and extramyocellular lipid signals in human myocardium. Sci Rep 2017;7(1):16898. https://doi.org/10.1038/s41598-017-16318-0.

[12] van Ewijk PA, Schrauwen-Hinderling VB, Bekkers SCAM, Glatz JFC, Wildberger JE, Kooi ME. MRS: a noninvasive window into cardiac metabolism. NMR Biomed 2015;28(7):747−66. https://doi.org/10.1002/nbm.3320.

[13] Loher H, Kreis R, Boesch C, Christ E. The flexibility of ectopic lipids. Int J Mol Sci 2016;17(9):1554. https://doi.org/10.3390/ijms17091554.

[14] Krogh A, Lindhard J. The relative value of fat and carbohydrate as sources of muscular energy: with appendices on the correlation between standard metabolism and the respiratory quotient during rest and work. Biochem J 1920;14(3−4):290−363.

[15] Goldberg IJ, Eckel RH, Abumrad NA. Regulation of fatty acid uptake into tissues: lipoprotein lipase- and CD36-mediated pathways. J Lipid Res 2009;50(Suppl. l):S86−90. https://doi.org/10.1194/jlr.R800085-JLR200.

[16] Kiens B. Skeletal muscle lipid metabolism in exercise and insulin resistance. Physiol Rev 2006;86(1):205−43.

[17] Martin WH, Dalsky GP, Hurley BF, Matthews DE, Bier DM, Hagberg JM, Rogers MA, King DS, Holloszy JO. Effect of endurance training on plasma free fatty acid turnover and oxidation during exercise. Am J Physiol 1993;265(5 Pt 1):E708−14.

[18] Romijn JA, Coyle EF, Sidossis LS, Gastaldelli A, Horowitz JF, Endert E, Wolfe RR. Regulation of endogenous fat and carbohydrate metabolism in relation to exercise intensity and duration. Am J Physiol 1993;265(3 Pt 1):E380−91.

[19] Badin P-M, Langin D, Moro C. Dynamics of skeletal muscle lipid pools. Trend Endocrinol Metabol 2013;24(12):607−15. https://doi.org/10.1016/j.tem.2013.08.001.

[20] Hansen TK, Gravholt CH, ØRskov H, Rasmussen MH, Christiansen JS, Jørgensen JOL. Dose dependency of the pharmacokinetics and acute lipolytic actions of growth hormone. J Clin Endocrinol Metabol 2002;87(10):4691−8.

[21] Møller N, Jørgensen JOL. Effects of growth hormone on glucose, lipid, and protein metabolism in human subjects. Endocr Rev 2009;30(2):152—77. https://doi.org/10.1210/er.2008-0027.

[22] Watt MJ, Spriet LL. Regulation and role of hormone-sensitive lipase activity in human skeletal muscle. Proc Nutr Soc 2004;63(2):315—22.

[23] Brechtel K, Niess AM, Machann J, Rett K, Schick F, Claussen CD, Dickhuth HH, Haering HU, Jacob S. Utilisation of intramyocellular lipids (IMCLs) during exercise as assessed by proton magnetic resonance spectroscopy (1H-MRS). Hormone Metabol Res 2001;33(2):63—6.

[24] Bucher J, Krüsi M, Zueger T, Ith M, Stettler C, Diem P, Boesch C, Kreis R, Christ E. The effect of a single 2 h bout of aerobic exercise on ectopic lipids in skeletal muscle, liver and the myocardium. Diabetologia 2014;57(5):1001—5. https://doi.org/10.1007/s00125-014-3193-0.

[25] De Bock K, Richter EA, Russell AP, Eijnde BO, Derave W, Ramaekers M, Koninckx E, Léger B, Verhaeghe J, Hespel P. Exercise in the fasted state facilitates fibre type-specific intramyocellular lipid breakdown and stimulates glycogen resynthesis in humans. J Physiol 2005;564(Pt 2):649—60.

[26] Hurley BF, Nemeth PM, Martin WH, Hagberg JM, Dalsky GP, Holloszy JO. Muscle triglyceride utilization during exercise: effect of training. J Appl Physiol 1986;60(2):562—7.

[27] Ith M, Huber PM, Egger A, Schmid J-P, Kreis R, Christ E, Boesch C. Standardized protocol for a depletion of intramyocellular lipids (IMCL). NMR Biomed 2010;23(5):532—8. https://doi.org/10.1002/nbm.1492.

[28] Krssak M, Petersen KF, Bergeron R, Price T, Laurent D, Rothman DL, Roden M, Shulman GI. Intramuscular glycogen and intramyocellular lipid utilization during prolonged exercise and recovery in man: a 13C and 1H nuclear magnetic resonance spectroscopy study. J Clin Endocrinol Metabol 2000;85(2):748—54.

[29] Larson-Meyer DE, Newcomer BR, Hunter GR. Influence of endurance running and recovery diet on intramyocellular lipid content in women: a 1H NMR study. Am J Physiol Endocrinol Metab 2002;282(1):E95—106.

[30] White LJ, Ferguson MA, McCoy SC, Kim H. Intramyocellular lipid changes in men and women during aerobic exercise: a (1)H-magnetic resonance spectroscopy study. J Clin Endocrinol Metabol 2003;88(12):5638—43.

[31] Zehnder M, Christ ER, Ith M, Acheson KJ, Pouteau E, Kreis R, Trepp R, Diem P, Boesch C, Décombaz J. Intramyocellular lipid stores increase markedly in athletes after 1.5 days lipid supplementation and are utilized during exercise in proportion to their content. Eur J Appl Physiol 2006;98(4):341—54.

[32] van Loon LJC, Koopman R, Stegen JHCH, Wagenmakers AJM, Keizer HA, Saris WHM. Intramyocellular lipids form an important substrate source during moderate intensity exercise in endurance-trained males in a fasted state. J Physiol 2003;553(Pt 2):611—25.

[33] van Loon LJC, Schrauwen-Hinderling VB, Koopman R, Wagenmakers AJM, Hesselink MKC, Schaart G, et al. Influence of prolonged endurance cycling and recovery diet on intramuscular triglyceride content in trained males. Am J Physiol Endocrinol Metab 2003;285(4):E804—11.

[34] Vermathen P, Saillen P, Boss A, Zehnder M, Boesch C. Skeletal muscle 1H MRSI before and after prolonged exercise. I. muscle specific depletion of intramyocellular lipids. Magn Reson Med 2012;68(5):1357—67. https://doi.org/10.1002/mrm.24168.

[35] Zehnder M, Ith M, Kreis R, Saris W, Boutellier U, Boesch C. Gender-specific usage of intramyocellular lipids and glycogen during exercise. Med Sci Sports Exerc 2005;37(9):1517—24.

[36] Christ ER, Egger A, Allemann S, Buehler T, Kreis R, Boesch C. Effects of aerobic exercise on ectopic lipids in patients with growth hormone deficiency before and after growth hormone replacement therapy. Sci Rep 2016;6:19310. https://doi.org/10.1038/srep19310.

[37] Trepp R, Flück M, Stettler C, Boesch C, Ith M, Kreis R, Hoppeler H, Howald H, Schmid J-P, Diem P, Christ ER. Effect of GH on human skeletal muscle lipid metabolism in GH deficiency. Am J Physiol Endocrinol Metab 2008;294(6):E1127—34. https://doi.org/10.1152/ajpendo.00010.2008.

[38] Loher H, Jenni S, Bucher J, Krüsi M, Kreis R, Boesch C, Christ E. Impaired repletion of intramyocellular lipids in patients with growth hormone deficiency after a bout of aerobic exercise. Growth Hormone IGF Res : Offic J Growth Hormone Res Soc Int IGF Res Soc 2018;42(43):32—9. https://doi.org/10.1016/j.ghir.2018.08.001.

[39] Egger A, Kreis R, Allemann S, Stettler C, Diem P, Buehler T, Boesch C, Christ ER. The effect of aerobic exercise on intrahepatocellular and intramyocellular lipids in healthy subjects. PLoS One 2013;8(8):e70865. https://doi.org/10.1371/journal.pone.0070865.

[40] Johnson NA, van Overbeek D, Chapman PG, Thompson MW, Sachinwalla T, George J. Effect of prolonged exercise and pre-exercise dietary manipulation on hepatic triglycerides in trained men. Eur J Appl Physiol 2012;112(5):1817—25. https://doi.org/10.1007/s00421-011-2158-y.

[41] Shulman GI. Ectopic fat in insulin resistance, dyslipidemia, and cardiometabolic disease. N Engl J Med 2014;371(12):1131—41. https://doi.org/10.1056/NEJMra1011035.

[42] Schrauwen-Hinderling VB, van Loon LJC, Koopman R, Nicolay K, Saris WHM, Kooi ME. Intramyocellular lipid content is increased after exercise in nonexercising human skeletal muscle. J Appl Physiol 2003;95(6):2328—32.

[43] Aengevaeren VL, Froeling M, van den Berg-Faay S, Hooijmans MT, Monte JR, Strijkers GJ, Nederveen AJ, Eijsvogels TMH, Bakermans AJ. Marathon running transiently depletes the myocardial lipid pool. Physiol Rep 2020;8(17):e14543. https://doi.org/10.14814/phy2.14543.

[44] Browning JD, Baxter J, Satapati S, Burgess SC. The effect of short-term fasting on liver and skeletal muscle lipid, glucose, and energy metabolism in healthy women and men. J Lipid Res 2012;53(3):577—86. https://doi.org/10.1194/jlr.P020867.

[45] Stannard SR, Thompson MW, Fairbairn K, Huard B, Sachinwalla T, Thompson CH. Fasting for 72 h increases intramyocellular lipid content in nondiabetic, physically fit men. Am J Physiol Endocrinol Metab 2002;283(6):E1185—91.

[46] Wietek BM, Machann J, Mader I, Thamer C, Häring H-U, Claussen CD, Stumvoll M, Schick F. Muscle type dependent increase in intramyocellular lipids during prolonged fasting of human subjects: a proton MRS study. Hormone Metabol Res 2004;36(9):639—44.

[47] Larson-Meyer DE, Borkhsenious ON, Gullett JC, Russell RR, Devries MC, Smith SR, Ravussin E. Effect of dietary fat on serum and intramyocellular lipids and running performance. Med Sci Sports Exerc 2008;40(5):892—902. https://doi.org/10.1249/MSS.0b013e318164cb33.

[48] Sakurai Y, Tamura Y, Takeno K, Kumashiro N, Sato F, Kakehi S, Ikeda S, Ogura Y, Saga N, Naito H, Katamoto S, Fujitani Y, Hirose T, Kawamori R, Watada H. Determinants of intramyocellular lipid accumulation after dietary fat loading in non-obese men. J Diab Invest 2011;2(4):310—7. https://doi.org/10.1111/j.2040-1124.2010.00091.x.

[49] Zderic TW, Davidson CJ, Schenk S, Byerley LO, Coyle EF. High-fat diet elevates resting intramuscular triglyceride concentration and whole body lipolysis during exercise. Am J Physiol Endocrinol Metab 2004;286(2):E217—25.

[50] Bachmann OP, Dahl DB, Brechtel K, Machann J, Haap M, Maier T, Loviscach M, Stumvoll M, Claussen CD, Schick F, Häring HU, Jacob S. Effects of intravenous and dietary lipid challenge on intramyocellular lipid content and the relation with insulin sensitivity in humans. Diabetes 2001;50(11):2579—84. https://doi.org/10.2337/diabetes.50.11.2579.

[51] Yost TJ, Jensen DR, Haugen BR, Eckel RH. Effect of dietary macronutrient composition on tissue-specific lipoprotein lipase activity and insulin action in normal-weight subjects. Am J Clin Nutr 1998;68(2):296—302.

[52] Lindeboom L, Nabuurs CI, Hesselink MKC, Wildberger JE, Schrauwen P, Schrauwen-Hinderling VB. Proton magnetic resonance spectroscopy reveals increased hepatic lipid content after a single high-fat meal with no additional modulation by added protein. Am J Clin Nutr 2015;101(1):65—71. https://doi.org/10.3945/ajcn.114.094730.

[53] Bortolotti M, Kreis R, Debard C, Cariou B, Faeh D, Chetiveaux M, Ith M, Vermathen P, Stefanoni N, Lê K-A, Schneiter P, Krempf M, Vidal H, Boesch C, Tappy L. High protein intake reduces intrahepatocellular lipid deposition in humans. Am J Clin Nutr 2009;90(4):1002—10. https://doi.org/10.3945/ajcn.2008.27296.

[54] van der Meer RW, Hammer S, Lamb HJ, Frölich M, Diamant M, Rijzewijk LJ, de Roos A, Romijn JA, Smit JWA. Effects of short-term high-fat, high-energy diet on hepatic and myocardial triglyceride content in healthy men. J Clin Endocrinol Metabol 2008;93(7):2702—8. https://doi.org/10.1210/jc.2007-2524.

[55] Kiens B, Essen-Gustavsson B, Gad P, Lithell H. Lipoprotein lipase activity and intramuscular triglyceride stores after long-term high-fat and high-carbohydrate diets in physically trained men. Clin Physiol 1987;7(1):1—9.

[56] Schrauwen-Hinderling VB, Kooi ME, Hesselink MK, Moonen-Kornips E, Schaart G, Mustard KJ, Hardie DG, Saris WH, Nicolay K, Schrauwen P. Intramyocellular lipid content and molecular adaptations in response to a 1-week high-fat diet. Obes Res 2005;13(12):2088—94. https://doi.org/10.1038/oby.2005.259.

[57] St-Onge MP, Newcomer BR, Buchthal S, Aban I, Allison DB, Bosarge A, Gower B. Intramyocellular lipid content is lower with a low-fat diet than with high-fat diets, but that may not be relevant for health. Am J Clin Nutr 2007;86(5):1316—22. https://doi.org/10.1093/ajcn/86.5.1316.

[58] van Herpen NA, Schrauwen-Hinderling VB, Schaart G, Mensink RP, Schrauwen P. Three weeks on a high-fat diet increases intrahepatic lipid accumulation and decreases metabolic flexibility in healthy overweight men. J Clin Endocrinol Metabol 2011;96(4):E691—5. https://doi.org/10.1210/jc.2010-2243.

[59] Lê K-A, Ith M, Kreis R, Faeh D, Bortolotti M, Tran C, Boesch C, Tappy L. Fructose overconsumption causes dyslipidemia and ectopic lipid deposition in healthy subjects with and without a family history of type 2 diabetes. Am J Clin Nutr 2009;89(6):1760—5. https://doi.org/10.3945/ajcn.2008.27336.

[60] Lecoultre V, Egli L, Carrel G, Theytaz F, Kreis R, Schneiter P, Boss A, Zwygart K, Lê K-A, Bortolotti M, Boesch C, Tappy L. Effects of fructose and glucose overfeeding on hepatic insulin sensitivity and intrahepatic lipids in healthy humans. Obesity 2013;21(4):782—5. https://doi.org/10.1002/oby.20377.

[61] Theytaz F, Noguchi Y, Egli L, Campos V, Buehler T, Hodson L, Patterson BW, Nishikata N, Kreis R, Mittendorfer B, Fielding B, Boesch C, Tappy L. Effects of supplementation with essential amino acids on intrahepatic lipid concentrations during fructose overfeeding in humans. Am J Clin Nutr 2012;96(5):1008—16. https://doi.org/10.3945/ajcn.112.035139.

[62] Simons N, Veeraiah P, Simons P, Schaper NC, Kooi ME, Schrauwen-Hinderling VB, Feskens E, van der Ploeg E, Van den Eynde M, Schalkwijk CG, Stehouwer C, Brouwers M. Effects of fructose restriction on liver steatosis (FRUITLESS); a double-blind randomized controlled trial. Am J Clin Nutr 2021;113(2):391—400. https://doi.org/10.1093/ajcn/nqaa332.

[63] Jacobs I, Lithell H, Karlsson J. Dietary effects on glycogen and lipoprotein lipase activity in skeletal muscle in man. Acta Physiol Scand 1982;115(1):85—90.

Chapter 7

Nonalcoholic fatty liver disease: from a benign finding to a life-threatening cardiometabolic liver disease

Koen C. van Son[1,2,3], A.G. (Onno) Holleboom[2] and Maarten E. Tushuizen[3]

[1]Department of Gastroenterology and Hepatology, Radboud University Medical Center, Nijmegen, the Netherlands; [2]Department of Internal Medicine, Amsterdam University Medical Center, Amsterdam, the Netherlands; [3]Department of Gastroenterology and Hepatology, Leiden University Medical Center, Leiden, the Netherlands

Introduction

Elevated liver enzymes are an increasingly common finding in routine medical blood testing. Often, a subsequently performed liver ultrasound shows signs of hepatic steatosis, more commonly known as fatty liver. The most common cause of hepatic steatosis is nonalcoholic fatty liver disease (NAFLD) [1−5]. NAFLD is defined as an accumulation of fat in the liver of > 5% found on imaging or by histology, in the absence of other causes of hepatic steatosis (such as excessive alcohol intake or use of certain medications, Table 7.1). The spectrum of NAFLD reaches from simple liver steatosis, also known as nonalcoholic fatty liver (NAFL), to nonalcoholic steatohepatitis (NASH), development of liver fibrosis, and eventually progression to cirrhosis and hepatocellular carcinoma (HCC) (Fig. 7.1) [1]. Currently, clinical care paths for patients with this potentially harmful disease are being developed [6,7].

NAFLD is mainly associated with obesity and is therefore increasingly common as a result of the "Western lifestyle," characterized by an unhealthy high-caloric diet and too little exercise. In 2016, the World Health Organization (WHO) showed a global prevalence of overweight (BMI $\geq$ 25 kg/m^2) of 36% within the general adult population and a global prevalence of obesity (BMI $\geq$ 30 kg/m^2) of 13%, with an estimated increasing trend [3].

In concert with strong increases in obesity and type 2 diabetes mellitus, the prevalence and severity of NAFLD are growing steadily [4]. At present, worldwide, over 25% of the adult population suffers from some stage of NAFLD [4]. In high-risk populations, such as patients with the metabolic syndrome or type 2 diabetes mellitus, the prevalence of NAFLD is over 60% [5]. Due to its strong association with obesity and type 2 diabetes mellitus, NAFLD is regarded as the hepatic component of the metabolic syndrome. Furthermore, NAFLD is increasingly diagnosed in children. In the period of 1988−1994, its prevalence in adolescents (12−19 years old) in the United States was calculated at 3.9%, which tripled to 10.7% in 2007−2010 [8]. More recently, the prevalence of NAFLD in nonobese children between 0 and 19 years old is estimated at almost 8% worldwide, while in obese children, this prevalence is even estimated to be over 34% [9].

Its high prevalence results in a large burden on healthcare, associated costs, a reduction of quality of life, and increased mortality rates [1,3−5]. Similar to the slowly progressive development of atherosclerosis that precedes overt cardiovascular disease, NAFLD-NASH usually only causes clinical signs of liver failure in patients after decades of exposure to metabolic risk factors, especially in case of concurrent risk factors such as excessive alcohol use or viral hepatitis [10].

TABLE 7.1 Causes of hepatic steatosis.

NAFLD	Most common concurrent diseases

• NAFL
  ○ Pure steatosis
  ○ Steatosis with mild lobular inflammation
	• AFLD—alcoholic fatty liver disease (alcohol in ♂ ≥ 30 g/day, in ♀ ≥ 20 g/day)
	
	• Drug-induced (amiodarone, MTX, tamoxifen, corticosteroids, valproate, antiretroviral)
	
	• Hepatitis C (genotype 3)

• NASH
  ○ Early NASH: none or mild (F0−F1) fibrosis
  ○ Fibrotic NASH: significant (≥F2) or advanced (≥F3, bridging) fibrosis
  ○ NASH cirrhosis (F4)
• Hepatocellular carcinoma
	• Other:
	  ○ Hemochromatosis
	  ○ Autoimmune hepatitis (AIH)
	  ○ Celiac disease
	  ○ Wilson's disease
	  ○ Acute fatty liver of the pregnancy (AFLP)
	  ○ Lipodystrophy
	  ○ Hormonal (hypopituitarism, hypothyroidism)
	  ○ Fasting/starvation
	  ○ Parental feeding
	  ○ Metabolic disease (LCAT deficiency, Wolman's disease (liposomal acid lipase deficiency)

*Associated with components of the metabolic syndrome (waist ♂≥94 and ♀≥80 cm; blood pressure ≥130/85 mmHg or treatment; fasting plasma glucose ≥5.6 mmol/L or treatment; fasting plasma triglycerides ≥1.7 mmol/L; HDL cholesterol ♂<1.0 and ♀<1.3 mmol/L).

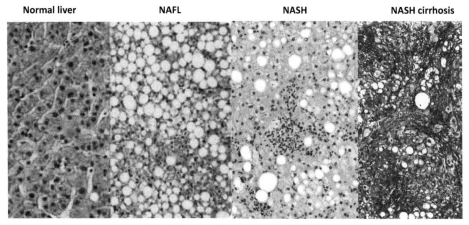

FIGURE 7.1 Different stages of NAFLD

Pathogenesis

Genetic and epigenetic determinants

Genetic variations, especially single nucleotide polymorphisms, exert an effect on all further mentioned pathophysiologic mechanisms, simplified in Fig. 7.2. Most important is the gene that codes for *patatin-like phospholipase 3* (PNPLA3), a protein homologous to enzymes involved in the lipid metabolism [11]. Single nucleotide polymorphisms within this gene are involved in the development and progression of NAFLD. The PNPLA3 I148M (rs738409 C/G-) variant is highly associated with an increase in hepatic steatosis and fibrosis and is responsible for circa 5.3% of total genetic variations in NAFLD susceptibility. Another gene of which variation is associated with NAFLD susceptibility is *transmembrane 6 superfamily member 2* (TM6SF2). The TM6SF2 protein stimulates hepatic secretion of very-low-density lipoprotein (VLDL)-cholesterol, which is limited in the rs58542926 variant. This causes VLDL to accumulate in the liver, resulting in steatosis, elevated plasma ALT values, and lower VLDL plasma concentrations. Two other genes that have emerged in this context are MBOAT7, a gene involved in the phospholipid remodeling cycle [12], and HSD17B13, a gene regulating uptake of lipid droplets within the liver [13].

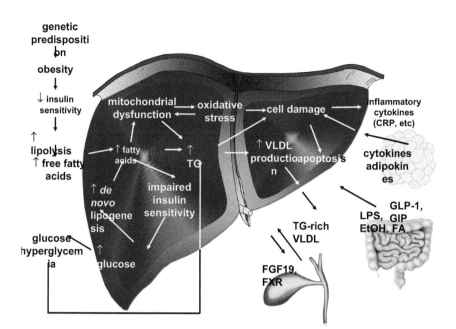

FIGURE 7.2 Pathogenesis of NAFLD

Nutrition

Excessive caloric intake is one of the major causes of the development of obesity, insulin resistance, and NAFLD. Studies have shown that doubling of the daily caloric intake with so-called fast foods in healthy volunteers results in elevated plasma ALT levels and increased steatosis within 4 weeks' time [14].

When studying the pathogenesis of NAFLD, it is important to take into account the effects of different types of nutrients. It has been shown that a diet high in carbohydrates is linked to NAFLD, as it stimulates insulin resistance and de novo lipogenesis. De novo lipogenesis of carbohydrates accounts for up to 26% of increased fatty acids in the liver. Notorious in this regard is fructose, which can be found in, for instance, sodas [15–17]. Studies in both animals and humans have shown that fructose stimulates de novo lipogenesis and blocks fatty acid oxidation in the liver, thus resulting in hepatic steatosis, increased oxidative stress, and hepatic fibrosis [18,19]. Additionally, fructose induces rapidly elevated blood glucose levels, followed by reactive hypoglycemia [20], and fructose inhibits leptin, thereby suppressing the sensation of hunger and resulting in overeating [21]. Yet, even with a normocaloric diet hepatic steatosis may develop if the diet is high in sugars such as fructose and sucrose [19].

Dietary lipids are involved in NAFLD to a lesser extent than dietary carbohydrates, as only about 15% of hepatic lipids in NAFLD patients are traced back to dietary fat [22]. High intake of saturated fats and cholesterol triggers lipolysis in adipocytes and increases free fatty acids (FFAs), resulting in reduced plasma adiponectin levels, attenuated lipid clearance from plasma, and increased beta-oxidation in muscles [21]. This causes increased uptake and storage of FFAs by the liver, resulting in hepatic steatosis.

On the other hand, the consumption of monounsaturated fatty acids (MUFAs) and polyunsaturated fatty acids (PUFAs) tends to have protective effects against NAFLD [17,20]. This is especially true for MUFAs, which can be found in foods such as peanuts and avocados, and omega-3 class PUFAs, which are mostly present in fish. PUFAs can improve insulin sensitivity, suppress de novo lipogenesis, and can enhance fatty acid oxidation. This is supported by various clinical nutritional interventions that indicate that the administration of omega-3 PUFAs reduces hepatic steatosis [20,23].

Diets characterized by a high intake of fast foods and rich in saturated fatty acids, transfats, simple sugars such as fructose and sucrose, red and processed meats, full-fat dairy products, and soft drinks have harmful effects on the liver [17]. This can be said for the so-called Western diet, which is particularly rich in saturated fat and added fructose. In contrast, the Mediterranean diet, which is low in saturated fat and cholesterol and rich in monounsaturated fats, omega-3 fatty acids, complicated carbohydrates, dietary fiber, and plant-based proteins, is beneficial to the liver and associated with lower rates of NAFLD [17].

Moreover, nutrition also plays a major role in the gut microbiome composition. Alterations in the gut microbiota influence the energy metabolism and nutrient absorption of the gut. Recent studies, both in humans and in mice, have shown specific gut microbiota to be associated to liver steatosis, obesity, and type 2 diabetes mellitus [24−28].

Insulin resistance and lipotoxicity

Insulin resistance plays a central role in the pathogenesis of NAFLD and NASH; however, the pathogenesis is complex with multiple factors playing an interactive role creating vicious circles [29,30]. Insulin resistance causes lipolysis in the peripheral adipose tissue, resulting in increased circulating FFAs [22]. These FFAs accumulate in the liver, where they stimulate the formation and accumulation of triglycerides within hepatocytes. This process leads to hepatic insulin insensitivity and hepatic gluconeogenesis, causing hyperglycemia and intrahepatic conversion of glucose into FFAs. The high plasma insulin levels, as part of systemic insulin resistance, amplify this process and simultaneously stimulate de novo lipogenesis, increasing the accumulation of FFAs. Subsequent upregulation of SREBP1c and ChREBP even further increases de novo lipogenesis, the production of triglycerides, and gluconeogenesis.

Ultimately, all these processes together cause an abundance of FFAs and triglycerides, to which the liver responds with four compensatory mechanisms: intracellular uptake in *lipid droplets*, resulting in the characteristic liver steatosis; secretion of lipids, leading to the characteristic mixed dyslipidemia seen in the majority of NAFLD patients; breakdown by mitochondrial beta-oxidation; and autophagia of lipid droplets (lipophagy). When these compensatory mechanisms fall short, lipotoxicity occurs. Lipotoxicity causes mitochondrial dysfunction that causes formation of reactive oxygen species (oxidative stress), resulting in inflammation and cell damage [31−33].

Inflammation and necroapoptosis

The overload of FFAs triggers two proinflammatory pathways: *c-jun terminal kinase* (JNK) via *apoptosis signal-regulating kinase 1* (ASK-1), and *nuclear factor kappa-light-chain-enhancer of activated B cells* (NF-kB). JNK induces inflammation and regulated cell death or apoptosis. The transcription factor NF-kB regulates acute inflammatory responses. Continuous activation of these pathways leads to the characteristic necroinflammation of hepatocytes found in liver biopsies, the differentiating factor between simple steatosis and NASH [34].

Adipocytokines

Another proinflammatory pathway is formed by cytokines from visceral fat tissue (so-called adipocytokines), such as IL-6 and TNF-α. These adipocytokines are directly transported to the liver through the portal system and lead to a proinflammatory hepatic environment [34−36]. High concentrations of leptin also contribute to this process by activating Kupffer cells and hepatic stellate cells. The anti-inflammatory and antifibrotic compound adiponectin is decreased as a result of excessive adipose tissue [37].

Formation of fibrosis

Lipotoxicity and oxidative stress trigger hepatocytes and Kupffer cells (intrahepatic macrophages) to form signal molecules that initiate fibrogenesis by converting resting hepatic stellate cells to active myofibroblasts. These myofibroblasts deposit collagen and other components of extracellular matrix within the liver; an essential step in the pathologic process of NASH-related fibrosis. The transcription factor *transcriptional coactivator with a PDZ-binding domain* (TAZ) has been identified as a NASH-specific pathway of fibrogenesis, sending paracrine profibrotic signals to hepatic stellate cells through the production of *Indian hedgehog ligand* [38].

Urea cycle dysregulation

The urea cycle takes place within the mitochondria and cytoplasm of hepatocytes and is an important process in which the toxic compound ammonia is catabolized into the nontoxic compound urea. Recent studies show a reduced expression of urea cycle enzymes in both animal studies and patients with NAFLD/NASH. Mitochondrial dysfunction in NASH is believed to underlie this decrease in the mitochondrial enzymes *carbamoylphosphate synthetase* (CPS1) and *ornithine transcarbamylase* (OTC), which causes dysregulation of the urea cycle process in the liver. The subsequent accumulation of ammonia may accelerate liver injury and fibrosis. Cell culture studies show that removal of ammonia from supernatants restores morphology and function of hepatic stellate cells, suggesting the process may be reversible [39,40].

Bile acids

Besides their function in absorbing lipids in the gut, there is accumulating evidence suggesting that bile acids also play a major role as signaling molecules in the liver and gut. Bile acids regulate the energy metabolism of lipids, sugars, and proteins by activating receptors like the farnesoid X-receptor (FXR) and Takeda G protein—coupled receptor 5 (TGR5). FXR is a transcription factor that decreases lipogenesis and gluconeogenesis and increases insulin sensitivity in the liver and gut. TGR5 is a membrane-bound receptor in muscle and adipose tissue that increases thermogenesis and energy expenditure [41,42]. There are multiple ongoing drug studies using bile acid derivatives and mimetics as possible treatments for NASH.

Microbiome

Like many other liver diseases, NASH is associated with a dysbiosis of gut bacteria. These alterations in the gut microbiome are most likely a result of dietary composition. A diet rich in lipids, animal-derived proteins, and sugars provides a more favorable culture medium for certain bacterial species (like Bacteroides) than for others [43,44]. However, the mechanisms that underlie the development of NASH through microbiome imbalance are not yet fully understood. One hypothesis is that certain bacterial compositions increase gut permeability, thereby exposing the portal vein and liver to (products of) gut bacteria that induce various inflammatory pathways. Another hypothesis is that gut bacteria may induce or protect against NASH by producing (anti-)inflammatory metabolites. Both harmful metabolites, such as alcohol, and protective microbes and their metabolites, such as *Eubacterium hallii* and butyrate, have been identified as possible mechanisms in the development of liver steatosis in recent mouse models [45]. A recent study showed that presence of high-alcohol-producing strains of *Klebsiella pneumoniae* in the gut was strongly associated with disease severity in a NAFLD cohort and could induce development of fatty liver disease in murine models. The endoalcohol production of these bacteria might activate similar molecular mechanisms as in fatty liver disease mediated by alcohol [46]. Finally, gut bacteria play an important role in the modification of bile acids. The dysbiosis of the microbiome can lead to alterations in bile acid composition, potentially decreasing the affinity of bile acid receptors for the absorption and metabolism of lipids, resulting in dysregulation of the energy metabolism [41,47].

Clinical consequences

Liver cirrhosis

Although NAFLD was previously considered to be relatively benign, increasing evidence has shown it can develop into a seriously harmful disease [48]. Especially in patients with NASH, the formation of fibrosis and cirrhosis adds not only to increased mortality but mainly also to increased morbidity. Data from the American Transplant Registry show that in 2018, NAFLD/NASH-related cirrhosis became the main indication for liver transplantation, overtaking other liver diseases such as hepatitis B/C and alcohol-related liver injury [49]. An additional problem is that the number of donors with signs of NAFLD is also rising, increasing the risk of posttransplantation complications for the recipient.

Hepatocellular carcinoma

HCC is often diagnosed in patients who were not yet known to have NAFLD and can even occur at the precirrhotic stage [50]. Patients with NAFLD who develop HCC have decreased survival rates compared with HCC patients with underlying alcoholic liver cirrhosis, potentially due to reduced susceptibility of NAFLD-HCC to immune surveillance [51]. Moreover, NAFLD has also been suggested as a risk factor for colon and breast cancer [52,53].

Cardiovascular disease

It is clear that patients with NAFLD have an increased risk to develop cardiovascular disease, considering the shared risk factors [54,55]. Recent research shows that the extent of hepatic steatosis (both measured by ultrasonography as measured by FibroScan with CAP) is associated with the amount of arterial stenosis on coronary angiography in patients after recent myocardial infarction [55]. A recent meta-analysis shows that NAFLD increases the risk of fatal and nonfatal cardiovascular disease (odds ratio 2.58 [1,78—3,75]). Moreover, the cumulative risk for mortality is increased in patients with coronary disease and stage 3 steatosis compared with patients with coronary disease and stage 1 and 2 steatosis [56,57]. Interestingly and as an expectation to the rule, patients who carry the TM6SF2 minor allele have a decreased risk of developing cardiovascular disease, likely due to the accumulation of harmful lipids within the liver and less within arterial atherosclerotic plaques [58]. Not only is the extent of fibrosis in patients with NAFLD associated with atherosclerosis, but it is also related to decreased left ventricular function [59]. Unfortunately, there are no data on the effect of treatment of NAFLD on "static endpoints" such as cardiovascular disease mortality; this open question is currently being addressed in ongoing multiple phase 3 drug trials.

Diagnostics

Most patients (but not all) with NAFLD express (slightly) elevated serum liver enzymes such as ALT, AST, and gamma-GT. Although they may serve as a diagnostic clue for the presence of liver disease, they fail to predict the presence and severity of hepatic steatosis, inflammation (NASH), and fibrosis. Therefore, various scores have been developed to estimate these aspects of NAFLD in a noninvasive way, such as the Fatty Liver Index [60] and the FIB4-score [61]. Various biomarkers and biomarker panels have also been proposed, such as procollagen CIII (pro-CIII) [62] and cytokeratin-18 fragments (CK-18) [63]; FibroTest (alpha2-macroglobulin, apolipoprotein A1, haptoglobin, GGT, bilirubin); and the Enhanced Liver Fibrosis (ELF-)test (hyaluronic acid, amino-terminal propeptide-of-type−III−collagen, tissue inhibitor of matrix metalloproteinase-1) [64]. However, the accuracy, validation, and availability of these scores and biomarkers are limited to date [61,65,66] and are currently being tested and validated in large-scale European (LITMUS) [67] and American (NIMBLE) biobank studies.

Ultrasonography, in which the reflection pattern of the liver is compared with the kidneys and/or spleen, is a tool often used to determine the presence and extent of hepatic steatosis [68]. This diagnostic test is widely available (especially in primary care) and of small cost, although its sensitivity is limited in patients with moderate steatosis (< 20%) and in those with a BMI ≥ 40 kg/m^2 [69]. Furthermore, ultrasonography cannot determine the presence and extent of inflammation (NASH) and fibrosis.

"Vibration-controlled" transient elastography, VCTE or FibroScan (brand name), is a noninvasive tool that can be used to measure the elasticity of the liver, thereby determining the presence and extent of steatosis [70]. This technique uses the simultaneous emission of both sonographic and electrical waves. Using the velocity of wave transmission through the tissue, it estimates liver elasticity: the faster the wave, the stiffer the tissue, as in fibrosis. By also using the extinguishment of the ultrasonography signal (the so-called *continued attenuation parameter*, or CAP), it estimates the amount of hepatic steatosis. This test was recently shown to be very accurate and easy to perform, and its availability in secondary care is expected to rise over the next few years [70].

The most accurate noninvasive method to diagnose and quantify liver steatosis is MRI, especially using the so-called PDFF (*proton density fat fraction*) technique [71]. This technique can be used to accurately assess the presence of fat in the liver and can thus be used to diagnose hepatic steatosis when hepatic triglyceride content ≥ 5.56%. Furthermore, liver fibrosis and inflammation can be assessed using specific MRI modalities, namely MRE 2D, MRE 3D, and cT1. Schaapman et al. proposed a multiparametric MR clinical algorithm that would allow diagnosis of hepatic steatosis as well as NASH and liver fibrosis using MRI modalities [72]. However, because this test is time-consuming, expensive, and of limited availability and its validity to measure fibrosis has not yet been confirmed, it is currently unsuitable for clinical use.

To date, the golden standard for diagnosing NASH remains a liver biopsy, in which the characteristic swelling of hepatocytes (ballooning) and lobular inflammation can be established (Fig. 7.1). An important additional benefit of liver biopsy is the possibility to assess the presence and extent of liver fibrosis. However, liver biopsy is an invasive procedure that can be painful, has a risk of postbiopsy bleeding (ca. 2%), and might convey a sampling error, due to only about 1/50.000th of the liver tissue being analyzed, while NAFLD is often not equally distributed throughout the liver [73].

Treatment

To date, there are no registered medical treatment options for NAFLD and NASH. However, the high healthcare burden of NAFLD has stimulated the research field, and the great variety of the described pathophysiological mechanisms involved in the development of NAFLD has resulted in many points of interest for potential treatment options. There are several ongoing phase 2 and phase 3 studies of which the results are to be evaluated in the upcoming years [74].

Obesity and lifestyle

The cornerstone of the treatment of NAFLD consists of lifestyle alterations [75,76]. A weight reduction of 8% has been shown to result in a 50% decrease in liver fat [76]. In patients undergoing bariatric surgery, a reduction in body weight of over 10% can even lead to regression of hepatic inflammation and fibrosis [77]. Yet, an increase in physical activity without any reduction in body weight also has a positive effect on hepatic steatosis [76]. Lifestyle changes and weight reduction are expected to remain centrally important within the treatment of NAFLD, since they exert positive effects not only on NAFLD but also on associated metabolic and cardiovascular diseases.

Nutrition

The Mediterranean diet, consisting of mainly single unsaturated fats derived from fish or olive oil, helps to reduce the amount of liver fat and insulin insensitivity, even without inducing body weight reduction [78]. Limiting the amount of free sugars in the diet has also been shown to have a positive effect on NAFLD [76]. Interestingly, the usage of three or more cups of coffee a day protects against NAFLD and the formation of fibrosis, possibly through an increase in autophagia of lipid droplets within hepatocytes [79].

Insulin sensitivity

Metformin, a treatment often used in patients with type 2 diabetes mellitus, has clearly positive effects on NASH, but not on fibrosis. The effect seems to be mainly connected to its induction of weight reduction [80]. In small studies, thiazolidinediones such as pioglitazone and rosiglitazone, which increase insulin sensitivity, have been shown to have a positive effect on NAFLD through the PPARgamma-agonism [81,82]. However, they come with disadvantages such as an increase in body weight, negative cardiovascular effects (mainly with rosiglitazone), and a possible association with the development of bladder cancer [83]. Recently, a phase 3 study on elafibranor, a combined PPAR-alfa-delta-agonist, failed to meet the predefined primary endpoint of NASH resolution without worsening of fibrosis in the intention to treat (ITT) population of 1070 patients. Although the secondary endpoint related to metabolic parameters did not achieve statistical significance, the study is being extended to reassess outcomes [84].

GLP1 receptor agonists and GLP1 analogs

GLP1 receptor agonists and analogs (liraglutide and semaglutide, respectively, exenatide) have direct effects on pancreatic insulin production but also impact the heart, brain, and gastrointestinal system [85]. There are no unambiguous data about a direct effect of these medications on the liver. Liraglutide seems to have a positive effect on NASH and even the formation of fibrosis by reducing body weight, even in patients without type 2 diabetes mellitus [86]. However, a phase 2 trial involving patients with NASH showed that treatment with semaglutide resulted in a significantly higher percentage of patients with NASH resolution than placebo. However, the trial did not show a significant between-group difference in the percentage of patients with an improvement in fibrosis stage [87].

SGLT2 inhibitors

SGLT2 inhibitors, including canagliflozine, dapagliflozine, and empaglifozine, target the sodium glucose cotransporter 2 in the kidneys. By selectively and reversibly blocking this cotransporter, they inhibit renal glucose reabsorption in the proximal tubule, which increases the excretion of glucose with the urine and reduces blood glucose levels in patients with type 2 diabetes mellitus. Because of safety concerns and the limited effects of the established drugs (only < 50% of serum glucose can be excreted via the urine), ongoing research is seeking novel/safer SGLT2 inhibitors. A potentially promising new SGLT2 inhibitor with partial suppression of SGLT1 has been proposed in recent murine studies [88].

Lipotoxicity

Although there have been safety concerns in the past about the prescription of statins in patients with elevated liver enzymes, these medications seem to have positive effects not only by decreasing risk of cardiovascular disease but also by inhibiting formation of hepatic fibrosis [89]. Moreover, multiple agents are being developed to block de novo lipogenesis within the liver (ACC inhibitors). There are, however, no results within this field yet [90].

Oxidative stress

Vitamin E is a well-known antioxidant and exerts a positive effect on the amount of liver fat when prescribed in high doses (800 IE a day) [91]. Unfortunately, no data is available on the effect of vitamin E on fibrosis, and high doses also seem to increase risk of developing prostate cancer and cerebrovascular accidents (CVAs). The European Liver Association guideline (developed in collaboration with the associations for diabetes and obesity) advises to consider vitamin E for patients with severe NAFLD in consultation with the patient [10].

Bile acids

Research shows that both ursodeoxycholic acid (a bile acid preparation) and colesevelam (a bile acid—binding resin) have no effect on the amount of liver fat [92,93]. However, in the phase 2 FLINT trial, the FXR-agonist obeticholic acid has been shown to induce in a histologic response of NASH in 46% of the participants who were given 25 mg of obeticholic acid a day (compared with 21% in the placebo group) [94]. Unfortunately, a commonly reported side effect (23%) was itching. The REGENERATE trial, a phase 3 trial concerning obeticholic acid, showed a small but significant reduction of fibrosis compared to the placebo group [95].

Apoptosis

Apoptosis signal-regulating kinase 1 (ASK1) is activated by extracellular TNF-α, intracellular oxidative stress, and ER stress and initiates the p38/JNK "pathway," resulting in apoptosis and fibrosis [96]. Selonsertib is an ASK1 inhibitor that was recently investigated in two phase 3 studies, one in F3 fibrosis, and one in F4 fibrosis. Both studies showed no significant effect of selonsertib on hepatic steatosis, inflammation, or fibrosis [84].

Inflammation and fibrosis

Cenicriviroc is a CCR2/5 antagonist, thereby inhibiting macrophages in the peripheral fat tissue, which improves insulin sensitivity and inhibits migration, activation, and proliferation of stellate cells. A phase 2 trial showed positive results of cenicriviroc on hepatic steatosis, inflammation, and fibrosis, and a phase 3 trial is currently being performed [97].

Thyroid hormone and thyroid mimetics have the potential to reduce NAFLD-NASH. There are signs that these hormones exert positive effects on hepatic steatosis by mediating the induction of autophagia of lipid droplets and mitochondrial beta-oxidation of fatty acids [98]. In 20 patients with type 2 diabetes mellitus and NAFLD, a low dose of thyroid hormone resulted in significant reduction of intrahepatic fat, measured by MRI-PDFF [99]. A phase 2 trial in which 78 patients with NASH were treated with a selective thyroid hormone receptor beta-agonist showed a significant reduction of intrahepatic fat measured by MRI-PDFF [100]. A phase 3 trial with this selective thyroid hormone receptor beta-agonist is currently ongoing [101].

Combination therapy

Because of the complex pathogenesis of the disease, future medical treatment of progressive NAFLD is expected to consist of combination therapy, not unlike the current multidimensional treatment of type 2 diabetes mellitus and hypertension. Different types of combination therapy are already being investigated in clinical trials, even before the first monotherapy for NASH has been registered. In the phase 2 ATLAS trial, selonsertib was combined with acetyl-CoA carboxylase (ACC) inhibition and an FXR-agonist over a period of 48 weeks. Although the primary endpoint of ≥ 1 fibrosis stage improvement without worsening of NASH was not met, significant improvement of various parameters including reduction in steatosis, lobular inflammation, and ballooning and significant improvements in ELF-score and liver stiffness by transient elastography (all $P \leq .05$) were shown [102]. Other combination strategies are awaited.

Probiotics and fecal microbiome transplantation

Animal model research suggests that influencing the microbiome by using probiotics has a positive effect on liver steatosis [43]. A placebo-controlled pilot study in 20 patients with biopsy-proven NAFLD showed a decrease in liver steatosis after 6 months of treatment with probiotics consisting of various species such as *Lactiplantibacillus plantarum*, *Lactobacillus delbrueckii* spp. *bulgaricus*, *Lactobacillus acidophilus*, *Lactobacillus rhamnosus*, and *Bifidobacterium bifidum*. A decrease in hepatic steatosis was found, which was associated with an increase in *Bacteroides* and a decrease of *Firmicutes* species [103].

Interestingly, a recent study demonstrated that allogenic fecal microbiome transplantation (FMT) using lean vegan donors in individuals with hepatic steatosis shows an effect on intestinal microbiota composition, which was associated with beneficial changes in plasma metabolites and markers of steatohepatitis, but not histology [104].

Development and implementation of clinical care paths and guidelines for NAFLD

Despite the rising prevalence and severity of NAFLD, there is still much room for improvement among healthcare professionals across the lines of care and also on the national guideline level. Lazarus et al. conducted an investigation assessing the NAFLD guidelines and strategies of 29 European countries [2]. The United Kingdom scored highest, mainly driven by a national guideline that focuses on early detection of NAFLD and associated comorbidities in primary care. None of the surveyed countries had written strategies for NAFLD assessment, 10 had clinical guidelines regarding NAFLD, and 11 recommended screening in patients with type 2 diabetes mellitus, obesity, and/or metabolic syndrome. This paper maps the challenges in health policy, guidelines, epidemiological grasp, and care management for NAFLD [2].

The unnoticed progression of NAFLD and limited awareness among healthcare professionals both lead to overreferrals and underdiagnoses. Most cases referred for assessment of NAFLD by the general practitioner or the internist to the hepatologist actually have mildly active and mildly progressive disease and could have been retained in primary care. On the other hand, patients with obesity and type 2 diabetes mellitus may progress to NAFLD with fibrosis stage 3 or 4 (F3—F4) while being under care of their general practitioner or internist, because the hepatic component of their metabolic syndrome is being overlooked [2]. The EASL-EASD-EASO guideline states that noninvasive tests (NITs) should aim to identify and assess NAFLD in individuals with increased metabolic risk in primary care and that NITs in secondary and tertiary care should identify those with worse liver prognosis [10].

Primary care

For primary care, Srivastava et al. published the Camden & Islington care path, using a two-tier system with FIB4-score and ELF plasma test to detect advanced stages of NASH fibrosis in primary care pracstices [105]. This pathway led to a profound reduction of referrals to the hepatologist by 80%, while at the same time significantly improving the detection of advanced fibrosis or cirrhosis by fourfold. In this care path, patients with steatosis hepatis on ultrasound and/or elevated ALT levels were included when excessive alcohol use or other liver diseases were excluded [105].

In addition to screening patients with elevated ALT or hepatic steatosis with ultrasound, several guidelines state that screening for advanced liver disease in patients with type 2 diabetes mellitus should be performed based on the high prevalence of NASH and liver fibrosis within this group of patients [10,70,106]. Additionally, according to the EASL-EASD-EASO guideline, this screening should be irrespective of liver enzyme levels, when risk factors for NAFLD such as type 2 diabetes mellitus and obesity are present [10]. A recent prospective study determined prevalence and severity of NAFLD by liver biopsy among patients with type 2 diabetes mellitus. The prevalence of significant ($\geq$F2) and advanced fibrosis ($\geq$F3) were 29.5% and 29.5%, respectively. Based on these results, more aggressive screening for NAFLD and fibrosis in patients with type 2 diabetes mellitus seems justified [106]. For the screening of this high-risk group attending primary care, the NAFLD Fibrosis Score (NFS), FIB4-score, and VCTE can be used to identify those at low or high risk of advanced fibrosis [107], since increased liver enzymes alone are insensitive for advanced fibrosis [108]. FIB4-score and NFS perform best at excluding severe fibrosis and cirrhosis, with negative predictive values of > 90%. Because of these high negative predictive values, these tests could be used in primary care to identify patients at low risk of severe fibrosis [107]. Unfortunately, due to low performance in patients with type 2 diabetes mellitus, noninvasive tests including the FIB4-score and NFS seem unsuitable for evaluating liver fibrosis in this group [109,110]. Moreover, the FIB4-score has been shown to underestimate the presence of advanced disease in elderly patients. Thus, higher cutoff points have been suggested for patients aged $\geq$ 65 years [111].

Secondary and tertiary care

In secondary and tertiary care, different guidelines recommend NITs to distinguish patients with NAFLD at low risk from those at high risk of advanced fibrosis [2,107]. To incorporate NITs into clinical practice, the simplest strategy is to start with a test with a high negative likelihood ratio to rule out high-risk cases [112]. In the European [10] and American [107] guidelines for the management of NAFLD in secondary and tertiary care, the NFS and FIB4-score are mentioned as possible NITs with intensive external validation in ethnically diverse NAFLD populations, with consistent results. These fibrosis scores and other biomarkers, as well as VCTE, are acceptable noninvasive procedures for the identification of patients at low risk of advanced fibrosis [113]. A recent meta-analysis showed that the ELF-test is an option in high prevalence settings such as secondary and tertiary care [114]. However, the ELF-test consists of three relatively complex assays and is patented and therefore comes at a higher cost than the FIB4-score. In a screening study with 1,000 patients with NAFLD, the ELF-test was even more costly than the combination of FIB4-score and VCTE for patients with an indeterminate FIB4-score. Detection of advanced fibrosis was comparable between the ELF-test and FIB4-score/VCTE [114]. Combination of an NIT with VCTE would increase diagnostic accuracy and might reduce the number of liver biopsies [107,113]. Yet, comparative care path studies with large sample sizes are required to determine the optimal two-tiered care path screening test combination.

In the evaluation of NAFLD, excessive alcohol consumption, and other, more sporadic liver diseases should be excluded. In addition, upon suspicion of NAFLD, associated comorbidities, such as obesity, type 2 diabetes mellitus, dyslipidemia, hypothyroidism, polycystic ovary syndrome, sleep apnea, and hypogonadism, should be assessed and treated [10,107]. Consideration of a liver biopsy is recommended when significant fibrosis is confirmed by screening with NITs and VCTE, and only if it impacts disease management [10,107]. In patients with indeterminate results upon screening (for example, positive autoimmune hepatitis serology) or increased risk of having NASH and when other liver disease cannot be excluded, a liver biopsy should be considered [105,113].

Conclusion

It is clear that NAFLD is an increasingly prevalent liver disease and that patients with NAFLD may present with a great variety of symptoms or even complications. In recognizing patients with a high-risk profile for the development of NASH, the collaboration of the general practitioner, assistant nurse, internist—endocrinologist, vascular internist, and gastroenterologist is highly important. Multidisciplinary care paths are currently being developed to aid this collaboration.

When patients are diagnosed with NAFLD, it is often hard to recognize which patients suffer from nonprogressive simple steatosis, which patients suffer from metabolically active steatohepatitis (NASH) with a high risk of development of cardiovascular disease, and which patients are at high risk of developing cirrhosis and HCC. Developing more accurate noninvasive diagnostic tools is necessary for a better capability for screening and differentiating between the different stages of liver disease, providing estimations for the chance of progression and the development of HCC.

Another area of concern in these patients is the high risk on the development of cardiovascular disease. Intensifying the support for improvement of lifestyle and treatment of comorbidities is essential to halt the progression of liver disease and prevent cardiovascular complications. This calls for a multidisciplinary approach to identify the patient population in need of additional care and to ensure it being delivered.

In conclusion, the increasing prevalence of NAFLD-NASH is worrisome and constitutes a major global problem. Solutions to face this challenge are to organize referral and care paths for NAFLD-NASH, as well as multidisciplinary treatment teams, to enhance awareness for this liver disease, to better identify and stage NAFL, NASH, and NASH fibrosis, and to offer optimal treatment options including potential pharmacotherapeutic options in the near future.

References

[1] Vernon G, Baranova A, Younossi ZM. Systematic review: the epidemiology and natural history of non-alcoholic fatty liver disease and non-alcoholic steatohepatitis in adults. Aliment Pharmacol Ther August 2011;34(3):274−85. Available from: https://pubmed.ncbi.nlm.nih.gov/21623852/.

[2] Lazarus Jv, Ekstedt M, Marchesini G, Mullen J, Novak K, Pericàs JM, et al. A cross-sectional study of the public health response to non-alcoholic fatty liver disease in Europe. J Hepatol January 1, 2020;72(1):14−24. Available from: https://pubmed.ncbi.nlm.nih.gov/31518646/.

[3] WHO. Obesity and overweight. 2021.

[4] Younossi Z, Anstee QM, Marietti M, Hardy T, Henry L, Eslam M, et al. Global burden of NAFLD and NASH: trends, predictions, risk factors and prevention. Nat Rev Gastroenterol Hepatol January 1, 2018;15(1):11−20. Available from: https://pubmed.ncbi.nlm.nih.gov/28930295/.

[5] Younossi ZM, Golabi P, de Avila L, Paik JM, Srishord M, Fukui N, et al. The global epidemiology of NAFLD and NASH in patients with type 2 diabetes: a systematic review and meta-analysis. J Hepatol October 1, 2019;71(4):793−801. Available from: https://pubmed.ncbi.nlm.nih.gov/31279902/.

[6] van Dijk A-M, Schattenberg JM, Holleboom AG, Maarten l, Tushuizen E. Referral care paths for non-alcoholic fatty liver disease-Gearing up for an ever more prevalent and severe liver disease. 2021.

[7] Lazarus Jv, Anstee QM, Hagström H, Cusi K, Cortez-Pinto H, Mark HE, et al. Defining comprehensive models of care for NAFLD. Nat Rev Gastroenterol Hepatol October 1, 2021;18(10):717−29. Available from: https://pubmed.ncbi.nlm.nih.gov/34172937/.

[8] Anderson EL, Howe LD, Jones HE, Higgins JPT, Lawlor DA, Fraser A. The prevalence of non-alcoholic fatty liver disease in children and adolescents: a systematic review and meta-analysis. PLoS One October 29, 2015;10(10). Available from: https://pubmed.ncbi.nlm.nih.gov/26512983/.

[9] Koot BGP, Nobili V. Screening for non-alcoholic fatty liver disease in children: do guidelines provide enough guidance? Obes Rev September 1, 2017;18(9):1050−60. Available from: https://pubmed.ncbi.nlm.nih.gov/28544608/.

[10] Marchesini G, Day CP, Dufour JF, Canbay A, Nobili V, Ratziu V, et al. EASL-EASD-EASO clinical practice guidelines for the management of non-alcoholic fatty liver disease. J Hepatol June 1, 2016;64(6):1388−402. Available from: https://pubmed.ncbi.nlm.nih.gov/27062661/.

[11] Anstee QM, Day CP. The genetics of NAFLD. Nat Rev Gastroenterol Hepatol November 2013;10(11):645−55. Available from: https://pubmed.ncbi.nlm.nih.gov/24061205/.

[12] Buch S, Stickel F, Trépo E, Way M, Herrmann A, Nischalke HD, et al. A genome-wide association study confirms PNPLA3 and identifies TM6SF2 and MBOAT7 as risk loci for alcohol-related cirrhosis. Nat Genet December 1, 2015;47(12):1443−8. Available from: https://pubmed.ncbi.nlm.nih.gov/26482880/.

[13] Abul-Husn NS, Cheng X, Li AH, Xin Y, Schurmann C, Stevis P, et al. A protein-truncating HSD17B13 variant and protection from chronic liver disease. N Engl J Med March 22, 2018;378(12):1096−106. Available from: https://pubmed.ncbi.nlm.nih.gov/29562163/.

[14] Kechagias S, Emersson Å, Dahlqvist O, Lundberg P, Lindström T, Nystrom FH. Fast-food-based hyper-alimentation can induce rapid and profound elevation of serum alanine aminotransferase in healthy subjects. Gut May 2008;57(5):649−54. Available from: https://pubmed.ncbi.nlm.nih.gov/18276725/.

[15] Chiu S, Sievenpiper JL, de Souza RJ, Cozma AI, Mirrahimi A, Carleton AJ, et al. Effect of fructose on markers of non-alcoholic fatty liver disease (NAFLD): a systematic review and meta-analysis of controlled feeding trials. Eur J Clin Nutr 2014;68(4):416−23. Available from: https://pubmed.ncbi.nlm.nih.gov/24569542/.

[16] Softic S, Stanhope KL, Boucher J, Divanovic S, Lanaspa MA, Johnson RJ, et al. Fructose and hepatic insulin resistance. Crit Rev Clin Lab Sci July 3, 2020;57(5):308−22. Available from: https://pubmed.ncbi.nlm.nih.gov/31935149/.

[17] Rives C, Fougerat A, Ellero-Simatos S, Loiseau N, Guillou H, Gamet-Payrastre L, et al. Oxidative stress in NAFLD: role of nutrients and food contaminants. Biomolecules December 1, 2020;10(12):1−69. Available from: https://pubmed.ncbi.nlm.nih.gov/33371482/.

[18] Roglans N, Vilà L, Farré M, Alegret M, Sánchez RM, Vázquez-Carrera M, et al. Impairment of hepatic Stat-3 activation and reduction of PPARalpha activity in fructose-fed rats. Hepatology March 2007;45(3):778−88. Available from: https://pubmed.ncbi.nlm.nih.gov/17326204/.

[19] Jensen T, Abdelmalek MF, Sullivan S, Nadeau KJ, Green M, Roncal C, et al. Fructose and sugar: a major mediator of non-alcoholic fatty liver disease. J Hepatol May 1, 2018;68(5):1063−75. Available from: https://pubmed.ncbi.nlm.nih.gov/29408694/.

[20] Yasutake K, Kohjima M, Kotoh K, Nakashima M, Nakamuta M, Enjoji M. Dietary habits and behaviors associated with nonalcoholic fatty liver disease. World J Gastroenterol February 21, 2014;20(7):1756−67. Available from: https://pubmed.ncbi.nlm.nih.gov/24587653/.

[21] Ullah R, Rauf N, Nabi G, Ullah H, Shen Y, Zhou YD, et al. Role of nutrition in the pathogenesis and prevention of non-alcoholic fatty liver disease: recent updates. Int J Biol Sci 2019;15(2):265−76. Available from: https://pubmed.ncbi.nlm.nih.gov/30745819/.

[22] Donnelly KL, Smith CI, Schwarzenberg SJ, Jessurun J, Boldt MD, Parks EJ. Sources of fatty acids stored in liver and secreted via lipoproteins in patients with nonalcoholic fatty liver disease. J Clin Invest 2005;115(5):1343−51. Available from: https://pubmed.ncbi.nlm.nih.gov/15864352/.

[23] Yu L, Yuan M, Wang L. The effect of omega-3 unsaturated fatty acids on non-alcoholic fatty liver disease: a systematic review and meta-analysis of RCTs. Pak J Med Sci July 1, 2017;33(4):1022−8. Available from: https://pubmed.ncbi.nlm.nih.gov/29067086/.

[24] Ley RE, Bäckhed F, Turnbaugh P, Lozupone CA, Knight RD, Gordon JI. Obesity alters gut microbial ecology. Proc Natl Acad Sci USA August 2, 2005;102(31):11070−5. Available from: https://pubmed.ncbi.nlm.nih.gov/16033867/.

[25] Ley RE, Turnbaugh PJ, Klein S, Gordon JI. Microbial ecology: human gut microbes associated with obesity. Nature December 21, 2006;444(7122):1022−3. Available from: https://pubmed.ncbi.nlm.nih.gov/17183309/.

[26] Haro C, Montes-Borrego M, Rangel-Zúñiga OA, Alcalä-Diaz JF, Gamez-Delgado F, Pérez-Martinez P, et al. Two healthy diets modulate gut microbial community improving insulin sensitivity in a human obese population. J Clin Endocrinol Metab January 1, 2016;101(1):233−42. Available from: https://pubmed.ncbi.nlm.nih.gov/26505825/.

[27] Muñoz-Garach A, Diaz-Perdigones C, Tinahones FJ. Gut microbiota and type 2 diabetes mellitus. Endocrinol Nutr: organo de la Sociedad Espanola de Endocrinologia y Nutricion December 1, 2016;63(10):560−8. Available from: https://pubmed.ncbi.nlm.nih.gov/27633134/.

[28] Leung C, Rivera L, Furness JB, Angus PW. The role of the gut microbiota in NAFLD. Nat Rev Gastroenterol Hepatol July 1, 2016;13(7):412−25. Available from: https://pubmed.ncbi.nlm.nih.gov/27273168/.

[29] Hardy T, Oakley F, Anstee QM, Day CP. Nonalcoholic fatty liver disease: pathogenesis and disease spectrum. Annu Rev Pathol May 23, 2016;11:451−96. Available from: https://pubmed.ncbi.nlm.nih.gov/26980160/.

[30] Isokuortti E, Zhou Y, Peltonen M, Bugianesi E, Clement K, Bonnefont-Rousselot D, et al. Use of HOMA-IR to diagnose non-alcoholic fatty liver disease: a population-based and inter-laboratory study. Diabetologia October 1, 2017;60(10):1873−82. Available from: https://pubmed.ncbi.nlm.nih.gov/28660493/.

[31] DeFronzo RA. Insulin resistance, lipotoxicity, type 2 diabetes and atherosclerosis: the missing links. Claude Bernard Lect 2009. Diabetologia July 1, 2010;53(7):1270−87. Available from: https://pubmed.ncbi.nlm.nih.gov/20361178/.

[32] Musso G, Cassader M, Paschetta E, Gambino R. Bioactive lipid species and metabolic pathways in progression and resolution of nonalcoholic steatohepatitis. Gastroenterology August 1, 2018;155(2):282−302.e8. Available from: https://pubmed.ncbi.nlm.nih.gov/29906416/.

[33] Hafizi Abu Bakar M, Kian Kai C, Wan Hassan WN, Sarmidi MR, Yaakob H, Zaman Huri H. Mitochondrial dysfunction as a central event for mechanisms underlying insulin resistance: the roles of long chain fatty acids. Diabetes Metab Res Rev July 1, 2015;31(5):453−75. Available from: https://pubmed.ncbi.nlm.nih.gov/25139820/.

[34] Musso G, Cassader M, Gambino R. Non-alcoholic steatohepatitis: emerging molecular targets and therapeutic strategies. Nat Rev Drug Discov April 1, 2016;15(4):249−74. Available from: https://pubmed.ncbi.nlm.nih.gov/26794269/.

[35] Rotundo L, Persaud A, Feurdean M, Ahlawat S, Kim HS. The Association of leptin with severity of non-alcoholic fatty liver disease: a population-based study. Clin Mol Hepatol December 1, 2018;24(4):392−401. Available from: https://pubmed.ncbi.nlm.nih.gov/30068065/.

[36] Saxena NK, Titus MA, Ding X, Floyd J, Srinivasan S, Sitaraman Sv, et al. Leptin as a novel profibrogenic cytokine in hepatic stellate cells: mitogenesis and inhibition of apoptosis mediated by extracellular regulated kinase (Erk) and Akt phosphorylation. Faseb J October 2004;18(13):1612−4. Available from: https://pubmed.ncbi.nlm.nih.gov/15319373/.

[37] Udomsinprasert W, Honsawek S, Poovorawan Y. Adiponectin as a novel biomarker for liver fibrosis. World J Hepatol October 1, 2018;10(10):708−18. Available from: https://pubmed.ncbi.nlm.nih.gov/30386464/.

[38] Wang X, Zheng Z, Caviglia JM, Corey KE, Herfel TM, Cai B, et al. Hepatocyte TAZ/WWTR1 promotes inflammation and fibrosis in nonalcoholic steatohepatitis. Cell Metab December 13, 2016;24(6):848−62. Available from: https://pubmed.ncbi.nlm.nih.gov/28068223/.

[39] de Chiara F, Heebøll S, Marrone G, Montoliu C, Hamilton-Dutoit S, Ferrandez A, et al. Urea cycle dysregulation in non-alcoholic fatty liver disease. J Hepatol October 1, 2018;69(4):905−15. Available from: https://pubmed.ncbi.nlm.nih.gov/29981428/.

[40] Jalan R, de Chiara F, Balasubramaniyan V, Andreola F, Khetan V, Malago M, et al. Ammonia produces pathological changes in human hepatic stellate cells and is a target for therapy of portal hypertension. J Hepatol April 1, 2016;64(4):823−33. Available from: https://pubmed.ncbi.nlm.nih.gov/26654994/.

[41] Trauner M, Claudel T, Fickert P, Moustafa T, Wagner M. Bile acids as regulators of hepatic lipid and glucose metabolism. Dig Dis May 2010;28(1):220−4. Available from: https://pubmed.ncbi.nlm.nih.gov/20460915/.

[42] de Aguiar Vallim TQ, Tarling EJ, Edwards PA. Pleiotropic roles of bile acids in metabolism. Cell Metab May 7, 2013;17(5):657−69. Available from: https://pubmed.ncbi.nlm.nih.gov/23602448/.

[43] Doulberis M, Kotronis G, Gialamprinou D, Kountouras J, Katsinelos P. Non-alcoholic fatty liver disease: an update with special focus on the role of gut microbiota. Metab Clin Exp June 1, 2017;71:182−97. Available from: https://pubmed.ncbi.nlm.nih.gov/28521872/.

[44] Wang B, Jiang X, Cao M, Ge J, Bao Q, Tang L, et al. Altered fecal microbiota correlates with liver biochemistry in nonobese patients with non-alcoholic fatty liver disease. Sci Rep August 23, 2016;6. Available from: https://pubmed.ncbi.nlm.nih.gov/27550547/.

[45] Udayappan S, Manneras-Holm L, Chaplin-Scott A, Belzer C, Herrema H, Dallinga-Thie GM, et al. Oral treatment with Eubacterium hallii improves insulin sensitivity in db/db mice. NPJ Biofilms Nicrobiom July 6, 2016;2. Available from: https://pubmed.ncbi.nlm.nih.gov/28721246/.

[46] Yuan J, Chen C, Cui J, Lu J, Yan C, Wei X, et al. Fatty liver disease caused by high-alcohol-producing *Klebsiella pneumoniae*. Cell Metab October 1, 2019;30(4):675−688.e7. Available from: https://pubmed.ncbi.nlm.nih.gov/31543403/.

[47] Vrieze A, Out C, Fuentes S, Jonker L, Reuling I, Kootte RS, et al. Impact of oral vancomycin on gut microbiota, bile acid metabolism, and insulin sensitivity. J Hepatol 2014;60(4):824−31. Available from: https://pubmed.ncbi.nlm.nih.gov/24316517/.

[48] Estes C, Razavi H, Loomba R, Younossi Z, Sanyal AJ. Modeling the epidemic of nonalcoholic fatty liver disease demonstrates an exponential increase in burden of disease. Hepatology January 1, 2018;67(1):123−33. Available from: https://pubmed.ncbi.nlm.nih.gov/28802062/.

[49] Flemming JA, Kim WR, Brosgart CL, Terrault NA. Reduction in liver transplant wait-listing in the era of direct-acting antiviral therapy. Hepatology March 1, 2017;65(3):804−12. Available from: https://pubmed.ncbi.nlm.nih.gov/28012259/.

[50] Hester D, Golabi P, Paik J, Younossi I, Mishra A, Younossi ZM. Among medicare patients with hepatocellular carcinoma, non-alcoholic fatty liver disease is the most common etiology and cause of mortality. J Clin Gastroenterol May 1, 2020;54(5):459−67. Available from: https://pubmed.ncbi.nlm.nih.gov/30672817/.

[51] Reddy SK, Steel JL, Chen HW, Demateo DJ, Cardinal J, Behari J, et al. Outcomes of curative treatment for hepatocellular cancer in nonalcoholic steatohepatitis versus hepatitis C and alcoholic liver disease. Hepatology June 2012;55(6):1809−19. Available from: https://pubmed.ncbi.nlm.nih.gov/22183968/.

[52] Mantovani A, Dauriz M, Byrne CD, Lonardo A, Zoppini G, Bonora E, et al. Association between nonalcoholic fatty liver disease and colorectal tumours in asymptomatic adults undergoing screening colonoscopy: a systematic review and meta-analysis. Metabol: Clin Experim October 1, 2018;87:1−12. Available from: https://pubmed.ncbi.nlm.nih.gov/29935236/.

[53] Kim GA, Lee HC, Choe J, Kim MJ, Lee MJ, Chang HS, et al. Association between non-alcoholic fatty liver disease and cancer incidence rate. J Hepatol January 1, 2017;68(1):140−6. Available from: https://pubmed.ncbi.nlm.nih.gov/29150142/.

[54] Gastaldelli A, Kozakova M, Höjlund K, Flyvbjerg A, Favuzzi A, Mitrakou A, et al. Fatty liver is associated with insulin resistance, risk of coronary heart disease, and early atherosclerosis in a large European population. Hepatology 2009;49(5):1537−44. Available from: https://pubmed.ncbi.nlm.nih.gov/19291789/.

[55] Targher G, Byrne CD, Lonardo A, Zoppini G, Barbui C. Non-alcoholic fatty liver disease and risk of incident cardiovascular disease: a meta-analysis. J Hepatol September 1, 2016;65(3):589−600. Available from: https://pubmed.ncbi.nlm.nih.gov/27212244/.

[56] Friedrich-Rust M, Schoelzel F, Maier S, Seeger F, Rey J, Fichtlscherer S, et al. Severity of coronary artery disease is associated with non-alcoholic fatty liver dis-ease: a single-blinded prospective mono-center study. PloS one October 1, 2017;12(10). Available from: https://pubmed.ncbi.nlm.nih.gov/29073252/.

[57] Keskin M, Hayıroğlu Mİ, Uzun AO, Güvenç TS, Şahin S, Kozan Ö. Effect of nonalcoholic fatty liver disease on in-hospital and long-term outcomes in patients with ST-segment elevation myocardial infarction. Am J cardiol November 15, 2017;120(10):1720–6. Available from: https://pubmed.ncbi.nlm.nih.gov/28867124/.

[58] Kahali B, Liu YL, Daly AK, Day CP, Anstee QM, Speliotes EK. TM6SF2: catch-22 in the fight against nonalcoholic fatty liver disease and cardiovascular disease? Gastroenterology April 1, 2015;148(4):679–84. Available from: https://pubmed.ncbi.nlm.nih.gov/25639710/.

[59] Canada JMN, Abbate A, Collen R, Billingsley H, Buckley LF, Carbone S, et al. Relation of hepatic fibrosis in nonalcoholic fatty liver disease to left ventricular diastolic function and exercise tolerance. Am J Cardiol February 1, 2019;123(3):466–73. Available from: https://pubmed.ncbi.nlm.nih.gov/30502049/.

[60] Bedogni G, Bellentani S, Miglioli L, Masutti F, Passalacqua M, Castiglione A, et al. The fatty liver index: a simple and accurate predictor of hepatic steatosis in the general population. BMC Gastroenterol November 2, 2006;6. Available from: https://pubmed.ncbi.nlm.nih.gov/17081293/.

[61] Shah AG, Lydecker A, Murray K, Tetri BN, Contos MJ, Sanyal AJ, et al. Comparison of noninvasive markers of fibrosis in patients with nonalcoholic fatty liver disease. Clin Gastroenterol Hepatol : The Offic Clin Pract J Am Gastroenterol Associat October 1, 2009;7(10):1104–12. Available from: https://pubmed.ncbi.nlm.nih.gov/19523535/.

[62] Daniels SJ, Leeming DJ, Eslam M, Hashem AM, Nielsen MJ, Krag A, et al. ADAPT: an algorithm incorporating PRO-C3 accurately identifies patients with NAFLD and advanced fibrosis. Hepatology March 1, 2019;69(3):1075–86. Available from: https://pubmed.ncbi.nlm.nih.gov/30014517/.

[63] Tsutsui M, Tanaka N, Kawakubo M, Sheena Y, Horiuchi A, Komatsu M, et al. Serum fragmented cytokeratin 18 levels reflect the histologic activity score of nonalcoholic fatty liver disease more accurately than serum alanine aminotransferase levels. J Clin Gastroenterol 2010;44(6):440–7. Available from: https://pubmed.ncbi.nlm.nih.gov/20104187/.

[64] Friedrich-Rust M, Rosenberg W, Parkes J, Herrmann E, Zeuzem S, Sarrazin C. Comparison of ELF, FibroTest and FibroScan for the non-invasive assessment of liver fibrosis. BMC Gastroenterol September 9, 2010;10. Available from: https://pubmed.ncbi.nlm.nih.gov/20828377/.

[65] Verhaegh P, Bavalia R, Winkens B, Masclee A, Jonkers D, Koek G. Noninvasive tests do not accurately differentiate nonalcoholic steatohepatitis from simple steatosis: a systematic review and meta-analysis. Clin Gastroenterol Hepatol June 1, 2018;16(6):837–61. Available from: https://pubmed.ncbi.nlm.nih.gov/28838784/.

[66] Vilar-Gomez E, Chalasani N. Non-invasive assessment of non-alcoholic fatty liver disease: clinical prediction rules and blood-based biomarkers. J Hepatol February 1, 2018;68(2):305–15. Available from: https://pubmed.ncbi.nlm.nih.gov/29154965/.

[67] Initiative IM. Liver investigation: testing marker utility in steatohepatitis. 2017.

[68] Hernaez R, Lazo M, Bonekamp S, Kamel I, Brancati FL, Guallar E, et al. Diagnostic accuracy and reliability of ultrasonography for the detection of fatty liver: a meta-analysis. Hepatology September 2, 2011;54(3):1082–90. Available from: https://pubmed.ncbi.nlm.nih.gov/21618575/.

[69] Saadeh S, Younossi ZM, Remer EM, Gramlich T, Ong JP, Hurley M, et al. The utility of radiological imaging in nonalcoholic fatty liver disease. Gastroenterology 2002;123(3):745–50. Available from: https://pubmed.ncbi.nlm.nih.gov/12198701/.

[70] Eddowes PJ, Sasso M, Allison M, Tsochatzis E, Anstee QM, Sheridan D, et al. Accuracy of FibroScan controlled attenuation parameter and liver stiffness measurement in assessing steatosis and fibrosis in patients with nonalcoholic fatty liver disease. Gastroenterology May 1, 2019;156(6):1717–30. Available from: https://pubmed.ncbi.nlm.nih.gov/30689971/.

[71] Caussy C, Reeder SB, Sirlin CB, Loomba R. Noninvasive, quantitative assessment of liver fat by MRI-PDFF as an endpoint in NASH trials. Hepatology August 1, 2018;68(2):763–72. Available from: https://pubmed.ncbi.nlm.nih.gov/29356032/.

[72] Schaapman JJ, Tushuizen ME, Coenraad MJ, Lamb HJ. Multiparametric MRI in patients with nonalcoholic fatty liver disease. J Magn Reson Imag June 1, 2021;53(6):1623–31. Available from: https://pubmed.ncbi.nlm.nih.gov/32822095/.

[73] Sanai FM, Keeffe EB. Liver biopsy for histological assessment: the case against. Saudi J Gastroenterol April 1, 2010;16(2):124–32. Available from: https://pubmed.ncbi.nlm.nih.gov/20339187/.

[74] Sumida Y, Yoneda M. Current and future pharmacological therapies for NAFLD/NASH. J Gastroenterol March 1, 2018;53(3):362–76. Available from: https://pubmed.ncbi.nlm.nih.gov/29247356/.

[75] Houghton D, Thoma C, Hallsworth K, Cassidy S, Hardy T, Burt AD, et al. Exercise reduces liver lipids and visceral adiposity in patients with nonalcoholic steatohepatitis in a randomized controlled trial. Clin Gastroenterol Hepatol January 1, 2017;15(1):96–102.e3. Available from: https://pubmed.ncbi.nlm.nih.gov/27521509/.

[76] Ratziu V. Non-pharmacological interventions in non-alcoholic fatty liver disease patients. Liver Int January 1, 2017;37(Suppl. 1):90–6. Available from: https://pubmed.ncbi.nlm.nih.gov/28052636/.

[77] Lassailly G, Caiazzo R, Buob D, Pigeyre M, Verkindt H, Labreuche J, et al. Bariatric surgery reduces features of nonalcoholic steatohepatitis in morbidly obese patients. Gastroenterology August 1, 2015;149(2):379–88. Available from: https://pubmed.ncbi.nlm.nih.gov/25917783/.

[78] Ryan MC, Itsiopoulos C, Thodis T, Ward G, Trost N, Hofferberth S, et al. The Mediterranean diet improves hepatic steatosis and insulin sensitivity in individuals with non-alcoholic fatty liver disease. J Hepatol July 2013;59(1):138–43. Available from: https://pubmed.ncbi.nlm.nih.gov/23485520/.

[79] Zelber-Sagi S, Salomone F, Webb M, Lotan R, Yeshua H, Halpern Z, et al. Coffee consumption and nonalcoholic fatty liver onset: a prospective study in the general population. Transl Res March 1, 2015;165(3):428–36. Available from: https://pubmed.ncbi.nlm.nih.gov/25468486/.

[80] Loomba R, Lutchman G, Kleiner DE, Ricks M, Feld JJ, Borg BB, et al. Clinical trial: pilot study of metformin for the treatment of non-alcoholic steatohepatitis. Aliment Pharmacol Ther January 2009;29(2):172–82. Available from: https://pubmed.ncbi.nlm.nih.gov/18945255/.

[81] Ratziu V, Giral P, Jacqueminet S, Charlotte F, Hartemann-Heurtier A, Serfaty L, et al. Rosiglitazone for nonalcoholic steatohepatitis: one-year results of the randomized placebo-controlled fatty liver improvement with rosiglitazone therapy (FLIRT) trial. Gastroenterology 2008;135(1):100—10. Available from: https://pubmed.ncbi.nlm.nih.gov/18503774/.

[82] Cusi K, Orsak B, Bril F, Lomonaco R, Hecht J, Ortiz-Lopez C, et al. Long-term pioglitazone treatment for patients with nonalcoholic steatohepatitis and prediabetes or type 2 diabetes mellitus: a randomized trial. Ann Intern Med September 6, 2016;165(5):305—15. Available from: https://pubmed.ncbi.nlm.nih.gov/27322798/.

[83] Tuccori M, Filion KB, Yin H, Yu OH, Platt RW, Azoulay L. Pioglitazone use and risk of bladder cancer: population based cohort study. BMJ March 30, 2016;352. Available from: https://pubmed.ncbi.nlm.nih.gov/27029385/.

[84] Guirguis E, Grace Y, Bolson A, DellaVecchia MJ, Ruble M. Emerging therapies for the treatment of nonalcoholic steatohepatitis: a systematic review. Pharmacotherapy March 1, 2021;41(3):315—28. Available from: https://pubmed.ncbi.nlm.nih.gov/33278029/.

[85] Drucker DJ. Mechanisms of action and therapeutic application of glucagon-like peptide-1. Cell Metab April 3, 2018;27(4):740—56. Available from: https://pubmed.ncbi.nlm.nih.gov/29617641/.

[86] Armstrong MJ, Gaunt P, Aithal GP, Barton D, Hull D, Parker R, et al. Liraglutide safety and efficacy in patients with non-alcoholic steatohepatitis (LEAN): a multicentre, double-blind, randomised, placebo-controlled phase 2 study. Lancet February 13, 2016;387(10019):679—90. Available from: https://pubmed.ncbi.nlm.nih.gov/26608256/.

[87] Newsome PN, Buchholtz K, Cusi K, Linder M, Okanoue T, Ratziu V, et al. A placebo-controlled trial of subcutaneous semaglutide in nonalcoholic steatohepatitis. N Engl J Med March 25, 2021;384(12):1113—24. Available from: https://pubmed.ncbi.nlm.nih.gov/33185364/.

[88] Chiang H, Lee JC, Huang HC, Huang H, Liu HK, Huang C. Delayed intervention with a novel SGLT2 inhibitor NGI001 suppresses diet-induced metabolic dysfunction and non-alcoholic fatty liver disease in mice. Br J Pharmacol January 1, 2020;177(2):239—53. Available from: https://pubmed.ncbi.nlm.nih.gov/31497874/.

[89] Eslami L, Merat S, Malekzadeh R, Nasseri-Moghaddam S, Aramin H. Statins for non-alcoholic fatty liver disease and non-alcoholic steatohepatitis. Coch Datab Syst Rev December 27, 2013;2013(12). Available from: https://pubmed.ncbi.nlm.nih.gov/24374462/.

[90] Loomba R, Kayali Z, Noureddin M, Ruane P, Lawitz EJ, Bennett M, et al. GS-0976 reduces hepatic steatosis and fibrosis markers in patients with nonalcoholic fatty liver disease. Gastroenterology November 1, 2018;155(5):1463—1473.e6. Available from: https://pubmed.ncbi.nlm.nih.gov/30059671/.

[91] Sanyal AJ, Chalasani N, Kowdley Kv, McCullough A, Diehl AM, Bass NM, et al. Pioglitazone, vitamin E, or placebo for nonalcoholic steatohepatitis. N Engl J Med May 6, 2010;362(18):1675—85. Available from: https://pubmed.ncbi.nlm.nih.gov/20427778/.

[92] Lindor KD, Kowdley KV, Heathcote EJ, Harrison ME, Jorgensen R, Angulo P, et al. Ursodeoxycholic acid for treatment of nonalcoholic steatohepatitis: results of a randomized trial. Hepatology March 2004;39(3):770—8. Available from: https://pubmed.ncbi.nlm.nih.gov/14999696/.

[93] Le TA, Chen J, Changchien C, Peterson MR, Kono Y, Patton H, et al. Effect of colesevelam on liver fat quantified by magnetic resonance in nonalcoholic steatohepatitis: a randomized controlled trial. Hepatology September 2012;56(3):922—32. Available from: https://pubmed.ncbi.nlm.nih.gov/22431131/.

[94] Neuschwander-Tetri BA, Loomba R, Sanyal AJ, Lavine JE, van Natta ML, Abdelmalek MF, et al. Farnesoid X nuclear receptor ligand obeticholic acid for non-cirrhotic, non-alcoholic steatohepatitis (FLINT): a multicentre, randomised, placebo-controlled trial. Lancet March 14, 2015;385(9972):956—65. Available from: https://pubmed.ncbi.nlm.nih.gov/25468160/.

[95] Younossi ZM, Ratziu V, Loomba R, Rinella M, Anstee QM, Goodman Z, et al. Obeticholic acid for the treatment of non-alcoholic steatohepatitis: interim analysis from a multicentre, randomised, placebo-controlled phase 3 trial. Lancet December 14, 2019;394(10215):2184—96. Available from: https://pubmed.ncbi.nlm.nih.gov/31813633/.

[96] Sano R, Reed JC. ER stress-induced cell death mechanisms. Biochimica et biophysica acta December 2013;1833(12):3460—70. Available from: https://pubmed.ncbi.nlm.nih.gov/23850759/.

[97] Friedman SL, Ratziu V, Harrison SA, Abdelmalek MF, Aithal GP, Caballeria J, et al. A randomized, placebo-controlled trial of cenicriviroc for treatment of nonalcoholic steatohepatitis with fibrosis. Hepatology May 1, 2018;67(5):1754—67. Available from: https://pubmed.ncbi.nlm.nih.gov/28833331/.

[98] Sinha RA, Singh BK, Yen PM. Direct effects of thyroid hormones on hepatic lipid metabolism. Nat Rev Endocrinol May 1, 2018;14(5):259—69. Available from: https://pubmed.ncbi.nlm.nih.gov/29472712/.

[99] Bruinstroop E, Dalan R, Cao Y, Bee YM, Chandran K, Cho LW, et al. Low-dose levothyroxine reduces intrahepatic lipid content in patients with type 2 diabetes mellitus and NAFLD. J Clin Endocrinol Metab July 1, 2018;103(7):2698—706. Available from: https://pubmed.ncbi.nlm.nih.gov/29718334/.

[100] Harrison S, Moussa S, Bashir M. MGL-3196, a selective thyroid hormone receptor-beta agonist significantly decreases hepatic fat in NASH-patients at 12 weeks, the primary endpoint in a 36 week serial liver biopsy study. J Hepatol 2018;68(S38).

[101] Harrison SA, Bashir M, Moussa SE, McCarty K, Pablo Frias J, Taub R, et al. Effects of resmetirom on noninvasive endpoints in a 36-week phase 2 active treatment extension study in patients with NASH. Hepatol Commun January 4, 2021;5(4):573—88.

[102] Loomba R, Noureddin M, Kowdley Kv, Kohli A, Sheikh A, Neff G, et al. Combination therapies including cilofexor and firsocostat for bridging fibrosis and cirrhosis attributable to NASH. Hepatology February 1, 2021;73(2):625—43. Available from: https://pubmed.ncbi.nlm.nih.gov/33169409/.

[103] Wong VWS, Wong GLH, Chim AML, Chu WCW, Yeung DKW, Li KCT, et al. Treatment of nonalcoholic steatohepatitis with probiotics. A proof-of-concept study. Ann Hepatol March 1, 2013;12(2):256—62.

[104] Witjes JJ, Smits LP, Pekmez CT, Prodan A, Meijnikman AS, Troelstra MA, et al. Donor fecal microbiota transplantation alters gut microbiota and metabolites in obese individuals with steatohepatitis. Hepatol Commun November 1, 2020;4(11):1578−90. Available from: https://pubmed.ncbi.nlm.nih.gov/33163830/.

[105] Srivastava A, Gailer R, Tanwar S, Trembling P, Parkes J, Rodger A, et al. Prospective evaluation of a primary care referral pathway for patients with non-alcoholic fatty liver disease. J Hepatol August 1, 2019;71(2):371−8. Available from: https://pubmed.ncbi.nlm.nih.gov/30965069/.

[106] Mikolasevic I, Domislovic V, Turk Wensveen T, Delija B, Klapan M, Juric T, et al. Screening for nonalcoholic fatty liver disease in patients with type 2 diabetes mellitus using transient elastography − a prospective, cross sectional study. Eur J Intern Med December 1, 2020;82:68−75. Available from: https://pubmed.ncbi.nlm.nih.gov/32839076/.

[107] Castera L, Yuen Chan HL, Arrese M, Afdhal N, Bedossa P, Friedrich-Rust M, et al. EASL-ALEH Clinical practice guidelines: non-invasive tests for evaluation of liver disease severity and prognosis. J Hepatol July 1, 2015;63(1):237−64. Available from: https://pubmed.ncbi.nlm.nih.gov/25911335/.

[108] Verma S, Jensen D, Hart J, Mohanty SR. Predictive value of ALT levels for non-alcoholic steatohepatitis (NASH) and advanced fibrosis in non-alcoholic fatty liver disease (NAFLD). Liver Int October 2013;33(9):1398−405. Available from: https://pubmed.ncbi.nlm.nih.gov/23763360/.

[109] Bril F, McPhaul MJ, Caulfield MP, Clark VC, Soldevilla-Pico C, Firpi-Morell RJ, et al. Performance of plasma biomarkers and diagnostic panels for nonalcoholic steatohepatitis and advanced fibrosis in patients with type 2 diabetes. Diabetes Care February 1, 2020;43(2):290−7. Available from: https://pubmed.ncbi.nlm.nih.gov/31604692/.

[110] Blank V, Petroff D, Beer S, Böhlig A, Heni M, Berg T, et al. Current NAFLD guidelines for risk stratification in diabetic patients have poor diagnostic discrimination. Sci Rep December 1, 2020;10(1). Available from: https://pubmed.ncbi.nlm.nih.gov/33110165/.

[111] Ishiba H, Sumida Y, Tanaka S, Yoneda M, Hyogo H, Ono M, et al. The novel cutoff points for the FIB4 index categorized by age increase the diagnostic accuracy in NAFLD: a multi-center study. J Gastroenterol November 1, 2018;53(11):1216−24. Available from: https://pubmed.ncbi.nlm.nih.gov/29744597/.

[112] Gleeson J, Barry J, O'Reilly S. Use of liver imaging and biopsy in clinical practice. N Engl J Med December 7, 2017;377(23):2296. Available from: http://www.ncbi.nlm.nih.gov/pubmed/29215220.

[113] Vali Y, Lee J, Boursier J, Spijker R, Löffler J, Verheij J, et al. Enhanced liver fibrosis test for the non-invasive diagnosis of fibrosis in patients with NAFLD: a systematic review and meta-analysis. J Hepatol August 1, 2020;73(2):252−62. Available from: https://pubmed.ncbi.nlm.nih.gov/32275982/.

[114] Srivastava A, Jong S, Gola A, Gailer R, Morgan S, Sennett K, et al. Cost-comparison analysis of FIB-4, ELF and fibroscan in community pathways for non-alcoholic fatty liver disease. BMC Gastroenterol July 11, 2019;19(1). Available from: https://pubmed.ncbi.nlm.nih.gov/31296161/.

Chapter 8

Myocardial lipids—techniques and applications of proton magnetic resonance spectroscopy of the human heart

Adrianus J. Bakermans
Department of Radiology and Nuclear Medicine, Amsterdam University Medical Centers, University of Amsterdam, Amsterdam, the Netherlands

The human heart requires a continuous supply of energy to maintain healthy contractile function of the myocardium. The majority of this biochemical energy is generated by oxidative phosphorylation in mitochondria, producing adenosine triphosphate (ATP) from energy substrates and oxygen (Fig. 8.1). Myocardial energy homeostasis relies on a well-regulated flexibility in substrate use. The breakdown of fatty acids via mitochondrial fatty acid β-oxidation provides 40%−60% of the total ATP production in a healthy adult heart. Dependent on oxygen and substrate availability, glucose, lactate, ketones, and amino acids can also serve as energy sources [1]. An adequate blood supply of oxygen and nutrients is essential for the heart, because cardiomyocytes only have a limited capacity to store such substrates intracellularly. Yet, in times of prolonged metabolic stress or excessive energy demand, the myocardium can resort to intracellular stores of triglycerides. Such ectopic storage of neutral lipid droplets is crucial for the heart to maintain myocardial energy homeostasis under physiological conditions. Ectopic myocardial lipids have become an important topic of clinical investigation, because excess lipid accumulation or myocardial steatosis has been linked to cardiomyopathy and cardiac dysfunction in obesity [2], type 2 diabetes [3], heart failure [4], and inherited metabolic disorders [5].

Biopsy access to the myocardium for a histological assessment of ectopic lipid storage is limited and risky, particularly compared with other organs and tissues, such as skeletal muscle, adipose tissue, and the liver. Instead, proton magnetic resonance spectroscopy (^{1}H-MRS) can provide nondisruptive quantitative data on myocardial lipid content in the beating heart (Fig. 8.2) in health and disease, but inherently comes with specific technical challenges that are different from ^{1}H-MRS of stationary tissues. This chapter discusses the techniques and applications of ^{1}H-MRS of the heart, which have contributed to our understanding of myocardial lipid metabolism in a unique, noninvasive way.

Localized proton magnetic resonance spectroscopy of the heart

With the heart safely hidden behind chest skeletal muscle and the rib cage, surrounded by pericardial and epicardial fat, in close proximity of the liver and the lungs, and with blood flowing at high velocity through its chambers and vessels, adequate localization of ^{1}H-MRS signal acquisitions is important for a noninvasive evaluation of the lipids within the myocardium. Besides anatomy, the heart's beating motion as well as respiration pose challenges to localized ^{1}H-MRS of the in vivo heart. The general principles of localized ^{1}H-MRS for noninvasive profiling of ectopic myocardial lipids are visualized in Fig. 8.3. Here, we address some aspects of localized ^{1}H-MRS that are particularly relevant for cardiac applications.

Typically, ^{1}H-MRS of the heart is conducted with single-shot single-voxel localization techniques, positioning a single volume of interest ("voxel") in the interventricular septum from which fully localized signal is acquired in each acquisition ("shot"). This location keeps the voxel clear from the pericardial and epicardial fat deposits that would otherwise contaminate the signals if the voxel were placed in the left-ventricular free wall [10] or anterior wall [11]. To ensure the

Visceral and Ectopic Fat. https://doi.org/10.1016/B978-0-12-822186-0.00007-9

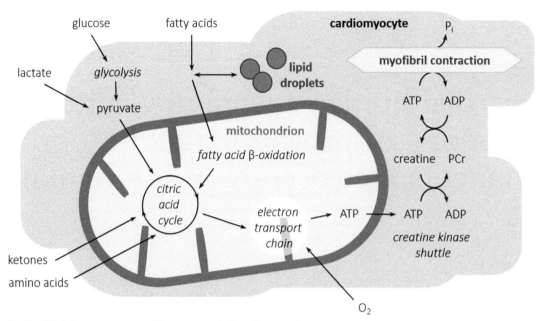

FIGURE 8.1 Simplified diagram of myocardial energy metabolism. Energy substrates (fatty acids, glucose, lactate, ketones, and amino acids) and oxygen are taken up by the cardiomyocyte. Glycolysis requires no oxygen to generate pyruvate and adenosine triphosphate (ATP) from glucose, accounting for ~5% of the myocardial ATP production. Fatty acids are transported into the mitochondrion to enter the fatty acid β-oxidation pathway for the production of acetyl-coenzyme A (CoA). Glucose-derived pyruvate, ketones, and branched-chain amino acids provide additional sources of acetyl-CoA production. Acetyl-CoA is oxidized by the citric acid cycle, in turn feeding the electron transport chain for the production of ATP through oxidative phosphorylation. Fatty acids can be stored intracellularly as triglycerides in lipid droplets. High-energy phosphate from ATP produced by the mitochondria is buffered and transported in the form of phosphocreatine (PCr) through the creatine kinase shuttle in the cytosol, and reconverted into ATP for use in energy-consuming processes such as contractile work by myofibrils. Myocardial lipid and creatine content can be quantified with proton magnetic resonance spectroscopy (^{1}H-MRS). Phosphorus-31 MRS (^{31}P-MRS) can interrogate high-energy phosphate metabolism through the direct detection of PCr, ATP, and inorganic phosphate (P_i). Myocardial contractility can be assessed with MRI. Substrate transporters and catalyzing enzymes are not shown in this diagram. For details, see Ref. [1].

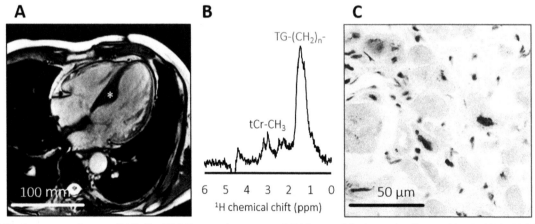

FIGURE 8.2 Assessment of myocardial lipids. (A) 3 T magnetic resonance (MR) image of the heart of a 69-year-old male (BMI, 22.0 kg/m^2) with obstructive hypertrophic cardiomyopathy scheduled for septal myectomy. Note the hypertrophied septal wall (*) that obstructs left ventricular outflow. (B) 3 T proton MR spectrum (^{1}H-MRS) obtained from the interventricular septum. Myocardial triglyceride (TG) content for this patient was 0.58% of the unsuppressed water signal. (C) 40× magnification photomicrograph of a sample from this patient's myocardium stained with Oil Red O and counterstained with hematoxyline, highlighting the presence of intracellular lipid droplets (red) in cardiomyocytes (nuclei in blue). The specimen was obtained intraoperatively via septal myectomy within the framework of a study that focused on validating noninvasive ^{1}H-MRS quantification of in vivo myocardial tissue metabolite content against ex vivo biochemical assays [6]. The myocardial triglyceride concentration determined via colorimetric assay in a myocardial tissue sample was 1.45 μmol/g wet weight for this patient. Whereas the triglycerides in intracellular lipid droplets are sufficiently mobile to be detected with ^{1}H-MRS, motion-restricted lipids such as those in cell and organelle membrane bilayers do not contribute to in vivo ^{1}H-MRS signal [7]. *Photomicrograph courtesy of J. de Vos, Biomedical Engineering and Physics, Amsterdam University Medical Centers, University of Amsterdam, Amsterdam, The Netherlands.*

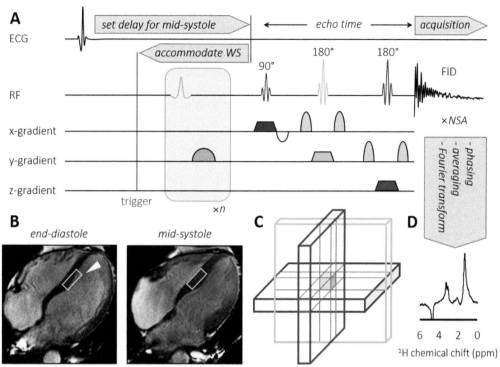

FIGURE 8.3   Single-shot single-voxel localization of proton magnetic resonance spectroscopy (^{1}H-MRS) using a point resolved spectroscopy (PRESS) sequence. (A) Timing diagram of ECG-triggered acquisition. A delay after R-wave detection in the ECG is inserted to ensure acquisition during mid-systole. A water suppression module (WS; orange) can be accommodated within this delay, e.g., with frequency-selective excitation of the water signal followed by a spoiler gradient. More effective water suppression can be achieved by repeating this block a number of times. With PRESS, three radiofrequency (RF) pulses subsequently excite (90 degrees; blue) and refocus (2 × 180 degrees; green, red) three orthogonal magnetic field gradient-selected slices to define the voxel of interest (C; ocher) at their intersection. The resultant echo signal (FID, free induction decay) is then recorded, representing the localized acquisition of one signal average in a single PRESS shot. Shots are repeated a number of times (NSA, number of signal averages) at repetition time (TR) intervals to increase the signal-to-noise ratio. In mice, the high heart rate may not allow sufficient time for both water suppression and localized acquisition within a single cardiac cycle, requiring a double-triggered approach over two heart beats [8]. (B) The interventricular septum moves into the prescribed voxel of interest (ocher) at mid-systole, while at end-diastole there is substantial contamination with ventricular blood (white arrow). (D) The FID is phase-corrected and averaged [9], and then Fourier-transformed to yield a spectrum with metabolite peaks.

correct positioning of this voxel, scout MR images are acquired to inform on subject anatomy. Left-ventricular long-axis and short-axis cinematographic MR images are acquired as part of a standard cardiac MR examination. These functional MR images can not only be used to quantify heart function (e.g., with stroke volumes, ejection fractions, strains) and morphology (e.g., with chamber volumes and myocardial mass) but also to guide positioning of the voxel within the desired phase of the cardiac cycle (Fig. 8.3). To restrict the acquired ^{1}H-MRS signal to the voxel of interest, either a point resolved spectroscopy (PRESS) [12] or a stimulated echo acquisition mode (STEAM) [13] single-shot single-voxel localization sequence is typically used. These sequences both employ radiofrequency (RF) excitation of three magnetic field gradient-selected orthogonal slices, with their intersection representing the voxel of interest (Fig. 8.3), but differ in the sense that PRESS requires two 180 degrees refocusing RF pulses that create the spin-echo signal instead of 90 degrees RF pulses that create a so-called stimulated echo in STEAM. The 90 degrees RF pulses for STEAM have a higher bandwidth than 180 degrees RF pulses, resulting in a smaller chemical shift displacement error between water and lipids for STEAM than for PRESS, particularly at higher magnetic field strengths. The signal amplitude of spin echoes in PRESS is twice as high as that of the stimulated echoes for STEAM, leading to a higher signal-to-noise ratio per acquisition for PRESS. Shorter echo times can be achieved with STEAM localization, which is particularly desirable for acquisitions in moving tissue. Indeed, to avoid motion artifacts, the "shot" length of a localized acquisition is ideally as short as possible. With STEAM, this shot length (i.e., echo time plus mixing time) can be as short at 17 ms [14] at 3 T. For PRESS, the shot length (i.e., echo time) is generally longer with reported values of approximately 20−25 ms at 1.5 T [11,15−17,18] to 35 ms at 3 T [19,20]. Whereas choosing long echo times for single-voxel spectroscopy can be a feasible approach to detect specific lipid species [21] or other metabolites [22], or to estimate metabolite-specific T_2 relaxation time constants [23] in relatively stationary tissue, the use of long echo times for ^{1}H-MRS of the heart has not been reported.

First PRESS [10] and later STEAM [24] were adopted in the 1990s for early studies with ^{1}H-MRS of the human heart at 1.5 T, and both have been used to establish measurement repeatability for myocardial lipid quantifications at 3 T [14,19,20] in the past decade. The suitability of alternatives to PRESS and STEAM localization has also been investigated. Another single-shot single-voxel localization sequence called sLASER (semi-adiabatic localization by adiabatic selective refocusing) [25] yields somewhat better measurement repeatability but requires long (>64 ms) echo times that decrease the signal-to-noise ratio compared with PRESS due to T_2 spin-spin decay [26]. A multi-voxel echoplanar spectroscopic imaging (EPSI) approach provides spatial information on myocardial lipid distribution but requires longer acquisition times and comes with a risk of signal contamination from epicardial fat [27]. Currently, STEAM and particularly PRESS with its higher sensitivity remain the localization methods that are predominantly used for ^{1}H-MRS of the heart.

Positioning the voxel of interest at the location of the interventricular septum essentially prescribes ^{1}H-MRS signal acquisition from a fixed position within the MR system's tube space, through which the interventricular septum moves rhythmically as the heart beats. Adequate signal acquisition from a septal voxel despite the beating of the heart can be ensured with what is called cardiac "triggering," i.e., the timed acquisition of signal from the voxel of interest triggered relative to an external reference signal that is typically the R-wave in the electrocardiogram (ECG). A delay after R-wave detection can be used to shift signal acquisitions to the desired phase of the cardiac cycle, e.g., to mid- [28,14] and end-diastole [26], more commonly, to mid- [10,19] and end-systole [11,15,17,29,18]. Compared with diastolic acquisitions, systolic acquisitions benefit from the thickened myocardial wall for voxel placement while suffering less from signal loss due to tissue motion and deformation [19,30], which can be further mitigated with advanced motion-compensated sequences [31] and signal processing [9].

Besides the cardiac cycle, the respiratory cycle imposes another periodical movement of the tissue of interest through the voxel of interest. The heart is transposed predominantly along the feet-head axis as it moves with the diaphragm. The heart's positions at inspiration and expiration can differ by several centimeters (Fig. 8.4), potentially leading to severe contamination of the spectra with signals originating from the liver or pericardial fat. Several approaches have been developed to compensate or mitigate the effects of respiratory motion in ^{1}H-MRS of the heart. The least demanding option from a technological perspective is to instruct subjects to hold their breath during signal acquisition. The breath hold is typically targeted to a comfortable position at end-expiration, during which several heart beats can then be used to trigger localized signal acquisition [14,28,32,33]. Although commonly employed for MR imaging of the heart and thorax, breath holding for ^{1}H-MRS applications may be undesirable. The many signal averages that are needed to achieve a signal-to-noise ratio that is sufficiently high for a quantitative analysis lead to long and/or many repeated breath holds. This can become a major hurdle for particular patients, e.g., those with congestive heart failure. Importantly, poor compliance with breath holding by the subject can lead to poor or unacceptable data quality [28]. As a practical alternative to breath holding, a synchronization approach has been adopted [29] by choosing a repetition time of approximately 4 s that matched the length of respiratory cycle, allowing essentially normal breathing for the subject.

To improve patient tolerance, and therewith the success rate of localized ^{1}H-MRS of the heart, additional triggering on the respiratory cycle has been introduced. This approach, more commonly referred to as "gating" requires a signal that informs on the breathing motion, e.g., derived from breathing-mediated fluctuations in the ECG signal amplitude [15], or from pressure changes in a respiratory belt positioned on the subject's abdomen or thorax [11]. This physiological signal informs on the acceptable end-expiratory window within the respiratory cycle during which a simultaneous ECG-derived trigger will initiate ^{1}H-MRS signal acquisition. This approach lowers scanning efficiency by potentially more than 50% [19] because only the cardiac triggered acquisitions within the defined respiratory gating window will be executed, but increases subject comfort and tolerance because no specific cooperation by the subject is required. Instead of using a physiology-derived external signal, a technique based on so-called "navigator" echo signals that are acquired with additional RF pulses preceding the actual ^{1}H-MRS acquisition has been developed [34]. These navigators are typically acquired from a volume positioned over the diaphragm at the liver dome, capturing the clear contrast of the liver-lung interface. After rapid reconstruction, the navigators then show the position of the diaphragm within the respiratory cycle. With a predefined window of acceptance corresponding to end-expiration, typically in the order of 5 mm, such navigator gating informs the decision to accept or discard ^{1}H-MRS data acquisition essentially in real time. In conjunction with respiratory navigator gating, navigators can be used for prospective volume tracking [34,35]. With volume tracking, the position of the voxel of interest is shifted within the MR's systems' tube space such that it follows the determined displacement of the heart from respiration. Still, respiratory gating is necessary in this approach, because typically the calibrations for water signal suppression and magnetic field shimming can only be optimized for a small window of the respiratory cycle [34]. Motion tracking can also be used to update the respiratory gating window to dynamically compensate for any drift of the end-expiration level of the liver-lung interface in the navigator signal throughout the duration of ^{1}H-MRS acquisition. This is particularly beneficial for patients with an irregular breathing pattern, and also

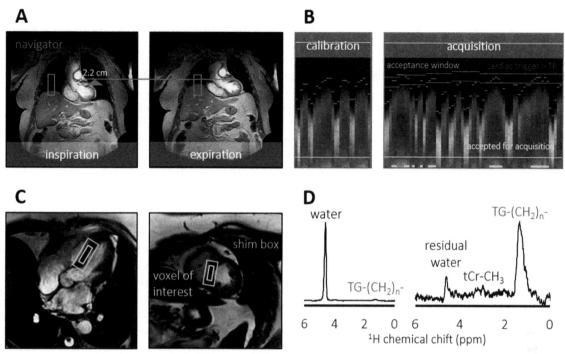

FIGURE 8.4 Motion compensation for localized ^{1}H-MRS of the human heart at 3 T. (A) Coronal MR images of a 66-year old female (BMI, 36.5 kg/m^2) with heart failure with preserved ejection fraction (HFpEF) acquired at end-inspiration and end-expiration, showing a 2.2 cm relative displacement of the heart. The position of the volume for respiratory navigator signal acquisition over diaphragm at the liver dome is indicated by the blue box. (B) Contrast in the navigator signal from the liver-lung interface is used to first calibrate the gating acceptance window (blue lines) that corresponds with end-expiration during a series of stable respiratory cycles, and then to inform on the decision to either accept acquisition of ^{1}H-MRS data (green bars) if a cardiac trigger (red bars) at at least the minimum repetition time (TR) occurs within the acceptance window, or to discard acquisition due to respiratory motion [18]. Note how the gating acceptance window slightly adjusts to accommodate a small drift in the end-expiration level of the liver-lung interface. (C) Long-axis and short-axis cinematographic MR images at mid-systole showing the position of the 8 × 20 × 25 mm^3 (4 mL) voxel of interest (ocher box) for localized ^{1}H-MRS in the interventricular septum with a point resolved spectroscopy (PRESS) sequence. The green box indicates the somewhat larger volume for shimming. (D) A ^{1}H-MR spectrum obtained from the interventricular septum without water suppression showing the dominant water signal at 4.7 ppm that is used as a quantification reference, and a water-suppressed ^{1}H-MR spectrum of eight signal averages at a scaling of 60× relative to the unsuppressed water signal, showing the signal for creatine-methyl (tCr-CH$_3$) at 3.0 ppm and triglyceride-methylene (TG−CH$_2$−)$_n$ at 1.3 ppm.

helps to compensate for movement of the subject. Such respiratory navigator gating has been developed and subsequently used successfully at 1.5 T [18] and later also at 3 T [19,20] magnetic field strengths with good measurement repeatability for myocardial lipid quantifications.

Combined, cardiac triggering and respiratory gating can be used to orchestrate the acquisition of localized ^{1}H-MRS signals from the beating heart. Variations in heart rate and breathing pattern may cause such experiments to become a lengthy procedure of more than 15 min, dependent on the number of signal averages, the chosen repetition time, the subject's heart rate, and the navigator efficiency [19,36]. To limit experimental time, a single breath hold approach has been developed that requires a single breath hold of 10 s to acquire 1 water reference signal and only three signal averages with water suppression [14]. A somewhat larger voxel was chosen to compensate for the lower signal-to-noise ratio that is achieved with only few signal averages. This quick assessment of myocardial lipid content was successfully applied and validated against histology in myocardial biopsy samples from patients with aortic stenosis [37], but yielded poor data quality in patients with heart failure [33]. Alternatively, retrospective gating on a fixed number of signal acquisitions has been proposed, allowing the subjects to breathe freely and limiting the acquisition time to a predefined duration [36]. Acquired spectra are accepted or rejected in a post-processing step based on thresholds for phase variations in the water and lipid signals, with large phase fluctuations between consecutive acquisitions reflecting poor signal stability due to motion. Such retrospective gating yielded a higher efficiency in terms of the achieved signal-to-noise ratio per unit time, allowing for a more than threefold shorter acquisition time relative to prospective respiratory navigator gating while obtaining similar spectral quality [38].

The dominant water signal is particularly suitable for evaluations of phase, frequency, and amplitude stability throughout data acquisition, but needs to be eliminated for a reliable detection of metabolite signals that can be a factor

1000 to 10,000 lower in amplitude (Fig. 8.4). In an approach called "metabolite cycling" the dominant water signal is preserved in all acquired spectra, but the metabolite signals are inverted with a frequency selective RF pulse alternatingly upfield or downfield from water, such that subtraction of the signals cancels the dominant water peak while leaving the metabolite peaks for analysis. Alternatively, summation yields the water peak as a quantification reference. Moreover, the preserved water signal in each acquisition allows for an evaluation and correction of signal stability for all acquisitions, and can be used for retrospective gating [38]. Water-suppression cycling is conceptually similar, but inverts the weakly suppressed water signal that can then still be used for spectral corrections as a reference signal while being fully eliminated upon averaging [28]. Most studies with successful ^{1}H-MRS acquisitions have employed (repeated) frequency-selective RF excitation pulses followed by "spoiler" gradients, nulling the water signal in water-suppressed spectra. Separate acquisitions with the water suppression RF pulses turned off are then used to obtain water spectra as a quantification reference. The water suppression module needs to be accommodated in the cardiac triggered and respiratory gated acquisitions, and adequate frequency-selective saturation of the water signal relies on a good homogeneity of the local magnetic field. Magnetic field shimming and RF pulse calibrations for water suppression can be performed using the same timing strategy to ensure optimization of the experimental parameters for the desired phases in the cardiac and respiratory cycles [14,15,19,34].

Despite all these approaches that are available to mitigate motion artifacts in ^{1}H-MRS of the heart, the acquisition of quantifiable data remains challenging. Compared with relatively stationary tissue such as skeletal muscle and the liver, the voxel of interest in the beating heart needs to be smaller to fit within the interventricular septum, and consequently yields a lower signal-to-noise ratio. Achieving homogeneity of the magnetic field ("shimming") within the septum is challenging due to the aforementioned motion, but also due to the high-velocity blood flow in the ventricles and the air-filled lungs that perturb the magnetic field. Poor magnetic field homogeneity hampers precise localization of signal acquisition, and deteriorates water suppression efficacy. Moreover, adequate shimming reduces the water line width, increases the signal-to-noise ratio, and benefits a quantitative analysis of tissue metabolite content [19]. Although typically done through iterative adjustments of the shim magnetic field gradients to minimize the water line width in spectra acquired with a single-voxel localization sequence, the required optimizations of magnetic field homogeneity and RF pulses can also be obtained through image-based calculations [39]. Finally, the need for cardiac triggering and breath holds or respiratory gating leads to variability in the effective repetition times, yielding complex modulations of the signal amplitudes due to metabolite-specific T_1-dependent partial saturation of magnetization effects, which may ultimately hamper a meaningful quantitative evaluation of the spectra [8].

Quantification of myocardial metabolite content

A quantitative evaluation of ^{1}H-MR spectra from the heart can yield valuable assessments of in vivo myocardial lipid metabolism, but is not trivial to perform [40]. In principle, ^{1}H-MRS is a quantitative method, because the amplitudes of the resonance signals in a ^{1}H-MR spectrum are proportional to the amount of the associated metabolite compounds that is present within the issue. These amplitudes can be estimated by fitting a biochemistry- and physics-informed model to the signals [40]. In practice, various (experimental) factors influence the signal amplitudes that prevent a straightforward quantification of tissue metabolite concentrations. First of all, the signal amplitudes depend on the number of hydrogen nuclei that contribute to the proton resonance signal of a certain compound. For water (H_2O), this is clear: two hydrogen nuclei per water molecule resonating at 4.7 ppm. For lipids or triglycerides, the number of hydrogen nuclei depends on the fatty acid chain lengths and degree of saturation, with saturated methylene $-(CH_2)_n-$ groups resonating at a different frequency (1.3 ppm) than other groups such as allylic methylene ($-CH_2-CH=CH-CH_2-$; 2.0 ppm) and methyl ($-CH_3$; 0.9 ppm). Secondly, in order to report concentrations, the tissue water fraction (e.g., in g water/g tissue) needs to be known or assumed. Thirdly, the signal amplitudes depend on the metabolite-specific T_2 relaxation time constants in relation to the echo time of the localization sequence. Finally, the signal amplitudes depend on partial saturation effects that are governed by metabolite-specific, tissue-specific, and magnetic field-strength dependent T_1 relaxation time constants and the effective repetition time of the acquisitions. Each of these factors can be corrected for to reach estimates of tissue lipid concentrations. These corrections are mostly based on assumptions that cannot be verified in vivo or determined for each subject individually.

The chemical composition of in vivo lipids differs per organ, and is influenced by factors such as nutritional status and diet (see Chapters 6 and 20). Although some insights can be obtained from relative quantifications of the different lipid-associated resonance signals [41,42], in vivo lipid composition will be unknown and requires assumptions on the average number of hydrogen nuclei within the triglyceride molecules that contribute to the signals in the ^{1}H-MR spectra [43]. The myocardial tissue water fraction is generally assumed to be constant, with a historical value of 72.7% being commonly used [11,16,26,28,44], even though the original source for that number refers to empirical data with a range of 63%—83% [45]. With a known and fixed echo time for the localization sequence, but without myocardial metabolite T_2 values reported in the literature, corrections for T_2 spin-spin signal decay are sometimes done by assuming T_2 relaxation time constants that have been reported for skeletal muscle [6,11,24,26,28]. For a straightforward correction of partial saturation effects, the T_1 relaxation time constants need to be known, and the effective repetition time needs to be constant. Both conditions are typically not met in practice. Metabolite T_1 values for the human heart are not available for any magnetic field strength in the literature. Instead, T_1 values reported for skeletal muscle can be assumed for myocardial metabolites [26—28].

Although some studies report an exact repetition time for their ^{1}H-MRS acquisitions, e.g., 3000 ms [32], 2 s [28], and even 550 ms [33,42], this cannot be reconciled with a cardiac-triggered sequence with inherent variations in heart rate and thus in repetition times. Correction for partial saturation effects with such modulations of magnetization becomes very complex if not impossible. The assumption of fully relaxed conditions for the lipid methylene signal may be valid at repetition times of more than 2 s [14,18] dependent on magnetic field strength, but does not hold at short repetition times [33,42] or for other metabolites of interest such as creatine or trimethylamine-containing compounds that have longer T_1 relaxation time constants [28]. Because the water T_1 relaxation time constant is much longer than for lipids, separate acquisitions at much longer repetition time are required for a fully relaxed water signal. The fluctuations in repetition times due to cardiac triggering and respiratory gating may be mitigated by employing "dummy excitations" to maintain a steady state of magnetization [46]. This approach has been successfully applied [47,48] and validated [49] in studies of the in vivo mouse heart (Fig. 8.5), where the time scale of the heart beat (R-R interval of ~ 100 ms) is short relative to the T_1 relaxation time constants [8]. Indeed, not adhering to steady state or fully relaxed conditions can lead to poor repeatability [42] and discrepancies between in vivo estimates with ^{1}H-MRS and biochemical assays on ex vivo tissue samples [28,52]. Methods to maintain a steady state of magnetization for ^{1}H-MRS of the human heart have not been reported. A practical solution to avoid partial saturation effects and the need to correct for them with assumed T_1 values is to acquire ^{1}H-MRS data at a long repetition time that ensures fully relaxed magnetization for all signals. This approach has been validated for myocardial lipid and creatine quantifications with ^{1}H-MRS of patients that were scheduled for open-heart surgery against biochemical assays in myocardial tissue obtained intraoperatively from the same patients [6].

With all, with only some, or without any of the corrections mentioned above, myocardial lipid content measured with ^{1}H-MRS is most commonly reported as a percentage of the unsuppressed water signal acquired from the same location. This approach allows for a straightforward comparison of results within a laboratory or study in which the experimental

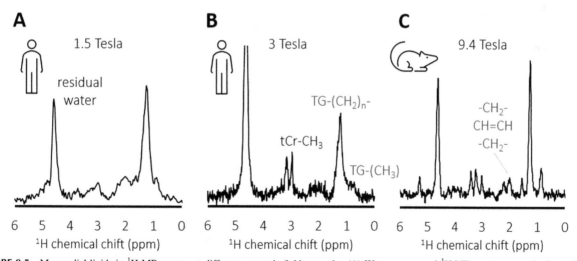

FIGURE 8.5 Myocardial lipids in ^{1}H-MR spectra at different magnetic field strengths. (A) Water-suppressed ^{1}H-MR spectrum acquired at 1.5 T in a healthy 62-year-old male volunteer, using a point resolved spectroscopy (PRESS) sequence for localized acquisition of signal from an 8 mL voxel at a repetition time (TR) of >3 s, an echo time (TE) of 26 ms, and 128 signal averages. The water line width at half maximum is 11.4 Hz and the reported myocardial lipid content for this subject is 0.82% of the unsuppressed water signal [50]. (B) Water-suppressed ^{1}H-MR spectrum acquired at 3 T in a healthy 53-year-old endurance-trained man (BMI, 25.0 kg/m^2), using PRESS (voxel, 4.8 mL; TR, >6 s; TE, 40 ms; 64 signal averages). Water line width was 15.8 Hz and the reported myocardial lipid content was 0.91% [51]. (C) Water-suppressed ^{1}H-MR spectrum acquired at 9.4 T in a 14-week-old male C57BL/6 mouse (body weight, 31.5 g), using PRESS (voxel, 4 μL; TR, 2 s; TE, 9.1 ms; 256 signal averages). Water line width was 25.4 Hz and the reported myocardial lipid content was 0.74% [49]. Note the increasing spectral resolution for higher magnetic field strengths that separates different metabolite signals, including creatine-methyl (tCr—CH$_3$) at 3.0 ppm, and triglyceride-methylene TG—(CH$_2$)$_n$— at 1.3 ppm, -methyl —(CH$_3$) at 0.9 ppm, and allylic methylene (—CH$_2$—CH=CH—CH$_2$—) at 2.0 ppm, particularly at 9.4 T.

conditions are the same. Still, results must be interpreted with caution if (patho-)physiological factors may induce a quantification bias, e.g., due to differences in heart rate and consequently repetition times between patient groups, or differences in myocardial water content or T_1 relaxation time constant due to myocardial fibrosis or scarring. Some studies included either multiple lipid resonance signals in estimating lipid content [26,32,53], both the methylene and methyl resonances [6,17,19,27,18,36], or only the prominent methylene signal [11,14,20,28]. The ratio of lipids over the creatine methyl signal instead of the water signal has also been used for measurements in healthy subjects [20], under the assumption that myocardial creatine content is stable in normal hearts, whereas it is known that creatine levels can be reduced in heart failure [16,54].

It is clear from above considerations that caution is warranted when comparing reported lipid levels between research groups and literature reports, and that results from a group of subjects in one study may not be transferable to a similar cohort in another. Even when tissue lipids concentrations (in µmol/g wet weight) are reported, the acquisition strategy, corrections, assumptions, and the quantification process may differ and yield different quantitative results [6,11,26,]. Given the complexity of ^{1}H-MRS data acquisition, processing, quantification, and interpretation in general, and for cardiac applications in particular, it is advisable that an experienced MR spectroscopist is consulted during study design, protocol development, and data evaluation. Complexity has been hampering the widespread use of ^{1}H-MRS in research and particularly in the clinic. Nonetheless, ^{1}H-MRS has contributed to our understanding of myocardial lipid metabolism in a unique, noninvasive way.

Lipids in the healthy human myocardium—effects of nutrition, fasting, and exercise

The reported myocardial lipid content in healthy adult humans is typically in the order of 0.5% of the unsuppressed water signal. It is imperative to note that such reported ratios are influenced by experimental conditions that can vary substantially between laboratories and between studies (see above), and that this number does not mean that 0.5% of the heart is composed of fat. Because standardization of data acquisition and quantification is lacking, reference values for ^{1}H-MRS estimates of myocardial lipid are currently not available. Several studies have used ^{1}H-MRS to investigate gender, age, and body mass index (BMI) as potential factors that mediate myocardial lipid content in healthy adults.

Gender

Gender has not convincingly been identified as a mediator of myocardial lipid content. Men (0.44 ± 0.11%) may harbor more myocardial lipids than women (0.26 ± 0.09%) [6], but the potentially confounding factors BMI and age were also slightly higher for the men in that study of healthy volunteers. A study of 40 age-matched healthy subjects [55] did not reveal a gender-mediated difference in myocardial lipid content (0.41 ± 0.47%). A study of 86 healthy participants [56] reported a myocardial lipid content of 12.3% in women and 6.7% in men, but experimental details were not provided that may explain these excessively high percentages that should thus be interpreted with caution. Differences in anatomy and physique between men and women may differentially contribute to any contamination with signal originating from tissue outside the voxel of interest, e.g., from chest skeletal muscle or breast tissue. Adequate localization of ^{1}H-MRS signal acquisition needs to be ensured to eliminate this potential source of bias in gender-focused studies.

Aging

Myocardial lipid content increases with age. Localized ^{1}H-MRS of 43 healthy men at an age range of 20−66 years revealed that physiological aging comes with higher levels of myocardial lipids, independent of BMI [50]. Importantly, this has an impact on heart function, even in healthy individuals. Elevated myocardial lipid levels were independently associated with an age-related decline in left ventricular diastolic function that was quantified as the E/A flow ratio of the early filling phase (E) and atrial contraction (A) with MRI measurements of blood flow across the mitral valve [50]. In healthy 20−29-year-olds, the myocardial lipid content was 0.25 ± 0.17%, and tripled in healthy 50−60 year olds (0.77 ± 0.70%), with no impact on systolic function and a weak positive correlation with BMI [57].

Body mass index

Besides gender and age, BMI seems a plausible mediator of myocardial lipid content in healthy subjects. Indeed, in a small study that compared five healthy lean (BMI, 22 ± 1 kg/m^2) with four moderately obese (30 ± 1 kg/m^2) men, plasma free fatty acid levels were twice as high in the obese men, and myocardial lipids were much higher (2.1 ± 0.5%) than in the lean subjects (0.8 ± 0.1%) [32]. In a large study of 153 nonobese healthy subjects aged 26−86 years, it was shown that myocardial lipid accumulation is associated with increased BMI, as well as with low aerobic fitness [58]. Again, early signs of diastolic but not systolic dysfunction were observed in subjects with higher myocardial lipid levels.

Athletes and exercise

The term "athlete's paradox" refers to the phenomenon that trained athletes, with high insulin sensitivity, harbor elevated levels of intracellular lipids in their skeletal muscles, similar to what is found in insulin-resistant patients with type 2 diabetes [59] (see Chapter 11). It is not known if this phenomenon also occurs in the myocardium. Only a few studies have investigated lipid content in the heart muscle of athletes. A small study found a lower myocardial lipid content in 10 male endurance athletes (0.60 ± 0.20%) compared to nonobese healthy men (0.89 ± 0.41%) [60]. Another study reported no apparent elevation of myocardial lipid levels in a small group of experienced male marathon runners, and found that running a single marathon depleted the myocardial lipid pool by nearly 30% [51]. Two weeks after completing the marathon, myocardial lipid levels had restored to baseline levels, demonstrating the dynamic nature of ectopic myocardial lipid storage in these athletes. The acute effect of physical exercise on myocardial lipid content has also been investigated in a laboratory setting. In 10 healthy men that were preloaded with a fat-rich diet for 3 days, myocardial lipid levels decreased by 17% after a 2-hour bout of moderate-intensity bicycling exercise [61]. In 11 male subjects that had performed a 2-hour bout of bicycling while fasted, the circulating plasma free fatty acid concentration elevated ninefold with a concomitant increase in myocardial lipid content of nearly 70% after 4 h of rest. This effect was absent when the subjects repeated the protocol in glucose-fed conditions [62]. In none of these studies, the observed acute changes in myocardial lipid content induced by physical exercise could be related to alterations in heart function.

Nutrition

Another important mediator of myocardial lipid content is the nutritional status and diet. Several studies in healthy volunteers have addressed the effect of various nutritional interventions on the myocardial lipid pools beyond diurnal variations [20]. Prolonged fasting in volunteers triggered a 37% decline in serum triglyceride concentration, while myocardial lipid content more than tripled [29]. Short-term caloric restriction in 14 healthy nonobese men on a very low-calorie diet for 3 days doubled the plasma concentration of free fatty acids, which was paralleled by an increase in myocardial lipid content from 0.38 ± 0.05% to 0.59 ± 0.06%. Left ventricular systolic function remained normal, but diastolic function, assessed via measurements of the early diastolic deceleration in blood flow across the mitral valve with velocity-encoded MRI, decreased and correlated negatively with increased myocardial lipid content after caloric restriction [63]. Progressive caloric restriction with 3 days of starvation in 10 lean, healthy men showed a similar effect, with plasma free fatty acids progressively increasing along with myocardial lipid content from 0.35 ± 0.14% at baseline to 1.26 ± 0.49% after 3 days of fasting [64]. Importantly, increasing myocardial lipid content with partial and complete starvation was paralleled by decreased left ventricular diastolic function but not systolic function. In 12 obese patients with type 2 diabetes that followed a very low-calorie diet for 16 weeks, their BMI was reduced, circulating free fatty acids dropped by more than 25%, and myocardial lipid content decreased from 0.88 ± 0.12% to 0.64 ± 0.14%, with a substantial improvement in cardiac performance and diastolic function in particular [65].

During endurance exercise or caloric restriction, fatty acids are released from the adipose tissue into the circulation for fueling oxidative metabolism in other organs. Some studies have investigated the acute effect of elevating the level of free fatty acids through the consumption of large amount of fat. A small study in three men and three women showed that the consumption of 50 g of fat induced a nearly 70% increase in serum triglyceride concentration, but myocardial lipid content remained unchanged [29]. In another study of 15 healthy men on a 3-day high fat high-caloric diet that included the consumption of 280 g of fat in 800 mL of cream per day, hepatic lipid levels more than doubled while no change in myocardial lipid levels was observed and diastolic function remained normal [66]. These results show that the elevation of free fatty acid concentrations through fat consumption represents a metabolic state that is distinctly different from caloric restriction, and that their influence on myocardial lipid metabolism and heart function differs. In the context of investigating the association between fructose consumption and nonalcoholic fatty liver disease (NAFLD; see Chapter 7), five healthy men and five healthy women followed a high-fructose diet (150 g/day) for 8 weeks [67]. Left ventricular function, heart morphology, nor myocardial lipid content were affected by high dietary fructose intake, suggesting that prolonged fructose intake does not affect myocardial lipid metabolism in healthy subjects.

The results from studies in healthy volunteers under various metabolically different physiological conditions illustrate that myocardial lipid storage is a highly dynamic process that can vary within individuals when conditions change. This implies that it is important to take standardization of factors that can have a short-term impact on myocardial lipid content, e.g., time of day, nutritional status, and physical activity, into account in the design of studies. The noninvasive and nondisruptive nature of ^{1}H-MRS of the human heart has allowed longitudinal studies in healthy volunteers that would not have been possible with other techniques or methods. Yet, most of the studies addressed above, and particularly those that involved longitudinal assessments, were conducted in small cohorts of less than 15 subjects. This may be related to the relatively long experimental time that is required for ^{1}H-MRS of the heart, and the potentially challenging logistical constraints due to limited MR system availability and associated high costs. Nonetheless, even in such small study cohorts, ^{1}H-MRS in combination with MRI has generally proven to be sufficiently sensitive to establish metabolic and functional changes of the healthy human heart under various physiological conditions.

Myocardial lipids in disease

Disturbed systemic and myocardial lipid metabolism and excess ectopic myocardial lipid accumulation or myocardial steatosis have been implicated in the pathogenesis of cardiomyopathy and heart failure in various diseases. The molecular mechanisms [3] and metabolic pathways [1,68] linking myocardial lipid accumulation with the development of cardiomyopathy have been reviewed elsewhere [69]. Localized ^{1}H-MRS of the human heart allows for noninvasive quantitative assessments of the intracellular neutral lipid droplets that store (excess) fatty acids as triglycerides. Such lipid droplets may be harmless themselves, but their presence and size may be a surrogate marker for tissue levels of other metabolites, such as ceramides, acylcarnitines, and diglycerides. Excess levels of these intermediate compounds can have toxic effects that disturb the normal biological processes in cardiomyocytes [70]. Myocardial lipid content, as a potential in vivo marker for such cardiac lipotoxicity, has been investigated extensively with ^{1}H-MRS to address the potential role for excess lipid accumulation in cardiomyopathy and cardiac dysfunction.

Insulin resistance and type 2 diabetes

Given the globally rising prevalence of obesity, type 2 diabetes, and metabolic syndrome, it is not surprising that the majority of studies that used ^{1}H-MRS over the past decades have focused on conditions of insulin resistance and type 2 diabetes. Obesity, in the absence of insulin resistance, is associated with a higher myocardial lipid content while systolic function in terms of the left ventricular ejection fraction is normal [29,71]. Myocardial lipid content in 14 healthy but obese men (BMI, 29.9 ± 0.01 kg/m^2) could be reduced almost twofold from $0.99 \pm 0.15\%$ to $0.54 \pm 0.04\%$ by a 12-week endurance and strength training program, and was paralleled by a small improvement in left ventricular ejection fraction [72]. Type 2 diabetes, with or without underlying obesity, was associated with more than twofold higher myocardial lipid levels compared to lean healthy subjects [73]. Likewise, myocardial lipid content was higher in 38 men with type 2 diabetes ($0.96 \pm 0.07\%$) compared to 28 age- and BMI-matched male volunteers ($0.65 \pm 0.05\%$), where elevated myocardial lipid levels were independently associated with impaired left ventricular diastolic function but not systolic function [74]. In a cross-sectional study that investigated the various stages in the development of type 2 diabetes in 34 women, it was shown that insulin resistance, impaired glucose tolerance, and ultimately type 2 diabetes were progressively associated with elevated myocardial lipid levels [75], although insulin resistance as such was not associated with high myocardial lipid levels in these women. A large study of 134 subjects that were subdivided in groups representing the progressive stages of type 2 diabetes found that glucose intolerance and type 2 diabetes are accompanied by excessive myocardial lipid accumulation [71]. A similar trend was found in 53 subjects, where the progression of cardiac steatosis was most pronounced in women with impaired glucose tolerance [76]. These in vivo data confirmed the presence of cardiac steatosis that was observed with histology in explanted hearts from patients with type 2 diabetes [77]. Notably, excessive myocardial lipid levels were present in absence of cardiac dysfunction or evident heart failure [71]. A physical exercise intervention with 12 weeks of endurance and strength training for 11 obese men with type 2 diabetes improved their aerobic fitness, insulin sensitivity, and systolic function, but did not lead to a consistent change in myocardial lipid content [78]. Similarly, 6 months of moderate-intensity training followed by a high-altitude trekking expedition lowered the visceral abdominal fat volume and hepatic lipid levels while improving exercise capacity in 12 patients with type 2 diabetes, but had no effect on their myocardial lipid content or heart function [79]. Within 10 days, insulin treatment acutely increased myocardial lipid levels by 80% in 10 patients with long standing type 2 diabetes, along with an increased myocardial wall thickness and mass but without changes in left ventricular systolic function [80]. After 6 months of insulin treatment, myocardial lipid content had returned to baseline levels, while left ventricular hypertrophy persisted. A study of 18 healthy volunteers that underwent a 6-hour hyperglycemic clamp showed that combined hyperglycemia and endogenous hyperinsulinemia induces an acute 34% elevation of myocardial lipid content along with higher left ventricular ejection fraction, despite low circulating levels of free fatty acids during the clamp. These results suggest that insulin release is the key mediator for increasing myocardial lipid levels in these healthy subjects, potentially due to increased uptake of free fatty acids by the myocardium and insulin-mediated inhibition of fatty acid β-oxidation [81]. An intervention with pioglitazone, an insulin-resistance and blood-glucose lowering agent, for 24 weeks in 34 men with type 2 diabetes improved left ventricular diastolic function and insulin sensitivity, but did not affect myocardial lipid content [82]. A different study of 16 subjects with type 2 diabetes treated with pioglitazone plus insulin for 6 months showed a reduction of myocardial lipid content by 33%, while cardiac performance did not change [83]. Other investigations of different therapeutic compounds have also benefited from the noninvasive nature of ^{1}H-MRS of the human heart in longitudinal studies, such as trimetazidine in obesity [84], and liraglutide [85] and metformin [82] in type 2 diabetes. Without a consistent relationship between increased myocardial lipid content and decreased cardiac performance, the results from these studies suggest that lipotoxicity through excess myocardial lipid accumulation is not the only mediator of impaired cardiac performance in insulin resistance and type 2 diabetes. Indeed, a deranged myocardial energy homeostasis [73] is an important contributor to the development cardiomyopathy and heart failure in type 2 diabetes [86].

Other diseases

Potential myocardial lipid overload has been investigated in various other diseases and disorders. In the hypertrophied heart, a shift in myocardial substrate utilization from fatty acid β-oxidation to glucose oxidation may induce excess ectopic storage of fatty acids [68]. In a longitudinal study of severe aortic valve stenosis, myocardial lipid content was higher in 25 symptomatic (0.89 ± 0.42%) as well as 14 asymptomatic patients (0.75 ± 0.36%) compared to age- and gender-matched control subjects (0.45 ± 0.17%), with myocardial lipid accumulation independently correlating with impaired left ventricular strain. Months after aortic valve replacement, both myocardial lipid content and left ventricular strain had recovered to normal values [37]. Such elevation of myocardial lipid content in severe aortic valve stenosis was confirmed in 13 patients, although myocardial lipid accumulation did not correlate with any cardiac dysfunction in that cross-sectional study [6]. Mitochondrial function and myocardial metabolism have been recognized as important therapeutic targets in heart failure, and metabolism-modulating treatments are emerging [1,87]. In a group of 27 patients with heart failure with preserved ejection fraction (HFpEF), pronounced cardiac steatosis was detected with ^{1}H-MRS (1.45 ± 0.25%) with respect to 14 age-, gender-, and BMI-matched control subjects (0.64 ± 0.16%), and correlated with decreased left ventricular diastolic circumferential strain rate [88]. In five women with subclinical HFpEF and impaired coronary microvascular function, myocardial lipid content was nearly twofold higher (0.83 ± 0.12%) than in their reference control group (0.43 ± 0.06%) of eight women with similar age and BMI, again demonstrating a reduced diastolic circumferential strain rate that was associated with cardiac steatosis [89].

Myocardial lipid overload has been implicated in the pathogenesis of cardiomyopathy and cardiac dysfunction that can occur in inherited metabolic disorders. A small study compared six patients with congenital lipodystrophy, a very rare condition that leads to extreme loss of subcutaneous fat, with six age-, gender-, and BMI-matched control subjects. Patients with lipodystrophy lack the capacity to store excess nutritional lipids in adipose tissue, which leads to elevated ectopic lipid deposition in liver and skeletal muscle. This study found that myocardial lipid content was almost threefold higher in parallel with left ventricular hypertrophy in patients with lipodystrophy [90]. Pharmacologically induced lipodystrophy, as can occur in subjects infected with the human immunodeficiency virus (HIV) that are treated with highly active antiretroviral therapy, led to substantial elevation of myocardial lipid levels, again paralleled by reduced circumferential strain and diastolic circumferential strain rate [91]. In Fabry disease, a lysosomal storage disease that is characterized by a progressive accumulation of sphingolipids, cardiac involvement leads to hypertrophy and conduction disorders and may be lethal. A comprehensive MR study in 30 patients with Fabry disease and 30 healthy control subjects revealed left ventricular hypertrophy in Fabry disease, in absence of myocardial lipid accumulation that was measured with ^{1}H-MRS [92]. A comprehensive MR examination was used for investigating the effect of inborn errors in long-chain fatty acid β-oxidation on myocardial lipid content and heart function [53]. In 14 adult patients with long-chain fatty acid β-oxidation disorders and 14 age-, gender-, and BMI-matched control subjects, subclinical differences in contractile function and mild left ventricular hypertrophy were revealed, while myocardial lipid levels were similar in both groups. Although severe fat infiltration has been reported for pediatric autopsy cases [5] and cardiac steatosis was found in mouse models of fatty acid β-oxidation deficiency [49], lipotoxic effects of ectopic lipid accumulation in the myocardium do not seem to play a major role in hypertrophic remodeling in these adult patients with long-chain fatty acid β-oxidation disorders, but rather a chronically compromised myocardial energy homeostasis [53]. Amyloidosis is characterized by extracellular deposition of misfolded amyloid proteins that may lead to organ failure, including the myocardium. A cross-sectional study in 11 patients with amyloidosis and 11 age- and gender-matched control subjects revealed a lower myocardial lipid content in amyloidosis (0.53 ± 0.23%) compared to the control group (0.80 ± 0.26%) that was associated with the degree of myocardial hypertrophy and systolic dysfunction [93].

In many studies, ^{1}H-MRS is part of a comprehensive MR examination of the heart that includes volumetric and functional imaging with cinematographic MRI, an assessment of diffuse fibrosis and interstitial expansion with myocardial T_1 mapping and extracellular volume fraction mapping, and tissue scarring with late gadolinium enhancement imaging after the administration of a gadolinium-based contrast agent. This unparalleled versatility in quantitative readouts makes MR a unique modality in the clinical workflow of disease diagnosis and follow-up. Inborn errors in metabolism are diseases that impact lipid utilization and storage on a systemic scale, similar to type 2 diabetes and metabolic syndrome. Indeed, with MRI and ^{1}H-MRS readily applicable in essentially all organs and tissues of the human body, MR should be regarded as the method of choice for a systemic or multi-organ evaluation of visceral and ectopic fat.

Concluding remarks and outlook

Localized ^{1}H-MRS of the human heart has proven to be a valuable tool to investigate myocardial lipid content in many different conditions and pathologies. A drawback of single-voxel MR spectroscopy is its low spatial resolution that typically only provides a single readout for the interventricular septum. Water-fat separation imaging, also referred to as Dixon MRI, may offer a solution to achieve a detailed regional analysis of myocardial steatosis and lipid deposition [94,95]. An MR imaging approach at high spatial resolution may shed light on the presence or absence of extracellular lipids that are commonly distinguished from intracellular lipid droplets with localized ^{1}H-MRS in skeletal muscle dependent on their macroscopic orientation with respect to the magnetic field of the MR system [96] (see Chapter 11), but not in the myocardium. Very few reports suggest the detection of extracellular myocardial lipids with ^{1}H-MRS. One study in 10 female volunteers used the interindividual difference in angles of the heart axis and voxel of interest orientation relative to the main magnetic field to separate extracellular lipids from intracellular myocardial lipid droplets [97], and another study in rats reported the detection of extracellular lipid deposits in animals that were fed a high-fat diet for 17 weeks [98]. Unlike myocytes in skeletal muscle, cardiomyocytes in the myocardium are not oriented in an elongated alignment, but are organized in a helical fashion with a gradually changing angle across the left ventricular wall [99]. A macroscopic homogeneous fiber orientation within the voxel of interest may therefore not be achieved in single-voxel localized ^{1}H-MRS of the heart, and any detection of quantification of extracellular lipids with ^{1}H-MRS in the myocardium should therefore be interpreted with caution.

Essentially all ^{1}H-MRS studies of the human heart have been conducted at magnetic field strengths of either 1.5 T or 3 T. Technological advancements for MR at 7 T theoretically hold promise for increased sensitivity with higher signal-to-noise ratios that can be exchanged for higher spatial resolution, and higher spectral resolution for improved separation of metabolite signals that may enable a quantitative assessment of lipid composition and degree of saturation (Fig. 8.5), and potentially the detection of extracellular lipid pools. However, at such ultrahigh magnetic field strengths, achieving magnetic field homogeneity and sufficient RF pulse bandwidths is a tremendous challenge. Improvements in image-based shimming [100] and RF pulse optimizations [101] are required to ensure adequate localization of signal acquisitions and water suppression efficacy, and to minimize the chemical shift displacement error, before the potential benefits of ^{1}H-MRS at ultrahigh magnetic field strengths can be exploited. Such improvements, together with increasing availability of ^{1}H-MRS techniques and expertise, will continue to contribute to meaningful applications of ^{1}H-MRS in investigations of human myocardial lipid metabolism in health and disease.

References

[1] Lopaschuk GD, Karwi QG, Tian R, Wende AR, Abel ED. Cardiac energy metabolism in heart failure. Circ Res 2021;128(10):1487−513. https://doi.org/10.1161/CIRCRESAHA.121.318241.

[2] Ren J, Wu NN, Wang S, Sowers JR, Zhang Y. Obesity cardiomyopathy: evidence, mechanisms and therapeutic implications. Physiol Rev 2021;101(4):1745−807. https://doi.org/10.1152/physrev.00030.2020.

[3] Nakamura M, Sadoshima J. Cardiomyopathy in obesity, insulin resistance and diabetes. J Physiol 2020;598(14):2977−93. https://doi.org/10.1113/JP276747.

[4] Marfella R, Di Filippo C, Portoghese M, Barbieri M, Ferraraccio F, Siniscalchi M, Cacciapuoti F, Rossi F, D'Amico M, Paolisso G. Myocardial lipid accumulation in patients with pressure-overloaded heart and metabolic syndrome. JLR (J Lipid Res) 2009;50(11):2314−23. https://doi.org/10.1194/jlr.P900032-JLR200.

[5] Bleeker JC, Visser G, Wijburg FA, Ferdinandusse S, Waterham HR, Nikkels PGJ. Severe fat accumulation in multiple organs in pediatric autopsies: an uncommon but significant finding. Pediatr Dev Pathol 2017;20(4):269−76. https://doi.org/10.1177/1093526617691708.

[6] Bakermans AJ, Boekholdt SM, de Vries DK, Reckman YJ, Farag ES, de Heer P, Uthman L, Denis SW, Zuurbier CJ, Houtkooper RH, Koolbergen DR, Kluin J, Planken RN, Lamb HJ, Webb AG, Strijkers GJ, Beard DA, Jeneson JAL, Nederveen AJ. Quantification of myocardial creatine and triglyceride content in the human heart: precision and accuracy of *in vivo* proton magnetic resonance spectroscopy. J Magn Reson Imag 2021;54(2):411−20. https://doi.org/10.1002/jmri.27531.

[7] Ruberg FL, Viereck J, Phinikaridou A, Qiao Y, Joseph Loscalzo J, Hamilton JA. Identification of cholesteryl esters in human carotid atherosclerosis by *ex vivo* image-guided proton MRS. JLR (J Lipid Res) 2006;47(2):310−7. https://doi.org/10.1194/jlr.M500431-JLR200.

[8] Bakermans AJ, Abdurrachim D, Geraedts TR, Houten SM, Nicolay K, Prompers JJ. *In vivo* proton T_1 relaxation times of mouse myocardial metabolites at 9.4 T. Magn Reson Med 2015;73(6):2069−74. https://doi.org/10.1002/mrm.25340.

[9] Gabr RE, Sathyanarayana S, Schär M, Weiss RG, Bottomley PA. On restoring motion-induced signal loss in single-voxel magnetic resonance spectra. Magn Reson Med 2006;56(4):754−60. https://doi.org/10.1002/mrm.21015.

[10] den Hollander JA, Evanochko WT, Pohost GM. Observation of cardiac lipids in humans by localized ^{1}H magnetic resonance spectroscopic imaging. Magn Reson Med 1994;32(2):175−80. https://doi.org/10.1002/mrm.1910320205.

[11] Szczepaniak LS, Dobbins RL, Metzger GJ, Sartoni-D'Ambrosia G, Arbique D, Vongpatanasin W, et al. Myocardial triglycerides and systolic function in humans: *in vivo* evaluation by localized proton spectroscopy and cardiac imaging. Magn Reson Med 2003;49(3):417−23. https://doi.org/10.1002/mrm.10372.

[12] Bottomley PA. Spatial localization in NMR spectroscopy *in vivo*. Ann N Y Acad Sci 1987;508:333−48. https://doi.org/10.1111/j.1749-6632.1987.tb32915.x.

[13] Frahm J, Merboldt K-D, Hänicke W. Localized proton spectroscopy using stimulated echoes. J Magn Reson (1969) 1987;72(3):502−8. https://doi.org/10.1016/0022-2364(87)90154-5.

[14] Rial B, Robson MD, Neubauer S, Schneider JE. Rapid quantification of myocardial lipid content in humans using single breath-hold ^{1}H MRS at 3 Tesla. Magn Reson Med 2011;66(3):619−24. https://doi.org/10.1002/mrm.23011.

[15] Felblinger J, Jung B, Slotboom J, Boesch C, Kreis R. Methods and reproducibility of cardiac/respiratory double-triggered ^{1}H-MR spectroscopy of the human heart. Magn Reson Med 1999;42(5):903−10. https://doi.org/10.1002/(sici)1522-2594(199911)42:5<903::aid-mrm10>3.0.co;2-n.

[16] Nakae I, Mitsunami K, Omura T, Yabe T, Tsutamoto T, Matsuo S, et al. Proton magnetic resonance spectroscopy can detect creatine depletion associated with the progression of heart failure in cardiomyopathy. J Am Coll Cardiol 2003;42(9):1587−93. https://doi.org/10.1016/j.jacc.2003.05.005.

[17] O'Connor RD, Xu J, Ewald GA, Ackerman JJH, Peterson LR, Gropler RJ, Bashir A. Intramyocardial triglyceride quantification by magnetic resonance spectroscopy: *in vivo* and *ex vivo* correlation in human subjects. Magn Reson Med 2011;65(5):1234−8. https://doi.org/10.1002/mrm.22734.

[18] van der Meer RW, Doornbos J, Kozerke S, Schär M, Bax JJ, Hammer S, et al. Metabolic imaging of myocardial triglyceride content: reproducibility of ^{1}H MR spectroscopy with respiratory navigator gating in volunteers. Radiology 2007;245(1):251−7. https://doi.org/10.1148/radiol.2451061904.

[19] de Heer P, Bizino MB, Lamb HJ, Webb AG. Parameter optimization for reproducible cardiac ^{1}H-MR spectroscopy at 3 Tesla. J Magn Reson Imag 2016;44(5):1151−8. https://doi.org/10.1002/jmri.25254.

[20] Ith M, Stettler C, Xu J, Boesch C, Kreis R. Cardiac lipid levels show diurnal changes and long-term variations in healthy human subjects. NMR Biomed 2014;27(11):1285−92. https://doi.org/10.1002/nbm.3186.

[21] Bredella MA, Ghomi RH, Thomas BJ, Miller KK, Torriani M. Comparison of 3.0 T proton magnetic resonance spectroscopy short and long echo-time measures of intramyocellular lipids in obese and normal-weight women. J Magn Reson Imag 2010;32(2):388−93. https://doi.org/10.1002/jmri.22226.

[22] Lindeboom L, Nabuurs CI, Hoeks J, Brouwers B, Phielix E, Kooi ME, Hesselink MKC, Wildberger JE, Stevens RD, Koves T, Muoio DM, Schrauwen P, Schrauwen-Hinderling VB. Long-echo time MR spectroscopy for skeletal muscle acetylcarnitine detection. J Clin Investig 2014;124(11):4915−25. https://doi.org/10.1172/JCI74830.

[23] Krššák M, Mlynárik V, Meyerspeer M, Moser E, Roden M. ^{1}H NMR relaxation times of skeletal muscle metabolites at 3 T. Magma 2004;16(4):155−9. https://doi.org/10.1007/s10334-003-0029-1.

[24] Bottomley PA, Weiss RG. Non-invasive magnetic-resonance detection of creatine depletion in non-viable infarcted myocardium. Lancet (London, England) 1998;351(9104):714−8. https://doi.org/10.1016/S0140-6736(97)06402-7.

[25] Garwood M, DelaBarre L. The return of the frequency sweep: designing adiabatic pulses for contemporary NMR. J Magn Reson 2001;153(2):155−77. https://doi.org/10.1006/jmre.2001.2340.

[26] Sourdon J, Roussel T, Costes C, Viout P, Guye M, Ranjeva J-P, Bernard M, Kober F, Rapacchi S. Comparison of single-voxel ^{1}H-cardiovascular magnetic resonance spectroscopy techniques for *in vivo* measurement of myocardial creatine and triglycerides at 3T. J Cardiovasc Magn Reson 2021;23(1):53. https://doi.org/10.1186/s12968-021-00748-x.

[27] Weiss K, Martini N, Boesiger P, Kozerke S. Metabolic MR imaging of regional triglyceride and creatine content in the human heart. Magn Reson Med 2012;68(6):1696−704. https://doi.org/10.1002/mrm.24178.

[28] Ding B, Peterzan M, Mózes FE, Rider OJ, Valkovič L, Rodgers CT. Water-suppression cycling 3-T cardiac ^{1}H-MRS detects altered creatine and choline in patients with aortic or mitral stenosis. NMR Biomed 2021;34(9):e4513. https://doi.org/10.1002/nbm.4513.

[29] Reingold JS, McGavock JM, Kaka S, Tillery T, Victor RG, Szczepaniak LS. Determination of triglyceride in the human myocardium by magnetic resonance spectroscopy: reproducibility and sensitivity of the method. Am J Physiol Endocrinol Metab 2005;289(5):E935−9. https://doi.org/10.1152/ajpendo.00095.2005.

[30] Weiss K, Summermatter S, Stoeck CT, Kozerke S. Compensation of signal loss due to cardiac motion in point-resolved spectroscopy of the heart. Magn Reson Med 2014;72(5):1201−7. https://doi.org/10.1002/mrm.25028.

[31] Fuetterer M, Stoeck CT, Kozerke S. Second-order motion compensated PRESS for cardiac spectroscopy. Magn Reson Med 2017;77(1):57−64. https://doi.org/10.1002/mrm.26099.

[32] Kankaanpää M, Lehto H-R, Pärkkä JP, Komu M, Viljanen A, Ferrannini E, et al. Myocardial triglyceride content and epicardial fat mass in human obesity: relationship to left ventricular function and serum free fatty acid levels. J Clin Endocrinol Metab 2006;91(11):4689−95. https://doi.org/10.1210/jc.2006-0584.

[33] Wu C-K, Lee J-K, Hsu J-C, Su M-YM, Wu Y-F, Lin T-T, Lan C-W, Hwang J-J, Lin L-Y. Myocardial adipose deposition and the development of heart failure with preserved ejection fraction. Eur J Heart Fail 2020;22(3):445−54. https://doi.org/10.1002/ejhf.1617.

[34] Schär M, Kozerke S, Boesiger P. Navigator gating and volume tracking for double-triggered cardiac proton spectroscopy at 3 Tesla. Magn Reson Med 2004;51(6):1091−5. https://doi.org/10.1002/mrm.20123.

[35] Kozerke S, Schär M, Lamb HJ, Boesiger P. Volume tracking cardiac ^{31}P spectroscopy. Magn Reson Med 2002;48(2):380−4. https://doi.org/10.1002/mrm.10182.

[36] Gastl M, Peereboom SM, Fuetterer M, Boenner F, Kelm M, Manka R, Kozerke S. Retrospective phase-based gating for cardiac proton spectroscopy with fixed scan time. J Magn Reson Imag 2019;50(6):1973−81. https://doi.org/10.1002/jmri.26802.

[37] Mahmod M, Bull S, Suttie JJ, Pal N, Holloway C, Dass S, Myerson SG, Schneider JE, De Silva R, Petrou M, Sayeed R, Westaby S, Clelland C, Francis JM, Ashrafian H, Karamitsos TD, Neubauer S. Myocardial steatosis and left ventricular contractile dysfunction in patients with severe aortic stenosis. Circ Cardiovasc Imaging 2013;6(5):808−16. https://doi.org/10.1161/CIRCIMAGING.113.000559.

[38] Peereboom SM, Gastl M, Fuetterer M, Kozerke S. Navigator-free metabolite-cycled proton spectroscopy of the heart. Magn Reson Med 2020;83(3):795−805. https://doi.org/10.1002/mrm.27961.

[39] Schär M, Vonken E-J, Stuber M. Simultaneous B_0- and B_1+-map acquisition for fast localized shim, frequency, and RF power determination in the heart at 3 T. Magn Reson Med 2010;63(2):419−26. https://doi.org/10.1002/mrm.22234.

[40] Near J, Harris AD, Juchem C, Kreis R, Marjańska M, Öz G, Slotboom J, Wilson M, Gasparovic C. Preprocessing, analysis and quantification in single-voxel magnetic resonance spectroscopy: experts' consensus recommendations. NMR Biomed 2021;34(5). https://doi.org/10.1002/nbm.4257. e4257.

[41] Hamilton G, Schlein AN, Middleton MS, Hooker CA, Wolfson T, Gamst AC, Loomba R, Sirlin CB. *In vivo* triglyceride composition of abdominal adipose tissue measured by ^{1}H MRS at 3T. J Magn Reson Imag 2017;45(5):1455−63. https://doi.org/10.1002/jmri.25453.

[42] Liao P-A, Lin G, Tsai S-Y, Wang C-H, Juan Y-H, Lin Y-C, Wu M-T, Yang L-Y, Liu M-H, Chang T-C, Lin Y-C, Huang Y-C, Huang P-C, Wang J-J, Ng S-H, Ng K-K. Myocardial triglyceride content at 3 T cardiovascular magnetic resonance and left ventricular systolic function: a cross-sectional study in patients hospitalized with acute heart failure. J Cardiovasc Magn Reson 2016;18:9. https://doi.org/10.1186/s12968-016-0228-3.

[43] Madden MC, Van Winkle WB, Kirk K, Pike MM, Pohost GM, Wolkowicz PE. ^{1}H-NMR spectroscopy can accurately quantitate the lipolysis and oxidation of cardiac triacylglycerols. Biochim Biophys Acta 1993;1169(2):176−82. https://doi.org/10.1016/0005-2760(93)90203-l.

[44] Bottomley PA, Atalar E, Weiss RG. Human cardiac high-energy phosphate metabolite concentrations by 1D-resolved NMR spectroscopy. Magn Reson Med 1996;35(5):664−70. https://doi.org/10.1002/mrm.1910350507.

[45] Snyder WS, Cook MJ, Nasset ES, Karhausen LR, Parry Howells G, Tipton IH. Report of the task group on reference man, vol. 23. Pergamon Press; 1975.

[46] Cassidy PJ, Schneider JE, Grieve SM, Lygate C, Neubauer S, Clarke K. Assessment of motion gating strategies for mouse magnetic resonance at high magnetic fields. J Magn Reson Imag 2004;19(2):229−37. https://doi.org/10.1002/jmri.10454.

[47] Bakermans AJ, van Weeghel M, Denis S, Nicolay K, Prompers JJ, Houten SM. Carnitine supplementation attenuates myocardial lipid accumulation in long-chain acyl-CoA dehydrogenase knockout mice. J Inherit Metab Dis 2013;36(6):973−81. https://doi.org/10.1007/s10545-013-9604-4.

[48] Schneider JE, Tyler DJ, ten Hove M, Sang AE, Cassidy PJ, Fischer A, et al. *In vivo* cardiac ^{1}H-MRS in the mouse. Magn Reson Med 2004;52(5):1029−35. https://doi.org/10.1002/mrm.20257.

[49] Bakermans AJ, Geraedts TR, van Weeghel M, Denis S, João Ferraz M, Aerts JMFG, Aten J, Nicolay K, Houten SM, Prompers JJ. Fasting-induced myocardial lipid accumulation in long-chain acyl-CoA dehydrogenase knockout mice is accompanied by impaired left ventricular function. Circ Cardiovasc Imaging 2011;4(5):558−65. https://doi.org/10.1161/CIRCIMAGING.111.963751.

[50] van der Meer RW, Rijzewijk LJ, Diamant M, Hammer S, Schär M, Bax JJ, Smit JWA, Romijn JA, de Roos A, Lamb HJ. The ageing male heart: myocardial triglyceride content as independent predictor of diastolic function. Eur Heart J 2008;29(12):1516−22. https://doi.org/10.1093/eurheartj/ehn207.

[51] Aengevaeren VL, Froeling M, van den Berg-Faay S, Hooijmans MT, Monte JR, Strijkers GJ, Nederveen AJ, Eijsvogels TMH, Bakermans AJ. Marathon running transiently depletes the myocardial lipid pool. Physiol Rep 2020;8(17):e14543. https://doi.org/10.14814/phy2.14543.

[52] Hankiewicz JH, Banke NH, Farjah M, Lewandowski ED. Early impairment of transmural principal strains in the left ventricular wall after short-term, high-fat feeding of mice predisposed to cardiac steatosis. Circ Cardiovasc Imaging 2010;3(6):710−7. https://doi.org/10.1161/CIRCIMAGING.110.959098.

[53] Knottnerus SJG, Bleeker JC, Ferdinandusse S, Houtkooper RH, Langeveld M, Nederveen AJ, Strijkers GJ, Visser G, Wanders RJA, Wijburg FA, Boekholdt SM, Bakermans AJ. Subclinical effects of long-chain fatty acid β-oxidation deficiency on the adult heart: a case-control magnetic resonance study. J Inherit Metab Dis 2020;43(5):969−80. https://doi.org/10.1002/jimd.12266.

[54] Cowan DW. The creatine content of the myocardium of normal and abnormal human hearts. Am Heart J 1934;9(3):378−85. https://doi.org/10.1016/S0002-8703(34)90224-6.

[55] Petritsch B, Köstler H, Gassenmaier T, Kunz AS, Bley TA, Horn M. An investigation into potential gender-specific differences in myocardial triglyceride content assessed by [1]H-magnetic resonance spectroscopy at 3 Tesla. J Int Med Res 2016;44(3):585−91. https://doi.org/10.1177/0300060515603884.

[56] Wu J, Yang L, Yang J, Yang CH, Zhang XH. Gender-specific normal levels of myocardial metabolites determined by localized [1]H-magnetic resonance spectroscopy. J Int Med Res 2012;40(4):1507−12. https://doi.org/10.1177/147323001204000430.

[57] Petritsch B, Gassenmaier T, Kunz AS, Donhauser J, Goltz JP, Bley TA, et al. Age dependency of myocardial triglyceride content: a 3T high-field [1]H-MR spectroscopy study. Röfo Fortschritte dem Geb Rontgenstrahlen Nukl 2015;187(11):1016−21. https://doi.org/10.1055/s-0035-1553350.

[58] Sarma S, Carrick-Ranson G, Fujimoto N, Adams-Huet B, Bhella PS, Hastings JL, Shafer KM, Shibata S, Boyd K, Palmer D, Szczepaniak EW, Szczepaniak LS, Levine BD. Effects of age and aerobic fitness on myocardial lipid content. Circ Cardiovasc Imaging 2013;6(6):1048−55. https://doi.org/10.1161/CIRCIMAGING.113.000565.

[59] Goodpaster BH, He J, Watkins S, Kelley DE. Skeletal muscle lipid content and insulin resistance: evidence for a paradox in endurance-trained athletes. J Clin Endocrinol Metab 2001;86(12):5755−61. https://doi.org/10.1210/jcem.86.12.8075.

[60] Sai E, Shimada K, Yokoyama T, Sato S, Miyazaki T, Hiki M, Tamura Y, Aoki S, Watada H, Kawamori R, Daida H. Association between myocardial triglyceride content and cardiac function in healthy subjects and endurance athletes. PLoS One 2013;8(4). https://doi.org/10.1371/journal.pone.0061604. e61604.

[61] Bucher J, Krüsi M, Zueger T, Ith M, Stettler C, Diem P, Boesch C, Kreis R, Christ E. The effect of a single 2 h bout of aerobic exercise on ectopic lipids in skeletal muscle, liver and the myocardium. Diabetologia 2014;57(5):1001−5. https://doi.org/10.1007/s00125-014-3193-0.

[62] Bilet L, van de Weijer T, Hesselink MKC, Glatz JFC, Lamb HJ, Wildberger J, Kooi ME, Schrauwen P, Schrauwen-Hinderling VB. Exercise-induced modulation of cardiac lipid content in healthy lean young men. Basic Res Cardiol 2011;106(2):307−15. https://doi.org/10.1007/s00395-010-0144-x.

[63] van der Meer RW, Hammer S, Smit JWA, Frölich M, Bax JJ, Diamant M, et al. Short-term caloric restriction induces accumulation of myocardial triglycerides and decreases left ventricular diastolic function in healthy subjects. Diabetes 2007;56(12):2849−53. https://doi.org/10.2337/db07-0768.

[64] Hammer S, van der Meer RW, Lamb HJ, Schär M, de Roos A, Smit JWA, et al. Progressive caloric restriction induces dose-dependent changes in myocardial triglyceride content and diastolic function in healthy men. J Clin Endocrinol Metab 2008;93(2):497−503. https://doi.org/10.1210/jc.2007-2015.

[65] Hammer S, Snel M, Lamb HJ, Jazet IM, van der Meer RW, Pijl H, Meinders EA, Romijn JA, de Roos A, Smit JWA. Prolonged caloric restriction in obese patients with type 2 diabetes mellitus decreases myocardial triglyceride content and improves myocardial function. J Am Coll Cardiol 2008;52(12):1006−12. https://doi.org/10.1016/j.jacc.2008.04.068.

[66] van der Meer RW, Hammer S, Lamb HJ, Frölich M, Diamant M, Rijzewijk LJ, et al. Effects of short-term high-fat, high-energy diet on hepatic and myocardial triglyceride content in healthy men. J Clin Endocrinol Metab 2008;93(7):2702−8. https://doi.org/10.1210/jc.2007-2524.

[67] Smajis S, Gajdošík M, Pfleger L, Traussnigg S, Kienbacher C, Halilbasic E, Ranzenberger-Haider T, Stangl A, Beiglböck H, Wolf P, Lamp T, Hofer A, Gastaldelli A, Barbieri C, Luger A, Trattnig S, Kautzky-Willer A, Krššák M, Trauner M, Krebs M. Metabolic effects of a prolonged, very-high-dose dietary fructose challenge in healthy subjects. Am J Clin Nutr 2020;111(2):369−77. https://doi.org/10.1093/ajcn/nqz271.

[68] Lopaschuk GD, Ussher JR, Folmes CDL, Jaswal JS, Stanley WC. Myocardial fatty acid metabolism in health and disease. Physiol Rev 2010;90(1):207−58. https://doi.org/10.1152/physrev.00015.2009.

[69] Wende AR, Brahma MK, McGinnis GR, Young ME. Metabolic origins of heart failure. JACC Basic Transl Sci 2017;2(3):297−310. https://doi.org/10.1016/j.jacbts.2016.11.009.

[70] Goldberg IJ, Trent CM, Schulze PC. Lipid metabolism and toxicity in the heart. Cell Metabol 2012;15(6):805−12. https://doi.org/10.1016/j.cmet.2012.04.006.

[71] McGavock JM, Lingvay I, Zib I, Tillery T, Salas N, Unger R, et al. Cardiac steatosis in diabetes mellitus: a [1]H-magnetic resonance spectroscopy study. Circulation 2007;116(10):1170−5. https://doi.org/10.1161/CIRCULATIONAHA.106.645614.

[72] Schrauwen-Hinderling VB, Hesselink MKC, Meex R, van der Made S, Schär M, Lamb H, Wildberger JE, Glatz J, Snoep G, Kooi ME, Schrauwen P. Improved ejection fraction after exercise training in obesity is accompanied by reduced cardiac lipid content. J Clin Endocrinol Metab 2010;95(4):1932−8. https://doi.org/10.1210/jc.2009-2076.

[73] Levelt E, Pavlides M, Banerjee R, Mahmod M, Kelly C, Sellwood J, Ariga R, Thomas S, Francis J, Rodgers C, Clarke W, Sabharwal N, Antoniades C, Schneider J, Robson M, Clarke K, Karamitsos T, Rider O, Neubauer S. Ectopic and visceral fat deposition in lean and obese patients with type 2 diabetes. J Am Coll Cardiol 2016;68(1):53−63. https://doi.org/10.1016/j.jacc.2016.03.597.

[74] Rijzewijk LJ, van der Meer RW, Smit JWA, Diamant M, Bax JJ, Hammer S, Romijn JA, de Roos A, Lamb HJ. Myocardial steatosis is an independent predictor of diastolic dysfunction in type 2 diabetes mellitus. J Am Coll Cardiol 2008;52(22):1793−9. https://doi.org/10.1016/j.jacc.2008.07.062.

[75] Krššák M, Winhofer Y, Göbl C, Bischof M, Reiter G, Kautzky-Willer A, Luger A, Krebs M, Anderwald C. Insulin resistance is not associated with myocardial steatosis in women. Diabetologia 2011;54(7):1871−8. https://doi.org/10.1007/s00125-011-2146-0.

[76] Iozzo P, Lautamaki R, Borra R, Lehto H-R, Bucci M, Viljanen A, Parkka J, Lepomaki V, Maggio R, Parkkola R, Knuuti J, Nuutila P. Contribution of glucose tolerance and gender to cardiac adiposity. J Clin Endocrinol Metab 2009;94(11):4472−82. https://doi.org/10.1210/jc.2009-0436.

[77] Sharma S, Adrogue JV, Golfman L, Uray I, Lemm J, Youker K, et al. Intramyocardial lipid accumulation in the failing human heart resembles the lipotoxic rat heart. FASEB (Fed Am Soc Exp Biol) J 2004;18(14):1692−700. https://doi.org/10.1096/fj.04-2263com.

[78] Schrauwen-Hinderling VB, Meex RCR, Hesselink MKC, van de Weijer T, Leiner T, Schär M, Lamb HJ, Wildberger JE, Glatz JFC, Schrauwen P, Kooi ME. Cardiac lipid content is unresponsive to a physical activity training intervention in type 2 diabetic patients, despite improved ejection fraction. Cardiovasc Diabetol 2011;10:47. https://doi.org/10.1186/1475-2840-10-47.

[79] Jonker JT, de Mol P, de Vries ST, Widya RL, Hammer S, van Schinkel LD, van der Meer RW, Gans ROB, Webb AG, Kan HE, de Koning EJP, Bilo HJG, Lamb HJ. Exercise and type 2 diabetes mellitus: changes in tissue-specific fat distribution and cardiac function. Radiology 2013;269(2):434−42. https://doi.org/10.1148/radiology.13121631.

[80] Jankovic D, Winhofer Y, Promintzer-Schifferl M, Wohlschläger-Krenn E, Anderwald CH, Wolf P, Scherer T, Reiter G, Trattnig S, Luger A, Krebs M, Krššák M. Effects of insulin therapy on myocardial lipid content and cardiac geometry in patients with type-2 diabetes mellitus. PLoS One 2012;7(12):e50077. https://doi.org/10.1371/journal.pone.0050077.

[81] Winhofer Y, Krssák M, Jankovic D, Anderwald C-H, Reiter G, Hofer A, Trattnig S, Luger A, Krebs M. Short-term hyperinsulinemia and hyperglycemia increase myocardial lipid content in normal subjects. Diabetes 2012;61(5):1210−6. https://doi.org/10.2337/db11-1275.

[82] van der Meer RW, Rijzewijk LJ, de Jong HWAM, Lamb HJ, Lubberink M, Romijn JA, Bax JJ, de Roos A, Kamp O, Paulus WJ, Heine RJ, Lammertsma AA, Smit JWA, Diamant M. Pioglitazone improves cardiac function and alters myocardial substrate metabolism without affecting cardiac triglyceride accumulation and high-energy phosphate metabolism in patients with well-controlled type 2 diabetes mellitus. Circulation 2009;119(15):2069−77. https://doi.org/10.1161/CIRCULATIONAHA.108.803916.

[83] Zib I, Jacob AN, Lingvay I, Salinas K, McGavock JM, Raskin P, Szczepaniak LS. Effect of pioglitazone therapy on myocardial and hepatic steatosis in insulin-treated patients with type 2 diabetes. J Invest Med 2007;55(5):230−6. https://doi.org/10.2310/6650.2007.00003.

[84] Bucci M, Borra R, Någren K, Pärkkä JP, Del Ry S, Maggio R, Tuunanen H, Viljanen T, Cabiati M, Rigazio S, Taittonen M, Pagotto U, Parkkola R, Opie LH, Nuutila P, Knuuti J, Iozzo P. Trimetazidine reduces endogenous free fatty acid oxidation and improves myocardial efficiency in obese humans. Cardiovasc Ther 2012;30(6):333−41. https://doi.org/10.1111/j.1755-5922.2011.00275.x.

[85] Paiman EHM, van Eyk HJ, van Aalst MMA, Bizino MB, van der Geest RJ, Westenberg JJM, Geelhoed-Duijvestijn PH, Kharagjitsingh AV, Rensen PCN, Smit JWA, Jazet IM, Lamb HJ. Effect of liraglutide on cardiovascular function and myocardial tissue characteristics in type 2 diabetes patients of South Asian descent living in The Netherlands: a double-blind, randomized, placebo-controlled trial. J Magn Reson Imag 2020;51(6):1679−88. https://doi.org/10.1002/jmri.27009.

[86] Karwi QG, Ho KL, Pherwani S, Ketema EB, Sun QY, Lopaschuk GD. Concurrent diabetes and heart failure: interplay and novel therapeutic approaches. Cardiovasc Res 2022;118(3):686−715. https://doi.org/10.1093/cvr/cvab120.

[87] Brown DA, Perry JB, Allen ME, Sabbah HN, Stauffer BL, Shaikh SR, Cleland JGF, Colucci WS, Butler J, Voors AA, Anker SD, Pitt B, Pieske B, Filippatos G, Greene SJ, Gheorghiade M. Expert consensus document: mitochondrial function as a therapeutic target in heart failure. Nat Rev Cardiol 2017;14(4):238−50. https://doi.org/10.1038/nrcardio.2016.203.

[88] Mahmod M, Pal N, Rayner J, Holloway C, Raman B, Dass S, Levelt E, Ariga R, Ferreira V, Banerjee R, Schneider JE, Rodgers C, Francis JM, Karamitsos TD, Frenneaux M, Ashrafian H, Neubauer S, Rider O. The interplay between metabolic alterations, diastolic strain rate and exercise capacity in mild heart failure with preserved ejection fraction: a cardiovascular magnetic resonance study. J Cardiovasc Magn Reson 2018;20(1):88. https://doi.org/10.1186/s12968-018-0511-6.

[89] Wei J, Nelson MD, Szczepaniak EW, Smith L, Mehta PK, Thomson LEJ, Berman DS, Li D, Bairey Merz CN, Szczepaniak LS. Myocardial steatosis as a possible mechanistic link between diastolic dysfunction and coronary microvascular dysfunction in women. Am J Physiol Heart Circ Physiol 2016;310(1):H14−9. https://doi.org/10.1152/ajpheart.00612.2015.

[90] Nelson MD, Victor RG, Szczepaniak EW, Simha V, Garg A, Szczepaniak LS. Cardiac steatosis and left ventricular hypertrophy in patients with generalized lipodystrophy as determined by magnetic resonance spectroscopy and imaging. Am J Cardiol 2013;112(7):1019−24. https://doi.org/10.1016/j.amjcard.2013.05.036.

[91] Nelson MD, Szczepaniak LS, LaBounty TM, Szczepaniak E, Li D, Tighiouart M, Li Q, Dharmakumar R, Sannes G, Fan Z, Yumul R, Hardy WD, Hernandez Conte A. Cardiac steatosis and left ventricular dysfunction in HIV-infected patients treated with highly active antiretroviral therapy. JACC Cardiovasc Imaging 2014;7(11):1175−7. https://doi.org/10.1016/j.jcmg.2014.04.024.

[92] Petritsch B, Köstler H, Weng AM, Horn M, Gassenmaier T, Kunz AS, et al. Myocardial lipid content in Fabry disease: a combined [1]H-MR spectroscopy and MR imaging study at 3 Tesla. BMC Cardiovasc Disord 2016;16(1):205. https://doi.org/10.1186/s12872-016-0382-4.

[93] Gastl M, Peereboom SM, Gotschy A, Fuetterer M, von Deuster C, Boenner F, Kelm M, Schwotzer R, Flammer AJ, Manka R, Kozerke S. Myocardial triglycerides in cardiac amyloidosis assessed by proton cardiovascular magnetic resonance spectroscopy. J Cardiovasc Magn Reson 2019;21(1):10. https://doi.org/10.1186/s12968-019-0519-6.

[94] Liu C-Y, Redheuil A, Ouwerkerk R, Lima JAC, Bluemke DA. Myocardial fat quantification in humans: evaluation by two-point water-fat imaging and localized proton spectroscopy. Magn Reson Med 2010;63(4):892−901. https://doi.org/10.1002/mrm.22289.

[95] Lu M, Zhao S, Jiang S, Yin G, Wang C, Zhang Y, Liu Q, Cheng H, Ma N, Zhao T, Chen X, Huang J, Zou Y, Song L, He Z, An J, Renate J, Xue H, Shah S. Fat deposition in dilated cardiomyopathy assessed by CMR. JACC Cardiovasc Imaging 2013;6(8):889−98. https://doi.org/10.1016/j.jcmg.2013.04.010.

[96] Boesch C, Kreis R. Dipolar coupling and ordering effects observed in magnetic resonance spectra of skeletal muscle. NMR Biomed 2001;14(2):140−8. https://doi.org/10.1002/nbm.684.

[97] Fillmer A, Hock A, Cameron D, Henning A. Non-water-suppressed ^{1}H MR spectroscopy with orientational prior knowledge shows potential for separating intra- and extramyocellular lipid signals in human myocardium. Sci Rep 2017;7(1):16898. https://doi.org/10.1038/s41598-017-16318-0.

[98] Nagarajan V, Gopalan V, Kaneko M, Angeli V, Gluckman P, Richards AM, Kuchel PW, Velan SS. Cardiac function and lipid distribution in rats fed a high-fat diet: *in vivo* magnetic resonance imaging and spectroscopy. Am J Physiol Heart Circ Physiol 2013;304(11):H1495–504. https://doi.org/10.1152/ajpheart.00478.2012.

[99] Streeter DD, Spotnitz HM, Patel DP, Ross J, Sonnenblick EH. Fiber orientation in the canine left ventricle during diastole and systole. Circ Res 1969;24(3):339–47. https://doi.org/10.1161/01.res.24.3.339.

[100] Hock M, Terekhov M, Stefanescu MR, Lohr D, Herz S, Reiter T, Ankenbrand M, Kosmala A, Gassenmaier T, Juchem C, Schreiber LM. B_0 shimming of the human heart at 7T. Magn Reson Med 2021;85(1):182–96. https://doi.org/10.1002/mrm.28423.

[101] Aigner CS, Dietrich S, Schaeffter T, Schmitter S. Calibration-free pTx of the human heart at 7T via 3D universal pulses. Magn Reson Med 2022;87(1):70–84. https://doi.org/10.1002/mrm.22289.

Chapter 9

Pancreas ectopic fat: imaging-based quantification

Alexandre Triay Bagur[1,2,a], Matthew Robson[2], Daniel Bulte[1] and Michael Brady[2,a]

[1]Department of Engineering Science, University of Oxford, Oxford, United Kingdom; [2]Perspectum Ltd, Oxford, United Kingdom

Introduction

The US Center for Disease Control estimates that in 2017—18, 42.4% of the US population was obese, defined as having a Body Mass Index (BMI) greater than 30. This amounts to 141 million people. Both the percentage and number have risen steadily from 30.5% in 1999—2000. As well, 14.4 million children and adolescents were reported as obese (19.3%), a number which has doubled in the past 30 years. The situation in Europe is more variable, but the World Health Organization (WHO) estimates that in 2020 up to 30% of adults are obese, while one-third of children aged 11 are overweight or obese. Worldwide, the WHO estimates that in 2016, more than 1.9 billion adults, 18 years and older, were overweight. Of these over 650 million were obese.

Obesity disrupts the normal metabolism in the body and, as a result, the inexorable rise in obesity has led to a corresponding increase in health-related complications. One widely reported and researched instance is **non-alcoholic fatty liver disease (NAFLD)**, where it is estimated that 27% of the US population (91m people) are living with NAFLD. Worse, approximately 23% of those with NAFLD, 21 million people, have progressed to the more severe form, nonalcoholic steatohepatitis (NASH). Left unchecked, NASH progresses to cirrhosis, hepatocellular carcinoma, and other manifestations of the metabolic syndrome.

A second instance is **type 2 diabetes mellitus (T2DM)**: already 30 million Americans have T2DM, while in Europe there are 60 million (approximately 10% of people aged at least 25 years). The WHO notes that the number of people with diabetes rose from 108 million in 1980 to 422 million in 2014. This is unsurprising, as the pancreas plays a key role in the development of obesity-related diseases. T2DM costs are currently projected to rise to $2 trillion by 2030 [1].

Indeed, the increasing incidence of NAFLD worldwide, strongly suggest that pancreatic fat will also become increasingly common. Conversely, pancreatic fat may induce local effects in the liver that affect the progression of NAFLD. Though there are several causes of accumulation of pancreatic fat (also known as pancreatic steatosis or pancreatic lipomatosis), there is increasing interest in **nonalcoholic fatty pancreas disease (NAFPD)**, defined as pancreatic steatosis in association with obesity and the metabolic syndrome [2]. This chapter discusses NAFPD and its effects.

The incidence of NAFPD is now already estimated to be 27%—33%, and it is present in nearly 70% of patients with NAFLD [3]; [4]. By analogy with NASH, the progressive form of NAFPD is called **nonalcoholic steatopancreatitis (NASP)** [5]. Owing primarily to incomplete definitions, NAFPD and NASP had been largely understudied until the past decade. It seems that Mathur et al. were the first to adopt the term NAFPD and showed using histology that leptin-deficient obese mice had heavier pancreata, higher pancreatic triglyceride levels and free fatty acids (FFA), and increased proinflammatory adipocytokines [6]. Recently, NAFPD has been shown to be reversible upon lifestyle- and bariatric surgery-induced weight loss [7—9].

Though there is a link between obesity and NAFLD/NASH and NAFPD/NASP, the situation is in fact quite complex. Recall that BMI is defined, for an adult, as weight (kg) divided by the square of height (m), though some adjustments are

---

a Authors contributed equally.

Visceral and Ectopic Fat. https://doi.org/10.1016/B978-0-12-822186-0.00026-2

made for age. "Normoweight" is equated to a BMI of up to 25 kg/m^2; "Overweight" as 25–30 kg/m^2; and "Obese" as greater than 30 kg/m^2. It has been shown that approximately 30% of obese adults are in fact "metabolically healthy" [10]. Conversely, significant metabolic abnormalities occur in 20%–30% of normoweight people. These facts remind us that BMI as a measure of metabolic health is both limited and potentially misleading.

An explanation of the discrepancies between BMI and metabolic health lies in the fact that there are several different kinds of fat, playing different metabolic roles, but all contributing to an individual's weight. Current data suggest that the **distribution of fat** is a better marker of metabolic risk than obesity per se. The most conspicuous is visceral fat, which gives rise to central obesity, and is composed of adipose tissue. Visceral fat is separate from subcutaneous fat and intramuscular fat. Most important for NAFLD/NASH and NAFPD/NASP, however, is **ectopic fat**, which is the storage of triglycerides in tissues other than adipose tissue in organs such as the liver, heart, and pancreas that normally contain only small amounts of fat. Evidently, BMI is a poor estimator for ectopic fat, and therefore for measuring the progression of NAFLD/NASH and NAFPD/NASP.

Though NAFLD/NASH and NAFPD/NASP frequently cooccur and are strongly interrelated, there are also major differences that complicate the picture. For example, the storage mechanism and impact of ectopic fat differs in the liver and the pancreas, reflecting the very different functions of these organs. Details are provided in Section Pancreas and ectopic fat, where the central importance of ectopic fat is highlighted. This in turn leads to the question of how the amount and progression of pancreatic fat, more especially pancreatic ectopic fat, can be measured, and this is the subject of Section Pancreas and ectopic fat and then in more detail in Section Information from MRI, which focuses on measurement using Magnetic Resonance Imaging (MRI). Though the complexity of the pancreas and the huge variability of the pancreas and its pathology challenge conventional image analysis methods, the increasing availability of large, well-curated databases such as the UK Biobank[1], the development of machine learning methods, and the increasing capabilities of cloud-based computing, outlined in Section Big data and AI, have enabled the image analysis methods outlined in Section Information from MRI. The chapter ends in Section Future Directions.

Pancreas and ectopic fat

The pancreas is one of the most complex (and least understood) organs in the human body. Here, we restrict ourselves to presenting the background required for Section Pancreas state assessment and Section Information from MRI.

Anatomically, the pancreas is situated between the liver, duodenum, and spleen, and behind the stomach. It is typically around 12–15 cm long and has two prominent ducts that run along the length of the pancreas: the main pancreatic duct and a smaller accessory pancreatic duct. These join with the common bile duct. The pancreas is generally divided into three parts, referred to as the head, body, and tail, as shown in Fig. 9.1. The head of the pancreas nestles into the duodenum, and it surrounds two major blood vessels: one artery and one vein. The longest linear length of the pancreas is the body, while the tail region abuts the spleen. Morphologically, the pancreas shape is variable across individuals, and this diversity is further amplified by pathology, not least fat infiltration and fibroinflammation. As we describe in Section Information from MRI, the pancreas is often difficult to locate, and even harder to delineate (segment). Nevertheless, automated pancreas segmentation methods have been developed, deploying methods from Big Data and Artificial Intelligence. We return to this issue in Section Big data and AI.

Physiologically, the liver and the pancreas are glands that are both endocrine and exocrine (Fig. 9.2). Exocrine glands secrete substances onto bodily surfaces by way of ducts. In this role, the pancreas secretes bile and pancreatic juice, by way of the pancreatic duct, into the duodenum. The endocrine system is a complex feedback system that uses hormones to regulate organs. As a part of the endocrine system, the pancreas regulates blood sugar levels by secreting insulin, glucagon, somatostatin, and pancreatic polypeptide. The endocrine tissues in the pancreas are distributed throughout the pancreas and take the form of clusters of cells known as the islets of Langerhans. These in turn are comprised of several kinds of cells, including beta cells that secrete insulin. In fact, adipose tissue has endocrine functions, producing a range of biochemicals including adipocytokines, tumor necrosis factor alpha (TNF-α), and interleukin-6 (IL-6) [11]. In contrast to endocrine pancreatic function, which is impacted adversely by fat accumulation, exocrine function is not affected until over 90% of its tissue is replaced by fat [12].

Pancreatic ectopic fat can be seen histologically as intralobular and interlobular accumulation of circular white adipocytes, whereas macroscopic evaluation shows an increasingly yellow appearance with higher steatosis gradings (Fig. 9.3). Small amounts of pancreatic fat are benign and are a relatively common finding in histology and imaging,

---

1. https://www.ukbiobank.ac.uk/.

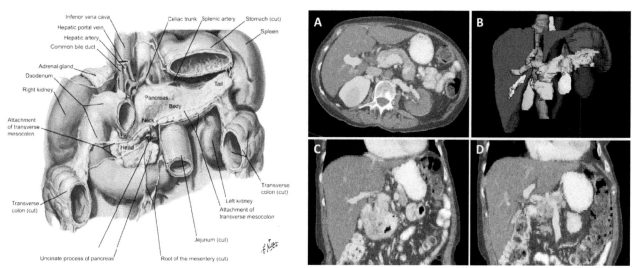

FIGURE 9.1 Illustration of the pancreas and surrounding duodenum and major vessels (left). The pancreatic duct is shown. Pancreatic head, body and tail have been outlined. CT scan with major structures outlined including the pancreas (dark green). (A) sagittal view; (B) 3D rendering of the outlines, structures anterior to the pancreas have been edited out; (C) coronal view showing the pancreas head sitting on the duodenum; (D) coronal view showing the pancreas curving around the portal vein (light brown). © *Elsevier, Inc., www.netterimages.com; "Multi-Atlas Labeling Beyond the Cranial Vault" dataset, https://doi.org/10.7303/syn3193805.*

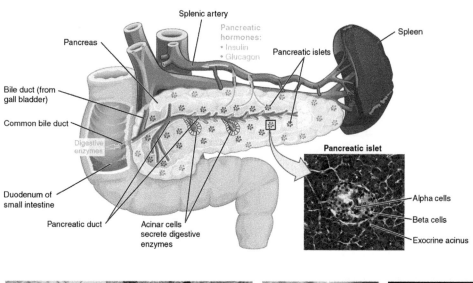

FIGURE 9.2 Physiologically, the pancreas has exocrine and endocrine functions. Acinar cells secrete digestive enzymes into the duodenum, whereas the pancreatic islets secrete hormones (insulin and glucagon) into the bloodstream to regulate blood sugar levels. © *OpenStax College [CC BY 3.0], via Wikimedia Commons.*

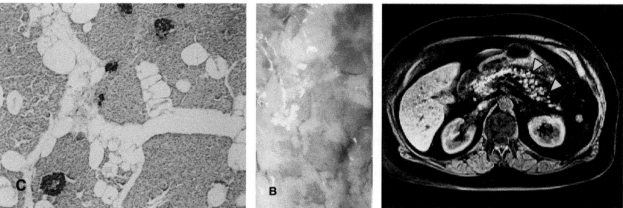

FIGURE 9.3 Pancreatic steatosis shown on different imaging modalities. (A) Histology shows intralobular and interlobular adipocyte infiltration (white cells) at 100x magnification.(B) Photograph of moderate steatosis shows yellow appearance and "marbling effect".(C) Abdominal Magnetic Resonance Imaging scan with pancreatic fat infiltration, fat appears dark and creates a granular tissue appearance. *Modified from Dholakia, S., E. J. Sharples, R. J. Ploeg, and P. J. Friend. Significance of steatosis in pancreatic transplantation. Transplant Rev 2017 31 (4): 225–231. https://doi.org/10.1016/j.trre.2017.08.001.*

associated with aging [13]. Greater amounts of pancreatic fat have been proposed to have health implications in obesity and the metabolic syndrome, diabetes type 2, acute and chronic pancreatitis, and pancreatic cancer. High amounts of pancreatic steatosis are also a contraindication for pancreatic transplantation [14].

Fat accumulation in the pancreas of obese versus lean subjects was described as early as 1933 by Ogilvie in a postmortem study [15]. Mathur et al. showed in histology that leptin-deficient obese mice had heavier pancreata, higher pancreatic triglyceride levels and free fatty acids (FFA), and increased proinflammatory adipocytokines [6]. Importantly, differences in fat deposition mechanisms exist between organs. While, for instance, liver fat is accumulated in hepatocytes, pancreatic fat accumulation can occur either as "fatty infiltration" by adipocytes or as "intracellular accumulation" in the parenchyma (exocrine and islet cells) [11,16,17]. Lipid composition in the pancreas has shown to be altered in relation with fat accumulation [18].

Pancreatic ectopic fat has been linked with insulin resistance [17,19—22]. Pancreatic fat accumulation is present in prediabetics, the amount of pancreatic fat increases before T2DM occurs, and pancreatic fat has been negatively associated with insulin secretion [17]. Studies showing no differences in pancreatic fat between diabetic status also exist [23]. There is still insufficient evidence to define a causal relationship between NAFPD and T2DM. This motivates accurate and robust measurement of pancreatic fat in the context of T2DM.

Ectopic fat accumulation and inflammation in the pancreas are among the early manifestations of chronic pancreas disease. Inflammation of the pancreas is known as pancreatitis, some of the main causes being gallstones; substantial and prolonged alcohol use; illnesses such as mumps; and prolonged exposure to very high levels of blood triglycerides. **Chronic pancreatitis** causes nonreversible morphology changes, for instance, the development of pancreatic fibrosis, which leads to the loss of exocrine and endocrine tissue and its function. The loss of endocrine tissue function may in turn lead to pancreatic diabetes.

Pancreatic cancer can also arise following chronic pancreatitis [24]. Adenocarcinoma is the most frequent pancreas tumor (95%) and originates in the exocrine portions of the gland. Most originate in the ducts, with the most frequent location being the pancreatic head (70%), followed by body (20%) and tail (10%). Pancreatic cancer is usually detected late, when it has spread to other parts of the body, and is one of the hardest to treat, with one of the lowest rates of survival. There has been an increase in pancreatic cancer over the past few decades, associated to obesity [25]. Cancer may also cause diabetes due to impairment of the endocrine function.

Regional assessment of pancreas pathology is important, for instance, by head, body, and tail. Uneven fat accumulation in the pancreas is very common and was observed and classified early on, arguing embryological differences [26,27]. Most pancreatic cancers are found in the head region, and it has been shown that there is a preferential loss of beta cells in the head region in patients with T2DM [28]. Those authors suggest that this may stem from the head being closest to the duodenum, so that pathology may progress from the duodenum or liver to the head, and then from head to tail. In an example of an early study, Patel et al. estimated using MRI the average pancreatic fat in NAFLD patients and found no significant variation between the fat content of the head, body, and tail of the pancreas [29]. Nevertheless, they noted that there was uneven accumulation of fat in the pancreas, which differs from the relatively homogenous liver steatosis in NAFLD. Unequal distribution of pancreatic fat was also reported by Kühn et al. using MRI [23]. A recent study by Nadarajah et al. showed that only pancreatic fat in the tail of the pancreas was significantly different between control group and those "at risk" for T2DM [5].

Pancreas state assessment

Ideally, we would make a series of measurements of the pancreas that satisfy the following criteria:

1. Noninvasive;
2. Reliably enable detection of pathology;
3. Reproducible; and
4. Enable staging of pathology;

There is such huge diversity in people and pathology that it is unlikely that a single kind of information will suffice in all cases, necessitating information "fusion."

Prior to the widespread availability of imaging, and recent developments in circulating biomarkers, assessment of visceral organs like the liver generally had recourse to **biopsy**. However, aside from being invasive, and often painful, biopsy only samples a small section (mm) of tissue, effectively ruling out regional assessment in hetero-geneous disease typical of the pancreas. It is evidently impractical to biopsy one-third of the population that is overweight, and also impractical to base routine monitoring of disease progression on biopsy. Endoscopic echography enables guided biopsy to stage fibrosis and to discard adenocarcinoma. Endoscopic retrograde cholangiopancreatography (ERCP) has been replaced and is only used for interventional procedures. Biopsy scores poorly on criterion 1.

The least invasive assessment of pancreas state is to use **circulating biomarkers**, as has been done routinely for the liver for over a decade. Asymptomatic T2DM is currently diagnosed using circulating biomarkers, via two out of three of (1) basal blood glucose $\geq$126 mg/dL, (2) glycemia $\geq$200 mg/dL after an oral glucose tolerance test (OGTT), and (3) glycated hemoglobin (HbA1c) $\geq$6.5%. In the specific case of pancreatic cancer, Zhang et al. have provided a recent review [30]. They note that "a variety of novel biomarkers from body fluids, including blood, urine, saliva, pancreatic juice, and stool, has been discovered in studies on the early detection of PC" and "Circulating biomarkers from blood have advantages in terms of stability, convenience, and abundance." Generally, circulating biomarkers have the advantage that they can detect minute quantities of pathology, so can signal early disease. However, there are generally several reasons why a biomarker may signal, with the increased likelihood of false positives and/or overdiagnosis. By themselves, circulating biomarkers score poorly on criterion 2. Importantly, the diagnosis of T2DM using circulating biomarkers means that symptoms as well as diagnosis of T2DM occur years after insulin resistance has begun, often already with complications. The combination of information from circulating biomarkers with the phenotypical information provided by imaging is increasing in prominence, particularly as machine learning straightforwardly enables the combination of these very different sources of information.

Pancreatic fat **imaging** has received increasing interest in the past few years. The location of the pancreas, together with the huge variation in pancreas shape and appearance, pose fundamental challenges for imaging methods.

Ultrasound imaging, in all its forms (B-mode, Doppler, Power, Elastography, etc.) has the advantage that it is relatively cheap and widely available at the point of care. Though the liver is considerably more accessible than the pancreas, even liver ultrasound has limited utility in part because the signal is attenuated by visceral adipose tissue, of which there may be a considerable amount. Ultrasound elastography has had most success in assessing liver elasticity, typical of late-stage NASH and cirrhosis. However, it is highly operator-dependent and challenging to perform in the pancreas due to its deep retroperitoneal location which make it inaccessible. It is also not specific to fat (e.g., fibrosis also increases stiffness) and has a high failure rate in overweight subjects, due to increased physical signal attenuation. Ultrasound scores poorly on criteria 2 and 3.

Computed Tomography (CT) is widely available and relatively cheap to perform. As well, it gives 3D reconstructions that are typically a factor of two in each dimension finer than MRI. However, there are two fundamental problems with CT for pancreas imaging. First, CT is based on ionizing radiation and so even though it continues to make massive contributions to medical imaging, its use should be avoided as far as practically possible. In particular, CT relies upon the attenuation by tissue of X-rays, and the more tissue the X-ray beam needs to traverse the more of the beam is attenuated. This is an issue for obese people, who, as we noted above, constitute one-third of the population. Second, while CT gives superb dense tissue contrast (e.g., bone, calcifications), it has poor contrast in soft tissues such as the pancreas. CT scores poorly on criteria 2, 4, and arguably 1.

Proton Magnetic Resonance Spectroscopy (MRS) has very high spectral resolution, meaning the ability to identify the different metabolites in a tissue. This is useful to separate tissue components such as water from fat, and even to evaluate the composition of fat [31,32]. This comes at the price of poor spatial resolution, since MRS only samples a single voxel of tissue typically of 2−8 mL in volume, ruling out regional assessment. MRS is also technically challenging to perform and scores poorly on criterion 3. It is also highly affected by artifacts such as breathing motion that may contaminate the voxel w, e.g., surrounding VAT fat [33], notably considering the small width and overall size and shape of the pancreas.

Magnetic Resonance Imaging (MRI) evidently satisfies criterion 1, and it can be applied to people of (almost) any size. MRI is a safe modality, especially when no intravenous contrast is used. MRI-based fat measurement is routinely used in organs like the liver. The key questions concern the extent to which MRI imaging and image analysis can satisfy criteria 2−4. This is the topic of Section Information from MRI.

As a result of the above, Magnetic Resonance (MR)-based methods are increasingly considered gold-standard for noninvasive pancreatic fat quantification.

Information from MRI

What information about pancreas state, particularly about the amount of ectopic fat, do we want to extract using MRI, possibly in tandem with circulating biomarkers? Here is a tentative list:

1. Pancreas volume assessment via segmentation of the entire pancreas, in part as a first step toward more detailed analysis;
2. Subsegmentation of the pancreas into head, body, and tail;
3. Section Introduction and Section Pancreas and ectopic fat highlighted the importance of pancreatic fat, particularly ectopic fat. This poses the challenge of estimating the amounts of ectopic and potentially other kinds of fat in the pancreas as a whole and in each of its subparts, and their spatial distributions;
4. The pancreas has a complex, but distinctive shape. Though pancreas shape varies considerably from individual to individual, it is reasonable to suppose that there are shape and texture *changes* that are characteristic of pathology;
5. Section Pancreas and ectopic fat noted that inflammation of the pancreas is one of the earliest manifestations of chronic pancreas disease. Inflammation can be qualitatively assessed on T1-weighted and T2-weighted images. MRI-based quantification of inflammation advanced over the past decade in part by the development of robust and repeatable T_1 relaxation time measurements. In the liver, cT_1, which corrects for iron content in tissue [34], has been shown to correlate closely with fibroinflammation.

We now discuss each of the above in more detail.

Pancreas volume

Volume was one of the earliest reported quantitative imaging biomarkers of the pancreas, since it does not require quantitative imaging per se. Normal pancreas volume is $71-83$ cm^3 higher in men than in women, and numerous studies have shown volume changes in disease [35]. Pancreas volume increases in overweight and obese subjects but is smaller in type 1 and type 2 diabetes [36]. For this reason, pancreas volume may be helpful to determine which overweight subjects may go on to develop T2DM.

Pancreas volumetry is generally performed through organ delineation on 3D scans, usually CT or MRI, by an expert radiologist. This is time-consuming and costly, and for these reasons it is not used in routine clinical practice. Semi- and fully automated organ segmentation methods have been developed over the past 20 years. Specifically, deep learning—based convolutional neural network (CNN) models have outperformed advanced approaches including (multi-)atlas-based segmentation. Medical image segmentation advanced with the introduction of the U-Net CNN architecture by Ronneberger et al. that achieved impressive results trained on a relatively small number of samples [37]; its 3D extension is still considered state-of-the-art in a wide range of applications [38].

Automated segmentation of the pancreas is a highly challenging segmentation task for three main reasons: (1) there is high intersubject variability of the organ, (2) it often presents itself with ill-defined boundaries, and (3) there is high "class imbalance," meaning there is much lower frequency of "pancreas" voxels than there is for "not pancreas" (i.e., "background"). Other technical and clinical factors like image resolution or the absence of peripancreatic visceral adipose tissue (VAT) affect automated pancreas segmentation methods negatively [39]. Alternatives to CNNs [40] or more efficient network architectures, for instance, self-adapting architectures [41], or those using attention mechanisms [42] have been proposed for pancreas segmentation.

Heterogeneity in how pancreatic fat deposits, as described in Section Pancreas and ectopic fat, motivates segmentation of the pancreas into main subregions, head, body, and tail, for regional assessment of pathology downstream. Many studies have reported clinically important differences in the head, body, and tail parts using manually drawn regions of interest [5,23,43]. Conversely, automated segmentation methods (including deep learning—based) have to date only aimed at delineating the whole pancreas. An automated method was recently proposed for delineating the pancreas into subregions by registration to a template [44]; an example of this method applied to one subject is shown in Fig. 9.4.

MRI-derived fat fraction

Recent studies using **MRI-derived proton density fat fraction (MRI-PDFF)** have shown the feasibility of the technique and have confirmed previous evidence that pancreatic fat increases with BMI [45] and that is elevated in T2DM subjects [19,46—48]. Confounder-corrected MRI-PDFF is now generally accepted in the liver literature, to the extent that it has been used as endpoint in many NASH drug trials [49] and is being adopted in the clinical management of liver disease

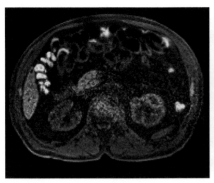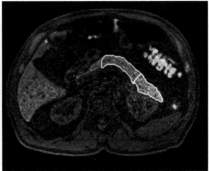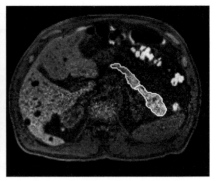

FIGURE 9.4 Automated 3D pancreas subsegmentation into head (blue), body (green), and tail (yellow) on a T_1-weighted MRI volumetric acquisition. Three axial slices of the same subject are shown at three distinct increasing heights.

patients. MRI-PDFF techniques exploit the fact that water and triglycerides have signals at different radio frequencies. By acquiring the MR signal at multiple delay times after signal excitation (echo time), and using an accepted physical signal model, we can quantify the proportion of signal that is due to fat and water. An illustration of the MRI-PDFF acquisition and reconstruction is shown in Fig. 9.5.

Ever since Dixon's seminal paper [50], MRI-PDFF methods may be classified as complex-based or magnitude-based, depending on whether they use the MRI phase images or not in the reconstruction procedure. Complex-based methods, including IDEAL (Iterative Decomposition of Water and Fat using Echo Asymmetry and Least squares estimation) [51], need a field inhomogeneity ("field map") estimation step, an ill-posed optimization problem with many local minima. Complex-based methods are sensitive to errors in the MRI phase data. Magnitude methods [52] are robust to phase availability and reliability but were widely believed to be able to estimate MRI-PDFF only up to 50% [53] until recently [54].

MRI-PDFF has been validated several times over for liver applications using a liver fat spectrum derived from MR spectroscopy [55]. It is unclear whether the "water plus fat" signal model from MRI-PDFF reconstruction is sufficient to explain pancreatic tissue, or whether other MR-visible chemical species should be considered. Furthermore, the liver spectrum may not be directly applicable to pancreas MRI-PDFF applications, and studies have shown differences in fat composition of liver and pancreas [18]. These differences might be explained by the different mechanisms for ectopic fat deposition in the two organs, discussed in Section Pancreas and ectopic fat. Currently no consensus pancreatic fat model exists in the literature for MRI-PDFF quantification. A broad single-peak model has been proposed using MRS, though it may reflect contamination from surrounding VAT [48,56]. **Fatty acid composition** methods stemming from MRI-PDFF may be able to shed light into this question, since they are not bound to the prior choice of a fat model [57,58]. Instead, fatty acid composition methods attempt to estimate triglyceride composition for each organ, additionally to MRI-PDFF, parameterizing composition by the number of double bonds, the number of methylene-interrupted double bonds, and the chain length of the triglyceride molecules [59,60]. Conversely, recent evidence in livers affected by NASH has suggested that the difference in MRI-PDFF from using models with different triglyceride compositions, for instance a tailored pancreatic model, is "unlikely to be clinically meaningful" [61].

Furthermore, most studies measuring pancreatic MRI-PDFF have used acquisitions designed for liver applications, including those that are commercially available, as well as a liver fat model and region-of-interest (ROI) sampling [23,46,62–68]. It is not clear whether conventional ROI sampling strategies are able to capture the heterogeneous fat deposition in the pancreas accurately, unlike pancreas subsegmentation, or whether the acquisition may need improvements to, e.g., increase SNR (for instance using multiple averages) and reduce signal contamination from VAT and the partial volume effect (PVE) (for example, using thinner slices) [56].

Pancreas morphology

Imaging markers based on pancreas shape may be informative and complementary to MRI-PDFF, especially in cases where there is substantial fat infiltration to allow region-of-interest sampling within the parenchyma. The observation that the pancreatic contour was more lobular (i.e., less smooth) in diabetic subjects was made as early as 1992 by Gilbeau et al. [69]. The quantification of pancreas morphology relied initially on manual, subjective binary scoring systems of surface "lobularity" or surface "smoothness" [69,70]. A "serrated" pancreas contour identified with CT has recently been proposed

1. Acquisition MRI Source Images

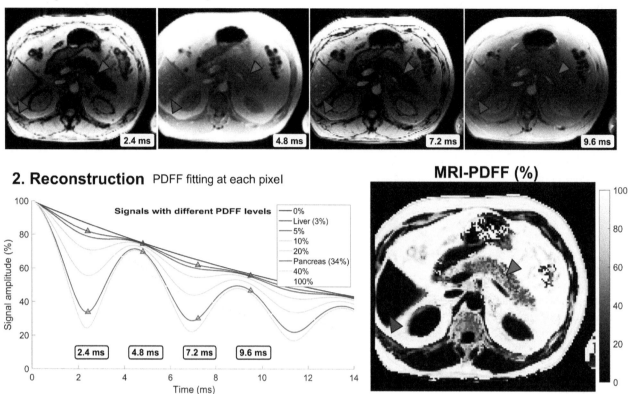

2. Reconstruction PDFF fitting at each pixel

MRI-PDFF (%)

FIGURE 9.5 Example of MRI source images acquired at distinct (echo) times at 1.5 T (top). The increasing presence of fat in a pixel amplifies the oscillatory patterns in the MR signal (bottom left). The MR signal is sampled at multiple times; in this example, every 2.4 ms. The quantity of fat with respect to water (i.e., MRI-PDFF) can be inferred from the sampled MR signal at every pixel, creating an MRI-PDFF image (bottom right). The MRI-PDFF of a type 2 diabetes subject shows increased ectopic fat in the pancreas (red arrowhead), and low levels of liver fat (magenta arrowhead).

as a predictor of postoperative pancreatic fistula after the Whipple procedure [70]. Fig. 9.6 shows examples of pancreata with smooth and lobular outlines. Manual scoring systems of surface "irregularity" have shown significant differences in the distributions of scores between type 2 diabetics and matched controls [71].

Hand-crafted, nonorgan-specific metrics such as curvature [72] or fractal dimension of the pancreas surface [73] has also been used. In a relatively small population, Al-Mrabeh et al. showed significant differences in pancreatic morphology between T2DM "responders" and "nonresponders" at 6 months in a diabetes remission trial, measured as the fractal dimension of two-dimensional projections of the pancreas surface [73]. More recently, the feasibility of a Pancreas Surface Lobularity metric, inspired in Liver Surface Nodularity measurement (used to evaluate liver cirrhosis) [74], has been

FIGURE 9.6 Examples of smooth (left) and lobular (right) pancreatic contours, indicated by the orange arrowheads. Pancreas surface lobularity is suggestive of fat infiltration by adipocytes.

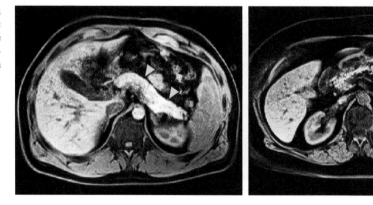

studied in a normal cohort [75]. Morphometry should be performed preferably on 3D acquisitions in CT or MRI for high reproducibility (vs. 2D acquisitions).

Pancreas fibroinflammation

The longitudinal relaxation time after MR excitation of a particular tissue is measured by the T_1 parameter. T_1 has received increased attention recently in liver applications for its ability to quantify fibroinflammation, particularly when corrected for the presence of iron, resulting in the corrected T_1 or cT_1 biomarker [34]. Increased values of cT_1 are associated with an increase in extracellular water at inflamed tissues because water has a long T_1 relaxation time compared to, e.g., fat or collagen.

T_1 has also recently been used in the context of chronic pancreas disease, in the presence of fibroinflammation. Notably, Tirkes et al. showed elevated pancreatic T_1 in chronic pancreatitis subjects in an early study [43]. While there are technical challenges in T_1 quantification [76], pancreatic T_1 could become an established pancreas imaging biomarker to quantify the degree of fibrosis and inflammation, complementary to direct and indirect pancreatic fat measurements, and also complementary to liver cT_1, for the assessment of downstream ectopic fat conditions.

Fig. 9.7 shows abdominal T_1 maps, for example, subjects, including low and high pancreatic T_1 cases.

Big Data and AI

Measuring pancreas state, including quantifying ectopic fat, is a challenging problem, made more difficult by the remarkable variability of the pancreas across individuals, the corresponding variability of (MRI) images, with the attendant image noise, the variety of pathologies that impact on the pancreas, and its physiological complexity. In the past, image analysis and information technology had struggled with such complexity. However, a set of interrelated developments offer

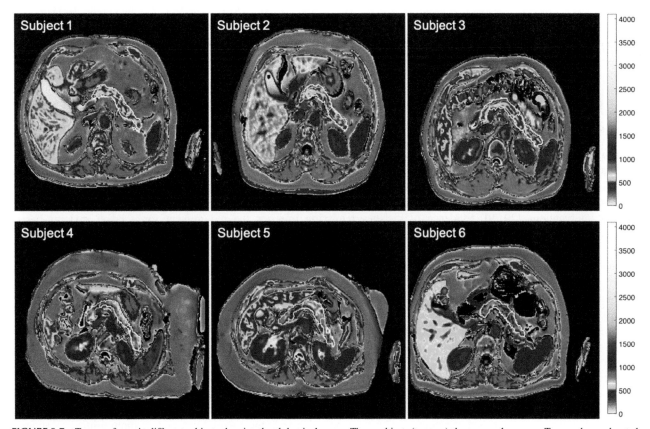

FIGURE 9.7 T_1 maps from six different subjects showing the abdominal organs Three subjects (top row) show normal pancreas T_1, one shows elevated liver T_1. Three subjects (bottom row) show elevated pancreas T_1, suggestive of fibroinflammation. Automated segmentations of the pancreas are shown (white outlines).

hope that these methods are starting to address this complexity, as evidenced by some of the examples presented in this chapter.

Fortuitously, over the past 25 years there have been a set of mutually reinforcing developments. First, the Internet, with ever-increasing bandwidth, has enabled large and growing datasets to be accumulated, associated with metadata, and carefully curated. Second, there have been a surge of innovations in **machine learning and artificial intelligence (AI)**, both for image analysis (e.g., deep convolution neural networks) and for the combination of information of different sorts (e.g., images plus circulating biomarker data). In fact, developments of the Internet have fueled applications of machine learning, while innovations in machine learning have fueled the need for novel datasets that can be provided by the Internet. And third, Cloud technology has provided not only "infinite" storage but increasingly "infinite" compute power. Machine learning, plus image analysis, has been the basis for many of the advances sketched in Section Information from MRI.

Still, there are generally orders of magnitude difference in the sizes of datasets of conventional visual images, for example, ImageNet which currently has 14,197,122 images, and those developed for medical image analysis. While computer-aided detection algorithms in areas such as mammography may aspire to training sets comprising a small number of millions of mammograms, most datasets available for clinical research count themselves lucky if they are able to amass a few hundred cases. Equally, it is often the case that image databases do not have corresponding data such as bloods or genomes.

Recognizing in 2006 that this would be an increasing requirement the UK Government, with the support of research councils and industry, established the **UK Biobank** study to investigate the respective contributions of genetic predisposition and environmental exposure (including nutrition, lifestyle, medications, etc.) to the development of disease. To this end, the UK Biobank aims to gather information on 500,000 nominally healthy volunteers. The imaging substudy of UK Biobank aims to acquire imaging data from 100,000 of those half a million subjects [77]. In particular, the abdominal quantitative MRI protocol enables development and validation of image reconstruction and image analysis methods for the quantification of pancreas fat, volume, morphology, and fibroinflammation, as well as for the detection of tumors and other lesions. Imaging data, including the pancreas, is being acquired at multiple centers across the UK. In addition to bulk imaging data, subjects' metadata—for instance their age, gender, BMI, information from medical records—are also available. Insights obtained from Biobank data may feed back into the design of novel acquisition methods as well as the development of novel imaging biomarkers of pancreas disease, including establishing the biomarker's (and organ's) normal variability and disease cut-offs.

Several examples described above in Section Information from MRI featured algorithms that were trained on UK Biobank data.

Future directions

A recent study using circulating biomarkers and age showed a cluster of five novel subgroups of adult-onset diabetes [78], where each of the groups may benefit from distinct lines of treatment. Novel imaging-based biomarkers could aid in early diagnosis and personalization of T2DM care, as well as providing new evidence disentangling T2DM heterogeneity. Pancreatic fat is one such image-based biomarker. There is now increasing evidence that T2DM may enter remission after lifestyle interventions [20,79]. Evidence of diabetes remission imposes the requirement for a novel imaging-based biomarker to be precise, so that it enables effective monitoring of disease progression. Imaging-based techniques are already being used to monitor diabetes progression in diabetes remission trials.

Importantly, trained CNN models are known to generalize poorly to different conditions or "domains," meaning there will likely be a performance drop when a previously trained system is applied to, for example, images acquired on a different MRI scanner model or field strength. This is one of the main reasons that currently precludes these models from being used routinely. Furthermore, obtaining labeled datasets is both costly and time-consuming. Recently proposed "self-supervised" models that remove the need for paired examples during model training may enhance learning efficiency and facilitate domain adaptation [80]. Advances in automated pancreas segmentation, including facilitating the training and transferability of models could make pancreas volume estimation part of clinical routine.

The availability of large datasets such as UK Biobank, with both imaging and nonimaging data, will further facilitate machine learning methods to be implemented in healthcare systems. The introduction of novel automated detection and routine abdominal imaging tests may also facilitate early diagnosis of pancreatic cancer. For instance, automated lesion detection and lesion volume measurement could be important in radiology workflows and in monitoring cancer progression. Novel techniques such as the combination of quantitative MRI and radiomics may elucidate distinct cancer types.

Advances in machine learning and pattern recognition facilitate improved data-driven approaches for pancreas shape characterization. Under the assumption that natural data falls into lower-dimensional manifolds [81], methods used in brain imaging for groupwise registration and computational anatomy [82], as well as representation learning methods based on deep unsupervised learning, may yield robust and useful imaging biomarkers for the pancreas. Preliminary results using manifold learning on UK Biobank subjects showed shape differences between genders, after normalizing for pancreas volume [83]. Shape characterization combined with parts segmentation into head, body, and tail, will enable regional morphometry, informing the different types of fat infiltration in disease.

In conclusion, imaging-based biomarkers of pancreatic fat accumulation and downstream manifestations of pancreatic steatosis like fibroinflammation, together with novel ways of determining them, have the potential to aid in early detection (and diagnosis), stratification of patient management (in heterogeneous, multiorgan diseases), and monitoring disease progression (where remission is possible), while saving costs to the healthcare system. Repurposing liver techniques for pancreas imaging as well as novel pancreas-specific techniques, and establishing their normal ranges, could prove useful in monitoring the progression and remission of nonalcoholic fatty pancreatic disease, diabetes type 2, chronic pancreatitis, and pancreatic cancer.

References

[1] Bommer C, Vera S, Heesemann E, Manne-Goehler J, Atun R, Bärnighausen T, Davies J, Vollmer S. Global economic burden of diabetes in adults: projections from 2015 to 2030. Diab Care 2018;41(5):963−70. https://doi.org/10.2337/dc17-1962.

[2] Smits MM, Erwin JM, Geenen van. The clinical significance of pancreatic steatosis. Nat Rev Gastroenterol Hepatol 2011;8(3):169−77. https://doi.org/10.1038/nrgastro.2011.4.

[3] Donnelly KL, Smith CI, Jose Jessurun SJS, Boldt MD, Parks EJ. Sources of fatty acids stored in liver and secreted via lipoproteins in patients with nonalcoholic fatty liver disease. J Clin Invest 2005;115(5):1343−51. https://doi.org/10.1172/JCI23621.

[4] Wang CY, Ou HY, Chen MF, Chang TC, Chang CJ. Enigmatic ectopic fat: prevalence of nonalcoholic fatty pancreas disease and its associated factors in a Chinese population. J Am Heart Assoc 2014;3(1):1−8. https://doi.org/10.1161/JAHA.113.000297.

[5] Nadarajah C, Fananapazir G, Cui E, Gichoya J, Thayalan N, Asare-Sawiri M, Menias CO, Sandrasegaran K. Association of pancreatic fat content with type II diabetes mellitus. Clin Radiol 2020;75(1):51−6. https://doi.org/10.1016/j.crad.2019.05.027.

[6] Mathur A, Marine M, Lu D, Deborah A, Swartz-Basile, Saxena R, Zyromski NJ, Pitt HA. Nonalcoholic fatty pancreas disease. HPB 2007;9(4):312−8. https://doi.org/10.1080/13651820701504157.

[7] Gaborit B, Abdesselam I, Kober F, Jacquier A, Ronsin O, Emungania O, Lesavre N, et al. Ectopic fat storage in the pancreas using 1 H-MRS: importance of diabetic status and modulation with bariatric surgery-induced weight loss. Int J Obes 2015;39(3):480−7. https://doi.org/10.1038/ijo.2014.126.

[8] Steven S, Hollingsworth KG, Small PK, Woodcock SA, Pucci A, Benjamin A, Al-Mrabeh A, Daly AK, Batterham RL, Taylor R. Weight loss decreases excess pancreatic triacylglycerol specifically in type 2 diabetes. Diabetes Care 2016;39(1):158−65. https://doi.org/10.2337/dc15-0750.

[9] Jiang Y, Spurny M, Ruth S, Tobias N, Schlett CL, Von Stackelberg O, Ulrich CM, et al. Changes in pancreatic fat content following diet-induced weight loss. Nutrients 2019;11(4):1−13. https://doi.org/10.3390/nu11040912.

[10] Wildman, R.P, Paul M., K. Reynolds, A.P Mcginn, S. Rajpathak, J. Wylie-Rosett, and Maryfran R Sowers. n.d. "The obese without cardiometabolic risk factor clustering and the normal weight with cardiometabolic risk factor clustering.".

[11] Gerst F, Wagner R, Barroso Oquendo M, Siegel-Axel D, Fritsche A, Martin H, Staiger H, Ulrich Häring H, Ullrich S. What role do fat cells play in pancreatic tissue? Mol Metabol 2019;25(May):1−10. https://doi.org/10.1016/j.molmet.2019.05.001.

[12] Psallas M, Vasileiadis T. Non-alcoholic fatty pancreas disease: a clinical entity we should not ignore any more ec gastroenterology and dõgestõve system special issue-2020" 03 (dm): 1−12. 2020.

[13] Saisho Y. Pancreas volume and fat deposition in diabetes and normal physiology: consideration of the interplay between endocrine and exocrine pancreas. Rev Diabet Stud 2016;13(2−3):132−47. https://doi.org/10.1900/RDS.2016.13.132.

[14] Dholakia S, Sharples EJ, Ploeg RJ, Friend PJ. Significance of steatosis in pancreatic transplantation. Transplant Rev 2017;31(4):225−31. https://doi.org/10.1016/j.trre.2017.08.001.

[15] Ogilvie RF. The islands of langerhans in 19 cases of obesity. J Pathol Bacteriol 1933;37(3):473−81. https://doi.org/10.1002/path.1700370314.

[16] Guglielmi V, Sbraccia P. Type 2 diabetes: does pancreatic fat really matter? Diabetes Metabol Res Rev 2018;34(2):1−8. https://doi.org/10.1002/dmrr.2955.

[17] Lee Y, Lingvay I, Szczepaniak LS, Ravazzola M, Orci L, Unger RH. Pancreatic steatosis: harbinger of type 2 diabetes in obese rodents. Int J Obes 2010;34(2):396−400. https://doi.org/10.1038/ijo.2009.245.

[18] Pinnick KE, Collins SC, Londos C, Gauguier D, Clark A, Barbara A, Fielding. Pancreatic ectopic fat is characterized by adipocyte infiltration and altered lipid composition. Obesity 2008;16(3):522−30. https://doi.org/10.1038/oby.2007.110.

[19] Tushuizen ME, Bunck MC, Pouwels PJ, Bontemps S, Van Waesberghe JHT, Schindhelm RK, Mari A, Heine RJ, Diamant M. Pancreatic fat content and β-cell function in men with and without type 2 diabetes. Diabetes Care 2007;30(11):2916−21. https://doi.org/10.2337/dc07-0326.

[20] Lim EL, Hollingsworth KG, Aribisala BS, Chen MJ, Mathers JC, Taylor R. Reversal of type 2 diabetes: normalisation of beta cell function in association with decreased pancreas and liver triacylglycerol. Diabetologia 2011;54(10):2506−14. https://doi.org/10.1007/s00125-011-2204-7.

[21] Wong VWS, Wong GLH, Wai Yeung DK, Abrigo JM, Shan Kong AP, Mei Chan RS, Chim AML, et al. Fatty pancreas, insulin resistance, and β-cell function: a population study using fat-water magnetic resonance imaging. Am J Gastroenterol 2014;109(4):589−97. https://doi.org/10.1038/ajg.2014.1.

[22] Dong Z, Luo Y, Cai H, Zhang Z, Peng Z, Jiang M, Li Y, Chang L, Li ZP, Shi Ting F. Noninvasive fat quantification of the liver and pancreas may provide potential biomarkers of impaired glucose tolerance and type 2 diabetes. Medicine 2016;95(23):1−7. https://doi.org/10.1097/MD.0000000000003858.

[23] Kühn J-P, Berthold F, Mayerle J, Henry V, Scott B, Reeder, Rathmann W, Lerch MM, Hosten N, Hegenscheid K, Peter J, Meffert. Pancreatic steatosis demonstrated at MR imaging in the general population: clinical relevance. Radiology 2015;276(1):129−36. https://doi.org/10.1148/radiol.15140446.

[24] Kleeff J, Whitcomb DC, Shimosegawa T, Esposito I, Lerch MM, Gress T, Mayerle J, et al. Chronic pancreatitis. Nat Rev Dis Prim 2017;3:1−18. https://doi.org/10.1038/nrdp.2017.60.

[25] Kyrgiou M, Kalliala I, Markozannes G, Gunter MJ, Paraskevaidis E, Gabra H, Martin-Hirsch P, Konstantinos K, Tsilidis. Adiposity and cancer at major anatomical sites: umbrella review of the literature. BMJ 2017;356:1−10. https://doi.org/10.1136/bmj.j477.

[26] Marchal G, Verbeken E, Steenbergen W, Baert A, Lauweryns J. Uneven lipomatosis: a pitfall in pancreatic sonography. Gastrointest Radiol 1989;14(1):233−7. https://doi.org/10.1007/BF01889205.

[27] Matsumoto S, Mori H, Miyake H, Takaki H, Maeda T, Yamada Y, Oga M. Uneven fatty replacement of the pancreas: evaluation with CT. Radiology 1995;194(2):453−8. https://doi.org/10.1148/radiology.194.2.7824726.

[28] Wang X, Misawa R, Zielinski MC, Cowen P, Jo J, Periwal V, Ricordi C, et al. Regional differences in islet distribution in the human pancreas - preferential beta-cell loss in the head region in patients with type 2 diabetes. PLoS One 2013;8(6):1−9. https://doi.org/10.1371/journal.pone.0067454.

[29] Patel NS, Peterson MR, Brenner DA, Heba E, Sirlin C, Loomba R. Association between novel MRI-estimated pancreatic fat and liver histology-determined steatosis and fibrosis in non-alcoholic fatty liver disease. Aliment Pharmacol Therapeut 2013;37(6):630−9. https://doi.org/10.1111/apt.12237.

[30] Zhang X, Shi S, Zhang B, Ni Q, Yu X, Xu J. Circulating biomarkers for early diagnosis of pancreatic cancer: facts and hopes. Am J Canc Res 2018;8(3):332−53.

[31] Ren J, Dimitrov I, Dean Sherry A, Malloy CR. Composition of adipose tissue and marrow fat in humans by 1H NMR at 7 tesla. J Lipid Res 2008;49(9):2055−62. https://doi.org/10.1194/jlr.D800010-JLR200.

[32] Hamilton G, Schlein AN, Middleton MS, Hooker CA, Wolfson T, Gamst AC, Loomba R, Sirlin CB. In vivo triglyceride composition of abdominal adipose tissue measured by 1H MRS at 3T. J Magn Reson Imag 2017;45(5):1455−63. https://doi.org/10.1002/jmri.25453.

[33] Hu HH, Kim HW, Nayak KS, Goran MI. Comparison of fat-water MRI and single-voxel MRS in the assessment of hepatic and pancreatic fat fractions in humans. Obesity 2010;18(4):841−7. https://doi.org/10.1038/oby.2009.352.

[34] Mojtahed A, Kelly CJ, Herlihy AH, Kin S, Wilman HR, McKay A, Kelly M, et al. Reference range of liver corrected T1 values in a population at low risk for fatty liver disease—a UK Biobank sub-study, with an appendix of interesting cases. Abdom Radiol 2019;44(1):72−84. https://doi.org/10.1007/s00261-018-1701-2.

[35] DeSouza SV, Singh RG, Rinki Murphy HDY, Plank LD, Petrov MS. Pancreas volume in health and disease: a systematic review and meta-analysis. Expet Rev Gastroenterol Hepatol 2018;12(8):757−66. https://doi.org/10.1080/17474124.2018.1496015.

[36] Garcia TS, Rech TH, Bauermann Leitão C. Pancreatic size and fat content in diabetes: a systematic review and meta-analysis of imaging studies. PLoS One 2017;12(7):1−15. https://doi.org/10.1371/journal.pone.0180911.

[37] Ronneberger O, Fischer P, Brox T. U-net: convolutional networks for biomedical image segmentation. Lect Notes Comput Sci 2015;9351:234−41. https://doi.org/10.1007/978-3-319-24574-4_28.

[38] Owler J, Irving B, Ridgeway G, Wojciechowska M, McGonigle J, Michael Brady S. Comparison of multi-atlas segmentation and U-net approaches for automated 3D liver delineation in MRI. In: Communications in computer and information science; 2020. p. 478−88. https://doi.org/10.1007/978-3-030-39343-4_41. vol. 1065 CCIS.

[39] Bagheri MH, Roth H, Kovacs W, Yao J, Farhadi F, Li X, Ronald M, Summers. Technical and clinical factors affecting success rate of a deep learning method for pancreas segmentation on CT. Acad Radiol 2020;27(5):689−95. https://doi.org/10.1016/j.acra.2019.08.014.

[40] Cai J, Lu Le, Xing F, Yang L. Pancreas segmentation in CT and MRI via task-specific network design and recurrent neural contextual learning. Advan in Comput Visi Patt Recognit 3−21 2019. https://doi.org/10.1007/978-3-030-13969-8_1.

[41] Isensee F, Jaeger PF, Simon A.A K, Petersen J, Maier-Hein KH. NnU-net: a self-configuring method for deep learning-based biomedical image segmentation. Nat Methods 2021;18(2):203−11. https://doi.org/10.1038/s41592-020-01008-z.

[42] Schlemper J, Oktay O, Michiel Schaap, Heinrich M, Kainz B, Glocker B, Rueckert D. Attention gated networks: learning to leverage salient regions in medical images. Med Image Anal 2019;53(April):197−207. https://doi.org/10.1016/J.MEDIA.2019.01.012.

[43] Tirkes T, Lin C, Cui E, Deng Y, Territo PR, Sandrasegaran K, Akisik F. Quantitative MR evaluation of chronic pancreatitis: extracellular volume fraction and MR relaxometry. Am J Roentgenol 2018;210(3):533−42. https://doi.org/10.2214/AJR.17.18606.

[44] Bagur, Alexandre T, Paul A, Ridgway GR, Brady M, Bulte DP. Pancreas MRI segmentation into head, body, and tail enables regional quantitative analysis of heterogeneous disease. medRxiv 2021. https://doi.org/10.1101/2021.11.30.21266158. 11.30.21266158.

[45] Lingvay I, Esser V, Legendre JL, Price AL, Wertz KM, Adams-Huet B, Zhang S, Unger RH, Szczepaniak LS. Noninvasive quantification of pancreatic fat in humans. J Clin Endocrinol Metab 2009;94(10):4070−6. https://doi.org/10.1210/jc.2009-0584.

[46] Sarma MK, Saucedo A, Hema Darwin C, Richard Felker E, Umachandran K, Kohanghadosh D, Xu E, Raman S, Albert Thomas M. Noninvasive assessment of abdominal adipose tissues and quantification of hepatic and pancreatic fat fractions in type 2 diabetes mellitus. Magn Reson Imag 2020;72(May):95−102. https://doi.org/10.1016/j.mri.2020.07.001.

[47] Majumder S, Philip NA, Takahashi N, Levy MJ, Singh VP, Chari ST. Fatty pancreas: should we Be concerned? Pancreas 2017;46(10):1251−8. https://doi.org/10.1097/MPA.0000000000000941.

[48] Begovatz P, Koliaki C, Weber K, Strassburger K, Nowotny B, Nowotny P, Müssig K, et al. Pancreatic adipose tissue infiltration, parenchymal steatosis and beta cell function in humans. Diabetologia 2015;58(7):1646−55. https://doi.org/10.1007/s00125-015-3544-5.

[49] Caussy C, Reeder SB, Sirlin CB, Loomba R. Noninvasive, quantitative assessment of liver fat by MRI-PDFF as an endpoint in NASH trials. Hepatology 2018. https://doi.org/10.1002/hep.29797.

[50] Dixon, Thomas W. Simple proton spectroscopic imaging. Radiology 1984;153(1):189−94. https://doi.org/10.1148/radiology.153.1.6089263.

[51] Reeder SB, Wen Z, Yu H, Angel RP, Garry E G, Markl M, Pelc NJ. Multicoil Dixon chemical species separation with an iterative least-squares estimation method. Magn Reson Med 2004;51(1):35−45. https://doi.org/10.1002/mrm.10675.

[52] Bydder M, Yokoo T, Hamilton G, Middleton MS, Chavez AD, Schwimmer JB, Lavine JE, Sirlin CB. Relaxation effects in the quantification of fat using gradient echo imaging. Magn Reson Imag 2008;26(3):347−59. https://doi.org/10.1016/j.mri.2007.08.012.

[53] Reeder SB, Cruite I, Hamilton G, Sirlin CB. Quantitative assessment of liver fat with magnetic resonance imaging and spectroscopy. J Magn Reson Imag 2011;34(4):729−49. https://doi.org/10.1002/jmri.22580.

[54] Bagur T, Alexandre CH, Irving B, Gyngell ML, Robson MD, Brady M. Magnitude-intrinsic water−fat ambiguity can Be resolved with multipeak fat modeling and a multipoint search method. Magn Reson Med 2019;82(1):460−75. https://doi.org/10.1002/mrm.27728.

[55] Hamilton G, Yokoo T, Bydder M, Cruite I, Schroeder ME, Sirlin CB, Middleton MS. In vivo characterization of the liver fat 1H MR spectrum. NMR Biomed 2011;24(7):784−90. https://doi.org/10.1002/nbm.1622.

[56] Sakai NS, Taylor SA, Chouhan MD. Obesity, metabolic disease and the pancreas-quantitative imaging of pancreatic fat. Br J Radiol 2018;91(1089):20180267. https://doi.org/10.1259/bjr.20180267.

[57] Bydder M, Girard O, Hamilton G. Mapping the double bonds in triglycerides. Magn Reson Imag 2011;29(8):1041−6. https://doi.org/10.1016/j.mri.2011.07.004.

[58] Peterson P, Månsson S. Simultaneous quantification of fat content and fatty acid composition using MR imaging. Magn Reson Med 2013;69(3):688−97. https://doi.org/10.1002/mrm.24297.

[59] Leporq B, Lambert SA, Ronot M, Vilgrain V, Bernard E, Van Beers. Quantification of the triglyceride fatty acid composition with 3.0 T MRI. NMR Biomed 2014;27(10):1211−21. https://doi.org/10.1002/nbm.3175.

[60] Trinh L, Peterson P, Leander P, Brorson H, Månsson S. In vivo comparison of MRI-based and MRS-based quantification of adipose tissue fatty acid composition against gas chromatography. Magn Reson Med 2020;84(5):2484−94. https://doi.org/10.1002/mrm.28300.

[61] Hong CW, Mamidipalli A, Hooker JC, Hamilton G, Wolfson T, Chen DH, Fazeli Dehkordy S, et al. MRI proton density fat fraction is robust across the biologically plausible range of triglyceride spectra in adults with nonalcoholic steatohepatitis. J Magn Reson Imag 2018;47(4):995−1002. https://doi.org/10.1002/jmri.25845.

[62] Fukui H, Hori M, Fukuda Y, Onishi H, Nakamoto A, Ota T, Ogawa K, et al. Evaluation of fatty pancreas by proton density fat fraction using 3-T magnetic resonance imaging and its association with pancreatic cancer. Eur J Radiol 2019;118(September):25−31. https://doi.org/10.1016/j.ejrad.2019.06.024.

[63] Kato S, Iwasaki A, Kurita Y, Arimoto J, Yamamoto T, Hasegawa S, Sato T, et al. Three-dimensional analysis of pancreatic fat by fat-water magnetic resonance imaging provides detailed characterization of pancreatic steatosis with improved reproducibility. PLoS One 2019;14(12):1−13. https://doi.org/10.1371/journal.pone.0224921.

[64] Idilman IS, Ali T, Berna S, Halil Elhan A, Celik A, Idilman R, Karcaaltincaba M. Quantification of liver, pancreas, kidney, and vertebral body MRI-PDFF in non-alcoholic fatty liver disease. Abdom Imag 2015;40(6):1512−9. https://doi.org/10.1007/s00261-015-0385-0.

[65] Boga S, Koksal AR, Sen İ, Kurul Yeniay M, Yilmaz Ozguven MB, Erdinc Serin, Mehmet Erturk S, Alkim H, Alkim C. Liver and pancreas: 'Castor and pollux' regarding the relationship between hepatic steatosis and pancreas exocrine insufficiency. Pancreatology 2020;20(5):880−6. https://doi.org/10.1016/j.pan.2020.04.020.

[66] Chai J, Liu P, Jin E, Su T, Zhang J, Shi K, Xu H, Yin J, Yu H. MRI chemical shift imaging of the fat content of the pancreas and liver of patients with type 2 diabetes mellitus. Exp Ther Med 2016;11(2):476−80. https://doi.org/10.3892/etm.2015.2925.

[67] Heber SD, Hetterich H, Lorbeer R, Bayerl C, Machann J, Auweter S, Storz C, et al. Pancreatic fat content by magnetic resonance imaging in subjects with prediabetes, diabetes, and controls from a general population without cardiovascular disease. PLoS One 2017;12(5):1−13. https://doi.org/10.1371/journal.pone.0177154.

[68] Al-Mrabeh, Ahmad KG, Hollingsworth, Sarah Steven, Tiniakos D, Taylor R. Quantification of intrapancreatic fat in type 2 diabetes by MRI. PLoS One 2017;12(4):1−19. https://doi.org/10.1371/journal.pone.0174660.

[69] Gilbeau JP, Poncelet V, Libon E, Derue G, Heller FR. The density, contour, and thickness of the pancreas in diabetics: CT findings in 57 patients. Am J Roentgenol 1992;159(3):527−31. https://doi.org/10.2214/ajr.159.3.1503017.

[70] Kusafuka T, Kato H, Iizawa Y, Noguchi D, Gyoten K, Hayasaki A, Fujii T, et al. Pancreas-visceral fat CT value ratio and serrated pancreatic contour are strong predictors of postoperative pancreatic fistula after pancreaticojejunostomy. BMC Surg 2020;20(1):1−12. https://doi.org/10.1186/s12893-020-00785-w.

[71] Macauley M, Percival K, Thelwall PE, Hollingsworth KG, Taylor R. Altered volume, morphology and composition of the pancreas in type 2 diabetes. PLoS One 2015;10(5):1−14. https://doi.org/10.1371/journal.pone.0126825.

[72] Asaturyan H, Thomas EL, Bell JD, Villarini B. A framework for automatic morphological feature extraction and analysis of abdominal organs in MRI volumes. J Med Syst 2019;43(12):334. https://doi.org/10.1007/s10916-019-1474-3.

[73] Al-Mrabeh, Ahmad KG, Hollingsworth, Steven S, Taylor R. Morphology of the pancreas in type 2 diabetes: effect of weight loss with or without normalisation of insulin secretory capacity. Diabetologia 2016;59(8):1753—9. https://doi.org/10.1007/s00125-016-3984-6.

[74] Smith AD, Branch CR, Kevin Z, Subramony C, Zhang H, Thaggard K, Hosch R, et al. Liver surface nodularity quantification from routine ct images as a biomarker for detection and evaluation of cirrhosis. Radiology 2016;280(3):771—81. https://doi.org/10.1148/radiol.2016151542.

[75] Sartoris R, Calandra A, Lee KJ, Gauss T, Vilgrain V, Ronot M. Quantification of pancreas surface lobularity on CT: a feasibility study in the normal pancreas. Korean J Radiol 2021;22. https://doi.org/10.3348/kjr.2020.1049.

[76] Stikov N, Boudreau M, Levesque IR, Tardif CL, Barral JK, Bruce Pike G. On the accuracy of T1 mapping: searching for common ground. Magn Reson Med 2015;73(2):514—22. https://doi.org/10.1002/mrm.25135.

[77] Littlejohns TJ, Holliday J, Gibson LM, Garratt S, Oesingmann N, Alfaro-Almagro F, Bell JD, et al. The UK Biobank imaging enhancement of 100,000 participants: rationale, data collection, management and future Directions. Nat Commun 2020;11(1):2624. https://doi.org/10.1038/s41467-020-15948-9.

[78] Ahlqvist E, Storm P, Käräjämäki A, Martinell M, Dorkhan M, Carlsson A, Vikman P, et al. Novel subgroups of adult-onset diabetes and their association with outcomes: a data-driven cluster Analysis of six variables. Lancet Diab Endocrinol 2018;6(5):361—9. https://doi.org/10.1016/S2213-8587(18)30051-2.

[79] Lean MEJ, Leslie WS, Barnes AC, Brosnahan N, George T, McCombie L, Peters C, et al. Primary care-led weight management for remission of type 2 diabetes (DiRECT): an open-label, cluster-randomised trial. Lancet 2018;391(10120):541—51. https://doi.org/10.1016/S0140-6736(17)33102-1.

[80] Yu EM, Iglesias JE, Dalca AV, Sabuncu MR. An auto-encoder strategy for adaptive image segmentation, vols. 1—11; 2020.

[81] Bengio Y, Courville A, Vincent P. Representation learning: a review and new perspectives. IEEE Trans Pattern Anal Mach Intell 2013;35(8):1798—828. https://doi.org/10.1109/TPAMI.2013.50.

[82] Ashburner J, Klöppel S. Multivariate models of inter-subject anatomical variability. Neuroimage 2011;56(2):422—39. https://doi.org/10.1016/j.neuroimage.2010.03.059.

[83] Bagur, Alexandre T, Ridgway G, McGonigle J, Michael Brady S, Bulte D. Pancreas segmentation-derived biomarkers: volume and shape metrics in the UK Biobank imaging study. Communications in computer and information science, vol. 1248; 2020. p. 131—42. https://doi.org/10.1007/978-3-030-52791-4_11. CCIS.

Chapter 10

Fat accumulation around and within the kidney

Ling Lin[1,2], Ilona A. Dekkers[3] and Hildo J. Lamb[3]

[1]The Eighth Affiliated Hospital of Sun Yat-sen University, Shenzhen, China; [2]Leiden University Medical Center, Leiden, the Netherlands; [3]Department of Radiology, Cardio Vascular Imaging Group (CVIG), Leiden University Medical Center, Leiden, the Netherlands

Introduction

The kidneys are surrounded by perirenal fat, which separates the kidney capsule and kidney fascia. Around the renal hilum, perirenal fat extends along renal arteries, veins, lymphatic vessels, nerve fibers, and collecting system, and fills the renal sinus with renal sinus fat. In addition, lipids can accumulate in the kidney parenchyma in obese status (also referred to as "fatty kidney"), mainly in the tubules and glomeruli. Fat accumulation around and within the kidney participates in the regulation of kidney function, energy metabolism, gluconeogenesis, and cardiovascular function through paracrine and endocrine pathways. Excessive kidney fat is associated with a number of clinical implications, such as chronic kidney disease, diabetes mellitus, hypertension, atherosclerosis, kidney neoplasm, etc. In this chapter, the anatomical, histological, and physiological characteristics of perirenal fat, renal sinus fat, and fat deposition in the renal parenchyma are described. Noninvasive quantification of these fat compartments using imaging modalities as well as their clinical implications is elaborated in this chapter.

Perirenal fat and renal sinus fat

Anatomical characteristics

Perirenal fat is located around the kidneys and the adrenal glands, and is separated from the pararenal fat in the retroperitoneal space by a condensed, membranous layer of renal fascia. Rena fascial encloses (except inferiorly) perirenal fat with the anterior fascia of Gerota [1] and the posterior fascia of Zuckerkandl [2] (Fig. 10.1). The anterior renal fascia is thin and on occasions elusive, while the posterior renal fascia is tough. Laterally the anterior fascia and the posterior fascia merge and form the lateroconal fascia. Medially the anterior fascia and the posterior fascia extend to midline, fuse with the vascular sheaths of the renal vessels, and at midline the left and right renal fascia fuse anterior to the aorta and the inferior vena cava (Fig. 10.2). However, this fusion has a defect below the level of renal hilum, which enables a potential communication across the midline between the two perirenal spaces [3]. There is a thin fascial plane between the adrenal gland and the kidney, but cranially the anterior fascia and the posterior fascia fuse above the adrenal gland and mix imperceptibly with the diaphragmatic fascia [4]. Unlike the lateral, medial, and superior part of the perirenal space, the inferior compartment is not completely closed. Part of the renal fascia merges with the ureteral sheath and part ends subtly within the retroperitoneal fat. A cadaver study using computed tomography (CT) found that contrast medium injected into the perirenal space tracked down to the pelvic extraperitoneal and presacral spaces, suggesting a communication between the caudal extremity of the perirenal space and the posterior pararenal space [3]. Inside the perirenal space, sparse strands of connective tissue exist in addition to adipose tissue [5]. In summary, the upper part of perirenal fat that is separated from pararenal fat and other retroperitoneal structures by a complete renal fascia, while the lower part of perirenal fat has the shape of an inverted cone but not completely enclosed by the renal fascia, with potential communication with the pelvis and the opposite side across the midline (Fig. 10.3).

Visceral and Ectopic Fat. https://doi.org/10.1016/B978-0-12-822186-0.00028-6

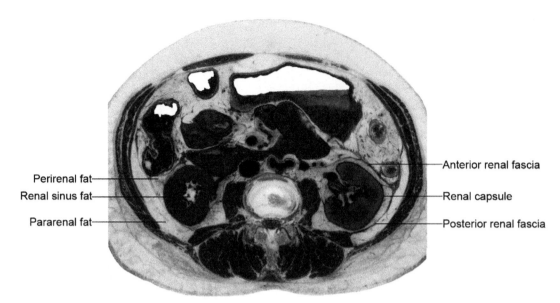

FIGURE 10.1   Cross-sectional view of the fat around the kidneys. *Adapted from a photo of a female cadaver from the Visible Human Project at https://www.nlm.nih.gov/research/visible/visible_human.html.*

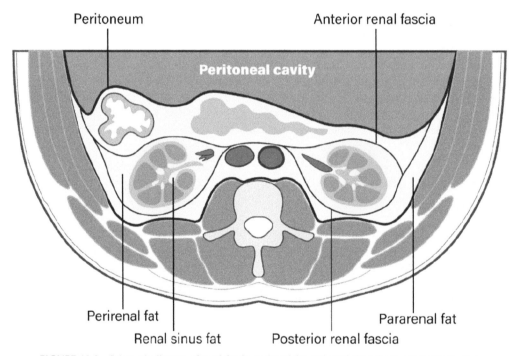

FIGURE 10.2   Schematic diagram of renal fascia, perirenal fat, and renal sinus fat in a transversal view.

Perirenal fat is well-vascularized by an anastomosing capillary network generated from the branches of the inferior suprarenal, left colic, renal, lumbar, and ovarian/testicular arteries [6,7]. Perirenal lymphatic vessels communicate extensively with renal subcapsular lymphatic vessels and eventually drain into the paraaortic lymph nodes [8]. Perirenal fat is also richly innervated. Animal studies have revealed that perirenal nerve fibers originate from the celiac-superior mesenteric ganglion, ipsilateral inferior mesenteric ganglion, adrenal ganglion, aorticorenal ganglion, gonadal ganglion, and L1−L3 ipsilateral sympathetic trunk ganglia [9,10].

Renal sinus fat is the extension of perirenal fat starting around the renal hilum and intrudes upon the renal parenchyma (Figs. 10.1−10.3). Renal sinus fat is separated from the renal parenchyma by the reflection of the renal capsule [11]. As there is no anatomical separation between renal sinus fat and perirenal fat, renal sinus fat is considered as a component of perirenal fat. Renal sinus fat is in close contact with the renal pelvis, calyces, renal vasculatures, lymphatic vessels, and

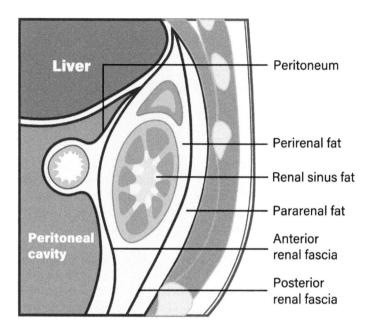

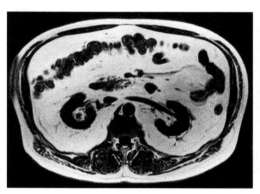
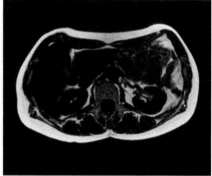

FIGURE 10.3 Schematic diagram of renal fascia, perirenal fat, and renal sinus fat in a sagittal view. The lower part of perirenal fat is not completely enclosed by the renal fascia, with potential communication with the pelvis.

FIGURE 10.4 Dixon fat-only images showing much larger amount of perirenal fat and renal sinus fat in an obese patient with diabetes (left) than that in a lean healthy volunteer (right).

nerve fibers. Therefore, renal sinus fat is also considered as a perivascular adipose tissue, which may contribute to the pathogenesis of cardiovascular diseases like other perivascular adipose tissue, such as epicardial fat [12]. However, it has not been confirmed whether renal sinus fat is physiologically and functionally different from the general perirenal fat, due to the lack of histological studies specific to sinus fat.

Both perirenal fat and renal sinus fat can be found in lean individuals [13−15]. The amount of perirenal fat and sinus fat varies with different individuals and metabolic conditions (Fig. 10.4). In a population aged 21−80 years old without renal diseases, renal sinus fat volume was found to increase with age, though it appeared to decrease in individuals older than 70 years of age [13]. Sex difference in the distribution of perirenal fat has been reported in previous studies, in which the thickness of perirenal fat measured on cross-sectional CT images was larger in men than that in women [16,17]. Another study found larger perirenal fat volume in men compared with women of comparable waist circumference [18]. Similarly, smaller renal sinus fat area was found in women than in men [18]. This study also found that the area of renal sinus fat derived from a single-slice CT image was correlated with the volume of perirenal fat, however not as strongly as the perirenal fat thickness correlated with perirenal fat volume [18]. Two studies found that renal sinus fat compartments distribute asymmetrically, with more fat accumulation in the left renal sinus than in the right [13,19]. Therefore, it is recommended to assess the left-side renal sinus fat for a more reliable observation [19].

Currently no standards or consensus is available for the definitions of excessive perirenal fat and renal sinus fat. In the general population, sinus fat volume in one kidney has been described to range from 0.07 to 11.23 cm^3 [19]. Perirenal fat thickness was found to be correlated with body mass index (BMI) [16]. However, it was also observed that obese individuals did not necessarily have proportionally increased perirenal fat when compared to the individuals with lower BMI [16]. In obese rabbits and humans, renal sinus fat is associated with kidney size [14,20,21]. In contrast to our recent findings that renal sinus fat volume derived from magnetic resonance imaging (MRI) was correlated with body size [14], no correlation was found between renal sinus fat area and any anthropometric measurements in a previous study [18]. Moreover, renal sinus fat volume was found to be positively associated with abdominal visceral adipose tissue (VAT) in individuals with prediabetes or diabetes [14,22] (Fig. 10.5).

Histological and pathophysiological characteristics

Currently the adipose tissue around the kidneys is considered as a special deposit of abdominal VAT, which shares the same developmental origin of VAT. However, the histological, physiological, and functional characteristics of renal adipose tissue are different from those of VAT in other anatomical locations [23]. Interestingly, a recent study of human adipose tissue found that the gene expression profile of perirenal adipose tissue was more analogous to that of subcutaneous adipose tissue (SAT) than VAT, but perirenal fat can still be distinguished from SAT according to different expression patterns [24].

Different from typical abdominal VAT which mainly consists of white adipocytes, perirenal adipose tissue is a mixture of white, brown, and beige adipocytes. In fetuses and infants (1−11 months of life), perirenal fat is predominantly composed of brown adipocytes [25]. After birth, the amount of brown adipose tissue decreases due to a progressive transition into white adipose tissue. Only a small portion of brown adipocytes with multilocular morphology remain active in perirenal fat in adults, mainly located in areas richly innervated by sympathetic nerve fibers, for instance, around the renal hilum and near the adrenal gland [26]. However, It has been observed that most of the perirenal fat in adults consists of unilocular dormant brown adipocytes, which are different from multilocular brown adipocytes and are evenly distributed in perirenal adipose tissue [26]. Gene analysis suggested that the majority of human perirenal adipocytes express the genes of uncoupling protein-1 (UCP1), a protein unique to brown adipocyte mitochondria [27]. However, there is a significant individual variability in the portion of UCP1-positive adipocytes in perirenal fat [27]. A study of a Siberia population who live in the coldest regions of the earth found higher percentage of brown adipocytes with more intensely expression of functional UCP1 in individuals living mainly outdoor, supporting the idea that perirenal adipose tissue can be converted to brown adipose tissue in cold conditions [28]. Sex difference in perirenal fat has also been reported by histological studies [29,30]. Mesenchymal stem cells derived from female perirenal adipose tissue express significantly more UCP1 mRNA than those from male perirenal adipose tissue, indicating that women have more potential to induce "browning" of perirenal fat than men [29]. The underlying mechanism could be the association between the number of X chromosomes and adiposity rather than the effects of sex hormones, as suggested by a murine study [30].

The unique component adipocytes form the basis of the physiological and functional characteristics that distinguish perirenal fat from other VAT deposits [31,32]. Perirenal fat functions as an active paracrine and endocrine organ,

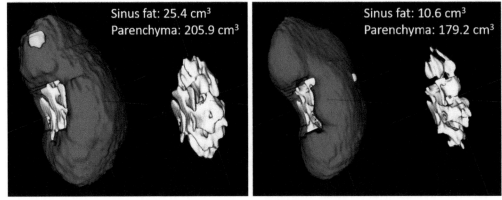

FIGURE 10.5 A patient with type 2 diabetes mellitus (left) had larger renal sinus fat volume than a healthy control (right) of similar body size. Renal parenchyma volume and sinus fat volume were obtained from Dixon images, where sinus fat was labeled yellow, and cysts (blue) were excluded from the calculation of parenchyma volume (red). Left: a 64-year-old male patient with type 2 diabetes mellitus whose height was 178.0 cm and weight was 86.9 kg. Right: a 61-year-old healthy male whose height was 178.5 cm and weight was 85.7 kg. *Adapted from Lin L., Dekkers I.A., Huang L., Tao Q., Paiman E.H.M., Bizino M.B., et al. Renal sinus fat volume in type 2 diabetes mellitus is associated with glycated hemoglobin and metabolic risk factors. J Diabetes Complicat 2021;107973; under a Creative Commons license.*

synthesizing and secreting a number of adipokines and inflammatory cytokines pertinent to energy metabolism and inflammation [33]. Perirenal fat participates in the regulation of kidney function, glucose and lipid metabolism, and cardiovascular homeostatic function by several physiological pathways including sympathetic activation, humoral regulation, renin-angiotensin system, and inflammation [33]. The underlying mechanisms of how perirenal fat contributes to chronic kidney disease, hyperglycemia, hypertension, and atherosclerosis have been summarized in recent publications [6,8,33,34].

Imaging-based quantification

Similar to other VAT compartments, accumulation of perirenal fat and renal sinus fat can be evaluated by imaging modalities including ultrasonography, CT, and MRI. Perirenal fat is mostly measured by ultrasonography and CT, while renal sinus fat is mainly quantified by CT and MRI. Table 10.1 provides a list of studies and the corresponding imaging modalities that were used for quantifying perirenal fat and sinus fat in humans.

Quantification of perirenal fat

While ultrasonography is most widely used in clinical studies to measure the thickness of perirenal fat, it is operator-dependent and the measurements are limited by the location of the acoustic window. The most frequently used acoustic window is the longitudinal scanning on the lateral aspect of the abdomen in the supine position, at which the surface of the kidney was almost parallel to the skin [15,35−43]. However, the problem of this method is that not only the thickness of perirenal fat is measured, but also the pararenal fat between the renal fascia and the inner side of abdominal musculature, which is retroperitoneal adipose tissue, is included (Fig. 10.6). Moreover, the pressure exerted by the probe might also impact the measurements. An alternative acoustic window adopted by a few studies was the longitudinal scanning along the midclavicular line, and the anterior distance from the border of the liver/spleen to the border of the inferior part the kidney was measured as the thickness of perirenal fat [44−46] (Fig. 10.7). This method can exclude the impact of pararenal

TABLE 10.1 Overview of human studies using imaging modalities for the quantification of perirenal fat and renal sinus fat.

| Imaging modality | Perirenal fat | | Renal sinus fat | |
	List of studies	Measurement	List of studies	Measurement
Ultrasound	Lamacchia et al. [35]; Sun et al. [36]; Sahin et al. [37]; De Pergola et al. [38]; Bassols et al. [15]; Geraci et al. [39]; Ricci et al. [40]; López Bermejo et al. [41]; Manno et al. [42]; Fang et al. [43]	Thickness of perirenal + pararenal fat	None	Not applicable
	Grima et al. [44,45]; D'Marco et al. [46]; Roever et al. [47]	Thickness		
CT	Favre et al. [18]; Eisner et al. [16]; Anderson et al. [17]; Koo et al. [48]; Chen et al. [49]; Ji et al. [50]	Thickness	Favre et al. [18]; Foster et al. [51]	Single-slice area
	Favre et al. [18]; Lama et al. [52]; Maimaituxun et al. [53]	Volume	Foster et al. [51]; Caglar et al. [13]; Krievina et al. [19]; Murakami et al. [54]; Lin et al. [55]	Volume
MRI	None	Not applicable	Wagner et al. [56]; Wagner et al. [57]; Zelicha et al. [58]; Spit et al. [59]	Single-slice area
			Chughtai et al. [20]	Single-slice volume
			Notohamiprodjo et al. [22]; Lin et al. [14]	Volume

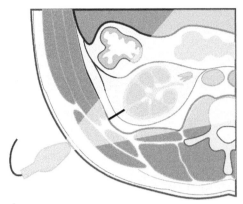

FIGURE 10.6 Schematic diagram showing the measurement of perirenal fat thickness on the lateral aspect of the abdomen using ultrasound. This method measures the sum of perirenal fat thickness plus pararenal fat thickness in the acoustic window (black line).

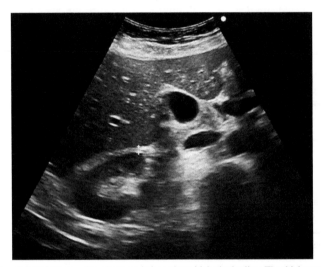

FIGURE 10.7 Measurement of perirenal fat thickness using ultrasound along the midclavicular line. The thickness of perirenal fat is the anterior distance from the border of the liver to the border of the inferior part of the kidney. *Reprinted from Grima P, Guido M, Zizza A, Chiavaroli R. Sonographically measured perirenal fat thickness: an early predictor of atherosclerosis in HIV-1-infected patients receiving highly active antiretroviral therapy? J Clin Ultrasound. 2010;38(4):190−195, under a Creative Commons license.*

fat, but has not been widely used. Intraobserver reproducibility of the ultrasonographic measurement of perirenal fat thickness was evaluated in several earlier studies, with coefficient of variance ranging from 3.2% to 6.5% [35−39,44,45]. Interobserver reproducibility was evaluated in only one study, presenting an interobserver intraclass correlation of 0.51 [40]. There was also one study placing the probe at the axillary midline in the longitudinal plain, where the posterior measurement of the lateral hypoechoic area was taken as the thickness of perirenal fat [47]. The reproducibility of this method was not evaluated, and this method has not been adopted by other studies.

CT and MRI images can also be used to evaluate perirenal fat. However, these imaging modalities are more expensive and less accessible than ultrasonography. Earlier studies using CT to quantify perirenal fat were mainly conducted in patients who underwent nephrectomy. The renal fascia is not always visible on CT images, especially the anterior fascia, which can be elusive or closely adjacent to pararenal structures, such as small intestines, colon, spleen, and liver. It is often impossible to accurately delineate the complete renal fascia, especially in less obese subjects. Therefore, the thickness of perirenal fat was measured in a number of studies instead of volumetric evaluation. However, the thickness of perirenal fat varies significantly with locations in different individuals (Fig. 10.8), and there is no expert consensus on where and how to measure the perirenal fat thickness. One previous study measured the anterior, posterior, lateral, anterolateral, postero-lateral, and medial perirenal fat thicknesses at the level of renal vein, among which the correlations with BMI and the gender differences were not consistent [16]. A recent study also measured the perirenal fat thickness at multiple locations on the slice passing through the renal vein, and the total perirenal fat thickness was defined as the sum of all the thicknesses

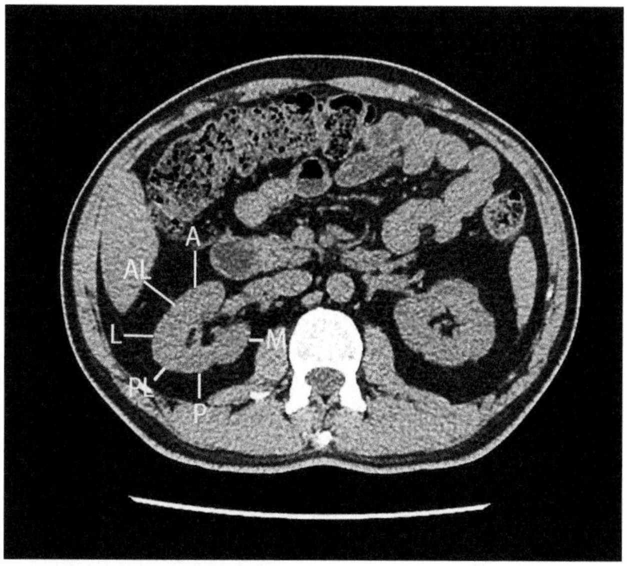

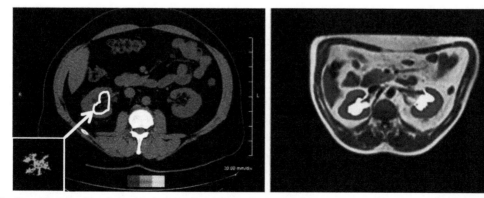

FIGURE 10.8   The thickness of perirenal fat varies significantly with the locations of measurements. *A*, anterior; *M*, medial; *L*, lateral; *AL*, anterolateral; *PL*, posterolateral; *P*, posterior.

on both sides [48]. Although one study suggested that perirenal thickness was a reliable estimate of perirenal mass, based on the Pearson's correlation coefficient (r = 0.86) between the posterior thickness and the volume of perirenal fat excluding renal sinus fat [18], the perirenal fat thickness in this study was the maximal distance between the posterior surface of the kidney and the inner margin of the abdominal wall, which also included the thickness of pararenal retroperitoneal fat.

Quantification of renal sinus fat

The ectopic accumulation of renal sinus fat was referred to as renal sinus lipomatosis in early studies [60,61]. Although ultrasonographical assessment of renal sinus fat is technically feasible, it has not been used in clinical studies regarding excessive sinus fat. Both CT and MRI have been adopted by previous studies for the quantification of the single-slice area or the volume of renal sinus fat based on Hounsfield Units in CT or signal intensity in MRI (Fig. 10.9). As aforementioned in this chapter, there is no anatomical separation between renal sinus fat and perirenal fat, thus the quantification of sinus fat requires an artificial border. A widely accepted border of renal sinus fat is defined by a straight line tangent to the parenchyma on both sides of the hilum at a transversal slice [13,14] (Fig. 10.10). Other definitions such as "a straight line

FIGURE 10.9   Quantification of renal sinus fat based on hounsfield units in CT (left) or signal intensity in T1-weighted MRI (right). *Images were adapted from published articles Foster MC, Hwang SJ, Porter SA, Massaro JM, Hoffmann U, Fox CS. Development and reproducibility of a computed tomography-based measurement of renal sinus fat. BMC Nephrol. 2011;12(1):52; Wagner R, Machann J, Guthoff M, Nawroth PP, Nadalin S, Saleem MA, et al. The protective effect of human renal sinus fat on glomerular cells is reversed by the hepatokine fetuin-A. Sci Rep. 2017;7(1):226 under a Creative Commons license.*

FIGURE 10.10 Quantification of renal sinus fat based on MRI. The left image shows the segmentation of renal sinus fat on a dixon-fat image. The border of renal sinus fat is defined by a straight line (white line) tangent to the parenchyma on both sides of the hilum at a transversal slice. The right image is the three-dimensional reconstruction of the sinus fat.

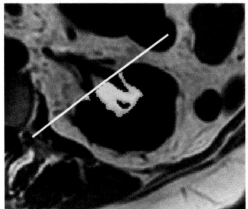
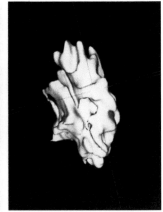

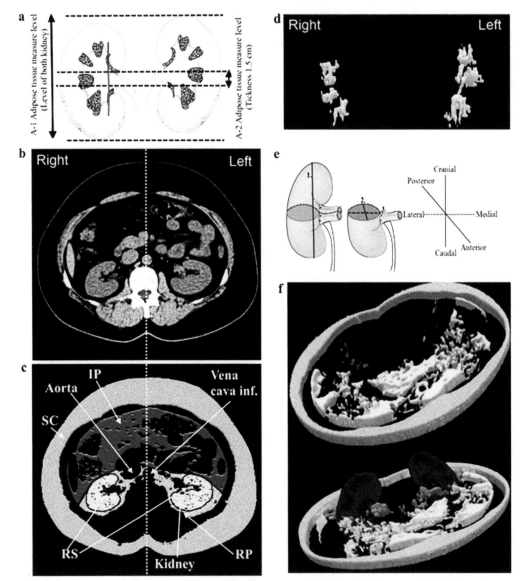

FIGURE 10.11 Volumetric analysis of renal sinus fat and the other adipose compartments by CT. Figure (B) and (C) show the segmentation of renal sinus fat (RS), intraperitoneal adipose tissue (IP), subcutaneous adipose tissue (SC), and retroperitoneal adipose tissue (RP). Figure (D) and (F) show the three-dimensional reconstruction of the left and right renal sinus fat (D) and the other adipose compartments (F). *Reprinted from a published article Krievina G, Tretjakovs P, Skuja I, Silina V, Keisa L, Krievina D, et al. Ectopic adipose tissue storage in the left and the right renal sinus is asymmetric and associated with serum kidney injury molecule-1 and fibroblast growth factor-21 levels increase. EBioMedicine. 2016;13:274–283 with permission.*

tracing across both dimples at the edge of the renal sinus [51,55], a space within the concavity of kidney" [20], and "within the curvature of the kidney" [59], have also been used. Due to the highly irregular shape and the small volume of renal sinus fat, it is preferable to exclude visible vasculatures and the collecting system within the renal sinus. The volume of renal sinus fat can be obtained by multiplying the area of renal sinus fat and thickness of each slice, and adding up the volumes of a series of consecutive slices covering the range of the renal sinus (Figs. 10.10 and 10.11).

The feasibility and high reproducibility of measuring single-slice area of renal sinus fat as well as sinus fat volume on CT were firstly presented in a sample from the Framingham cohort [51]. In this study the single-slice area and the volume of renal sinus fat were similarly correlated with BMI, waist circumference, and abdominal VAT. Renal sinus fat quantification based on MRI was firstly performed in a study of 205 participants with cardiovascular risk factors, in which the volume of a single-slice renal sinus fat was obtained at the level of the second lumbar vertebra [20]. Another study measured the area of renal sinus fat at the level of the entry of the renal arteries [56]. MRI quantification of single-slice area of sinus fat is most frequently performed on T1-weighted image, in which the hyperintense sinus fat can be differentiated from the isointense kidney parenchyma [57] (Fig. 10.9).

Volumetric evaluation of renal sinus fat on CT has been studied in a population aged 21−80 years old without renal diseases [13], as well as in a group of asymptomatic middle age (30−45 years old) participants [19]. With the increased application of high-resolution Dixon imaging in clinical MRI [62], accurate measurement of sinus fat volume based on Dixon images has been feasible (Fig. 10.10) with high intra- and interrater reproducibility [14,22] (Fig. 10.12).

Based on previous studies and the features of each imaging modality, there are a few considerations for future studies regarding imaging-based quantification of perirenal fat and renal sinus fat. Perirenal fat is frequently quantified by thickness due to the challenge of delineating the renal fascia, and ultrasonography is the most widely used imaging modality. However, the interobserver reproducibility is largely unknown and may be impacted by operator-dependence, which is one of the major disadvantages of ultrasonography. Moreover, significant variance of the perirenal fat thickness and the involvement of pararenal fat in the measurement further compromises the accuracy of this quantification method. As for renal sinus fat, volumetric measurement is recommended due to its small size and highly irregular shape, and high intra- and interobserver reproducibility using CT and MRI has been reported. Considering the radiation risk from CT, renal sinus fat volume quantified by MRI might be preferable over other methods in evaluating the fat accumulation around the kidneys.

Renal parenchyma triglyceride

Excessive adipose tissue not only accumulates around the kidney but also increases the amount of lipid droplets inside the renal parenchymal cells. The infiltration of lipids in the kidney, also known as "fatty kidney" or renal steatosis, has been recognized for more than a century [63]. Intrarenal fat deposits in the glomeruli and proximal tubules interfere with the metabolism of lipids and glucose, and contribute to kidney injury as well as insulin resistance [34].

Histological characteristics and pathophysiological relevance

Nonesterified fatty acids (NEFA) produced by abdominal adipose tissue play a key role in the accumulation of lipids in renal cells. More than 99% circulating NEFA is bounded with plasma albumin, and is carried to the liver where synthesis

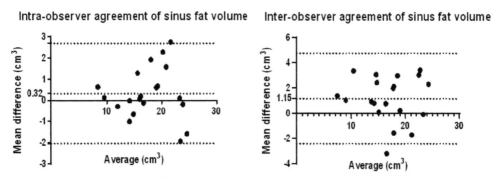

FIGURE 10.12 Intra- and interobserver reproducibility of sinus fat volume was high based on high-resolution MRI. *Adapted from Lin L, Dekkers IA, Huang L, Tao Q, Paiman EHM, Bizino MB, et al. Renal sinus fat volume in type 2 diabetes mellitus is associated with glycated hemoglobin and metabolic risk factors. J Diabetes Complicat. 2021:107973; under the terms of the Creative Commons.*

of very low density lipoprotein is stimulated. Intracellular reesterification results in the production of excessive tri-glycerides that can be delivered to nonadipose peripheral tissue [64]. During this process, modified low density lipoprotein (LDL) (small dense LDL or oxidized LDL) is generated and can lead to intracellular accumulation of cholesteryl esters in cells with scavenger receptors [65]. Both triglycerides and cholesteryl esters can be stored in kidney cells by means of lipid droplets, which are coated with a monolayer of phospholipid and regulatory proteins such as adipophilin [66]. Extensive lipid droplets can accumulate in mesangial cells, podocytes, and proximal epithelial tubular cells, as revealed by histo-logical studies of renal samples from patients with obesity-related glomerulopathy or metabolically unhealthy obesity [66]. The impact of lipids accumulation on renal cellular structure and function varies with the types of renal cells, which has been thoroughly elucidated in a previous review (Fig. 10.13) [67], and is briefly summarized below.

Mesangial cells are the specialized microvascular pericyte in the renal glomerulus and are in direct contact with li-poproteins, as there is no basal membrane between mesangium and glomerular endothelium. Obesity-induced endothelial dysfunction can lead to increased lipoprotein leakage, which results in the accumulation of lipids in mesangial cells [68,69]. Moreover, normal feedback regulation in mesangial cells is disrupted by inflammation, which leads to the

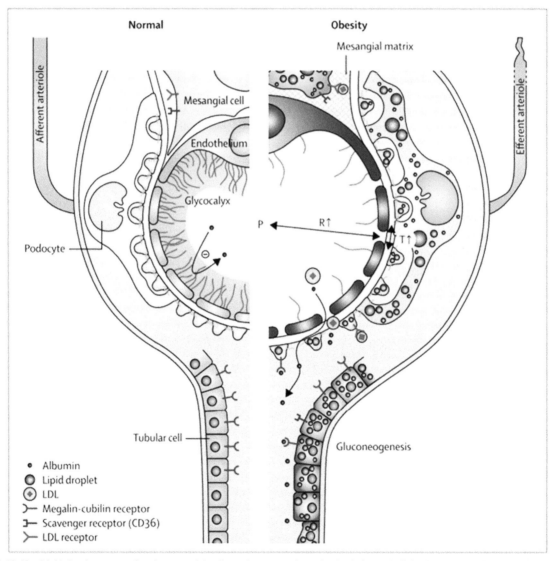

FIGURE 10.13 Lipid droplets accumulate in mesangial cells, podocytes, and proximal tubular epithelial cells and contribute to glomerulomegaly, glomerulosclerosis, and enhanced gluconeogenesis. *Reprinted from a published article De Vries AP, Ruggenenti P, Ruan XZ, Praga M, Cruzado JM, Bajema IM, et al. Fatty kidney: emerging role of ectopic lipid in obesity-related renal disease. Lancet Diabetes Endocrinol. 2014;2(5):417−426, with permission from Elsevier.*

transformation of mesangial cells to lipid-laden foam cells [70,71]. This transformation of mesangial cells results in the loss of contractile function and contributes to glomerulomegaly [67].

Accumulation of ectopic lipids including NEFA, cholesteryl esters, and fatty acids in podocytes has been linked to podocyte-specific insulin resistance [67,72] and apoptosis of podocytes [73]. Podocyte insulin resistance can impact the morphological adjustment of podocytes in response to postprandial alterations of glomerular filtration rate (GFR) [67]. Podocytes apoptosis is prevalent in patients with obesity-related glomerulopathy and can cause further loss of podocytes and segmental glomerulosclerosis due to increased mechanical strain on remaining podocytes [74,75].

Hypertrophy of proximal tubular epithelial cells has been observed in obesity, probably in response to increased hemodynamic and metabolic load [76]. Moreover, increased absorption of luminal NEFA-bound albumin and basolateral plasma NEFA in obesity leads to the accumulation of NEFA in proximal epithelial tubular cells [67]. The tubular NEFA overload enhances renal gluconeogenesis by interfering with tubular insulin signaling and eventually induces tubulointerstitial injury [77,78].

Imaging-based quantification

Currently proton magnetic resonance spectroscopy (^{1}H-MRS) is the only noninvasive technique to quantify lipid content in vivo, and has been applied to measure the content of triglyceride in liver [79], muscle [80], and myocardium [81] with sufficient accuracy for clinical assessment [82]. Unlike MRI, which provides anatomical information based on signals of water, ^{1}H-MRS provides a biochemical assay of tissue in selected regions based on spatially encoded chemical information [83]. The feasibility and reproducibility of renal triglyceride content measurement in human with ^{1}H-MRS has been shown at 1.5T [84] and 3.0T [85], respectively. In addition, the ^{1}H-MRS measured renal triglyceride content has been validated in a porcine study against gold-standard enzymatic assay [86].

Dixon fat/water images in three directions are usually obtained for better planning before the ^{1}H-MRS scan. A single voxel is placed in the renal parenchyma carefully avoiding perirenal fat and sinus fat (Fig. 10.14). The kidney is an organ with low lipids content. Overall lipid content only comprises 0.6%–1.64% of normal kidney weight [87]. Pathological studies have estimated that in normal human kidney, 1/5 of the lipid content is triglyceride, 1/10 is NEFA, and cholesterol concentration is 1/20 or less [87,88]. Renal spectra obtained by ^{1}H-MRS mainly originate from the proton resonances of methylene (CH_2) groups of triglyceride (Fig. 10.14). Cholesterol also contains CH_2 groups, but is less magnetic susceptible and results in resonance loss in clinical ^{1}H-MRS. Therefore, the lipid content quantified by ^{1}H-MRS is predominantly triglyceride content. In healthy young volunteers, total cortical triglyceride content is around 0.44% [84]. The percentage of renal triglyceride varies with different scanners and scan protocols, and studies of larger scale are needed to determine the normal references.

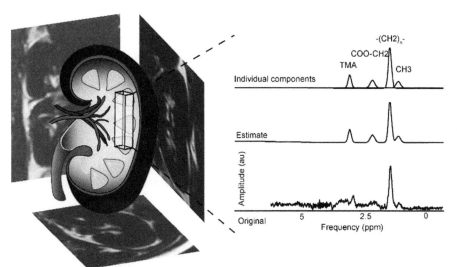

FIGURE 10.14 Single-voxel ^{1}H-MRS is planned in renal parenchyma avoiding perirenal and sinus fat (left). Corresponding spectra with methylene—$(CH_2)_n$—peak between 1.2 and 1.4 ppm (right). TMA, trimethylamines. *Reprinted from a published article Dekkers IA, Bizino MB, Paiman EHM, Smit JW, Jazet IM, de Vries APJ, et al. The effect of glycemic control on renal triglyceride content assessed by proton spectroscopy in patients with type 2 diabetes mellitus: a single-center parallel-group trial. J Ren Nutr. 2020 under a Creative Commons license.*

Clinical implications of excessive kidney fat

Fat around the kidney has been helpful in conventional diagnostic radiology for localizing renal lesions and staging of renal tumors. In the past decade, the research interests in kidney fat have been shifted to its association with chronic kidney disease, insulin resistance, and cardiovascular diseases in the context of obesity. In addition, the clinical implications of perirenal fat have been studied in urological operations, nephrolithiasis, and cancer.

Association with chronic kidney disease and insulin resistance

Obesity and diabetes mellitus developed in the context of obesity have become the leading causes of chronic kidney disease [90]. The clinical and pathologic characteristics and pathogenesis of obesity-related glomerulopathy have been thoroughly illustrated in a previous review article [90]. Accumulation of perirenal fat, renal sinus fat and renal triglyceride content has been found in obese patients with or without type 2 diabetes mellitus (T2DM) [14,22,42,89]. Studies of the tissue samples collected from patients who underwent urological surgeries suggested that perirenal fat may contribute locally to the regulation of kidney function through chronic inflammation [53]. In nonhypertensive and nondiabetic obese patients, larger perirenal fat thickness was found in patients with microalbuminuria than those with normoalbuminuria [36]. Moreover, perirenal fat thickness was independently associated with urinary albumin/creatinine ratio, indicating its potential utility in predicting early kidney damage [36]. Excessive perirenal fat was found to be associated with reduced GFR in patients with T2DM [35,43] as well as in patients with hypertension [39]. Furthermore, perirenal fat thickness showed a higher predictive value for chronic kidney disease than subcutaneous and visceral fat in patients with T2DM [49].

Similar results have been reported in regard to renal sinus fat. In a nondiabetic cohort at diabetic risk, excessive renal sinus fat was found to be associated with exercise-induced albuminuria, independent of age, sex, and VAT [56]. In a mixed cohort of lean and obese participants, renal sinus fat volume was positively associated with the level of kidney injury factor (KIM)-1 and fibroblast growth factor (FGF)-21, which are serum biomarkers of kidney injury [19]. Another study showed that in the presence of nonalcoholic fatty liver disease, the elevated hepatokine fetuin-A may impair renal function through increased renal sinus fat [57]. In the Framingham Study, "fatty kidney" defined by renal sinus fat larger than 90% of a healthy reference sample, was associated with higher odds ratio of chronic kidney disease and diabetes mellitus, even after adjustment for VAT [91]. A recent study reported that renal sinus fat volume was negatively associated with gold-standard GFR, but positively associated with renal vascular resistance in patients with T2DM [59]. Our own study also found that sinus fat volume was positively associated with glycated hemoglobin and urinary albumin/creatinine ratio in patients with T2DM [14].

Association with cardiovascular diseases

Both perirenal fat and sinus fat have been associated with hypertension [40,92] and calcified atherosclerosis [48,54]. It is proposed that excessive perirenal fat and sinus fat can induce mechanical compression of the renal parenchyma, vasculatures, nerve fibers, and the collecting system, which subsequently stimulates the renin-angiotensin-aldosterone system and sympathetic nerves system. All these mechanisms lead to increased sodium reabsorption and contribute to hyperfiltration and hypertension [93]. In addition, perirenal adipose tissue can secrete all components of renin-angiotensin-aldosterone system, as well as a number of adipokines and cytokines directly linked to vasoactivity and endothelial function [6]. As aforementioned, excessive perirenal fat and sinus fat are also associated with microalbuminuria, which is a robust risk factor for cardiovascular diseases.

A positive association between para- and perirenal fat thickness measured by ultrasonography and 24-hour diastolic blood pressure has been reported in a cohort of overweight and obese subjects, independent of anthropometric, hormonal, and metabolic parameters [38]. A study of 284 morbidly obese patients reported a larger thickness of perirenal fat in hypertensive patients than in nonhypertensive ones [40]. In a cohort of 3929 participants, perirenal fat thickness derived from CT was associated with arterial calcification in renal artery and abdominal aorta after adjustment for multiple confounders [48]. Moreover, studies in healthy [41] and overweight children [15] have reported a positive association between perirenal fat size and carotid intima-media thickness.

In the Framingham Study, renal sinus fat was associated with higher odds ratio of hypertension, even after adjustment for BMI or VAT [91]. Renal sinus fat was significantly associated with the number of prescribed antihypertensive medications and stage II hypertension in participants at risk for cardiovascular events, even after accounting for several potential confounders including intraperitoneal fat [20]. The ratio of renal sinus fat versus VAT was proposed as an independent risk indicator of coronary artery calcification in a study of middle-aged patients with suspected coronary artery disease [54].

Implications for other diseases

The quantification of perirenal fat can also be beneficial for preoperational evaluations of nephrectomy, nephrolithiasis, and cancer. The thickness of perirenal fat measured on CT images can be used to calculate the Mayo adhesive probability score [94], which has been helpful in predicting adherent perinephric fat in partial nephrectomy [50,94–96]. A study of laparoscopic donor nephrectomy found that CT-measured perirenal fat was positively associated with operative complexity as reflected by operative time [17]. A recent study reported that the posterior thickness of perirenal fat measured on transversal CT was an independent predictor of postoperative complications after laparoscopic distal gastrectomy for patients with gastric cancer [97]. Larger volume of perirenal fat was found around calcium oxalate stone-bearing kidneys than kidneys without stones in a cohort of 40 patients with nephrolithiasis [52]. Due to the proximity of perirenal fat to the kidney and its paracrine function, there might be unique impact of prerenal fat on renal parenchymal tumors. It was demonstrated in 174 patients with clear cell renal carcinoma that perirenal fat size was correlated with local progression and life expectancy [98] (Fig. 10.15). This potential utility of perirenal fat measurement in decision-making for renal tumors might be extended to ovarian cancer, as a study in 258 patients demonstrated the association between perirenal adiposity and lower progression-free survival from ovarian cancer [99].

Changes of excessive kidney fat after intervention

Most previous clinical studies of excessive kidney fat were cross-sectional in design. Longitudinal studies regarding the changes of kidney fat after intervention are scarce and in relatively small sample size [19,58,89]. In the aforementioned study of morbidly obese patients, 89 patients who underwent sleeve-gastrectomy showed a significant decrease of perirenal fat thickness as well as antihypertensive medications needed [40]. Interestingly, controversial results have been reported regarding the change of renal sinus fat after antiobesity intervention. One study found no significant reduction of renal sinus fat when VAT significantly (> 5%) decreased [19], while another study demonstrated a decrease in renal sinus fat after an 18-month weight loss trial [58]. As for intrarenal fat, a recent study demonstrated decreased renal triglyceride content quantified by ^{1}H-MRS after 26-week glycemic control in patients with T2DM [89].

Summary and perspectives

Perirenal fat and renal sinus fat are much smaller in size than the general visceral and subcutaneous adipose compartments. Lipid accumulation in renal parenchyma is also lower than other organs capable of storing ectopic fat, such as liver. However, fat accumulation around and within the kidney directly participate in the regulation of kidney function, lipids

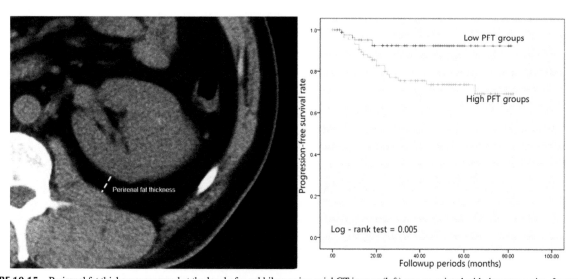

FIGURE 10.15 Perirenal fat thickness measured at the level of renal hilum using axial CT images (left) was associated with the progression-free survival in patients with localized clear cell renal cell carcinoma (right). High perirenal fat thickness (green line) predicted a poorer progression-free survival than low perirenal fat thickness (blue line). *Reprinted from a published article Huang H, Chen S, Li W, Wu X, Xing J, editors. High perirenal fat thickness predicts a poor progression-free survival in patients with localized clear cell renal cell carcinoma. Urol Oncol: seminars and original investigations. 2018;36(4):157.e1–157.e6, with permission from Elsevier.*

metabolism, gluconeogenesis, and cardiovascular homeostasis, which may have a unique role in the development of obesity-related diseases independent of the general VAT. There has been a lack of early-onset biomarkers for the clinical management of obesity-related chronic kidney disease and cardiovascular diseases. Excessive kidney fat may have a role in the pathogenesis of obesity-related diseases and is potentially reversible after intervention. Therefore, imaging-based quantification of perirenal fat, renal sinus fat, and renal triglyceride content may bring new opportunities for early diagnosis and prognosis of obesity-related diseases. However, large-scale and longitudinal studies are required before these imaging biomarkers can be implemented in clinical practice. Furthermore, it remains unclear whether excessive fat around the kidney (perirenal and sinus fat) is associated with intrarenal lipid accumulation and to what degree they contribute to different disease entities.

Perirenal fat thickness measured by ultrasonography might be preferable for large-scale population studies; however, the interobserver reproducibility remains to be validated. CT or MRI-based quantification is more accurate and reproducible, especially for longitudinal studies. Considering the challenge of delineating renal fascia and the radiation risk from CT, volumetric quantification of renal sinus fat based on high-resolution MRI might be preferable for the evaluation of the fat accumulation around the kidneys in future studies. Finally, the utility of ^{1}H-MRS for the quantification of renal triglyceride content might gradually increase with the rising interests in intrarenal lipid, similar to that for the liver and the heart. With the development of artificial intelligence, imaging-based quantification of kidney fat might be simplified via deep-learning algorithms. Interdisciplinary collaboration among endocrinologists, nephrologists, and radiologists is essential for further investigations of excessive kidney fat, and may contribute to improved clinical management of obesity-related diseases in the future.

References

[1] Gerota D. Beitrage zur kenntnis des befestigungsapparates der niere. Arch Anat Entwicklungsgesch 1895;19:265–86.

[2] Zuckerkandl E. Uber den Fixationsapaparat der Nieren. Med Jahrb 1883:59–67.

[3] Thornton FJ, Kandiah SS, Monkhouse WS, Lee MJ. Helical CT evaluation of the perirenal space and its boundaries: a cadaveric study. Radiology 2001;218(3):659–63.

[4] Marx WJ, Patel SK. Renal fascia: its radiographic importance. Urology 1979;13(1):1–7.

[5] Raptopoulos V, Touliopoulos P, Lei Q, Vrachliotis T, Marks Jr S. Medial border of the perirenal space: CT and anatomic correlation. Radiology 1997;205(3):777–84.

[6] Liu B-X, Sun W, Kong X-Q. Perirenal fat: a unique fat pad and potential target for cardiovascular disease. Angiology 2019;70(7):584–93.

[7] Meyers MA, Friedenberg RM, King MC, Meng C-H. The significance of the renal capsular arteries. Br J Radiol. 1967;40(480):949–56.

[8] Grigoraş A, Balan RA, Căruntu I-D, Giuşcă SE, Lozneanu L, Avadanei RE, et al. Perirenal adipose tissue—current knowledge and future opportunities. J Clin Med 2021;10(6):1291.

[9] Czaja K, Kraeling R, Klimczuk M, Franke-Radowiecka A, Sienkiewicz W, Lakomy M. Distribution of ganglionic sympathetic neurons supplying the subcutaneous, perirenal and mesentery fat tissue depots in the pig. Acta Neurobiol Exp 2002;62(4):227–34.

[10] Czaja K, Lakomy M, Kaleczyc J, Barb C, Rampacek G, Kraeling R. Leptin receptors, NPY, and tyrosine hydroxylase in autonomic neurons supplying fat depots in a pig. Biochemical and biophysical research communications 2002;293(3):1138–44.

[11] Kaissling B. Structural analysis of the rabbit kidney. 1979.

[12] Montani J-P, Carroll JF, Dwyer TM, Antic V, Yang Z, Dulloo AG. Ectopic fat storage in heart, blood vessels and kidneys in the pathogenesis of cardiovascular diseases. Int J Obes 2004;28(4):S58–65.

[13] Caglar V, Songur A, Acar M, Uygur R, Alkoc OA, Acar T. Volumetric evaluation of fat in the renal sinus in normal subjects using stereological method on computed tomography images and its relationship with body composition. Folia Morphol 2014;73(3):302–8.

[14] Lin L, Dekkers IA, Huang L, Tao Q, Paiman EHM, Bizino MB, et al. Renal sinus fat volume in type 2 diabetes mellitus is associated with glycated hemoglobin and metabolic risk factors. J Diabetes Complicat 2021:107973.

[15] Bassols J, Martinez-Calcerrada JM, Prats-Puig A, Carreras-Badosa G, Xargay-Torrent S, Lizarraga-Mollinedo E, et al. Perirenal fat is related to carotid intima-media thickness in children. Int J Obes 2018;42(4):641–7.

[16] Eisner BH, Zargooshi J, Berger AD, Cooperberg MR, Doyle SM, Sheth S, et al. Gender differences in subcutaneous and perirenal fat distribution. Surg Radiol Anat 2010;32(9):879–82.

[17] Anderson KM, Lindler TU, Lamberton GR, Baron PW, Ojogho OK, Baldwin DD. Laparoscopic donor nephrectomy: effect of perirenal fat upon donor operative time. J Endourol 2008;22(10):2269–74.

[18] Favre G, Grangeon-Chapon C, Raffaelli C, Francois-Chalmin F, Iannelli A, Esnault V. Perirenal fat thickness measured with computed tomography is a reliable estimate of perirenal fat mass. PLoS One 2017;12(4):e0175561.

[19] Krievina G, Tretjakovs P, Skuja I, Silina V, Keisa L, Krievina D, et al. Ectopic adipose tissue storage in the left and the right renal sinus is asymmetric and associated with serum kidney injury molecule-1 and fibroblast growth factor-21 levels increase. EBioMedicine 2016;13:274–83.

[20] Chughtai HL, Morgan TM, Rocco M, Stacey B, Brinkley TE, Ding J, et al. Renal sinus fat and poor blood pressure control in middle-aged and elderly individuals at risk for cardiovascular events. Hypertension 2010;56(5):901–6.

[21] Dwyer TM, Banks SA, Alonso-Galicia M, Cockrell K, Carroll JF, Bigler SA, et al. Distribution of renal medullary hyaluronan in lean and obese rabbits. Kidney Int 2000;58(2):721—9.

[22] Notohamiprodjo M, Goepfert M, Will S, Lorbeer R, Schick F, Rathmann W, et al. Renal and renal sinus fat volumes as quantified by magnetic resonance imaging in subjects with prediabetes, diabetes, and normal glucose tolerance. PLoS One 2020;15(2):e0216635.

[23] Chau Y-Y, Bandiera R, Serrels A, Martínez-Estrada OM, Qing W, Lee M, et al. Visceral and subcutaneous fat have different origins and evidence supports a mesothelial source. Nat Cell Biol 2014;16(4):367—75.

[24] Schleinitz D, Krause K, Wohland T, Gebhardt C, Linder N, Stumvoll M, et al. Identification of distinct transcriptome signatures of human adipose tissue from fifteen depots. Eur J Hum Genet 2020;28(12):1714—25.

[25] Tanuma Y, Ohata M, Ito T, Yokochi C. Possible function of human brown adipose tissue as suggested by observation on perirenal brown fats from necropsy cases of variable age groups. Arch Histol Jpn 1976;39(2):117—45.

[26] Jespersen NZ, Feizi A, Andersen ES, Heywood S, Hattel HB, Daugaard S, et al. Heterogeneity in the perirenal region of humans suggests presence of dormant brown adipose tissue that contains brown fat precursor cells. Mol Metabol 2019;24:30—43.

[27] Svensson PA, Lindberg K, Hoffmann JM, Taube M, Pereira MJ, Mohsen-Kanson T, et al. Characterization of brown adipose tissue in the human perirenal depot. Obesity 2014;22(8):1830—7.

[28] Efremova A, Senzacqua M, Venema W, Isakov E, Di Vincenzo A, Zingaretti MC, et al. A large proportion of mediastinal and perirenal visceral fat of Siberian adult people is formed by UCP1 immunoreactive multilocular and paucilocular adipocytes. J Physiol Biochem 2020;76(2):185—92.

[29] Van den Beukel JC, Grefhorst A, Hoogduijn MJ, Steenbergen J, Mastroberardino PG, Dor FJ, et al. Women have more potential to induce browning of perirenal adipose tissue than men. Obesity 2015;23(8):1671—9.

[30] Chen X, McClusky R, Chen J, Beaven SW, Tontonoz P, Arnold AP, et al. The number of x chromosomes causes sex differences in adiposity in mice. PLoS Genet 2012;8(5):e1002709.

[31] Foster MT, Pagliassotti MJ. Metabolic alterations following visceral fat removal and expansion: beyond anatomic location. Adipocyte 2012;1(4):192—9.

[32] Hartman AD. Adipocyte fatty acid mobilization in vivo: effects of age and anatomical location. Lipids 1985;20(5):255—61.

[33] Hammoud SH, AlZaim I, Al-Dhaheri Y, Eid AH, El-Yazbi AF. Perirenal adipose tissue inflammation: novel insights linking metabolic dysfunction to renal diseases. Front Endocrinol 2021;12(942).

[34] Mende CW, Einhorn D. Fatty kidney disease: a new renal and endocrine clinical entity? Describing the role of the kidney in obesity, metabolic syndrome, and type 2 diabetes. Endocr Pract 2019;25(8):854—8.

[35] Lamacchia O, Nicastro V, Camarchio D, Valente U, Grisorio R, Gesualdo L, et al. Para- and perirenal fat thickness is an independent predictor of chronic kidney disease, increased renal resistance index and hyperuricaemia in type-2 diabetic patients. Nephrol Dial Transplant 2010;26(3):892—8.

[36] Sun X, Han F, Miao W, Hou N, Cao Z, Zhang G. Sonographic evaluation of para-and perirenal fat thickness is an independent predictor of early kidney damage in obese patients. Int Urol Nephrol 2013;45(6):1589—95.

[37] Sahin SB, Durakoglugil T, Ayaz T, Sahin OZ, Durakoglugil E, Sumer F, et al. Evaluation of para-and perirenal fat thickness and its association with metabolic disorders in polycystic ovary syndrome. Endocr Pract 2015;21(8):878—86.

[38] De Pergola G, Campobasso N, Nardecchia A, Triggiani V, Caccavo D, Gesualdo L, et al. Para- and perirenal ultrasonographic fat thickness is associated with 24-hours mean diastolic blood pressure levels in overweight and obese subjects. BMC Cardiovasc Disord 2015;15(1):108.

[39] Geraci G, Zammuto MM, Mattina A, Zanoli L, Geraci C, Granata A, et al. Para-perirenal distribution of body fat is associated with reduced glomerular filtration rate regardless of other indices of adiposity in hypertensive patients. J Clin Hypertens 2018;20(10):1438—46.

[40] Ricci MA, Scavizzi M, Ministrini S, De Vuono S, Pucci G, Lupattelli G. Morbid obesity and hypertension: the role of perirenal fat. J Clin Hypertens 2018;20(10):1430—7.

[41] López-Bermejo A, Prats-Puig A, Osiniri I, Martínez-Calcerrada J-M, Bassols J. Perirenal and epicardial fat and their association with carotid intima-media thickness in children. Ann Pediatr Endocrinol Metab 2019;24(4):220.

[42] Manno C, Campobasso N, Nardecchia A, Triggiani V, Zupo R, Gesualdo L, et al. Relationship of para- and perirenal fat and epicardial fat with metabolic parameters in overweight and obese subjects. Eat Weight Disord 2019;24(1):67—72.

[43] Fang Y, Xu YC, Yang YX, Liu C, Zhao D, Ke J. The relationship between perirenal fat thickness and reduced glomerular filtration rate in patients with type 2 diabetes. J Diabetes Res 2020:2020.

[44] Grima P, Guido M, Chiavaroli R, Zizza A. Ultrasound-assessed perirenal fat is related to increased ophthalmic artery resistance index in HIV-1 patients. Cardiovasc Ultrasound 2010;8(1):1—9.

[45] Grima P, Guido M, Zizza A, Chiavaroli R. Sonographically measured perirenal fat thickness: an early predictor of atherosclerosis in HIV-1-infected patients receiving highly active antiretroviral therapy? J Clin Ultrasound 2010;38(4):190—5.

[46] D'Marco L, Salazar J, Cortez M, Salazar M, Wettel M, Lima-Martínez M, et al. Perirenal fat thickness is associated with metabolic risk factors in patients with chronic kidney disease. Kidney Res Clin Pract 2019;38(3):365.

[47] Roever L, Resende ES, Veloso FC, Diniz ALD, Penha-Silva N, Casella A, et al. Perirenal fat and association with metabolic risk factors the uberlandia heart study. Medicine 2015;94(38):e1105.

[48] Koo BK, Denenberg JO, Wright CM, Criqui MH, Allison MA. Associations of perirenal fat thickness with renal and systemic calcified atherosclerosis. Endocrinol Metab (Seoul) 2020;35(1):122—31.

[49] Chen X, Mao Y, Hu J, Han S, Gong L, Luo T, et al. Perirenal fat thickness is significantly associated with the risk for development of chronic kidney disease in diabetic patients. Diabetes 2021;70(10):2322—32.

[50] Ji C, Tang S, Yang K, Xiong G, Fang D, Zhang C, et al. Analysis of factors influencing Mayo adhesive probability score in partial nephrectomy. Med Sci Monit 2017;23:6026−32.

[51] Foster MC, Hwang SJ, Porter SA, Massaro JM, Hoffmann U, Fox CS. Development and reproducibility of a computed tomography-based measurement of renal sinus fat. BMC Nephrol 2011;12(1):52.

[52] Lama DJ, Safiullah S, Yang A, Okhunov Z, Landman J, Clayman RV. Three-dimensional evaluation of perirenal fat volume in patients with nephrolithiasis. Urolithiasis 2018;46(6):535−41.

[53] Maimaituxun G, Fukuda D, Izaki H, Hirata Y, Kanayama HO, Masuzaki H, et al. Levels of adiponectin expression in peri-renal and subcutaneous adipose tissue and its determinants in human biopsied samples. Front Endocrinol 2019;10:897.

[54] Murakami Y, Nagatani Y, Takahashi M, Ikeda M, Miyazawa I, Morino K, et al. Renal sinus fat volume on computed tomography in middle-aged patients at risk for cardiovascular disease and its association with coronary artery calcification. Atherosclerosis 2016;246:374−81.

[55] Lin P, Min Z, Wei G, Lei H, Feifei Z, Yunfei Z. Volumetric evaluation of renal sinus adipose tissue on computed tomography images in bilateral nephrolithiasis patients. Int Urol Nephrol 2020;52(6):1027−34.

[56] Wagner R, Machann J, Lehmann R, Rittig K, Schick F, Lenhart J, et al. Exercise-induced albuminuria is associated with perivascular renal sinus fat in individuals at increased risk of type 2 diabetes. Diabetologia 2012;55(7):2054−8.

[57] Wagner R, Machann J, Guthoff M, Nawroth PP, Nadalin S, Saleem MA, et al. The protective effect of human renal sinus fat on glomerular cells is reversed by the hepatokine fetuin-A. Sci Rep 2017;7(1):2261.

[58] Zelicha H, Schwarzfuchs D, Shelef I, Gepner Y, Tsaban G, Tene L, et al. Changes of renal sinus fat and renal parenchymal fat during an 18-month randomized weight loss trial. Clin Nutr 2018;37(4):1145−53.

[59] Spit KA, Muskiet MHA, Tonneijck L, Smits MM, Kramer MHH, Joles JA, et al. Renal sinus fat and renal hemodynamics: a cross-sectional analysis. Magma 2020;33(1):73−80.

[60] Rha SE, Byun JY, Jung SE, Oh SN, Choi YJ, Lee A, et al. The renal sinus: pathologic spectrum and multimodality imaging approach. Radiographics 2004;24(Suppl. 1)):S117−31.

[61] Nikolaidis P, Gabriel H, Khong K, Brusco M, Hammond N, Yagmai V, et al. Computed tomography and magnetic resonance imaging features of lesions of the renal medulla and sinus. Curr Probl Diagn Radiol 2008;37(6):262−78.

[62] Ma J. Dixon techniques for water and fat imaging. J Magn Reson Imaging 2008;28(3):543−58.

[63] Rickards E. Remarks on the fatty transformation of the kidney. Br Med J 1883;2(1175):2.

[64] Björntorp P. Portal" adipose tissue as a generator of risk factors for cardiovascular disease and diabetes. Arteriosclerosis: An Official Journal of the American Heart Association, Inc. 1990;10(4):493−6.

[65] Steinberg D, Parthasarathy S, Carew TE, Khoo JC, Witztum JL. Beyond cholesterol. N Engl J Med 1989;320(14):915−24.

[66] Straub BK, Gyoengyoesi B, Koenig M, Hashani M, Pawella LM, Herpel E, et al. Adipophilin/perilipin-2 as a lipid droplet-specific marker for metabolically active cells and diseases associated with metabolic dysregulation. Histopathology 2013;62(4):617−31.

[67] De Vries AP, Ruggenenti P, Ruan XZ, Praga M, Cruzado JM, Bajema IM, et al. Fatty kidney: emerging role of ectopic lipid in obesity-related renal disease. Lancet Diabetes Endocrinol 2014;2(5):417−26.

[68] Ruan XZ, Varghese Z, Powis SH, Moorhead JF. Human mesangial cells express inducible macrophage scavenger receptor. Kidney Int 1999;56(2):440−51.

[69] Li J, Li H, Wen Y-b, Li X-w. Very-low-density lipoprotein-induced triglyceride accumulation in human mesangial cells is mainly mediated by lipoprotein lipase. Nephron Physiol 2008;110(1):p1−10.

[70] Chen Y, Ruan XZ, Li Q, Huang A, Moorhead JF, Powis SH, et al. Inflammatory cytokines disrupt LDL-receptor feedback regulation and cause statin resistance: a comparative study in human hepatic cells and mesangial cells. Am J Physiol Ren Physiol 2007;293(3):F680−7.

[71] Ruan XZ, Varghese Z, Powis SH, Moorhead JF. Dysregulation of LDL receptor under the influence of inflammatory cytokines: a new pathway for foam cell formation. Kidney Int 2001;60(5):1716−25.

[72] Lennon R, Pons D, Sabin MA, Wei C, Shield JP, Coward RJ, et al. Saturated fatty acids induce insulin resistance in human podocytes: implications for diabetic nephropathy. Nephrol Dial Transplant 2009;24(11):3288−96.

[73] Sieber J, Lindenmeyer MT, Kampe K, Campbell KN, Cohen CD, Hopfer H, et al. Regulation of podocyte survival and endoplasmic reticulum stress by fatty acids. Am J Physiol Ren Physiol 2010;299(4):F821−9.

[74] Verani RR. Obesity-associated focal segmental glomerulosclerosis: pathological features of the lesion and relationship with cardiomegaly and hyperlipidemia. Am J Kidney Dis 1992;20(6):629−34.

[75] Fukuda A, Chowdhury MA, Venkatareddy MP, Wang SQ, Nishizono R, Suzuki T, et al. Growth-dependent podocyte failure causes glomerulosclerosis. J Am Soc Nephrology 2012;23(8):1351−63.

[76] Tobar A, Ori Y, Benchetrit S, Milo G, Herman-Edelstein M, Zingerman B, et al. Proximal tubular hypertrophy and enlarged glomerular and proximal tubular urinary space in obese subjects with proteinuria. PLoS One 2013;8(9):e75547.

[77] Tiwari S, Singh RS, Li L, Tsukerman S, Godbole M, Pandey G, et al. Deletion of the insulin receptor in the proximal tubule promotes hyperglycemia. J Am Soc Nephrol 2013;24(8):1209−14.

[78] Yamahara K, Kume S, Koya D, Tanaka Y, Morita Y, Chin-Kanasaki M, et al. Obesity-mediated autophagy insufficiency exacerbates proteinuria-induced tubulointerstitial lesions. J Am Soc Nephrol 2013;24(11):1769−81.

[79] Thomas EL, Hamilton G, Patel N, O'dwyer R, Doré CJ, Goldin RD, et al. Hepatic triglyceride content and its relation to body adiposity: a magnetic resonance imaging and proton magnetic resonance spectroscopy study. Gut 2005;54(1):122−7.

[80] Boesch C, Machann J, Vermathen P, Schick F. Role of proton MR for the study of muscle lipid metabolism. NMR Biomed: Int J Devot Develop Appl 2000;11(3):330–5.

[81] Van der Meer RW, Lamb HJ, Smit JW, de Roos A. MR imaging evaluation of cardiovascular risk in metabolic syndrome. Radiology 2012;264(1):21–37.

[82] Kamba M, Meshitsuka S, Iriguchi N, Koda M, Kimura K, Ogawa T. Measurement of relative fat content by proton magnetic resonance spectroscopy using a clinical imager. J Magn Reson Imag: An Offic J Int Soci Mag Res Med 2000;11(3):330–5.

[83] Preul MC, Caramanos Z, Collins DL, Villemure J-G, Leblanc R, Olivier A, et al. Accurate, noninvasive diagnosis of human brain tumors by using proton magnetic resonance spectroscopy. Nat Med 1996;2(3):323–5.

[84] Hammer S, de Vries AP, de Heer P, Bizino MB, Wolterbeek R, Rabelink TJ, et al. Metabolic imaging of human kidney triglyceride content: reproducibility of proton magnetic resonance spectroscopy. PLoS One 2013;8(4):e62209.

[85] Dekkers IA, de Heer P, Bizino MB, de Vries APJ, Lamb HJ. (1) H-MRS for the assessment of renal triglyceride content in humans at 3T: a primer and reproducibility study. J Magn Reson Imag 2018;48(2):507–13.

[86] Jonker JT, de Heer P, Engelse MA, van Rossenberg EH, Klessens CQF, Baelde HJ, et al. Metabolic imaging of fatty kidney in diabesity: validation and dietary intervention. Nephrol Dial Transplant 2018;33(2):224–30.

[87] Druilhet RE, Overturf ML, Kirkendall WM. Cortical and medullary lipids of normal and nephrosclerotic human kidney. Int J Biochem 1978;9(10):729–34.

[88] Druilhet R, Overturf M, Kirkendall W. Structure of neutral glycerides and phosphoglycerides of human kidney. Int J Biochem 1975;6(12):893–901.

[89] Dekkers IA, Bizino MB, Paiman EHM, Smit JW, Jazet IM, de Vries APJ, et al. The effect of glycemic control on renal triglyceride content assessed by proton spectroscopy in patients with type 2 diabetes mellitus: a single-center parallel-group trial. J Ren Nutr 2020;31(6):611–19.

[90] D'Agati VD, Chagnac A, de Vries AP, Levi M, Porrini E, Herman-Edelstein M, et al. Obesity-related glomerulopathy: clinical and pathologic characteristics and pathogenesis. Nat Rev Nephrol 2016;12(8):453–71.

[91] Foster MC, Hwang SJ, Porter SA, Massaro JM, Hoffmann U, Fox CS. Fatty kidney, hypertension, and chronic kidney disease: the Framingham Heart Study. Hypertension 2011;58(5):784–90.

[92] Mazairac AH, Joles JA. Renal sinus adiposity and hypertension. Am Heart Assoc; 2010.

[93] Hall ME, do Carmo JM, da Silva AA, Juncos LA, Wang Z, Hall JE. Obesity, hypertension, and chronic kidney disease. Int J Nephrol Renovascular Dis 2014;7:75.

[94] Davidiuk AJ, Parker AS, Thomas CS, Leibovich BC, Castle EP, Heckman MG, et al. Mayo adhesive probability score: an accurate image-based scoring system to predict adherent perinephric fat in partial nephrectomy. Eur Urol 2014;66(6):1165–71.

[95] Martin L, Rouviere O, Bezza R, Bailleux J, Abbas F, Schott-Pethelaz A-M, et al. Mayo adhesive probability score is an independent computed tomography scan predictor of adherent perinephric fat in open partial nephrectomy. Urology 2017;103:124–8.

[96] Prospective assessment and histological analysis of adherent perinephric fat in partial nephrectomiesDariane C, Le Guilchet T, Hurel S, Audenet F, Beaugerie A, Badoual C, et al., editors. Urol Oncol: sem and orig investigat 2017;35(2):39.e9–39.e17.

[97] Eto K, Ida S, Ohashi T, Kumagai K, Nunobe S, Ohashi M, et al. Perirenal fat thickness as a predictor of postoperative complications after laparoscopic distal gastrectomy for gastric cancer. BJS open 2020;4(5):865–72.

[98] Huang H, Chen S, Li W, Wu X, Xing J. High perirenal fat thickness predicts a poor progression-free survival in patients with localized clear cell renal cell carcinoma. Urol Oncol: seminars and original investigat 2018;36(4):157.e1–6.

[99] Zhang Y, Coletta AM, Allen PK, Parikh AM, Cox-Mattin M, Meyer LA, et al. Perirenal adiposity is associated with lower progression-free survival from ovarian cancer. Int J Gynecol Cancer 2018;28(2):285–92.

Chapter 11

Skeletal muscle fat

Ivica Just[1,2] and Martin Krššák[1,2]

[1]*Division of Endocrinology and Metabolism, Department of Medicine III, Medical University of Vienna, Vienna, Austria;* [2]*High-Field MR Centre, Department of Biomedical Imaging and Image-guided Therapy, Medical University of Vienna, Vienna, Austria*

Introduction

Skeletal muscle is the main tissue responsible for body posture and movement. To accomplish this function, skeletal muscle requires a major part of whole-body energy metabolism. Even at rest the musculature is responsible for approximately 30% of the metabolic rate of human body. With this metabolic and physiologic function in focus and being accessible to early magnetic resonance (MR) equipment, skeletal muscle was one of the first targets of examinations by in vivo ^{31}P magnetic resonance spectroscopy (MRS). In vivo ^{1}H MRS examinations of human muscle followed with the advent of volume-selective MRS methods. [1]H MR Imaging (MRI) and computed tomography (CT) measurement can provide an assessment of macroscopic skeletal muscle fat infiltration, which is an important marker of metabolic, mobility, and overall muscle dysfunction. Over the years, the in vivo measurement of intramyocellular lipids (IMCL) by ^{1}H-MRS has found its way into academic and clinical research in the fields of metabolism, diabetology, mitochondrial disorders, skeletal muscle dystrophy, and sports physiology. In this chapter, we will describe the role of muscular lipids in sports physiology, the pathogenesis of insulin resistance, as well as in neuromuscular disease and skeletal muscle dystrophy. We will also describe the basics of the ^{1}H MRS/I and CT assessment of skeletal muscle fat infiltration and intramyocellular lipid accumulation.

Skeletal muscle fat infiltration

Fat infiltration can be defined in its broadest description as a storage of lipids underneath the deep fascia of muscle. This consists of adipocytes located between the muscle fibers, termed intramuscular fat (IMC) and also between muscle groups, separated by fascia from subcutaneous fat, and called, literally, intermuscular adipose tissue (IMAT) [1] (Fig. 11.1) There is also a special depot of IMCL, which is discussed separately later. In addition, based on this definition, all other lipids except from IMCL can be referred to as extramyocellular lipids (EMCL) and exhibit different characteristics in relation to magnetic resonance imaging (MRI) and spectroscopy (Table 11.1).

IMAT is considered to be an ectopic fat depot similar to visceral adipose tissue (VAT) found in the abdomen [2] (Chapter 1, VAT) and due to their particular position close to muscle fibers, it is possible to hypothesize that the biology of intermuscular adipocytes may differ from that of adipocytes from other sites [3]. Although IMAT is a relatively small fat depot accounting for as little as 8% of the adipose tissue in the thigh [4], it has been linked to systemic markers of inflammation [5]. It also is positively associated with insulin resistance and an increased risk of developing a type 2 diabetes [4], but unlike IMCLs, IMAT remains low in insulin-sensitive, endurance-trained athletes [6], consistent with a negative relationship of IMAT to insulin sensitivity. It is currently unknown whether IMAT acts merely as a marker of metabolic dysfunction or whether it may have an intermediary or modifying role in insulin resistance. Since IMAT sits near the muscle fibers, it is possible that IMAT may interact with muscle fibers through a yet unknown pathway leading to muscle dysfunction and insulin resistance [5].

Increased levels of IMAT were found in various skeletal muscle groups, for example, in the paraspinal muscles of patients with chronic back pain, and in the locomotor muscles of individuals diagnosed with HIV, spinal cord injury, cerebrovascular accidents, diabetes, and chronic obstructive pulmonary disease [2]. An increase in IMAT is usually observed with progressive loss of contractile mass [7]. Multiple pathological conditions are characterized by relative or absolute

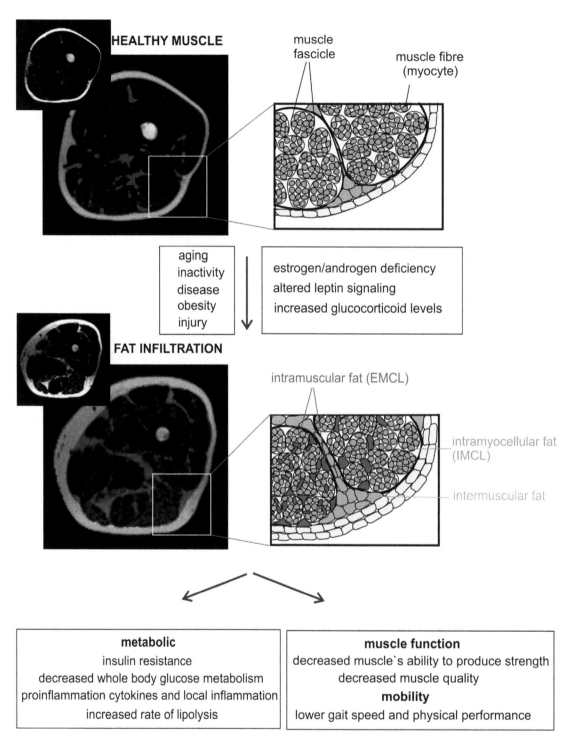

FIGURE 11.1 Skeletal muscle fat infiltration. Causes of fat infiltration and its consequences for the whole-body metabolism and muscle function and mobility.

muscle atrophy due to various reasons—impairment in the restoration process after injuries, inherited muscle genetic defect (mitochondrial or metabolic), or degenerative process during aging or in the presence of cancer [8]. In all of these conditions, a replacement of the functional muscle tissue with white adipose tissue is a well-established phenomenon [9].

TABLE 11.1 Overview of skeletal muscle fat depots and methods for their identification.

Morphology/Histology	Subcutaneous adipose tissue (SAT)	Intramuscular fat	Intermuscular fat	Intramyocellular lipids
Noninvasive imaging/CT & MRI	Subcutaneous adipose tissue (SAT)	Intramuscular & intermuscular & (intramyocellular) adipose tissue (IMAT)		
¹H Magnetic resonance spectroscopy	Subcutaneous adipose tissue (SAT)	Extramyocellular Lipids (EMCL)		Intramyocellular lipids (IMCL)

IMAT seems to be a significant predictor of both muscle function and mobility function in older adults. The increase in IMAT contributes to the process of loss of muscle strength, mobility and muscle activation, most probably also due to high levels of proinflammatory cytokines in fatty infiltrated muscles that are associated with poor muscle function [2].

One specific group of conditions with muscle fat infiltration are neuromuscular diseases (NMD). These are genetically determined, individually rare diseases characterized by progressive muscle degeneration and weakness that lead, ultimately, to functional disabilities. More than 70 forms have been identified with different causes and pathogenic mechanisms. Some forms are detected in early childhood with rapid progression, leading to deterioration of respiratory function and cardiomyopathy, while others are not detected until adulthood and progress very slowly [10−12].

Frequently observed histological features are edema, fibrosis, immune cell infiltration, fat and connective tissue deposition, and eventually, replacement of the myofibers (Fig. 11.2). Muscle fat infiltration differs between muscles and diseases, with nonuniform fat distribution patterns along the proximodistal muscle axis highly associated with disease progression, while functional and strength measures are correlated to the fat fraction in NMD [13−15].

Flexibility of IMAT fatty infiltration

As stated above skeletal muscle fat infiltration, no matter the main cause (aging, injury, disease), has a deleterious effect on muscle homeostasis [2,4,5,16−21]. Any possibility to reverse or stabilize the process could bring improvement in quality of life in elderly or immobile people, but is also a secret to mitigate effects of aging.

Multiple studies have examined the effects of diet, exercise, or their combination on the IMAT volume. In general, most of them showed that exercise alone, or in combination with caloric restriction, influenced IMAT depots [22−34]. This decrease is usually associated with weight loss. However, when comparing protocols leading to weight loss, study by Murphy et al. [27] showed that training intervention resulted in the twofold reduction of IMAT in comparison to that one caused by caloric restriction and also correlated with improvement of insulin sensitivity. Possible explanation of this stronger effect of exercise could be preferable utilization of lipids from IMAT while exercising [35]. We should also note

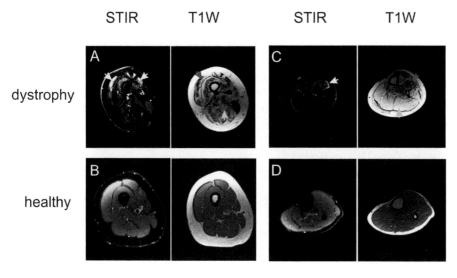

FIGURE 11.2 Examples of MRI of dystrophy. Various changes in the thigh (A) and calf (C) muscles in dysferlinopathic type of dystrophy, measured by T_1-weighted (T_1w) and STIR (short-T_I inversion recovery) sequences. *Red arrows* indicate fat infiltration, *green arrows* indicate replacement of muscle with fat tissue, both visible in T_1w and *yellow arrows* in the STIR image point to area of inflammation or edema. (B, D) Second row with the same images from healthy volunteer for comparison.

that caloric restriction also often leads to the reduction of lean mass and muscle volume [36,37], not only fat. Regarding form of exercise, Tunon-Suarez et al. [38] showed that for IMAT reduction aerobic training is more effective than resistance training. Resistance training can increase muscle mass but does not necessarily result in decrease of IMAT [36,37,39]. The meta-analysis of effects of exercise on people with chronic diseases [38] showed the importance of the level of exercise intensity, with negative response to high intensity of exercise, regardless its modality (aerobic or resistance) [40−45]. Moreover, resistance training in people with end-stage disease, or in advanced age, resulted paradoxically in increase of IMAT [40,46]. The reason is unclear, but it is possible that accumulation of adipose tissue was prompted by exercise-induced anabolic milieu within the muscle.

In the group of obese and overweight people with T2DM, effect of exercise on IMAT was only marginal [38]. Although study by Gallagher et al. [47] applying one-year-long moderate intensity aerobic training showed no effect on IMAT depots, significant difference appeared when comparing with control group, whose IMAT content increased during this time period up to 60%. Similar results were confirmed by Goodpaster et al. [48] and Keating [49], proving effectiveness of exercise for sedentary overweight and obese older adults.

Even though weight loss is often necessary for IMAT reduction, it may not be desirable for frail people with already low BMI, or older adults. As a possible solution, it was shown that in case of injured, immobile, or elderly patients, prevention or reduction of fat accumulation in the muscle can be accomplished by mechanical stimulation in the form of whole body vibration [50,51]. Explanation is offered by interfering with the bias of mesenchymal stem cells, which are diverted by mechanical stimulation from its fat differentiation pathway.

In short we can say that age, obesity, inactivity, injury, and/or neuromuscular disease are linked to increase of IMAT with increased markers of metabolic disease (insulin resistance, inflammation), muscle dysfunction (decreased muscle strength, quality and activation), and overall mobility dysfunction (decreased gait speed and physical performance, increased mobility risk and fractures) (Fig. 11.1). However, levels of IMAT appear to be to certain extent a modifiable risk factor. Exercise, physical activity, and caloric restriction as a part of intentional weight loss (in contrary to weight loss due to illness) appear to be effective countermeasures against increases of IMAT [25,27−29].

Intramyocellular lipids

An overabundance of plasma triglycerides and free fatty acids is frequently associated with pathophysiology of insulin resistance and diabetes mellitus [52]. Early hypothesis of substrate competition as the major mechanism involved in the impairment of glucose uptake by free fatty acids [53] was revised in the late 1990s. At that time, research demonstrated direct impairment of the insulin signaling cascade [54], glucose transport/phosphorylation [55−58], as well as glycogen synthesis [59] by circulating free fatty acids.

Other metabolically active sources of triglycerides that could influence cellular glucose uptake are the lipids stored in the myocytes. These fat depots are not released into the circulation but may influence glucose utilization directly. Early evidence from histological and biochemical skeletal muscle biopsy analysis has shown a correlation between the skeletal muscle triglyceride aggregation and insulin resistance [60−62]. These techniques, however, could not sufficiently discriminate between intramyocellular (IMCL) and extramyocellular (EMCL) lipid stores, and thus, the question about the direct effect of intracellular lipids remained open. Consequent correlative studies, using localized ^{1}H MRS of skeletal muscle, have shown increased IMCL content in different insulin-resistant, lean, obese, adolescent, type 1 and type 2 diabetic population [63−68].

These findings are also supported by the results of the studies that used CT for the assessment of skeletal muscle fat content [4,69]. Further experiments have revealed differences in IMCL content in different muscle groups [63,66,70−74] and point toward specific relations between insulin sensitivity and IMCL content in predominantly oxidative and glycolytic muscles. These studies showed a higher IMCL content in the predominantly oxidative, type I fiber—soleus (SOL) muscle than in the predominantly glycolytic, type II-fiber tibialis anterior (TA) muscle [63,66,70−73,75], the latter one being a better predictor of peripheral insulin resistance than IMCL content in SOL muscle. Taken together, these studies suggested the hypothesis that IMCLs, especially in glycolytic TA muscle, influence directly skeletal muscle glucose uptake and so it's content is a good marker of insulin resistance.

However, increased IMCL content was observed also in endurance-trained athletes [76−78], who are also highly insulin-sensitive. Revealing this paradox rendered the above-mentioned hypothesis questionable for sedentary and obese population and mandated a systematic explanation. Papers that reported results of histochemical analysis of muscle biopsies focusing on muscle fiber type-specific triglyceride content and fiber type distribution in insulin-sensitive, insulin-resistant, and endurance-trained states showed a shift in muscle fiber distribution toward oxidative type I muscle fibers [79−82], increased type I fiber-specific IMCL content in trained individuals, and increased skeletal muscle and whole-body oxidative capacity with the endurance training [83–85]. In addition, the observation of IMCL depletion during prolonged sub-maximal exercise [86–88], suggesting that increased IMCL stores could be of substantial benefit for endurance runners, sparked the question of whether the increased muscular triglycerides concentrations in the skeletal muscle of insulin-resistant individuals caused insulin resistance or were, rather, the results of impaired oxidative capacity.

Subsequently, further studies were designed to assess the regulation of IMCL stores in various conditions. Part of these studies is reviewed in Chapter 6, but here we would like to point out those that were essential in understanding the role of IMCL in human physiology.

First, it was hypothesized that an experimental elevation of IMCL content would cause, or at least be associated with, increased insulin resistance, and diet, or a pharmacologically induced increase in insulin sensitivity would be mirrored by a decrease of IMCL content. This was confirmed in studies using a short-term (3–7 days) high fat diet [89,90] or experimental protocols with intralipid [91] or amino acids infusion [56]. IMCL content also decreased with increasing insulin sensitivity due to the 8–10 month of leptin replacement in patients with generalized lipodystrophy [92] and 6 months of caloric restriction with or without exercise in overweight population [67].

Nevertheless, similar [89,91] but shorter intralipid infusion in young healthy men decreased glucose uptake, but did not increase the IMCL content in the SOL muscle [93,94]. Another study showed that increased plasma FFA, elevated by 3 days of fasting, induced increase of IMCL level in vastus lateralis muscle [95] of young healthy males. IMCL stores also increased due to an endurance exercise training program despite an obvious increase of insulin sensitivity [96], and remain stable despite improving insulin sensitivity by dietary intervention in young healthy humans [97] or 3 months of glitazone treatment in T2DM patients [98].

These, to some extent, controversial findings shifted the focus back to the skeletal muscle lipid oxidation pathway, as it was hypothesized that mitochondrial oxidative and phosphorylation capacity might be a contributing factor to insulin resistance and increased IMCL content [99]. One of the key intermediate metabolites of lipid oxidation, long chain acyl-CoA, was found to be involved in the regulation of skeletal muscle glucose transport and utilization [100–102], and the intracellular content of this metabolite was negatively correlated with whole-body insulin sensitivity [103]. In vitro studies have also found that accelerated beta-oxidation in muscle cells employs an insulin-sensitizing effect independently of changes in intracellular lipid content [104] and that increased stearoyl-CoA desaturase 1 activity protects against fatty acid–induced skeletal muscle insulin resistance [105]. Further studies also found that skeletal muscle mitochondrial phosphorylation capacity and/or demand is associated with decrease of peripheral insulin sensitivity and an increased IMCL content in elderly sedentary individuals [106], as well as insulin-resistant offspring of T2DM patients [107]. Skeletal muscle oxidative capacity was identified as a better predictor of insulin sensitivity than either IMCL concentration or long-chain fatty acyl CoA content in a population that spanned older T2DM patients to young, well-trained athletes [108]. This was also the case in another slightly overweight (BMI $\sim$ 29 kg/m^2) type 2 diabetic population [109]. It was also shown that experimental elevation of circulating FFA diminishes the effect of insulin stimulation on skeletal muscle ATP synthesis in parallel with the effect on glucose transport and phosphorylation without having an influence on IMCL content in skeletal muscle [93,94]. Physical activity induced enhancement of lipid oxidation is also associated with improvements in insulin sensitivity in overweight and obese, sedentary humans [67,84,110].

Thus, it seems to be clear that dynamics of IMCL metabolism plays greater role in the physiology of muscle action and pathophysiology of insulin resistance than the IMCL amount itself. As already stated, lipids within the myocells are organized into droplets. The deregulated dynamics of lipid droplets might result in increased, toxic, free fatty acids in the cytosol and/or increased intracellular lipid storage, which is associated with metabolic diseases. Droplet size, protein decoration, location within the cell, and interaction with mitochondria might play major roles [111,112]. A histopathological analysis of biopsy samples showed that athletes primarily store lipids in numerous small lipid droplets in the intermyofibrillar space in oxidative type I muscle fibers, whereas T2DM patients store lipids in fewer LDs that are significantly larger and are primarily found in the sub-sarcolemmal space of glycolytic type II muscle fibers [113]. Furthermore, recent data suggests that differences in the composition of proteins that decorate lipids may functionally translate into a higher lipid droplet turnover and a more efficient mitochondrial fat oxidation in athletes, while myocellular lipids in T2DM patients are less accessible for lipolysis, thus favoring storage of lipids [114].

As already pointed out, ^{1}H MRS demonstrated the ability to detect IMCL [115]. With the addition of diffusion weighting (DW), further micro-environmental differences between EMCL and IMCL, for example, the space restrictions of lipid compartments, could be elaborated [116]. Subsequent experiments employed the measurement of the apparent diffusion coefficient of IMCL to assess the skeletal muscle lipid droplet size and its alteration in an animal model of streptozotocin-induced diabetes and high fat diet–induced obesity [117]. Despite a similar total IMCL content, differences in diffusion restrictions confirmed increased lipid droplet size in high fat diet–induced obesity and streptozotocin-induced diabetes. Differences in energy and lipid metabolism are also connected to the saturation profile of ingested and stored lipids. Traditional analysis of biopsy extracts cannot distinguish between membrane-, extracellular-, and intracellular-lipids, which hampers the physiological interpretation of these analysis. In addition to total IMCL content, ^{1}H MRS can assess the ratio between methylene and methyl-protons, which provides a surrogate saturation index of IMCL accessible [118]. An initial study researching the value of the surrogate marker revealed differences between insulin-resistant, lipodystrophic patients and insulin-sensitive athletes [118].

Flexibility of IMCL

The accumulation of IMCL reacts to various factors. Among long-term effects, endurance training was proven to increase its level already after 4−6 weeks of intervention [119,120], but it was not the case with high intensity training [121]. Long-term caloric restriction led to decreased IMCL in obese patients [67].

Short-term variations in IMCL are physiological and can change quite dynamically, proving high metabolic activity of IMCL. It was observed that their level changes diurnally between morning and evening [122]. Even a single bout of submaximal exercise or moderate hiking results in depletion of IMCL through stimulated fat oxidation, and increased usage of IMCL [87,122−126]. This especially applies to submaximal exercise [127,128]. After depletion of the IMCL pool was observed, replenishment followed [87,88,129,130], which is dependent on the fat content of the diet during recovery period [88,131]. What is interesting, due to higher exposure to free fatty acids in plasma during exercise, levels of IMCL increase in the nonexercising muscles [96].

Another well-documented modulator of IMCL is a fat-rich diet, which generally results in an elevated IMCL content [89,90,123,132]; however, 1 day exposure to high fat diet did not really affect IMCL levels, although 24 h low fat diet resulted in their slight decrease [122]. Similarly, an elevation of plasma fatty acids, either after prolonged fasting due to the stimulation of lipolysis in adipose tissue [95,133], or due to intravenous lipid infusion, increased exposure of muscle to free fatty acids [89,129], and was followed by pronounced elevations of IMCL content. It is also not surprising that IMCL levels and repletion/depletion vary between different muscles [89,134]. This could be attributed to differences in muscle fiber composition and different loading of various muscle groups in daily life and exercise challenges.

To briefly summarize, recent studies suggest that increased IMCL content in sedentary and insulin-resistant individuals is a result of defects in lipid oxidation and/or lipid oversupply rather than a direct cause of insulin resistance, and that IMCL stores are efficient energy storage pools, which are increased and highly accessible in endurance-trained individuals (Fig. 11.3).

With that in mind, there are several aspects to be considered in process of planning a study involving measurements of IMCL. Concentrations of IMCL in skeletal muscle are affected by the long-term metabolic phenotype (insulin sensitivity, mitochondrial activity, training status) and by short-term influences, such as exercise and diet (see also Chapter 6 and [135]).

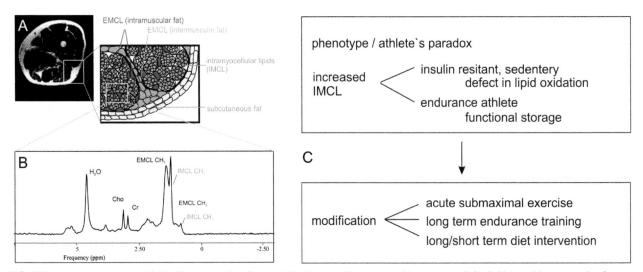

FIGURE 11.3 Intramyocellular lipids. Illustration of IMCL deposition in myocells, together with extramyocellular lipid (A) with an example of spectra from the muscle (B), containing signal from EMCL and IMCL main peaks. Summarization of athlete/s paradox and possible modification of the volume of IMCL storage (C).

Careful standardization of studies on resting IMCL levels is mandatory, as short-term variations in IMCL content may be of magnitude like that of the effect being investigated (e.g., a cross-sectional comparison of metabolic phenotypes or the effect of an intervention). It is, therefore, vital that confounding factors (e.g., diet or activity level) are accounted for in the study design. Also, strenuous exercise should be omitted and an energy-balanced diet is recommended in the 2−3 days preceding IMCL investigation. To avoid diurnal changes in activity, measurements should be performed at the same time of day.

Methods to assess lipids in the muscle

In skeletal muscle, fat infiltration, intra- and intermuscular adipose tissue (IMAT), and IMCL represent different forms of lipid storage with distinctly different physiological function and imaging features. While the discrete localization and high concentration of IMAT make imaging methods (CT, MRI) most appropriate [12,136], IMCL which are stored in droplets within the cells can be directly measured only by ^{1}H-MRS [115,125,134,137,138].

Computed tomography—CT

Signal intensity in the conventional CT images correspond to the linear attenuation coefficient, which depends on physical properties (including density) of tissue within the volume of interest. Signal intensity is expressed in so-called CT numbers or Hounsfield units, which can range from −1000 to +3095 (4096 values). Based on their density and resulting differences in X-ray attenuation, muscle and fat tissue display different ranges of Hounsfield units—(−190 to −30 HU for fat and 0 to 100 HU for muscle), resulting in muscle-to-fat contrast on the CT image. Measurements of fat accumulation are thus based on volumetric measurements in the case of subcutaneous and visceral fat depots [139−141] (Fig. 11.4). In the case of ectopic (intrahepatic, IMAT) lipid accumulation, measurements are based on comparison of the X-ray attenuation between liver tissue and spleen or between muscle and fat tissue (bone marrow or an external phantom) [142]. Measurements in intrahepatic and intramuscular fat accumulation have been validated against histological and biochemical measurements from the biopsy [142,143] yielding satisfactory correlation. New approaches to CT technologies have emerged to overcome limitation of traditional CT—radiation exposure, limitations in distinguishing between various soft tissue and necessity to use iodine contrast agents. Already in clinical practice, dual energy CT, also known as dual source CT or spectral CT, is used. In contrast to conventional single energy CT, dual energy CT uses two separate X-ray energy proton spectra which create two different images based on the attenuation properties of the tissues for different energies [144,145]. Good correlation between dual-energy and conventional CT applied for fat fractions assessment in rotator cuff muscle was reported [146] as well as between multi-echo Dixon MRI and dual-energy CT in the assessment of intrahepatic and intramuscular fat [147]. It is also interesting to mention photon counting CT, a new approach which is currently under development and would result in even higher differentiation and image resolution, less artifacts, and less radiation [148].

The main advantage of imaging methods (CT and MRI) is the ability to quantify localized adipose tissue or ectopic fat. The request for localized information can be, to some extent, answered by DXA measurement, where images of specific body segments can be separated for the analysis, but it cannot provide the differentiation of subcutaneous and deeper fat or intracellular fat depots directly. Investigators are strongly advised to apply multi-slice or whole-body CT scans for correct assessment of fat distribution. However, this highlights the single safety limitation of CT scans related to relative high

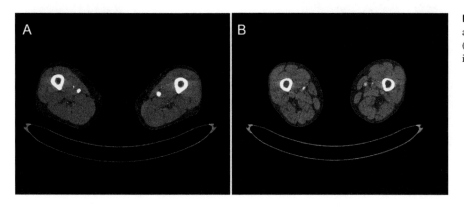

FIGURE 11.4 CT of skeletal muscle. Images from dual energy CT of healthy (A) and dystrophic (B) patient, showing fat infiltrating into the muscle.

radiation dose applied during the whole body measurements, restricting the use of CT scans for measurement purposes, particularly in children.

MRI of skeletal muscle

Positioning of a measured sample in a strong homogeneous magnetic field forces protons within the sample to align according to the direction of the magnetic field and creates a macroscopic magnetization of the sample. Interaction of the spins with externally applied radiofrequency (RF) waves at resonant frequency changes the magnitude and direction of this macroscopic magnetization in a process called excitation. After switching off the RF waves, magnetization returns to the thermal equilibrium in a time- and direction-dependent manner. This process is called relaxation and the changing magnetization induces electric signal in the receiver coil. Signal intensity in MRI is dependent not only on the proton density in the volume of interest, but also on the interaction between tissue protons and externally applied RF waves during the excitation, and on the interaction between nuclei within the tissue during the relaxation. Different physical properties of protons within water and fatty acid molecules result in strong differences in time- and phase-dependent behavior of these nuclei during the relaxation, producing relaxation- and phase-dependent contrast for MRI.

Spin-lattice- or T_1-relaxation-based contrast can be used for volumetric measurements of subcutaneous, intraabdominal and intramuscular fat accumulation. Multisegment, multi-lice 2D images or real 3D datasets are acquired [149] and areas of fat volume can be segmented and divided into separate compartments in a more or less automated fashion [150,151]. Initially, the acquisition of multisegment, multislice 2D datasets required about 30 min, but the improvements in MRI hardware, data acquisition, and reconstruction now allow for continuous whole-body data acquisition during defined movement of the patient table in the magnet [152−155]. This procedure can reduce scanning time to less than 3 min and make the whole-body MRI measurement of fat distribution highly desirable and affordable even for the clinical praxis [156,157].

T_1-weighted images are often used for visual semiquantitative assessment of fat infiltration of the muscle [158−162], but quantitative methods, especially Dixon techniques (see below), proved to be much more precise [163], and showed that a simple T_1-weighting approach often overestimates fatty infiltration [164].

Phase behavior−based contrast can be used for the quantitation of the intramuscular fat accumulation. In basic version, images with water and fat signal contribution "in phase" and "out-of-phase" are added or subtracted in order to obtain pure water and pure fat images [165,166] (Fig. 11.5A). While separate water and fat images remain qualitative, fat fraction,

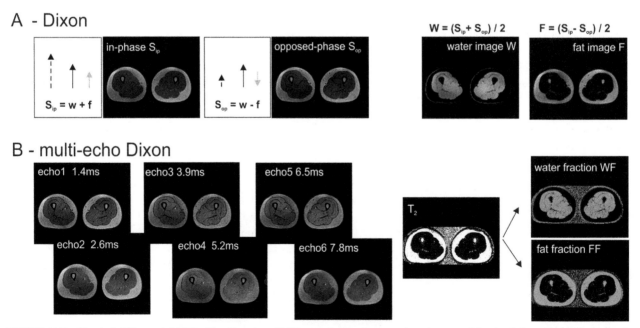

FIGURE 11.5 Chemical shift encoded MRI—Dixon imaging. (A) Dixon technique for separation of water and fat signal. Image is acquired when fat and water signal is in phase Sip and their signal is cumulated, and when water and fat signal is in opposed phase Sop and is subtracted. Pure water and fat images are reconstructed based on arithmetic operations expressed by equations for W and F. (B) Multiecho Dixon technique is based on acquisition of multiple images in different echo time points (in this case 6), applies advanced spectral mode for fitting the fat signal and takes T_2 values into account. Sequence usually results directly into water (WF) and fat (FF) fraction images.

which comes from combining these two, becomes quantitative. It is generally defined as $FF = f/(f + w)$ where w is water signal and fat signal [13]. Modern version of Dixon-MRI acquires multiple echo images and applies advanced fat spectral model (Fig. 11.5B). To define techniques that would be comparable across studies and independent of protocol and MR system used, working group around Strijkers and Kan [13] suggested optimal approach for Dixon technique for muscles. In general, to address confounding factors, the Dixon sequence should acquire at least three echoes to compensate for field inhomogeneities and to be able to account for T2* relaxation [167,168], apply a long enough TR and low flip angles to minimize T_1-weighting, and should implement a complex spectral model of fat consisting of multiple peaks [169−171]. An iterative decomposition method that yielded water and fat images from one image acquisition was also reported [172,173]. With these approaches, accurate estimation of lower fat fraction/infiltration (e.g., in skeletal muscle) is possible and can be referred to as the proton density fat fraction (PDFF) [13]. Spatial resolution of T_1w or Dixon MR images is provided by system hardware performance and can be lower than 1 mm in-plane.

Other MR techniques using conventional imaging technology, but exciting only the fat signal or water and fat multibands separately are water/fat-selective MRI approaches [174,175]. These methods can produce fat distribution maps of muscle with excellent spatial resolution (< 1 mm in plane) [176,177], but also cannot separate extra- and intramyocellular signal contributions directly (see below ^{1}H MRS for IMCL). A similar disadvantage features also CT quantification of muscle fat by overall signal attenuation. CT measurement was correlated with total intramuscular lipid concentration measured by MRS (EMCL + IMCL) [178]. Splitting the MRS measure into extra- and intracellular compartment yielded to preferential prediction of EMCL in the TA muscle, while the CT measurement predicted IMCL in the SOL muscle [178]. Nevertheless, indirect threshold-based differentiation of MRI pixels containing IMCL only was also introduced and successfully tested [162,179].

Here, we would like to mention special imaging of neuromuscular dystrophies. Techniques used in this group of rare diseases, in large part, overlap with methods for fat infiltration imaging and skeletal muscle spectroscopy, but, as the focus is also on other biomarkers of disease progression, which can precede fatty infiltration, a more comprehensible list of MR-based methods can be found elsewhere [13].

Comparative studies of MRI and CT have demonstrated that MRI has a higher sensitivity than CT in the identification of early fatty replacement in muscle, and that MRI, because it is not density-based, provides better anatomical details of soft tissue than CT [1,158]. Studies comparing CT and MRI measurements have generally shown good agreement and both methods are acceptably precise measures of IMAT [147,180,181]. Both CT and MRI appear to be appropriate and advanced techniques for measuring IMAT; however, drawing conclusions concerning absolute amounts of IMAT across studies may be difficult if different methods of measurement are employed. Many studies have also used slightly different definitions of IMAT (i.e., adipose tissue in a muscle, adipose tissue between muscles, or adipose tissue under the fascia of the thigh), and conclusions drawn across studies should be interpreted within this context [2]. Thus the same IMAT definition and measurement method should be used in time-course studies.

From the safety point of view, magnetic resonance techniques represent no radiation risk, but the presence of strong magnetic field and switching of the magnetic field gradients make metallic objects (splinters, tattoos, colored contact lenses, piercing, uterus coil), different medical devices (pace makers, cardiac valves, clips, electrodes, neurostimulators), implants, prostheses, shunts, and stents contraindicated for an MR examination. Another practical point of view is the restricted space in the clear bore of the magnet. Usual clear diameter of $\sim 60-70$ cm excludes morbidly obese patients from the examination. Nevertheless, the advantages and the versatility of the method, as well as wider availability of MR systems predetermine broad applications in future clinical praxis.

Postprocessing and assessment of fat infiltration imaging

For quantitative evaluation of fat infiltration, multiple approaches can be applied. Fat fraction can be evaluated in various ways, e.g., whole muscle fat fraction, muscle group fat fraction, specific volume fat fraction of individual muscle or muscle groups, or related to contractile part of the muscle as contractile cross-sectional area [13]. For these analyses, it is necessary to outline individual muscles or muscle groups and segment them into meaningful compartments [163]. This task can be quite challenging due to the high variability of the shape of the muscles. In cases with high fat infiltration or muscular dystrophies, visibility of the borders between individual muscles is often hampered. Coregistration of fat fraction maps with morphological images is helpful and often necessary. Manual segmentation is, at the moment, the gold standard, but is very time consuming and operator dependent [182]. As an emerging technology, semiautomated and automated methods have been introduced based on propagation of manually drawn masks [183] or other algorithms [184−186]. Various approaches use templates from databases or atlas-based registration [187,188]. These methods, although tested only on healthy subjects so far, can bring efficient improvements with an 85% reduction of segmentation time [183] and a proven volume error of up to approximately 18% [187,189].

One of the novel approaches for the assessment of water/fat distribution, especially interesting for muscular dystrophies, was published by Nasel et al. [190]. Based on water and fat images acquired by the Dixon technique, the approach applies a robust separation of regular from nonregular muscle image components and performs principal and individual component analyses. Compared to muscle group—based fat fraction analysis, preliminary results suggest a higher power to detect subtle shifts of water/fat signal relation [190].

MRS of skeletal muscle

Additionally to imaging techniques, magnetic resonance can also be applied in a spectroscopic fashion. Different electron clouds within the molecule result in different resonance frequencies of protons in water and fatty acid. This effect is called chemical shift of resonant frequencies and it does not depend on the magnetic field strength applied. In praxis, it is given in relative units—parts per million (ppm). The main advantage of spectroscopic measurement is the direct separation and quantitation of water and fat fraction of diverse soft tissues.

Localization of the spectroscopic signal can be done in single voxel—(volume pixel) or in a matrix-based, multivoxel fashion. In the latter case, the method is called chemical shift imaging (CSI) or spectroscopic imaging (SI), in which the signal intensities of different chemical entities can be used to produce distribution maps of metabolites of interest. Current best achievable geometric resolution currently is $\sim 1\ cm^3$ for single voxel spectroscopy and $\sim 0.5\ cm^3$ for the spectroscopic imaging [74,191]. Most studies use single-voxel localization; much fewer studies have introduced CSI methods or higher-dimensional, correlated spectroscopic localization techniques [192]. While CSI methods offer the advantage of increased spatial coverage and resolution, the technical issues (longer acquisition times, acquisition-type dependence on relaxation times, large datasets, water referencing, need of sophisticated knowledge of techniques) limit their widespread application [73,74].

For single-voxel spectroscopy, the voxel should be selected in homogeneous tissue, that is, in one specific muscle. Next to unambiguous physiological interpretation of the results, specific features of anisotropic muscle tissue are of major concern. Differences in magnetic properties of a bulk cylinder, such as EMCL and spheric vesicle-accumulated IMCL, even give the potential to separate these two compartments (Fig. 11.6). Macro- and microscopic susceptibility differences cause local magnetic fields to vary strongly, such that lipid peaks of different compartments can be shifted in resonance frequency by up to ~ 0.2 ppm. The IMCL resonances are unaffected by these susceptibility effects while EMCL resonances are shifted downfield relative to IMCL depending on the pennation angle [115,125,134], which can differ in neighboring muscle groups. This phenomenon was observed for the first time in early 1990s [115] and was subsequently confirmed by theory and model experiments [137] later on. Successful validation against histological and biochemical analyses of biopsies [193] and the increasing accessibility of the MR equipment led to a number of metabolic studies ever since. Recently, acquisition and processing methods have been reviewed and recommendations for robust protocols have been provided [191].

Regarding the hardware used, magnetic fields of 3T and higher are more favorable for sufficient signal separation and various combinations of transmit and receive RF coils are common. Local volume coils, such as knee- or extremity coils, are efficient for spectroscopy of the lower leg and knee-adjacent portions of upper leg since this approach combines relatively strong RF fields with a homogeneous excitation. Any motion of the examined body part (leg) should be restricted. The selection of a specific muscle is mostly determined by the physiological aim of a study (e.g., comparison with biopsy data, dominant fiber types); however, the selection should, whenever possible, also take into account that some muscles are more suited for ^{1}H-MRS. Due to the orientation dependence of the EMCL/IMCL separation, the best separation of signals will be achieved in fusiform muscles with a uniform fiber orientation along the axis of the muscle, for example, the m. TA or m. vastus intermedius. If the study design involves feathered muscles with varying fiber orientations (e.g., m. SOL), the separation of EMCL/IMCL is smaller, and thus, contamination of the IMCL resonance by EMCL is more likely. Regardless of the orientation of the leg relative to the direction of the magnetic field, if EMCL content in the voxel is high, the EMCL signal covers the IMCL signal and a reliable fitting of IMCL is hampered [134]. In general, voxel size for IMCL acquisition should be as small as SNR allows, approximately 10×10 mm in the transversal image plane. If necessary, the voxel size should be enlarged preferentially along the muscle axis (typically to less than 20 mm). Quantitative measurement of EMCL in the musculature is hampered by its inhomogeneous distribution. Single-voxel ^{1}H-MRS is inappropriate for EMCL since even small voxel shifts lead to almost arbitrary variations. For a quantification of EMCL, fat-selective imaging approaches (see above) should be considered.

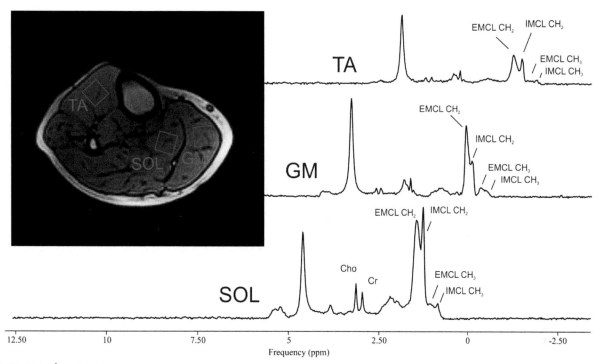

FIGURE 11.6 ^{1}H MRS of skeletal muscle—intramyocellular lipids (IMCL). Anatomical scout image (left) with the depiction of signal acquisition volumes (red boxes) and short echo time (STEAM, $T_E = 20$ ms) single voxel MR spectra of soleus—(SOL), gastrocnemius medialis—(GM), and tibialis anterior (TA) muscles. Please note differences in the line splitting between EMCL and IMCL resonances caused by orientational dependence of bulk magnetic susceptibility as well as differences in the signal intensity of IMCL—CH$_2$ resonance caused by differences in the muscle specific IMCL amount.

Two versions of single voxel spectroscopy are usually considered. Spin echo—based method (PRESS) applies a 90 degree RF pulse for excitation and two 180 degrees RF pulses refocusing the MR signal. Stimulated echo-based method (STEAM) applies a sequence of three 90 degrees RF pulses. Compared to PRESS, STEAM yields only half the possible signal-to-noise, but the nature of the RF-sequence and shorter pulses applied allow for a shorter echo time (T_E) of acquisition. Furthermore, J-modulation effects, which can influence the echo time evolution of the MR signal, are less pronounced in STEAM acquisition. In both cases, an efficient water signal suppression scheme should precede MRS signal excitation. Separate acquisition of the water signal is mandatory for the quantification of IMCL.

While the choice of echo time (T_E) and repetition time (T_R) is dictated by the T_1 and T_2 of lipids and water [191], a rather short T_E ($< 30–40$ ms) and moderate T_R of ≥ 2000 ms are recommended. Differences between T_2 of EMCL and IMCL can be exploited through long T_E acquisition approaches ($T_E \geq 150$ ms) to improve line-splitting between EMCL and IMCL peaks [194–196]. However, such spectra are heavily T_2-weighted and even exact knowledge of T_2 relaxation times cannot avoid quantification errors.

Postprocessing and quantitation of 1H-MR spectra from skeletal muscle

Most MR systems are equipped with vendor-specific software for postprocessing; however, external software packages for offline postprocessing offer more advanced algorithms.

Spectral processing for IMCL quantitation begins with a visual inspection of the spectra. Several fitting procedures are available, yet it cannot be sufficiently emphasized that clearly visible line-splitting of IMCL and EMCL in the methyl and methylene region (0.9–1.5 ppm) is necessary for reliable fitting. If the EMCL CH$_2$-signal is strong, small uncertainties of the EMCL line width and shape can influence the adjacent IMCL—CH$_2$ signal substantially. In general, strong prior knowledge input into the fitting algorithms is recommended. This includes fixed or at least related line-widths of the contributing peaks. LCModel [197] provides a commercially available algorithm with IMCL and EMCL signals included in the basis dataset. If jMRUI [198,199] or fitting algorithms embedded in the scanner software are used, an extended set of prior knowledge is required to make IMCL/EMCL separation robust (Fig. 11.7). Most fitting and quantification approaches [125] use an average composition of lipids in IMCL to estimate the chain length and unsaturation (i.e., the number of CH$_2$

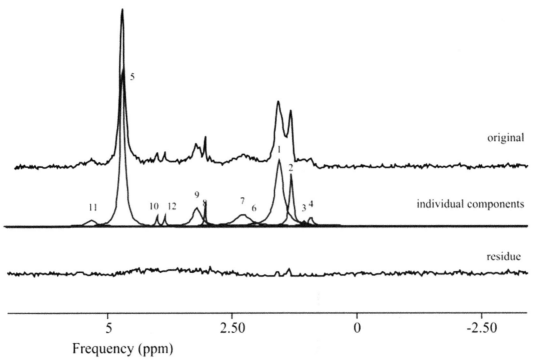

FIGURE 11.7 Fitting in jMRUI. Example of spectral fitting procedure by AMARES algorithm in jMRUI. Original acquired spectrum is at the top, individual components that are fitted based on the predefined parameters of the peaks are below, and the residue left from the spectrum after subtracting fitted components are at the bottom.

per fatty acid chain in the methylene peak). This is reasonable, yet not fully accurate, since it has been shown that lipids in other adipose tissue compartments can change saturation and chain length with diet [200]. More recently, similar variations between groups have been reported for IMCL during a fasting protocol [201] and different ratios of CH_2-CH_3 signal have been found in lipodystrophic, trained, and untrained population [118].

To compare MR spectra from different acquisitions (e.g., different volunteers), normalization of the spectra must be performed. IMCL content can be quantified with respect to a concentration reference. Using the tissue water signal as an internal concentration reference is the most common way to accomplish this; however, it involves several assumptions: (i) constant tissue water content between individuals, (ii) no change in water tissue content with nutritional or hydration status. While these assumptions are relatively robust for homogeneous populations under standard conditions, they need to be considered for the particular study being conducted [202,203].

Corrections for signal decay (T_2) and signal saturation (T_1) of metabolites and reference signals are necessary for an absolute quantitation [115,194,204–209]. Appropriate T_1 correction should be performed if T_R is less than 5 times the longest T_1 of interest, while a signal correction for T_2 relaxation is generally necessary [115,194–196,204–206,209]. The reproducibility of IMCL measurements has been assessed, and the results showed intraday variations of less than 12% for the TA and the SOL muscle [195,196,210] which are low compared to interindividual differences (several hundred percentage points).

Summary

Ectopic lipid deposits in skeletal muscle play a major role in pathophysiology of metabolic disease, skeletal muscle atrophy, and neuromuscular disorders. An increased amount of IMAT can be quantified using CT and MRI. The accumulation of IMCL, which is important not only for endurance performance, but also accompanies insulin-resistant states, can be measured by ^{1}H magnetic resonance spectroscopy (MRS). The combination of noninvasive imaging methods and classical histopathological examination of tissue biopsy, as well as assessment of muscle physiology, molecular biology, and biochemistry, can improve the knowledge, identify therapeutic targets, and accompany lifestyle or medication interventions.

References

[1] Karampinos DC, et al. Characterization of the regional distribution of skeletal muscle adipose tissue in type 2 diabetes using chemical shift-based water/fat separation. J Magn Reson Imag 2012;35(4):899−907.

[2] Addison O, et al. Intermuscular fat: a review of the consequences and causes. Int J Endocrinol 2014;2014:309570.

[3] Pond CM, Mattacks CA. The effects of noradrenaline and insulin on lipolysis in adipocytes isolated from nine different adipose depots of Guinea-pigs. Int J Obes 1991;15(9):609−18.

[4] Goodpaster BH, Thaete FL, Kelley DE. Thigh adipose tissue distribution is associated with insulin resistance in obesity and in type 2 diabetes mellitus. Am.J.Clin.Nutr. 2000;71(4):885−92.

[5] Beasley LE, et al. Inflammation and race and gender differences in computerized tomography-measured adipose depots. Obesity 2009;17(5):1062−9.

[6] Kim J, et al. Intermuscular adipose tissue-free skeletal muscle mass: estimation by dual-energy X-ray absorptiometry in adults. J Appl Physiol 2004;97(2):655−60.

[7] Dulor JP, et al. Expression of specific white adipose tissue genes in denervation-induced skeletal muscle fatty degeneration. FEBS Lett 1998;439(1−2):89−92.

[8] Prado CM, et al. Prevalence and clinical implications of sarcopenic obesity in patients with solid tumours of the respiratory and gastrointestinal tracts: a population-based study. Lancet Oncol 2008;9(7):629−35.

[9] Vettor R, et al. The origin of intermuscular adipose tissue and its pathophysiological implications. Am J Physiol Endocrinol Metab 2009;297(5):E987−98.

[10] Burakiewicz J, et al. Quantifying fat replacement of muscle by quantitative MRI in muscular dystrophy. J Neurol 2017;264(10):2053−67.

[11] Hooijmans MT, et al. Non-uniform muscle fat replacement along the proximodistal axis in Duchenne muscular dystrophy. Neuromuscul Disord 2017;27(5):458−64.

[12] Prompers JJ, et al. Dynamic MRS and MRI of skeletal muscle function and biomechanics. NMR Biomed 2006;19(7):927−53.

[13] Strijkers GJ, et al. Exploration of new contrasts, targets, and MR imaging and spectroscopy techniques for neuromuscular disease - a workshop report of working group 3 of the biomedicine and molecular biosciences COST action BM1304 MYO-MRI. J Neuromuscul Dis 2019;6(1):1−30.

[14] Blake DJ, et al. Function and genetics of dystrophin and dystrophin-related proteins in muscle. Physiol Rev 2002;82(2):291−329.

[15] Ljubicic V, Burt M, Jasmin BJ. The therapeutic potential of skeletal muscle plasticity in Duchenne muscular dystrophy: phenotypic modifiers as pharmacologic targets. FASEB J 2014;28(2):548−68.

[16] Ryan AS, et al. Atrophy and intramuscular fat in specific muscles of the thigh: associated weakness and hyperinsulinemia in stroke survivors. Neurorehabil Neural Repair 2011;25(9):865−72.

[17] Ryan AS, Nicklas BJ. Age-related changes in fat deposition in mid-thigh muscle in women: relationships with metabolic cardiovascular disease risk factors. Int J Obes Relat Metab Disord 1999;23(2):126−32.

[18] Goodpaster BH, et al. Association between regional adipose tissue distribution and both type 2 diabetes and impaired glucose tolerance in elderly men and women. Diabetes Care 2003;26(2):372−9.

[19] Miljkovic-Gacic I, et al. Adipose tissue infiltration in skeletal muscle: age patterns and association with diabetes among men of African ancestry. Am J Clin Nutr 2008;87(6):1590−5.

[20] Leskinen T, et al. Physically active vs. inactive lifestyle, muscle properties, and glucose homeostasis in middle-aged and older twins. Age 2013;35(5):1917−26.

[21] Solomon AM, Bouloux PM. Modifying muscle mass - the endocrine perspective. J Endocrinol 2006;191(2):349−60.

[22] Prior SJ, et al. Reduction in midthigh low-density muscle with aerobic exercise training and weight loss impacts glucose tolerance in older men. J Clin Endocrinol Metab 2007;92(3):880−6.

[23] Durheim MT, et al. Relationships between exercise-induced reductions in thigh intermuscular adipose tissue, changes in lipoprotein particle size, and visceral adiposity. Am J Physiol Endocrinol Metab 2008;295(2):E407−12.

[24] Ryan AS, et al. Dietary restriction and walking reduce fat deposition in the midthigh in obese older women. Am J Clin Nutr 2000;72(3):708−13.

[25] Ryan AS, Ortmeyer HK, Sorkin JD. Exercise with calorie restriction improves insulin sensitivity and glycogen synthase activity in obese post-menopausal women with impaired glucose tolerance. Am J Physiol Endocrinol Metab 2012;302(1):E145−52.

[26] Marcus RL, et al. Comparison of combined aerobic and high-force eccentric resistance exercise with aerobic exercise only for people with type 2 diabetes mellitus. Phys Ther 2008;88(11):1345−54.

[27] Murphy JC, et al. Preferential reductions in intermuscular and visceral adipose tissue with exercise-induced weight loss compared with calorie restriction. J Appl Physiol 2012;112(1):79−85.

[28] Ryan AS, Nicklas BJ, Berman DM. Aerobic exercise is necessary to improve glucose utilization with moderate weight loss in women. Obesity 2006;14(6):1064−72.

[29] Goodpaster BH, et al. Effects of weight loss on regional fat distribution and insulin sensitivity in obesity. Diabetes 1999;48(4):839−47.

[30] Santanasto AJ, et al. Impact of weight loss on physical function with changes in strength, muscle mass, and muscle fat infiltration in overweight to moderately obese older adults: a randomized clinical trial. J Obes 2011;2011.

[31] Taaffe DR, et al. Alterations in muscle attenuation following detraining and retraining in resistance-trained older adults. Gerontology 2009;55(2):217−23.

[32] Lee S, et al. Exercise without weight loss is an effective strategy for obesity reduction in obese individuals with and without Type 2 diabetes. J Appl Physiol 2005;99(3):1220−5.

[33] Avila JJ, et al. Effect of moderate intensity resistance training during weight loss on body composition and physical performance in overweight older adults. Eur J Appl Physiol 2010;109(3):517–25.

[34] Mazzali G, et al. Interrelations between fat distribution, muscle lipid content, adipocytokines, and insulin resistance: effect of moderate weight loss in older women. Am J Clin Nutr 2006;84(5):1193–9.

[35] Stallknecht B, Dela F, Helge JW. Are blood flow and lipolysis in subcutaneous adipose tissue influenced by contractions in adjacent muscles in humans? Am J Physiol Endocrinol Metab 2007;292(2):E394–9.

[36] Nicklas BJ, et al. Effects of resistance training with and without caloric restriction on physical function and mobility in overweight and obese older adults: a randomized controlled trial. Am J Clin Nutr 2015;101(5):991–9.

[37] Manini TM, et al. Effect of dietary restriction and exercise on lower extremity tissue compartments in obese, older women: a pilot study. J Gerontol A Biol Sci Med Sci 2014;69(1):101–8.

[38] Tunon-Suarez M, et al. Exercise training to decrease ectopic intermuscular adipose tissue in individuals with chronic diseases: a systematic review and meta-analysis. Phys Ther 2021;101(10).

[39] Walts CT, et al. Do sex or race differences influence strength training effects on muscle or fat? Med Sci Sports Exerc 2008;40(4):669–76.

[40] Cheema B, et al. Progressive exercise for anabolism in kidney disease (PEAK): a randomized, controlled trial of resistance training during hemodialysis. J Am Soc Nephrol 2007;18(5):1594–601.

[41] Janssen I, et al. Effects of an energy-restrictive diet with or without exercise on abdominal fat, intermuscular fat, and metabolic risk factors in obese women. Diabetes Care 2002;25(3):431–8.

[42] Mavros Y, et al. Changes in insulin resistance and HbA1c are related to exercise-mediated changes in body composition in older adults with type 2 diabetes: interim outcomes from the GREAT2DO trial. Diabetes Care 2013;36(8):2372–9.

[43] Jung JY, et al. Effects of aerobic exercise intensity on abdominal and thigh adipose tissue and skeletal muscle attenuation in overweight women with type 2 diabetes mellitus. Diabetes Metab J 2012;36(3):211–21.

[44] Sipila S, Suominen H. Effects of strength and endurance training on thigh and leg muscle mass and composition in elderly women. J Appl Physiol 1995;78(1):334–40.

[45] Taaffe DR, et al. The effect of hormone replacement therapy and/or exercise on skeletal muscle attenuation in postmenopausal women: a yearlong intervention. Clin Physiol Funct Imag 2005;25(5):297–304.

[46] Cadore EL, et al. Multicomponent exercises including muscle power training enhance muscle mass, power output, and functional outcomes in institutionalized frail nonagenarians. Age 2014;36(2):773–85.

[47] Gallagher D, et al. Changes in adipose tissue depots and metabolic markers following a 1-year diet and exercise intervention in overweight and obese patients with type 2 diabetes. Diabetes Care 2014;37(12):3325–32.

[48] Goodpaster BH, et al. Effects of physical activity on strength and skeletal muscle fat infiltration in older adults: a randomized controlled trial. J Appl Physiol 2008;105(5):1498–503.

[49] Keating SE, et al. Effect of resistance training on liver fat and visceral adiposity in adults with obesity: a randomized controlled trial. Hepatol Res 2017;47(7):622–31.

[50] Novotny SA, et al. Low intensity, high frequency vibration training to improve musculoskeletal function in a mouse model of Duchenne muscular dystrophy. PLoS One 2014;9(8):e104339.

[51] Frechette DM, et al. Diminished satellite cells and elevated adipogenic gene expression in muscle as caused by ovariectomy are averted by low-magnitude mechanical signals. J Appl Physiol 2015;119(1):27–36.

[52] DeFronzo RA. Pathogenesis of type 2 diabetes mellitus. Med Clin North Am 2004;88(4):787–835 [ix].

[53] Randle PJ, et al. The glucose fatty-acid cycle. Its role in insulin sensitivity and the metabolic disturbances of diabetes mellitus. Lancet 1963;1:785–9.

[54] Griffin ME, et al. Free fatty acid-induced insulin resistance is associated with activation of protein kinase C theta and alterations in the insulin signaling cascade. Diabetes 1999;48(6):1270–4.

[55] Cline GW, et al. Impaired glucose transport as a cause of decreased insulin-stimulated muscle glycogen synthesis in type 2 diabetes. N Engl J Med 1999;341(4):240–6.

[56] Krebs M, et al. Free fatty acids inhibit the glucose-stimulated increase of intramuscular glucose-6-phosphate concentration in humans. J Clin Endocrinol Metab 2001;86(5):2153–60.

[57] Roden M, et al. Rapid impairment of skeletal muscle glucose transport/phosphorylation by free fatty acids in humans. Diabetes 1999;48(2):358–64.

[58] Roden M, et al. The roles of insulin and glucagon in the regulation of hepatic glycogen synthesis and turnover in humans. J Clin Invest 1996;97(3):642–8.

[59] Roden M, et al. Mechanism of free fatty acid-induced insulin resistance in humans. J Clin Invest 1996;97(12):2859–65.

[60] Ebeling P, et al. Intramuscular triglyceride content is increased in IDDM. Diabetologia 1998;41(1):111–5.

[61] Pan DA, et al. Skeletal muscle triglyceride levels are inversely related to insulin action. Diabetes 1997;46(6):983–8.

[62] Phillips DI, et al. Intramuscular triglyceride and muscle insulin sensitivity: evidence for a relationship in nondiabetic subjects. Metabolism 1996;45(8):947–50.

[63] Jacob S, et al. Association of increased intramyocellular lipid content with insulin resistance in lean nondiabetic offspring of type 2 diabetic subjects. Diabetes 1999;48(5):1113–9.

[64] Krssak M, et al. Intramyocellular lipid concentrations are correlated with insulin sensitivity in humans: a 1H NMR spectroscopy study. Diabetologia 1999;42(1):113−6.

[65] Perseghin G, et al. Insulin resistance, intramyocellular lipid content, and plasma adiponectin in patients with type 1 diabetes. Am J Physiol Endocrinol Metab 2003;285(6):E1174−81.

[66] Perseghin G, et al. Intramyocellular triglyceride content is a determinant of in vivo insulin resistance in humans: a 1H-13C nuclear magnetic resonance spectroscopy assessment in offspring of type 2 diabetic parents. Diabetes 1999;48(8):1600−6.

[67] Larson-Meyer DE, et al. Effect of calorie restriction with or without exercise on insulin sensitivity, beta-cell function, fat cell size, and ectopic lipid in overweight subjects. Diabetes Care 2006;29(6):1337−44.

[68] Sinha R, et al. Assessment of skeletal muscle triglyceride content by (1)H nuclear magnetic resonance spectroscopy in lean and obese adolescents: relationships to insulin sensitivity, total body fat, and central adiposity. Diabetes 2002;51(4):1022−7.

[69] Goodpaster BH, et al. Intramuscular lipid content is increased in obesity and decreased by weight loss. Metabolism 2000;49(4):467−72.

[70] Anderwald C, et al. Effects of insulin treatment in type 2 diabetic patients on intracellular lipid content in liver and skeletal muscle. Diabetes 2002;51(10):3025−32.

[71] Hwang JH, et al. Regional differences in intramyocellular lipids in humans observed by in vivo 1H-MR spectroscopic imaging. J.Appl.Physiol 2001;90(4):1267−74.

[72] Kautzky-Willer A, et al. Increased intramyocellular lipid concentration identifies impaired glucose metabolism in women with previous gestational diabetes. Diabetes 2003;52(2):244−51.

[73] Vermathen P, Kreis R, Boesch C. Distribution of intramyocellular lipids in human calf muscles as determined by MR spectroscopic imaging. Magn Reson Med 2004;51(2):253−62.

[74] Just Kukurova I, et al. Two-dimensional spectroscopic imaging with combined free induction decay and long-TE acquisition (FID echo spectroscopic imaging, FIDESI) for the detection of intramyocellular lipids in calf muscle at 7 T. NMR Biomed 2014;27(8):980−7.

[75] Klepochova R, et al. Muscle-specific relation of acetylcarnitine and intramyocellular lipids to chronic hyperglycemia: a pilot 3-T (1)H MRS study. Obesity 2020;28(8):1405−11.

[76] Klepochova R, et al. Differences in muscle metabolism between triathletes and normally active volunteers investigated using multinuclear magnetic resonance spectroscopy at 7T. Front Physiol 2018;9:300.

[77] Goodpaster BH, et al. Skeletal muscle lipid content and insulin resistance: evidence for a paradox in endurance-trained athletes. J.Clin.Endocrinol.Metab 2001;86(12):5755−61.

[78] Thamer C, et al. Intramyocellular lipids: anthropometric determinants and relationships with maximal aerobic capacity and insulin sensitivity. J.Clin.Endocrinol.Metab 2003;88(4):1785−91.

[79] Anderson PJ, et al. Visceral fat and cardiovascular risk factors in Chinese NIDDM patients. Diabetes Care 1997;20(12):1854−8.

[80] Clore JN, et al. Skeletal muscle phosphatidylcholine fatty acids and insulin sensitivity in normal humans. Am J Physiol 1998;275(4 Pt 1):E665−70.

[81] Hickey MS, et al. The insulin action-fiber type relationship in humans is muscle group specific. Am J Physiol 1995;269(1 Pt 1):E150−4.

[82] Nyholm B, et al. Evidence of an increased number of type IIb muscle fibers in insulin-resistant first-degree relatives of patients with NIDDM. Diabetes 1997;46(11):1822−8.

[83] Essen B, et al. Metabolic characteristics of fibre types in human skeletal muscle. Acta Physiol Scand 1975;95(2):153−65.

[84] Goodpaster BH, Katsiaras A, Kelley DE. Enhanced fat oxidation through physical activity is associated with improvements in insulin sensitivity in obesity. Diabetes 2003;52(9):2191−7.

[85] He J, Watkins S, Kelley DE. Skeletal muscle lipid content and oxidative enzyme activity in relation to muscle fiber type in type 2 diabetes and obesity. Diabetes 2001;50(4):817−23.

[86] Brechtel K, et al. Fast elevation of the intramyocellular lipid content in the presence of circulating free fatty acids and hyperinsulinemia: a dynamic 1H-MRS study. Magn Reson Med 2001;45(2):179−83.

[87] Krssak M, et al. Intramuscular glycogen and intramyocellular lipid utilization during prolonged exercise and recovery in man: a 13C and 1H nuclear magnetic resonance spectroscopy study. J Clin Endocrinol Metab 2000;85(2):748−54.

[88] Larson-Meyer DE, Newcomer BR, Hunter GR. Influence of endurance running and recovery diet on intramyocellular lipid content in women: a 1H NMR study. Am J Physiol Endocrinol Metab 2002;282(1):E95−106.

[89] Bachmann OP, et al. Effects of intravenous and dietary lipid challenge on intramyocellular lipid content and the relation with insulin sensitivity in humans. Diabetes 2001;50(11):2579−84.

[90] Schrauwen-Hinderling VB, et al. Intramyocellular lipid content and molecular adaptations in response to a 1-week high-fat diet. Obes Res 2005;13(12):2088−94.

[91] Boden G, et al. Effects of acute changes of plasma free fatty acids on intramyocellular fat content and insulin resistance in healthy subjects. Diabetes 2001;50(7):1612−7.

[92] Simha V, et al. Effect of leptin replacement on intrahepatic and intramyocellular lipid content in patients with generalized lipodystrophy. Diabetes Care 2003;26(1):30−5.

[93] Brehm A, et al. Acute elevation of plasma lipids does not affect ATP synthesis in human skeletal muscle. Am J Physiol Endocrinol Metab 2010;299(1):E33−8.

[94] Brehm A, et al. Increased lipid availability impairs insulin-stimulated ATP synthesis in human skeletal muscle. Diabetes 2006;55(1):136−40.

[95] Stannard SR, et al. Fasting for 72 h increases intramyocellular lipid content in nondiabetic, physically fit men. Am J Physiol Endocrinol Metab 2002;283(6):E1185−91.

[96] Schrauwen-Hinderling VB, et al. The increase in intramyocellular lipid content is a very early response to training. J.Clin.Endocrinol.Metab 2003;88(4):1610—6.

[97] Frost GS, et al. Carbohydrate-induced manipulation of insulin sensitivity independently of intramyocellular lipids. Br J Nutr 2003;89(3):365—75.

[98] Mayerson AB, et al. The effects of rosiglitazone on insulin sensitivity, lipolysis, and hepatic and skeletal muscle triglyceride content in patients with type 2 diabetes. Diabetes 2002;51(3):797—802.

[99] Shulman GI. Cellular mechanisms of insulin resistance. J Clin Invest 2000;106(2):171—6.

[100] Faergeman NJ, Knudsen J. Role of long-chain fatty acyl-CoA esters in the regulation of metabolism and in cell signalling. BiochemJ 1997;323(Pt 1):1—12.

[101] Tippett PS, Neet KE. An allosteric model for the inhibition of glucokinase by long chain acyl coenzyme A. J Biol Chem 1982;257(21):12846—52.

[102] Wititsuwannakul D, Kim KH. Mechanism of palmityl coenzyme A inhibition of liver glycogen synthase. J Biol Chem 1977;252(21):7812—7.

[103] Ellis BA, et al. Long-chain acyl-CoA esters as indicators of lipid metabolism and insulin sensitivity in rat and human muscle. Am J Physiol Endocrinol Metab 2000;279(3):E554—60.

[104] Perdomo G, et al. Increased beta-oxidation in muscle cells enhances insulin-stimulated glucose metabolism and protects against fatty acid-induced insulin resistance despite intramyocellular lipid accumulation. J Biol Chem 2004;279(26):27177—86.

[105] Pinnamaneni SK, et al. Stearoyl CoA desaturase 1 is elevated in obesity but protects against fatty acid-induced skeletal muscle insulin resistance in vitro. Diabetologia 2006;49(12):3027—37.

[106] Petersen KF, et al. Mitochondrial dysfunction in the elderly: possible role in insulin resistance. Science 2003;300(5622):1140—2.

[107] Petersen KF, Dufour S, Shulman GI. Decreased insulin-stimulated ATP synthesis and phosphate transport in muscle of insulin-resistant offspring of type 2 diabetic parents. PLoS Med 2005;2(9):e233.

[108] Bruce CR, et al. Muscle oxidative capacity is a better predictor of insulin sensitivity than lipid status. J.Clin.Endocrinol.Metab 2003;88(11):5444—51.

[109] Schrauwen-Hinderling VB, et al. Impaired in vivo mitochondrial function but similar intramyocellular lipid content in patients with type 2 diabetes mellitus and BMI-matched control subjects. Diabetologia 2007;50(1):113—20. https://doi.org/10.1007/s00125-006-0475-1. Epub 2006 Nov 9.

[110] Gan SK, et al. Changes in aerobic capacity and visceral fat but not myocyte lipid levels predict increased insulin action after exercise in overweight and obese men. Diabetes Care 2003;26(6):1706—13.

[111] Geltinger F, et al. Friend or foe: lipid droplets as organelles for protein and lipid storage in cellular stress response. Aging Dis Mole 2020;25(21).

[112] Kahn D, et al. Subcellular localisation and composition of intramuscular triacylglycerol influence insulin sensitivity in humans. Diabetologia 2021;64(1):168—80.

[113] Daemen S, et al. Distinct lipid droplet characteristics and distribution unmask the apparent contradiction of the athlete's paradox. Mol Metab 2018;17:71—81.

[114] Gemmink A, et al. Decoration of myocellular lipid droplets with perilipins as a marker for in vivo lipid droplet dynamics: a super-resolution microscopy study in trained athletes and insulin resistant individuals. Biochim Biophys Acta Mol Cell Biol Lipids 2021;1866(2):158852.

[115] Schick F, et al. Comparison of localized proton NMR signals of skeletal muscle and fat tissue in vivo: two lipid compartments in muscle tissue. Magn Reson Med 1993;29(2):158—67.

[116] Brandejsky V, Kreis R, Boesch C. Restricted or severely hindered diffusion of intramyocellular lipids in human skeletal muscle shown by in vivo proton MR spectroscopy. Magn Reson Med 2012;67(2):310—6.

[117] Cao P, et al. Diffusion magnetic resonance monitors intramyocellular lipid droplet size in vivo. Magn Reson Med 2015;73(1):59—69.

[118] Savage DB, et al. Accumulation of saturated intramyocellular lipid is associated with insulin resistance. J Lipid Res 2019;60(7):1323—32.

[119] Phillips SM, et al. Progressive effect of endurance training on metabolic adaptations in working skeletal muscle. Am J Physiol 1996;270(2 Pt 1):E265—72.

[120] Morgan TE, Short FA, Cobb LA. Effect of long-term exercise on skeletal muscle lipid composition. Am J Physiol 1969;216(1):82—6.

[121] Bergman BC, et al. Evaluation of exercise and training on muscle lipid metabolism. Am J Physiol 1999;276(1):E106—17.

[122] Machann J, et al. Morning to evening changes of intramyocellular lipid content in dependence on nutrition and physical activity during one single day: a volume selective 1H-MRS study. Magma 2011;24(1):29—33.

[123] Decombaz J, et al. Postexercise fat intake repletes intramyocellular lipids but no faster in trained than in sedentary subjects. Am J Physiol Regul Integr Comp Physiol 2001;281(3):R760—9.

[124] van Loon LJ, et al. Influence of prolonged endurance cycling and recovery diet on intramuscular triglyceride content in trained males. Am J Physiol Endocrinol Metab 2003;285(4):E804—11.

[125] Boesch C, et al. In vivo determination of intra-myocellular lipids in human muscle by means of localized 1H-MR-spectroscopy. Magn Reson Med 1997;37(4):484—93.

[126] Ith M, et al. Standardized protocol for a depletion of intramyocellular lipids (IMCL). NMR Biomed 2010;23(5):532—8.

[127] Romijn JA, et al. Regulation of endogenous fat and carbohydrate metabolism in relation to exercise intensity and duration. Am J Physiol 1993;265(3 Pt 1):E380—91.

[128] van Loon LJ, et al. The effects of increasing exercise intensity on muscle fuel utilisation in humans. J Physiol 2001;536(Pt 1):295—304.

[129] Brechtel K, et al. Utilisation of intramyocellular lipids (IMCLs) during exercise as assessed by proton magnetic resonance spectroscopy (1H-MRS). Horm Metab Res 2001;33(2):63—6.

[130] Zehnder M, et al. Gender-specific usage of intramyocellular lipids and glycogen during exercise. Med Sci Sports Exerc 2005;37(9):1517—24.

[131] Stettler R, et al. Interaction between dietary lipids and physical inactivity on insulin sensitivity and on intramyocellular lipids in healthy men. Diabetes Care 2005;28(6):1404—9.

[132] Watt MJ, Heigenhauser GJ, Spriet LL. Intramuscular triacylglycerol utilization in human skeletal muscle during exercise: is there a controversy? J Appl Physiol 2002;93(4):1185—95.

[133] Wietek BM, et al. Muscle type dependent increase in intramyocellular lipids during prolonged fasting of human subjects: a proton MRS study. Horm Metab Res 2004;36(9):639—44.

[134] Boesch C, et al. Role of proton MR for the study of muscle lipid metabolism. NMR Biomed 2006;19(7):968—88.

[135] Loher H, et al. The flexibility of ectopic lipids. Int J Mol Sci 2016;17(9).

[136] Goodpaster BH. Measuring body fat distribution and content in humans. Curr Opin Clin Nutr Metab Care 2002;5(5):481—7.

[137] Szczepaniak LS, et al. Bulk magnetic susceptibility effects on the assessment of intra- and extramyocellular lipids in vivo. Magn Reson Med 2002;47(3):607—10.

[138] Machann J, et al. In vivo proton NMR studies in skeletal musculature. Annu Rep NMR Spectrosc 2003;50:1—74.

[139] Busetto L, et al. Assessment of abdominal fat distribution in obese patients: anthropometry versus computerized tomography. Int J Obes Relat Metab Disord 1992;16(10):731—6.

[140] Dixon AK. Abdominal fat assessed by computed tomography: sex difference in distribution. Clin Radiol 1983;34(2):189—91.

[141] Tokunaga K, et al. A novel technique for the determination of body fat by computed tomography. Int J Obes 1983;7(5):437—45.

[142] Goodpaster BH, et al. Skeletal muscle attenuation determined by computed tomography is associated with skeletal muscle lipid content. J.Appl.Physiol 2000;89(1):104—10.

[143] Ricci C, et al. Noninvasive in vivo quantitative assessment of fat content in human liver. J.Hepatol. 1997;27(1):108—13.

[144] Hsu, C.V., Z Dual energy CT. Radiopaedia. Radiopaedia 2014 17.2.2022 [cited 2022 20.2.]; Available from: https://doi.org/10.53347/rID-31353.

[145] Patino M, et al. Material separation using dual-energy CT: current and emerging applications. Radiographics 2016;36(4):1087—105.

[146] Baillargeon AM, et al. Fat quantification of the rotator cuff musculature using dual-energy CT-A pilot study. Eur J Radiol 2020;130:109145.

[147] Gassenmaier S, et al. Quantification of liver and muscular fat using contrast-enhanced Dual Source Dual Energy Computed Tomography compared to an established multi-echo Dixon MRI sequence. Eur J Radiol 2021;142:109845.

[148] Willemink MJ, et al. Photon-counting CT: technical principles and clinical prospects. Radiology 2018;289(2):293—312.

[149] Thomas EL, et al. Magnetic resonance imaging of total body fat. J.Appl.Physiol 1998;85(5):1778—85.

[150] Positano V, et al. An accurate and robust method for unsupervised assessment of abdominal fat by MRI. J.Magn Reson.Imaging 2004;20(4):684—9.

[151] Thomas EL, Bell JD. Influence of undersampling on magnetic resonance imaging measurements of intra-abdominal adipose tissue. Int J Obes Relat Metab Disord 2003;27(2):211—8.

[152] Aldefeld B, Bornert P, Keupp J. Continuously moving table 3D MRI with lateral frequency-encoding direction. Magn Reson Med 2006;55(5):1210—6.

[153] Kruger DG, et al. Continuously moving table data acquisition method for long FOV contrast-enhanced MRA and whole-body MRI. Magn Reson Med 2002;47(2):224—31.

[154] Kruger DG, et al. Dual-velocity continuously moving table acquisition for contrast-enhanced peripheral magnetic resonance angiography. Magn Reson Med 2005;53(1):110—7.

[155] Sommer G, et al. Multicontrast sequences with continuous table motion: a novel acquisition technique for extended field of view imaging. Magn Reson Med 2006;55(4):918—22.

[156] Ludescher B, et al. Correlation of fat distribution in whole body MRI with generally used anthropometric data. Invest Radiol 2009;44(11):712—9.

[157] Wurslin C, et al. Topography mapping of whole body adipose tissue using A fully automated and standardized procedure. J Magn Reson Imag 2010;31(2):430—9.

[158] Mercuri E, et al. Muscle MRI in inherited neuromuscular disorders: past, present, and future. J Magn Reson Imag 2007;25(2):433—40.

[159] Fischer D, et al. Diagnostic value of muscle MRI in differentiating LGMD2I from other LGMDs. J Neurol 2005;252(5):538—47.

[160] Fuchs B, et al. Fatty degeneration of the muscles of the rotator cuff: assessment by computed tomography versus magnetic resonance imaging. J Shoulder Elbow Surg 1999;8(6):599—605.

[161] Kinali M, et al. Muscle histology vs MRI in Duchenne muscular dystrophy. Neurology 2011;76(4):346—53.

[162] Boettcher M, et al. Intermuscular adipose tissue (IMAT): association with other adipose tissue compartments and insulin sensitivity. J Magn Reson Imag 2009;29(6):1340—5.

[163] Fischer MA, et al. Quantification of muscle fat in patients with low back pain: comparison of multi-echo MR imaging with single-voxel MR spectroscopy. Radiology 2013;266(2):555—63.

[164] Alizai H, et al. Comparison of clinical semi-quantitative assessment of muscle fat infiltration with quantitative assessment using chemical shift-based water/fat separation in MR studies of the calf of post-menopausal women. Eur Radiol 2012;22(7):1592—600.

[165] Dixon WT. Simple proton spectroscopic imaging. Radiology 1984;153(1):189—94.

[166] Reeder SB, et al. Multicoil Dixon chemical species separation with an iterative least-squares estimation method. Magn Reson Med 2004;51(1):35—45.

[167] Glover GH, Schneider E. Three-point Dixon technique for true water/fat decomposition with B0 inhomogeneity correction. Magn Reson Med 1991;18(2):371—83.

[168] Loughran T, et al. Improving highly accelerated fat fraction measurements for clinical trials in muscular dystrophy: origin and quantitative effect of R2* changes. Radiology 2015;275(2):570–8.

[169] Yu H, et al. Multiecho water-fat separation and simultaneous R2* estimation with multifrequency fat spectrum modeling. Magn Reson Med 2008;60(5):1122–34.

[170] Hamilton G, et al. In vivo characterization of the liver fat (1)H MR spectrum. NMR Biomed 2011;24(7):784–90.

[171] Ren J, et al. Composition of adipose tissue and marrow fat in humans by 1H NMR at 7 Tesla. J Lipid Res 2008;49(9):2055–62.

[172] Fuller S, et al. Iterative decomposition of water and fat with echo asymmetry and least-squares estimation (IDEAL) fast spin-echo imaging of the ankle: initial clinical experience. AJR Am J Roentgenol 2006;187(6):1442–7.

[173] Reeder SB, et al. Iterative decomposition of water and fat with echo asymmetry and least-squares estimation (IDEAL): application with fast spin-echo imaging. Magn Reson Med 2005;54(3):636–44.

[174] Schick F, et al. MRI of muscular fat. Magn Reson Med 2002;47(4):720–7.

[175] Bachrata B, et al. Simultaneous Multiple Resonance Frequency imaging (SMURF): fat-water imaging using multi-band principles. Magn Reson Med 2021;85(3):1379–96.

[176] Machann J, et al. Lipid content in the musculature of the lower leg assessed by fat selective MRI: intra- and interindividual differences and correlation with anthropometric and metabolic data. J.Magn Reson.Imag 2003;17(3):350–7.

[177] Goodpaster BH, et al. Skeletal muscle lipid concentration quantified by magnetic resonance imaging. Am J Clin Nutr 2004;79(5):748–54.

[178] Larson-Meyer DE, et al. Muscle-associated triglyceride measured by computed tomography and magnetic resonance spectroscopy. Obesity 2006;14(1):73–87.

[179] Kiefer LS, et al. Distribution patterns of intramyocellular and extramyocellular fat by magnetic resonance imaging in subjects with diabetes, prediabetes and normoglycaemic controls. Diabetes Obes Metab 2021;23(8):1868–78.

[180] Klopfenstein BJ, et al. Comparison of 3 T MRI and CT for the measurement of visceral and subcutaneous adipose tissue in humans. Br J Radiol 2012;85(1018):e826–30.

[181] Mitsiopoulos N, et al. Cadaver validation of skeletal muscle measurement by magnetic resonance imaging and computerized tomography. J Appl Physiol 1998;85(1):115–22.

[182] Barnouin Y, et al. Manual segmentation of individual muscles of the quadriceps femoris using MRI: a reappraisal. J Magn Reson Imag 2014;40(1):239–47.

[183] Ogier A, et al. Individual muscle segmentation in MR images: a 3D propagation through 2D non-linear registration approaches. Annu Int Conf IEEE Eng Med Biol Soc 2017;2017:317–20.

[184] Baudin PY, et al. Discriminative parameter estimation for random walks segmentation. Med Image Comput Comput Assist Interv 2013;16(Pt 3):219–26.

[185] Baudin PY, et al. Prior knowledge, random walks and human skeletal muscle segmentation. Med Image Comput Comput Assist Interv 2012;15(Pt 1):569–76.

[186] Gilles B, Magnenat-Thalmann N. Musculoskeletal MRI segmentation using multi-resolution simplex meshes with medial representations. Med Image Anal 2010;14(3):291–302.

[187] Karlsson A, et al. Automatic and quantitative assessment of regional muscle volume by multi-atlas segmentation using whole-body water-fat MRI. J Magn Reson Imag 2015;41(6):1558–69.

[188] Prescott JW, et al. Anatomically anchored template-based level set segmentation: application to quadriceps muscles in MR images from the Osteoarthritis Initiative. J Digit Imag 2011;24(1):28–43.

[189] Le Troter A, et al. Volume measurements of individual muscles in human quadriceps femoris using atlas-based segmentation approaches. Magma 2016;29(2):245–57.

[190] Nasel C, et al. Advanced analysis of the water/fat distribution in skeletal muscle tissue using magnetic resonance imaging in patients with neuromuscular disease. Front Physiol 2020;8:195.

[191] Krssak M, et al. Proton magnetic resonance spectroscopy in skeletal muscle: experts' consensus recommendations. NMR Biomed 2021;34(5):e4266.

[192] Furuyama JK, et al. A pilot validation of multi-echo based echo-planar correlated spectroscopic imaging in human calf muscles. NMR Biomed 2014;27(10):1176–83.

[193] Howald H, et al. Content of intramyocellular lipids derived by electron microscopy, biochemical assays, and (1)H-MR spectroscopy. J.Appl.-Physiol 2002;92(6):2264–72.

[194] Ren J, Sherry AD, Malloy CR. 1H MRS of intramyocellular lipids in soleus muscle at 7 T: spectral simplification by using long echo times without water suppression. Magn Reson Med 2010;64(3):662–71.

[195] Skoch A, et al. Intramyocellular lipid quantification from 1H long echo time spectra at 1.5 and 3 T by means of the LCModel technique. J.Magn Reson.Imag 2006;23(5):728–35.

[196] Bredella MA, et al. Comparison of 3.0 T proton magnetic resonance spectroscopy short and long echo-time measures of intramyocellular lipids in obese and normal-weight women. J Magn Reson Imag 2010;32(2):388–93.

[197] Provencher SW. Automatic quantitation of localized in vivo 1H spectra with LCModel. NMR Biomed 2001;14(4):260–4.

[198] Naressi A, et al. Java-based graphical user interface for the MRUI quantitation package. Magma 2001;12(2–3):141–52.

[199] Vanhamme L, van den Boogaart A, Van Huffel S. Improved method for accurate and efficient quantification of MRS data with use of prior knowledge. J Magn Reson 1997;129(1):35–43.

[200] Machann J, et al. Intra- and interindividual variability of fatty acid unsaturation in six different human adipose tissue compartments assessed by (1) H-MRS in vivo at 3 T. NMR Biomed 2017;30(9).

[201] Thankamony A, et al. Compositional marker in vivo reveals intramyocellular lipid turnover during fasting-induced lipolysis. Sci Rep 2018;8(1):2750.

[202] Forsberg AM, et al. Muscle composition in relation to age and sex. Clin Sci (Lond) 1991;81(2):249−56.

[203] Mingrone G, et al. Unreliable use of standard muscle hydration value in obesity. Am J Physiol Endocrinol Metab 2001;280(2):E365−71.

[204] Krssak M, et al. 1H NMR relaxation times of skeletal muscle metabolites at 3 T. Magma 2004;16(4):155−9.

[205] Lindeboom L, et al. Long-echo time MR spectroscopy for skeletal muscle acetylcarnitine detection. J Clin Invest 2014;124(11):4915−25.

[206] Baguet A, et al. Important role of muscle carnosine in rowing performance. J Appl Physiol 2010;109(4):1096−101.

[207] Klepochova R, et al. Detection and alterations of acetylcarnitine in human skeletal muscles by 1H MRS at 7 T. Invest Radiol 2017;52(7):412−8.

[208] Just Kukurova I, et al. Improved spectral resolution and high reliability of in vivo (1) H MRS at 7 T allow the characterization of the effect of acute exercise on carnosine in skeletal muscle. NMR Biomed 2016;29(1):24−32.

[209] Ren J, et al. Dynamic monitoring of carnitine and acetylcarnitine in the trimethylamine signal after exercise in human skeletal muscle by 7T 1H-MRS. Magn Reson Med 2013;69(1):7−17.

[210] Machann J, et al. Intramyocellular lipids and insulin resistance. Diab Obes.Metab 2004;6(4):239−48.

Chapter 12

Bone marrow adipose tissue

Bénédicte Gaborit[1,2], Sonia Severin[3] and Philippe Valet[4]

[1]Aix Marseille Univ, INSERM, INRAE, C2VN, Marseille, France; [2]Department of Endocrinology, Metabolic Diseases and Nutrition, Pôle ENDO, APHM, Marseille, France; [3]INSERM U1048 and Paul Sabatier University, Institute of Cardiovascular and Metabolic Diseases, Toulouse, France; [4]Restore UMR 1301 Inserm, 5070 CNRS, Université Paul Sabatier, Toulouse, France

Abbreviations

ALL Acute lymphocytic leukemia
AMARES Advanced Method for Accurate, Robust and Efficient Spectral fitting
AML Acute Myeloid Leukemia
AN Anorexia Nervosa
BADGE Bisphenol A DiGlycidyl Ether
BM Bone Marrow
BMAT Bone Marrow Adipose Tissue
BMD Bone Mineral Density
BMFF Bone Marrow Fat Fraction,
c/EBP CCAAT-Enhancer-Binding Protein
CLL Chronic Lymphocytic Leukemia
CML Chronic Myeloid Leukemia
CMP Common Myeloid Progenitors
CV Coefficient of Variation
CXCL C-X-C Motif Chemokine Ligand
DECT Dual-energy Computed Tomography
DPP4 Dipeptidyl peptidase-4
EV Extracellular Vesicles
FABP4 Fatty Acid Binding Protein-4
GFP Green Fluorescence Protein
^{1}H-MRS Proton magnetic resonance spectroscopy
HFD High Fat Diet
HSC Hematopoietic Stem Cell
ICC Interclass Correlation Coefficient
IDEAL Iterative Decomposition with Echo Asymmetry and Least squares estimation
IDL Interactive Data Language
IL Interleukin
LSK Lin-Sca+Kit+
MALP Mesenchymal cell population-marrow Adipogenic Lineage Precursors
MEP Megakaryocyte-Erythroid Progenitors
MIP Macrophage Inflammatory Protein
MM Multiple Myeloma
MPP MultiPotent Progenitors
MRI Magnetic Resonance Imaging
MSC Mesenchymal Stromal Cell
PPAR Peroxisome Proliferator-activated Receptor
PRESS PointResolved Spectroscopy
PTH1R ParaThyroid Hormone Receptor 1

169

PTHR ParaThyroid Hormone Receptor
RANKL Receptor Activator of Nuclear factor- κB Ligand
RNA RiboNucleotide Acid
SCF Stem Cell Factor
SECT Single-Energy Computed Tomography
STEAM Stimulated Echo Acquisition Mode
STIRShort Tau Inversion Recovery
T1D Type 1 Diabetes
T2D Type 2 Diabetes
TNF Tumor Necrosis Factor
UCP Uncoupling Protein

Introduction

Bone marrow adipose tissue (BMAT) has been considered for a long time as a silent bystander that fills the bone marrow (BM) cavity when bone mass was low or hematopoiesis impaired. Over the past decades, interest in the functional role of BMAT has gradually increased and recently new findings revealed this adipose tissue as a secretory and metabolically active organ distinct from extramedullary adipose depots. Indeed, BM adipocytes (BMAs) reside in the BM in close contact with bone, hematopoietic cells, marrow stromal cells, nerves, and blood vessels. BMAT thus refers to BM areas where BMA are the predominant cell type [1−3]. Within BM, osteoblasts and adipocytes arise from a common mesenchymal stem cell. BMAs have been shown to play an active role in the support of neoplastic cells in the BM niche and have been shown to increase with aging, osteoporosis, metabolic diseases, and in anorexia nervosa. BMAT is now recognized as an actor within bone microenvironment, implicated in whole-body energy metabolism, hematopoiesis, skeletal health, and bone homeostasis [4,5]. Noninvasive imaging techniques, such as magnetic resonance imaging (MRI) or proton magnetic resonance spectroscopy (^{1}H-MRS), have considerably increased the understanding of this ectopic fat depot and opened new horizons to predict bone fragility and anemia development [6,7]. Nevertheless, as species-specific differences in BMAT exist, caution needs to be taken when extrapolating information across species.

Bone marrow fat origin

In 1976, Tavassoli revealed, by ultrastructural analysis, that BMA develop from a medullar perivascular progenitor that differs from the "fibroblast-like" phenotype of the extramedullary adipocyte progenitor [8]. Because of the medullar location of those adipocytes, it has been difficult to directly study their characteristics compared to extramedullar adipocytes. BMA originate from a multipotent mesenchymal stromal cell that resides in the perivascular compartment at the endosteal surface in the bone marrow (BM) space. BM MSCs represent a heterogeneous cell population with regard to their cell surface marker expression and differentiation potential toward the osteoblast, adipocyte, or chondrocyte lineages [9] (Fig. 12.1). MSC differentiation into adipocytes is specifically controlled by several regulatory factors, including transcription factors (such as Peroxisome Proliferator-activated Receptor (PPAR) γ and CCAAT-enhancer-binding protein (c/EBP) α) and soluble mediators (as adiponectin and leptin, for example) (see section "Secretory profile and endocrine regulation of BMAT") [10].

Recently, lineage tracing analysis (by fluorescence-activated cell sorting or fluorescence imaging using transgenic mouse models displaying the fluorescent *mT/mG* reporter driven by the cre-recombinase under the control of lineage-specific promoters) has been key to understanding the origin of BMA. The *Vav1-cre:mT/mG* mice model after BM reconstitution subsequent to a sublethal irradiation allows to show that BMA progenitors are radio-resistant and non-hematopoietic cells that reside in bones and do not come from the circulation [11−14]. Also, it is becoming clearer that BMA arise from a different lineage from that of extramedullar white and brown adipocytes. BMA fail to express the cell surface marker profile of white adipocyte progenitors (Lin$^-$; CD29$^+$; CD34$^+$; Sca1$^+$; PdgfRα$^+$; with or without CD24) [15]. In *Pdgrβ-cre: mT/mG* mice in which all white adipocytes were eGFP-traced, only half of the BMA are eGFP-labeled [15]. *Myf5-cre:mT/mG* mice that display a brown adipocyte eGFP-tracing do not express eGFP in all BM [13,16]. However, RNA-seq analysis shows that several genes enriched in BM-resident adipocyte precursors are also expressed in committed brown pre-adipocytes (e.g., Ebf2, Entpd2, Fam129a, and *Acy3*), which would support at least some potential similarities to the brown adipose tissue lineage [17−19]. Inversely, knowing that Prrx1 and Osterix 1 are markers of early mesenchymal progenitors, in *Prrx1-cre:mT/mG* or *Osx-cre:mT/mG* mouse models, all BMA were eGFP-labeled whereas at the periphery only few peripheral white adipocytes were eGFP-traced [13,20,21]. Schulz laboratory identified by cell

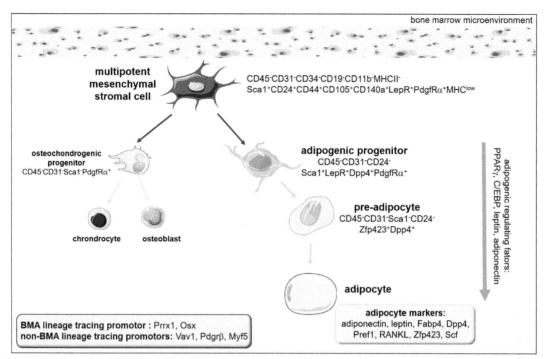

FIGURE 12.1 Bone marrow adipocyte origin. In the bone marrow, multipotent mesenchymal stromal cells have the capacity to differentiate both into osteochondrogenic progenitors and adipogenic progenitors. $CD45^-CD31^-Sca1^-PdgfR\alpha^+$ osteochondrogenic progenitors differentiate into chondrocytes or osteoblasts. $CD45^-CD31^-CD24^-Sca1^+LepR^+Dpp4^+PdgfR\alpha^+$ adipocyte progenitors give rise to $CD45^-CD31^-Sca1^-CD24^-Zfp423^+Dpp4^+$ pre-adipocytes that finally differentiate in adipocytes under the influence of transcriptional factors (PPARγ et C/EBP) and soluble factors (as leptin and adiponectin). Transgenic mouse models expressing the fluorescent mT/mG reporter drived by the cre-recombinase under the control of lineage-specific promoters) allow the BMA and non-BMA lineage tracing.

sorting lineage tracing a developmental hierarchy pattern composed of three different populations of BM adipocyte progenitor cells: a multipotent perivascular osteogenic/adipocyte stem cell-like cell population ($CD45^-CD31^-Sca1^+PdgfR\alpha^+CD24^+$) that unilaterally commit to either adipogenic or osteoblastic lineage, a fate-committed progenitor cell population toward adipogenic lineage ($CD45^-CD31^-Sca1^+PdgfR\alpha^+CD24^-$), and a subsequent mature $CD45^-CD31^-Sca1^-Zfp423^+$ preadipocyte precursor cells [19] (Fig. 12.1). Moreover, BMA can derive from a Osterix$^+$, LrpR$^+$, Nestin$^+$ MSC population that do not express Gremlin 1, a marker of MSCs which give rise to osteoblasts, chondrocytes, myofibroblasts, or reticular marrow stromal cells but not adipocytes [22−28]. Further characterization related to BMA origin is needed in view of the apparent heterogeneous profiles.

Main characteristics in physiology

Main characteristics

BMAT is situated within the marrow cavity in an organized manner, constituting 70% of BM volume and accounting for approximately 5%−10% of total fat mass in healthy adult humans [29−31]. BMAT show a similar distribution in rodents and other animals, predominating in the arms and legs but being scarce in the spine and more central skeleton [30]. Remarkably, women display less BMAT compared with age-matched men prior the menopause age, while the following period is associated with a marked increase of BM adiposity [32,33].

Variation during growth

BM adiposity development has been shown to be age, bone site, and gender dependent [29]. At birth, bone cavities are mainly filled with red hematopoietic marrow. Red marrow comprises 60% hematopoietic cells and 40% fat cells whereas yellow marrow contains approximately 95% fat cells and 5% nonfat cells [34]. BMAT formation then occurs in a centripetal way shortly before birth and the replacement of hematopoietic marrow by adipose marrow is initiated in the terminal phalanges. However, in the femur and the tibia the appearance of BMAT starts later around the age of seven and is complete by the age of 18 (Fig. 12.2A). In the vertebrae and ribs, BMAT is not detected until late. By the age of 25 years, BMAT is considered to represent 70% of the BM volume while hematopoietic BM is mainly restricted to the axial skeleton, ribs, sternum, and proximal metaphysis of long bones. Afterward, the BM conversion into BMAT slowly progresses throughout the adulthood. In a given long bone, yellow marrow is preferentially located in the diaphysis and epiphysis whereas red marrow is mainly localized in the metaphysis [35] (Fig. 12.2A).

The development pattern in rodents is similar to that in humans. Histological studies of femur or tibia show the presence of BMAT at adult age, which further increases with aging [36]. Of note, the percentage of BM adiposity appears low in rodents when compared with humans and varies according to the mouse strain.

Variation with aging

In healthy adults, marrow adiposity increases with aging. MRI studies in healthy adults have shown that the marrow adiposity of the lumbar spine increases approximately 7% per decade from 30% at age 30 to >50% at the age of 60 years [33,37]. During these years BMAT is 10% greater in men than in women but this difference reverses after menopause [38,39] (Fig. 12.2B). Indeed, an accelerated fatty conversion of BM was observed in females with increasing age particularly evident after menopause. Baum et al., using chemical shift encoding-based water−fat MRI, showed that these relative age-related vertebral proton density fat fraction (PDFF) changes displayed an anatomical variation with most pronounced modifications at lower lumbar vertebral levels in both sexes [40]. In the femur, marrow adiposity also increases with age but is higher at younger age starting at 60% in the diaphysis and 67% in the femoral neck in women at age 20−30, increasing to 76% and 81%, respectively, at age 50−60 [32]. After reaching a peak between the age of 15−30 years, bone mass declines with aging. In men, this decline is gradual whereas in women the decline accelerates post-menopause. The increase in BMA with age correlates with age-related bone loss (see Section "BMAT and skeletal health").

All in all, BMAT appears in the BM cavity shortly before birth and expands during skeleton growth in childhood and adolescence in a distal-to-proximal way, replacing the hematopoietic marrow almost completely in the long bones when reaching peak bone mass by the age of 20−30. During aging, vertebral BMAT continues to increase but bone mass decreases (Fig. 12.2B). Men have higher marrow adiposity than women, but this difference reverses after menopause, implying that marrow adiposity is, at least partially, hormonally controlled. Further studies are needed to elucidate the exact role of marrow adiposity in growth and development [2].

Regional specific differences in BMAT composition

Historic and recent observations in rabbits, mice, and humans support the concept that BMAT undergoes differential development and regulation depending on where it is located in the skeleton [41,42]. Using osmium tetroxide staining and microcomputed tomography Scheller et al. nicely reported the first characterization of two BMAT subpopulations in rodents (Fig. 12.3):

− constitutive BMAT (cBMAT) which arises first and early in life in distal tibia and caudal vertebrae has low hematopoiesis, contains large adipocytes, and remains preserved upon systemic challenges.
− regulated BMAT (rBMAT) whose formation is late, increases with age, and occurs in a more scattered way (as single adipocytes interspersed with active hematopoiesis) in the proximal tibia, distal femur, and lumbar vertebrae [42].

FIGURE 12.2 (A) Physiological replacement of hematopoietic marrow by adipose marrow in the femur. (B) Sex related changes in bone mass and BM adiposity with aging.

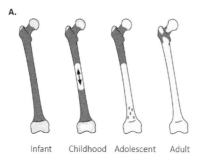

Infant   Childhood   Adolescent   Adult

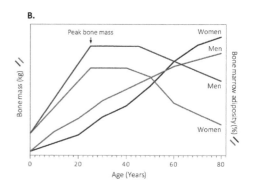

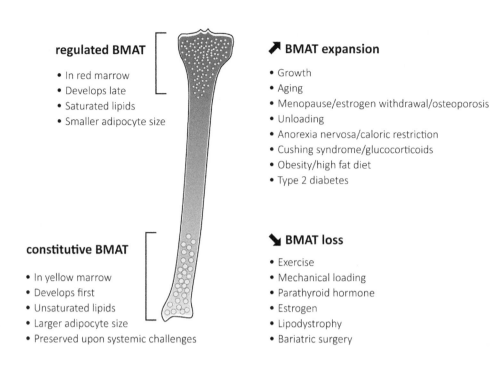

regulated BMAT

- In red marrow
- Develops late
- Saturated lipids
- Smaller adipocyte size

constitutive BMAT

- In yellow marrow
- Develops first
- Unsaturated lipids
- Larger adipocyte size
- Preserved upon systemic challenges

↗ BMAT expansion

- Growth
- Aging
- Menopause/estrogen withdrawal/osteoporosis
- Unloading
- Anorexia nervosa/caloric restriction
- Cushing syndrome/glucocorticoids
- Obesity/high fat diet
- Type 2 diabetes

↘ BMAT loss

- Exercise
- Mechanical loading
- Parathyroid hormone
- Estrogen
- Lipodystrophy
- Bariatric surgery

FIGURE 12.3 Two components of bone marrow fat and factors associated with bone marrow adipose tissue expansion or loss.

Experiments in mice and/or rats have shown that rBMAT adipocytes preferentially develop within the red marrow throughout life, are smaller in size (31–33 mm diameter), contain more saturated lipids, and express lower levels of the adipogenic transcription factors CCAAT/enhancer binding protein alpha and beta (*Cebpa* and *Cebpb*). Conversely, cMAT adipocytes develop shortly after birth, are larger in size (38–39 mm diameter), contain more unsaturated lipids, and have elevated *Cebpa* and *Cebpb*. Although they appear to be developmentally distinct, it is unclear whether they derive from distinct progenitors or instead represent a different state of maturation of the BM adipocyte from a common lineage. How such classification can be extrapolated to humans remains still uncertain.

Effect of exercise and caloric restriction

Voluntary running exercise in rodents was found to lower BMAT and increase bone mass in eucaloric and hypercaloric states while degrading bone mass in caloric restriction states, suggesting differential modulation of BMAT and bone depending on whole-body energy status [43,44]. Liu et al. compared in vitro proliferative, differential, and antiapoptosis abilities of both BM and adipose-derived mesenchymal stromal cells (MSC) derived from exercised and sedentary rats under normal and hypoxia/serum deprivation conditions, and observed that exercise may enhance proliferative ability and decrease adipogenic ability of both MSCs [45]. In vivo studies evidenced decreased adipocyte differentiation and increased preosteoblast formation in the BM of climbing mice and running rats [46–48]. In humans, Bertheau et al. showed using a 2-point T1-weighted VIBE Dixon sequence in 385 subjects without known cardiovascular diseases that exercise was inversely correlated with L1 and L2 vertebral BMAT fat fraction (FF) but not hip BMAT-FF, when exercising for more than 2 h per week [49]. The decrease of BMAT with exercise training in humans was also reported in professional wrestlers compared to untrained men [50]. Recently, Attané et al. showed that BMA displays distinct lipid metabolic properties compared to extramedullar adipocytes, with a cholesterol-orientated metabolism and a decreased lipolytic function due to a decreased monoacylglycerol lipase expression [51]. This could explain the preservation or even the expansion of BMAT under caloric restriction in mice [36,52], rabbits [53,54], and human patients suffering from anorexia nervosa [55,56] except in severe nutrient deprivation [57] and late stages of anorexia nervosa, associated with gelatinous transformation of the BM [55,58].

Impact of unloading

Human studies in women cosmonauts have shown that extended bed rest drives an increased marrow adipogenesis which persists 1 year after the resumption of regular activities (Fig. 12.3) [59]. In the absence of mechanical cues, PPARγ and receptor activator of nuclear factor-Kappa-B ligand (RANKL), which promotes osteoclast-mediated bone resorption, are both elevated indicating an effect that could be stopped upon reintroduction of mechanical stimuli [48]. In animal models, skeletal unloading is also associated with high BMAT and low bone mass [60,61]. Rats exposed to spaceflight or hindlimb unloading (i.e., to simulate the weightlessness experienced during spaceflight) showed impaired bone mineral acquisition and greater BMAT that returned to normal upon reloading. In immunocompromised model of mice, treatment with sclerostin-neutralizing antibody, a bone anabolic agent, prevented rosiglitazone-induced bone loss and reduced BMAT in some but not all BMAT locations [62].

Microscopic aspect

BMA are not grouped in lobules as in the other ectopic fat depots, but they are dispersed within the hematopoietic tissue. Adipocytes often appear as distinct, translucent, yellow elliptical cells in the marrow cavity. Their diameter can vary from 40 to 65 μm according to the fat infiltration, the site, or the age (hypertrophia increasing with age) [29,63]. Their size is in general smaller than that of subcutaneous and visceral adipocytes in humans and rodents and rBMAT being smaller than cBMA (Fig. 12.3) [64]. In usual optic microscopy of undecalcified bone, the preparation of the sample removes lipid content, then the shapes of adipocytes appear as cellular "ghosts." BMA can be also studied with confocal microscopy or on frozen slides or by microtomography after labeling with osmium [35,65]. Indeed, osmium tetroxide is a heavy metal which stains lipid in the adipocytes [66].

In vivo imaging

Because BMAT is inside bone, it makes it is much more difficult to study than other adipose tissues. Historically, bone biopsies were performed at the iliac crest to assess bone health and these biopsies included the marrow space in which adipocytes ghosts were seen. This difficulty contributes to the scarcity of data and has prompted the development of new noninvasive imaging tools to study BMAT. Recently, the international BM adiposity Society has created a Nomenclature and a Methodologies Working Group to standardize the terminology and methods used in the BMAT research literature [3,67]. To date, MRI is considered as the gold standard to evaluate in vivo BMAT and the best method to distinguish yellow fat marrow from hematopoietic red marrow [3,68]. A summary of imaging modalities available for BMAT quantification is presented in Table 12.1.

Computed tomography

Low resolution and consequent partial voluming, beam hardening artifacts, and high radiation doses are the limitations of CT-based quantification of BM fat.

Single-energy CT (SECT)

Computed tomography (CT) uses X-rays to obtain images based on tissue attenuation. The tissue density passed by the X-ray beam is defined by the attenuation coefficient, a measure of how easily a material can be penetrated by an X-ray beam. The CT density of tissue is expressed in Hounsfield Units (HU), obtained from a linear transformation of attenuation coefficients based on the arbitrary definitions of air (−1000 HU) and water (0 HU). On this scale, fat density ranged from −60 to −120 HU [6,69,70]. The BM cavity has three components: the trabecular bone, the hematopoietic tissue, and the adipose tissue. Hence, CT density assessment does not allow for specific quantification of BMAT or bone mineral density (BMD) [71]. Besides, beam hardening and the preferential loss of lower-energy photons from a polychromatic X-ray beam cause SECT to underestimate the amount of fat in the marrow cavity of long bones, and create alterations of the attenuation profile of the medullary cavity [72]. Bean hardening leads to BMAT not being seen by the X-rays hardened by surrounding radio-dense bone [7]. However, the lower the HU is, the higher fat content is [6]. SECT is most helpful when applied in specific anatomic locations, devoid of trabecular bone such as the mid-diaphysis of long bone. Indeed, CT density measurement provides a better approximation of BMAT in this location [72−74].

Dual-energy CT (DECT)

In DECT, element-specific energy-dependent attenuation coefficients can be used to differentiate elements with different atomic numbers from one another [75]. It is also possible to quantify fat compared to other tissues in this manner. The various energy spectra that are needed can be generated by sequential scans with a high and low tube voltage, by two

TABLE 12.1 Summary of imaging modalities available for BMAT quantification.

Technique	Advantages	Limitations	Artifacts and technical considerations	Clinical applications
Single energy CT	– Relatively widely available	– Ionizing radiation – CT density does not distinguish the 3 components (yellow, red or bone)	– Beam hardening	– Marrow replacing disorders – Radiation therapy follow-up
Dual-energy CT	– Good agreement with histology and ¹H-MRS – Assessment of BMD and BMAT in a single examination	– Ionizing radiation	B-eam hardening	– Bone health after cancer therapy
Conventional T1-weighted MRI	– Part of routine clinical care – Reliable and accurate – No ionizing radiation	– Limited availability – Mainly qualitative assessment – Unable to assess BMAT composition	– Partial volume effects	– Diseases of BM
Water-fat imaging	- No ionizing radiation – Multiple-site assessment (spine, femur) – Great agreement with ¹H-MRS for quantification of BMAT – Relatively short acquisition	– No qualitative assessment of BMAT – Requires post-processing assessment	– Multiple peaks in the fat spectrum – *T1 bias – Susceptibility artifact from trabecular bone T2* decay effects	– Emerging technique for BMAT composition all clinical applications (metabolic, bone, malignancies)
¹H-MRS	– Gold standard for in vivo BMAT quantification – Both qualitative (saturated/unsaturated) and quantitative – Excellent agreement with histology – No ionizing radiation	– Requires post-processing analysis – Limited area of evaluation (single voxel) – Relatively long acquisition for multiple skeletal regions	– Susceptibility artifact from trabecular bone (water and fat peaks overlap) specially in case of a strong water peak	– Emerging technique for BMAT composition all clinical applications (metabolic, bone, skeletal integrity, fracture risk assessment)

separate tube detector systems (dual-source DECT), or with an X-ray tube that switches in milliseconds between high and low voltage (fast-kVp-switching DECT). In BM, DECT fat quantification allows more valid quantification of BMD than conventional methods. The differences in attenuation between the high and low energy beams are the basis for which DECT identifies the composition of different tissues [6]. Recent studies in healthy volunteers and necropsies have quantified marrow adipose tissue content which correlated closely with BMAT quantified by histology and ^{1}H-MRS [76,77]. An advantage of DECT is the assessment of BMD and BMAT content in a single examination [6]. Moreover, studies have suggested that intravertebral BMAT can affect the accuracy of BMD measurements obtained by SECT, therefore, the assessment of MAT by DECT is important for the accurate assessment of BMD in states of increased marrow adiposity by correcting the BMD with BMAT [77]. Complementary studies regarding DECT fat quantification by split-filter DECT or dual-layer spectral CT should be conducted [78].

Magnetic resonance imaging

MRI has become the preferred imaging method for evaluating diseases of or associated with BM [3,7,79]. MRI-based BMAT quantification techniques are noninvasive and facilitate imaging of large volumes of interest in different anatomical regions. It has thus been proposed as a reliable and accurate method to investigate the association between bone loss and BM adiposity.

T1-weighted MRI

MRI images are typically acquired based on the proportion of hydrogen atoms within a tissue. Therefore, the major determinants of the MRI appearance of BM are its fat and water content. T1-weighted spin-echo or fast spine-echo sequences are most suitable to assess BMAT given the high fat content of BM. Most fat protons within BM are residing in aliphatic (-CH2-) chains of triglycerides, facilitating T1-relaxation and resulting in T1 shortening [80]. Therefore, BMAT appears hyperintense (bright) on T1-weighted images and follows the signal intensity of the subcutaneous adipose tissue. On fat-suppressed or fluid-sensitive sequences (short tau inversion recovery (STIR) sequences, fat-suppressed T2-, or proton density-weighted) BMAT is lower in signal intensity than muscle [6]. While T1-weighted MRI is primarily used in clinical practice to assess the physiologic or pathologic appearance of BM, and to rule out BM replacement in patients with cancer, it has been used for semiquantitative measurements of BMAT volume [81]. The intra- and interobserver reproducibility for the assessment of BM fat volume in T1-weighted images were reported to be 1% (intraobserver) and 2.6% (interobserver) [82]. The main source of error for the calculation of BM fat volume based on T1-weighted MRI results from partial volume effects and threshold selection, especially in regions with red marrow [83]. However, T1-weighted MRI measurements of BMAT were found to correlate with different water fat imaging techniques, such as the iterative decomposition with echo asymmetry and least squares estimation (IDEAL) technique, and the Dixon method in adults and children [82,84].

Water-fat imaging

Water-fat imaging, also referred to as chemical shift-encoding-based water-fat imaging, Dixon, IDEAL or fat fraction method, represents an MRI-based method that generates water and fat images. Separation of water and fat signal is based on the chemical shift difference between water and fat resonance frequencies and can provide a quantitative measurement of the signal fraction of both water and fat [40,85]. Chemical shift encoding-based water-fat imaging allows the spatially resolved assessment of the BM fat fraction (BMFF), allowing for assessment of multiple vertebrae, pelvis or proximal femurs in a single acquisition [83]. High-resolution BMFF mapping is highly beneficial in regions with heterogeneous distribution of BMAT (proximal femur, spine) [68]. An advantage of water-fat imaging is its short acquisition time and widely availability, with a good 10-times reproducibility (coefficient of variance from 0.69% to 1.70%) [86]. However, several confounding factors have to be considered when measuring BMFF by using water-fat imaging, including the presence of multiple peaks in the fat spectrum, T1-bias, and T2*-decay effects [83]. The presence of trabecular bone most importantly shortens the T2* of water and fat components, inducing a rapid decay of the measured gradient echo signal with echo time [87]. After correcting for T2* decay effects, a good agreement was reported in vivo between ^{1}H-MRS-based and imaging-based BMFF in both spine and the proximal femur [87,88]. Ex vivo studies comparing water-fat imaging with phantoms or trabecular bone specimens have shown excellent agreement between BMFF quantification and histology [89−91].

Proton magnetic resonance spectroscopy ^{1}H-MRS

Proton magnetic resonance spectroscopy (^{1}H-MRS) is considered as the gold standard for in vivo BM fat quantification [6,83]. It can provide both quantitative (BMFF) and qualitative (BMAT composition) information and has proven to be reliable and accurate in different regions including the spine and the hip [70,92]. Point-resolved spectroscopy (PRESS) and stimulated echo acquisition mode (STEAM) single-voxel ^{1}H-MRS pulse sequences are the two commonly used sequences to obtain fat spectra at various skeletal sites [68] (Fig. 12.4). The BMFF can be calculated as a fat/water ratio and expressed as a percentage using the formula BMFF (%) = Ifat/(Ifat + Iwater) × 100, where I refers to the fat or water peak area under the curve obtained from postprocessing software such as Advanced Method for Accurate, Robust and Efficient Spectral fitting (AMARES) [93]. BMAT measured by ^{1}H-MRS has been shown to correlate closely with BMAT content from biopsies [94] and showed excellent short-term (baseline, 6 weeks CV = 9.9% interclass correlation coefficient (ICC = 0.97 (95% CI 0.94−099)) and long-term reproducibilities (baseline, 6 months CV = 12% ICC = 0.95) (95% CI 0.88 to 0.98) for follow-up [95]. Furthermore, 7T studies provide promising results by improving chemical shift dispersion compared to 1.5 or 3.0 T [96].

^{1}H-MRS can not only quantify the amount of BMAT but also assess its composition, such as the amount of unsaturated and saturated lipids, which may serve as biomarkers of skeletal integrity [96−98]. BM fatty acids can be quantified based on the number of double bonds that they carry. Higher magnetic field strengths allow the visualization of additional lipid peaks of fatty acid saturation and unsaturation estimates: olefinic protons at 5.3 ppm (−CH=CH−), an estimate of fatty acid unsaturated bonds; bulk methylene protons at 1.3 ppm [(−CH$_2$−)n], an estimate of fatty acids saturated bonds [6,70]. The degree of unsaturation can be determined by the unsaturation index, a ratio between the olefinic resonance and total lipid content [97,98]. However, susceptibility effects from the trabecular bone can cause significant overlapping of water and olefinic peaks, presenting a technical challenge for quantification of lipid unsaturation, especially in the presence of a strong water peak (i.e., in the spine) [83]. Nevertheless, ^{1}H-MRS remains an emerging noninvasive technique for BMAT composition assessment.

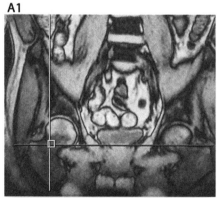

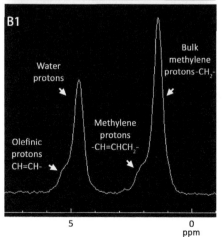

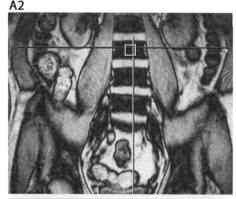

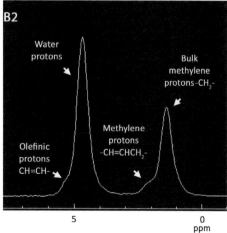

FIGURE 12.4 Quantitative and qualitative BM fat assessment using proton magnetic resonance spectroscopy 1H-MRS. Representative images of voxel location within the proximal femur (A), and the third lumbar vertebral body (B). Representative spectra of water and lipid peaks (B1 (femur) -B2 (spine)). The area under the curve of the lipid and water peaks are used to calculate the lipid to water ratio using semi-automatic method (AMARES) Advanced Method for Accurate, Robust and Efficient Spectral fitting) implemented under an Interactive Data Language (IDL) environment. Unsaturated lipids corresponding to olefinic protons (double bond −CH=CH−); Residual lipids corresponding to methylene protons (α-to a double bond −CH=CHCH2−) and saturated lipids corresponding to bulk methylene protons (CH2−).

Secretory profile and endocrine regulation of BMAT

The secretory profile of BMAT and its functional endocrine and paracrine implications remain largely undetermined. However, there is no evidence from gene expression studies that any of the adipokines secreted from white adipose tissue are not expressed by BMAT [29,99]. However, differences in relative expression and/or secretion of proteins from white adipose tissue and BMAT exist, and likely reflect the distinctive functions and properties of each ectopic fat depot. The adipokines, adiponectin, and leptin are detected in isolated mature BMAT [52,100,101]. Nevertheless, their mRNA expression levels were found low compared with extramedullary adipocytes in healthy adult bone marrow donors or 6-month healthy mice [102,103]. Regarding leptin, this may simply reflect the smaller size of BMA [99]. Alternatively, this could reflect that BMA are in an earlier stage of differentiation as suggested by an increase in the expression of C/EBPb, regulator of G-protein signaling 2 (RGS2), and perilipin 2 (Plin2) [103] compared to epididymal adipocytes [103]. Remarkably, BMAT explants from rabbits or human patients were shown to secrete more adiponectin than other white adipose tissue depots. Caloric restriction in rodents and humans showed elevation of circulating adiponectin despite white adipose tissue loss [52]. However, this could be explained by BMAT expansion during caloric restriction [57]. To determine whether BMAT contributes to circulating adiponectin with caloric restriction, Cawthorn et al. inhibited BMAT expansion by overexpressing the Wnt10b transgene (which potently inhibits adipogenesis) from the osteocalcin promoter in mice (OCN−Wnt10b) and showed that inhibition of BMAT expansion was sufficient to suppress caloric restriction-associated hyperadiponectinemia [52]. These observations support the ability of BMAT to function as an endocrine organ and to modulate metabolism at the systemic level in the context of caloric restriction (Fig. 12.5).

Very recently, adipsin has been evidenced as the most upregulated adipokine during BMAT expansion in mice and humans in a PPARγ acetylation-dependent manner [104]. Genetic ablation of adipsin in mice specifically inhibited BMAT expansion, and improved bone mass during caloric restriction, thiazolidinedione treatment, and aging. These effects were mediated through its downstream effector, complement component C3, to prime common progenitor cells toward adipogenesis rather than osteoblastogenesis through inhibiting Wnt/β-catenin signaling [104] (Fig. 12.5).

BMAT secreted factors have been analyzed in conditioned media from three types of cell preparations: isolated bone MSC that are in vitro differentiated to adipocytes, primary BMA purified by collagenase digestion, and whole BMAT explants [105]. In vitro, human adipocytes derived from sternal MSC and primary human adipocytes have been found to secrete the cytokines interleukin (IL)-6, tumor necrosis factor (TNFα), macrophage inflammatory protein (MIP)-1/, G-CSF,

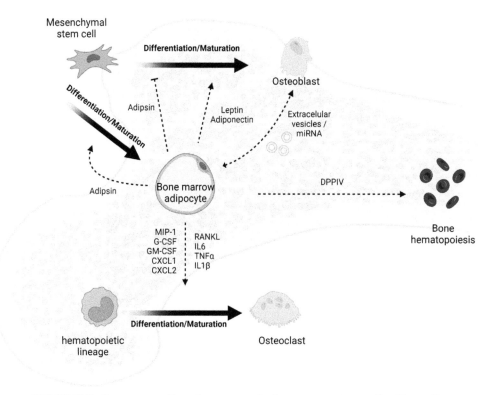

FIGURE 12.5 Bone marrow adipose tissue as an endocrine organ, secretory profile of bone adipocytes.

and GM-CSF [106,107]. In mice, in vitro MSC-derived adipocytes also produce chemokines such as CXCL1 and CXCL2, ligands of CXCR2 receptor, that could accelerate osteoclast maturation and progression of skeletal tumors in bone [108]. BMAT is also sensitive to a proinflammatory environment, as BMA were reported to express inflammatory genes, such as TNFα, IL-6, and IL-1β at higher levels than visceral adipocytes [103]. In this context, IL-1β, IL-6, TNFα, and interferon γ significantly inhibit gene expression and secretion of leptin by BMA [109]. The receptor activator of nuclear factor-kB (NF-kB) ligand (RANKL) has been defined as a protein produced by osteoblasts. Recently it has been shown to be also expressed by BMAT and contributes to ovariectomized-induced bone loss and activation of osteoclasts [110]. Blocking of RANKL production by mesenchymal cell population-marrow adipogenic lineage precursors (MALP) prevented bone loss [111] (Fig. 12.5).

More recently, adipocytes have been described to release extracellular vesicles (EVs) that could influence MSC differentiation routes. Martin et al., in a coculture model of MSC-derived adipocytes and MSC-derived osteoblasts, showed RNA and miRNA transfer from MSc-derived adipocytes to osteoblasts through EVs, i.e., PPARγ, leptin, CEBPα, and CEBPδ transcripts as well as the antiosteoblastic miR-138, miR30c, miR125a, miR-125b, miR-31 miRNAs [112] (Fig. 12.5).

Recent transcriptomic analyses revealed that BMAT is functionally distinct from white and brown adipose tissues, does not express uncoupling protein (UCP) 1 and is not activated by cold [113], has impaired glucose metabolism, and decreased insulin responsiveness [31]. Besides, in humans, positron emission tomography-computed tomography (PET/CT) with 18F-fluorodeoxyglucose interestingly revealed that basal glucose uptake in BMAT was greater than in axial bones, subcutaneous fat, or skeletal muscle, underscoring the potential of BMAT to influence systemic glucose homeostasis [31]. Furthermore, Ambrosi et al. reported that BMAT secretes dipeptidyl peptidase-4 (DPP4), a protease that is a target of diabetes therapies that increase with aging and obesity and causes impairment of bone healing and hematopoietic stem cell (HSC) restoration [19] (Fig. 12.5).

From an endocrine point of view, bone and BMAT metabolism are tightly linked (see section "BMAT and skeletal health"). BMAT is under extensive hormonal regulation. Estradiol is an important regulator of BMAT, and early animal studies have demonstrated that ovariectomy increases BMAT [114]. Ovariectomy is thus commonly used in experimental studies to induce BMAT expansion. These observations have been extended to humans, as BMAT increases during aging and this increase is accelerated in women after menopause (Fig. 12.3) [40]. Postmenopausal hormonal replacement therapy with oral 17-β or transdermal estradiol decreases BMAT in women showing that indeed estradiol is a key player in BMAT endocrine regulation [115,116]. In addition to sex hormones, glucocorticoids have a profound effect on body fat distribution. Using ^{1}H-MRS, we first demonstrated that patients with Cushing syndrome that results from chronic exposure to excess glucocorticoids have increased BMAT in the femoral neck and L3 vertebrae compared to healthy controls and cured patients (average remission time 43 months) matched for age and sex [93]. Parathyroid hormone, an important regulator of calcium metabolism and potent osteoanabolic drug, also influences BMAT. Teriparatide treatment in osteopenic women and in ovariectomized and tail-suspended rats reduces BMAT [117,118] and other studies showed that this effect can be induced by genetic deletion of the parathyroid hormone PTH receptor (PTH1R) in MSC (Fig. 12.3) [119].

BMAT and skeletal health

In humans, cross-sectional studies using different methods show an inverse correlation between marrow adipose tissue mass and bone quality, with high medullar adipocyte content resulting in bone density loss. In healthy young people, MAT was found to be negatively correlated with the amount of bone in the axial and appendicular skeleton [73,74]. In African, American, and Caucasian healthy adults, a negative relationship existed between MRI-measured BMAT and hip and lumbar bone density [120,121]. In aging, obesity, menopause, anorexia, or glucocorticoid treatment, osteoporosis and fracture risk were often inversely associated to diffuse or local BM fat accumulation (Fig. 12.3) [122–126]. In postmenopausal women, bone fractures were associated to a low unsaturation and a high saturation of marrow fat whereas a switch toward unsaturated fatty acids is observed in BM serum [97,98,127]. This is correlated with the observation that saturated fatty acids impair osteoblastogenesis and enhance adipogenesis [128,129]. Therefore, the correlation between BMAT and BMD is often cited as a negative regulator of bone mass and BMAT expansion appears to be a relevant marker of a compromised bone integrity.

However, this correlation does not uniformly hold as for subjects with metabolic disorders such obesity and type 2 diabetes (T2D) that have higher MAT but also higher femoral neck bone density [130] or for rodents. For instance, C3H/HeJ mice have high bone density and a high number of BMA, whereas B6 mice have very low trabecular and cortical bone densities and very low number of marrow adipocytes in their long bones [66,131]. However, increased marrow adiposity induced by glucocorticoids or thiazolidinedione treatment in C57BL/6 mice strain is associated to bone loss [132–134].

Caloric restriction or starvation in growing mice leads to an increased accumulation of BM fat and a decreased bone density and increased bone resorption [36]. Inversely, exercise has been shown to increase bone density and decrease bone adiposity [135]. The influence of the medullar adipose tissue on bone mass in a context of high-fat diet (HFD) in rodents also remain controversial and depends on strain, gender, age and the diet composition and duration. A majority of studies associate BMAT expansion to a decreased bone quality with a reduction in bone mass and impaired bone strength in obese mice on HFD [136–140]. However, Scheller et al. show that this increased BMAT that contributes to bone deterioration is not necessary for HFD-induced bone loss [136]. Lecka-Czernik et al. also report that diet-induced obesity is responsible for an initial increase in bone mass followed by an impaired bone formation [141,142]. Meanwhile, Doucette et al. also reported that MAT expansion during diet-induced obesity occurred without any changes in bone phenotype [143]. In lactating mice or mice exposed to cold, high adiposity in the BM does not systematically correlate to bone density loss [144,145]. Also, blocking BMAT expansion in mice does not have any effect on bone integrity [146,147] and a subsequent dietary weight loss after MAT expansion due to obesity does not completely improve the defective skeletal morphology and biomechanics induced by obesity [136].

The link between BMA and bone could be attributed to the common origin of their BM progenitors [9]. The conditional PTH1R deficient mice (*Prx1-Cre:PTH1R^{fl/fl}*) that exhibited a significantly reduced bone mass, high bone resorption, and increased MAT revealed that in the absence of PTH1R signaling, MSCs are prone to differentiate into MAT adipocytes and produce RANKL that results in bone density loss [119]. Leptin/LepR signaling appears to be also a regulator of the balance between adipogenesis and osteogenesis by increasing BM adiposity and inducing low bone mass [26,148,149]. BMA also secrete factors to directly regulate bone remodeling, even without gross changes in BMAT quantity as EVs, adipokines (leptin, adiponectin, etc.), inflammatory factors (IL-6, TNFα, etc.) (see Section "Secretory profile and endocrine regulation of BMAT" and Fig. 12.5). In vitro studies revealed that BMAT can directly inhibit osteoblast proliferation due to the lipotoxicity of fatty acids delivered from adipocytes to osteoblasts and induce osteoblast apoptosis [150–152]. BMAT also contribute to osteoclast differentiation of primary BM cells and secrete chemokines C-X-C Motif Chemokine Ligand (CXCL) 1 and 2, which promoted osteoclast maturation in metastatic prostate cancer [108,153]. In mice treated with rosiglitazone, the increased BM adipose tissue mass enhances osteoclastic activity [133].

BMAT and hematopoiesis

Recent three-dimensional electron microscopy analysis revealed that BMAs are closely associated with erythroblast islands and that a single BM adipocyte interacts with more than 100 hematopoietic cells through direct cell–cell contact and indirect signals [154]. In a pioneer study, Naveiras et al. identified BMAT as a negative regulator of hematopoiesis. In adipocyte-rich BM, Lin-Kit + Sca1 + hematopoietic stem cells (LSK HSCs) and multipotent progenitors (MPP) are reduced in numbers and in their cycling capacity, as also the case for common myeloid progenitors (CMPs), granulocyte-macrophage progenitors (GMPs), and megakaryocyte-erythroid progenitors (MEPs). In a genetically modified lipoatrophic A-ZIP/F1 "fatless" mice, which are incapable of forming adipocytes and in mice treated with PPARγ inhibitor, Bisphenol A DiGlycidyl Ether (BADGE) that inhibits adipogenesis, the loss of BM adipose tissue improved hematopoietic recovery by enhancing LSK engraftment in marrow transplantation experiment after lethal irradiation or chemotherapy [155,156]. In line with these observations, aging and obesity reduced hematopoietic reconstitution capacity following BM transplant whereas a reduced marrow adiposity due to exercise restores hematopoiesis [157]. Indeed, adipocytes might impair hematopoietic repopulation by the secretion of DPP4, an important antidiabetic target [19,158,159] (Fig. 12.5). More recently, in vitro studies show that primary human adipocytes derived from MSCs induced a decline and a subsequent long-term maintenance of HSCs [160] and primary human BMA purified from the iliac crest have the ability to support differentiation of CD34+ hematopoietic progenitor cells [102]. Spindler et al. also observed that adipocytes can support primitive hematopoietic cells in vitro, but thiazolidinedione-induced BMAT overgrowth does not have any impact in HSC frequencies in vivo [161]. Some other studies revealed that BMA are positive regulators for HSC maintenance and hematopoietic regeneration in steady-state hematopoiesis and in metabolic stress contexts as obesity and aging as a source of stem cell factor (SCF) [162–164] Ambrosi et al. also observed that adipogenic transplants of adipogenic-committed progenitor cells (CD45⁻CD31⁻Sca1⁺PdgfRα⁺CD24⁻) or mature CD45⁻CD31⁻Sca1⁻Zfp423⁺ preadipocyte precursor cells into irradiated mice reduced LSK frequencies and impaired hematopoietic repopulation. However, transplantation of the multipotent CD45⁻CD31⁻Sca1⁺CD24⁺ cells to generate adipocytes increases LSK BM recovery, suggesting that the different stage of adipocyte precursors can exert distinct effect on hematopoiesis [19]. Therefore, whether BMAT plays beneficial or detrimental roles in hematopoiesis requires further attention but appears to be experimental model-, differentiation state-, location-, and disease-dependent.

Myelopoiesis and lymphopoiesis are two branches of hematopoiesis besides HSC. It remains controversial regarding the protective or inhibitory role of BMAT in myelopoiesis and lymphopoiesis. By secreting soluble factors, BMAT inhibit B lymphopoiesis [165–167]. In particular, in vitro culture of BM cells with adiponectin, a BMAT-secreted hormone [168], results in a strong inhibitory effect on B lymphopoiesis and a slight enhancement of myelopoiesis [169]. In rodents, obesity also rapidly suppresses B lymphopoiesis by disrupting the supportive capacity of the BM niche and upregulates myelopoiesis [157,170,171]. Indeed, HFD in mice induces a shift of lymphoid to myeloid cell differentiation with an enhanced canonical myeloid gene (*Csf1r*, *Spi1*, *Runx1*) expression and a decreased lymphoid gene (*Flt3*, *Tcf3*, *Ebf1*) expression [172]. An enhancement of lymphopoietic functions has however been observed in an obesity context [173]. Recently, Valet and colleagues showed a role for BMA in megakaryopoiesis and platelet production. Indeed, in vitro coculture of adipocytes with BM hematopoietic progenitors shows that delipidation of adipocytes directly support different maturation stages of the megakaryocyte, the precursors of blood platelets. In a high fat diet mouse model, increased adiposity mass in the BM is associated to an enhanced megakaryocytic maturation and ectopic platelet release [174].

BMAT in cancer

There is accumulating evidence that BMAT plays an active role in generation of a metabolic niche suitable for the proliferation and the survival of malignant blasts in the BM. Both in patients and in rodents, PPARγ agonist therapy that induces adipogenesis rescued healthy hematopoietic output and repressed leukemic growth [175,176]. Meta-analysis of human cohort studies revealed that obesity, inducing a higher BM adiposity mass, is associated with an increased risk of developing acute myeloid leukemia (AML), acute lymphocytic leukemia (ALL), chronic myeloid leukemia (CML), chronic lymphocytic leukemia (CLL), and multiple myeloma (MM) leukemia and relapse [177,178]. In AML, medullar adipocytes within and around the tumor support the proliferation and survival of malignant cells, through a fatty acid transfer from adipocytes to AML blasts via an adipocyte lipolysis activation and the fatty acid binding protein-4 (FABP4) expressed by AML cells [179]. This is correlated to the presence of small adipocytes in the BM predicting poor prognoses in AML [180]. Disturbance of BMAT function by AML cells impaired the myelo-erythropoiesis [176] and chemotherapy that inhibit BM adipogenesis reinforce the efficacy of chemotherapy in AML patients during complete remission [181]. MAT affects T cell-ALL proliferation in vitro and in vivo thereby mediating chemoresistance [182]. Obesity increases the probability of relapse in ALL patients and impairs the efficacy of the chemotherapy as shown in obese mice injected with ALL malignant cells [183], and caloric restriction improves the outcome of B cell-ALL and T cell-ALL [184]. In vitro, BMA from MM femoral biopsies support the proliferation and migration of MM cells and inhibit their apoptosis to protect MM cells from chemotherapy [185,186] by secreting soluble molecules [187]. BMA support the survival of acute monocytic leukemia cells by regulating their fatty acid β oxidation [188].

In breast and prostate cancer, BMAT can be utilized by cancer cells as a lipid source to promote proliferation, migration, and invasion [189,190]. Increasing marrow adipose tissue promotes the progression of osteolytic prostate cancer growth within bone [191]. BMA promote Warburg phenotype of metastatic prostate cancer cells by a metabolic reprogramming of tumor cells via HIF-1α activation [192]. Marrow adipocytes also induce expression of lipid chaperone FABP4, proinflammatory IL-1β, and oxidative stress protein Heme Oxygenase 1 (HMOX-1) in prostatic tumor cells to stimulate their growth and invasiveness [189]. Human primary BMA are able to support the directed migration and homing of prostatic cancer cells to bone in a CCR3-dependent manner by secreting CCL7 [193].

BMAT and metabolic diseases

It has been recognized for a long time that weight loss is associated with bone loss. In anorexia nervosa (AN), a psychiatric disorder characterized by self-induced starvation and low BMI, lumbar and femoral BMAT unexpectedly develops, while other adipose tissues (subcutaneous and visceral) are extremely depleted, along with suppressed bone acquisition (Fig. 12.3) [194]. In early biopsied BM series, BM appeared to be either normal, hypoplastic, or with gelatinous degeneration [55] that correlate with the amount of weight loss. Hypoplastic or aplastic BM showed an increase in BM fat fraction due to an increase in adipocyte diameters, while in complete gelatinous degeneration of the BM, fat fraction and adipocyte diameters decreased [55]. This suggests that BMAT may initially accumulate as an accommodation for surviving in less severe phases of starvation, but upon terminal illness BMAT could be utilized as a last fuel [195]. More recently, noninvasive imaging modalities have shown that BMAT is increased in AN patients compared to healthy age-matched controls and that the relative contribution of BMAT to total body fat in this disease is multiplied by 2.4 [52,194]. Importantly, after recovery from AN (defined as normal weight and achievement of eumenorrhea), levels of BMAT normalize, implying a reversible effect [196]. Interestingly, AN patients with amenorrhoea exhibited higher BMAT than

AN patients with normal menstrual cycles, which might be related to the additive effect of estrogen deficiency on marrow adiposity [194]. Bone loss and increased incidence of fracture are well-established hallmarks of AN, and indeed the inverse association between BMD and marrow adiposity was confirmed in clinical studies of AN patients [2].

By contrast, rodent models of caloric restriction report conflicting results. In some models marrow adiposity indeed increases, whereas in others BMAT does not change [36,197]. These differences might be partly explained by differences in age, sex, genetics of the rodents, the degree of caloric restriction, or the amount of weight loss.

Obesity is characterized by low-grade inflammation, challenging the immune cell responses in peripheral tissues. Further, the obesogenic condition increases BM cellularity by 20%−30%, affects HSC differentiation capacity, and increases white and red blood cell counts [198]. Bone mineral density is normal or increased in obesity, which might be due to the higher load on bones, but bone quality is generally impaired leading to increased fracture risk. Increased BMAT could contribute to this impaired bone quality. Many studies using bone biopsies or MRI except one [199] have proven an increase in BMAT in obese pre- and postmenopausal women and in young and older men [56,200,201]. In these studies, BMAT was inversely related to bone mass and measures of skeletal fragility and increased marrow adiposity were associated with a decrease in bone formation. Di Iorgi et al. using SECT attenuation measurements of the mid-femoral diaphysis in young healthy adults showed that BMAT was neither associated with visceral or subcutaneous adipose tissue nor with metabolic, lipid profile or cardiovascular risk factors. These findings support the notion that the negative metabolic health outcomes known to be associated to obesity are independent of BMAT [72].

On the other hand, weight loss in clinically obese patients decreases BMAT [202]. After gastric bypass, all obese patients lost weight and BMAT. Interestingly, patients with a lower content of BMAT preoperatively lost less BMAT in comparison to patients with a higher BMAT at baseline who lost more BMAT in the postoperative period [203]. However, the BMAT reduction after bariatric procedures depends on the type of procedure used and the initial diabetes status [204−207], suggesting that factors other than weight loss alone may play a role in BMAT homeostasis. Also in rodents, HFD-induced obesity increases BMAT, independent of sex and genetic background [140,143,208].

By contrast, patients with type 1 congenital generalized lipodytrophy and BSCL2-linked lipodystrophy or adipocyte-specific loss of the *Lmna* gene models of familial partial lipodystrophy type 2 display decreased BMAT [30,209].

Diabetes, both type 1 (T1D) and type 2 (T2D), is associated with increased fragility fracture risk and marrow adiposity is considered as a potential contributing factor to this increased risk [210]. Although BMD is decreased in T1D, BMD in T2DM is often normal or even slightly elevated compared with an age-matched control population. However, in both T1DM and T2DM, bone turnover decreases, and bone material properties and microstructure of bone are impaired [210]. Regarding T1D, genetically or streptozotocin-induced insulin deficiency results in increased BMAT in the long bones of mice [134]. However, preventing BMAT formation does not impact on bone loss [211]. Moreover, in imaging clinical studies BMAT content measured at different bone sites was unchanged in T1D patients compared with control subjects [212,213]. Thus, the involvement of BMAT in T1D remains unclear and deserves further explorations. Several studies investigated BMAT in T2D with conflicting results. In the Osteoporotic Fractures in Men Study, an increased adiposity in the vertebral marrow was found in the self-reported diabetic patients compared to nondiabetic subjects using ^{1}H-MRS [214]. But other authors did not find an association between BMAT volume and diabetes [199,215,216]. Nevertheless, BMAT was positively related to glycated hemoglobin HbA1c levels and lower lipid unsaturation in patients with diabetes [199,216]. Studies in mouse models showed consistently increased marrow adiposity with diabetes [134,217].

Concluding remarks

Bone marrow adipose tissue appears shortly after birth and increases during growth and aging. Bone marrow adipocytes reside in the bone marrow with bone and hematopoietic cells and growing evidence suggests that the BMA are actively involved in skeletal health, metabolic diseases, and hematopoiesis. Besides, BMA secrete active molecules and adipokines which can have local paracrine, but perhaps also systemic, effects. The exact role of the BMA in local and systemic energy metabolism will become clear from future studies. In addition, BMAT can now be measured noninvasively with new noninvasive multiple imaging modalities such as MRI and ^{1}H-MRS, and this could add to the better understanding of this hidden and deep ectopic fat. Over the last decades BMA has evolved from gap-filler to key player in the BM niche and many investigators are now exploring its characteristics, function, and origin. These studies will provide more insight into its role in health and disease. Future research should address optimal windows for personalized medicine in relation with patient-specific BMAT profile.

References

[1] Cawthorn WP, Scheller EL. Editorial: bone marrow adipose tissue: formation, function, and impact on health and disease. Front Endocrinol 2017;8:112.

[2] Veldhuis-Vlug AG, Rosen CJ. Clinical implications of bone marrow adiposity. J Intern Med 2018;283(2):121–39.

[3] Tratwal J, Labella R, Bravenboer N, Kerckhofs G, Douni E, Scheller EL, et al. Reporting guidelines, review of methodological standards, and challenges toward harmonization in bone marrow adiposity research. Report of the methodologies working Group of the international bone marrow adiposity society. Front Endocrinol 2020;11:65.

[4] Muruganandan S, Govindarajan R, Sinal CJ. Bone marrow adipose tissue and skeletal health. Curr Osteoporos Rep 2018;16(4):434–42.

[5] Tencerova M, Ferencakova M, Kassem M. Bone marrow adipose tissue: role in bone remodeling and energy metabolism. Best Pract Res Clin Endocrinol Metab 2021:101545.

[6] Singhal V, Bredella MA. Marrow adipose tissue imaging in humans. Bone 2019;118:69–76. https://doi.org/10.1016/j.bone.2018.01.009. Epub 2018 Jan 10.

[7] Bani Hassan E, Ghasem-Zadeh A, Imani M, Kutaiba N, Wright DK, Sepehrizadeh T, et al. Bone marrow adipose tissue quantification by imaging. Curr Osteoporos Rep 2019;17(6):416–28.

[8] Tavassoli M. Ultrastructural development of bone marrow adipose cell. Acta Anat 1976;94(1):65–77.

[9] Sivasubramaniyan K, Lehnen D, Ghazanfari R, Sobiesiak M, Harichandan A, Mortha E, et al. Phenotypic and functional heterogeneity of human bone marrow- and amnion-derived MSC subsets. Ann N Y Acad Sci 2012;1266:94–106.

[10] Tencerova M, Kassem M. The bone marrow-derived stromal cells: commitment and regulation of adipogenesis. Front Endocrinol September 21, 2016;7:127.

[11] Majka SM, Fox KE, Psilas JC, Helm KM, Childs CR, Acosta AS, et al. De novo generation of white adipocytes from the myeloid lineage via mesenchymal intermediates is age, adipose depot, and gender specific. Proc Natl Acad Sci 2010;107(33):14781–6.

[12] Berry R, Rodeheffer MS. Characterization of the adipocyte cellular lineage in vivo. Nat Cell Biol 2013;15(3):302–8.

[13] Horowitz MC, Berry R, Holtrup B, Sebo Z, Nelson T, Fretz JA, et al. Bone Marrow Adipocyt 2017;6(3):193–204.

[14] Berry R, Rodeheffer MS, Rosen CJ, Horowitz MC. Adipose tissue-residing progenitors (adipocyte lineage progenitors and adipose-derived stem cells (ADSC)). Curr Mol Biol Rep 2015;1(3):101–9.

[15] Rodeheffer MS, Birsoy K, Friedman JM. Identification of white adipocyte progenitor cells in vivo. Cell October 17 , 2008;135(2):240–9.

[16] Seale P, Bjork B, Yang W, Kajimura S, Chin S, Kuang S, et al. PRDM16 controls a brown fat/skeletal muscle switch. Nature 2008;454(7207):961–7.

[17] Wang W, Kissig M, Rajakumari S, Huang L, Lim H, Won K-J, et al. Ebf2 is a selective marker of brown and beige adipogenic precursor cells. Proc Natl Acad Sci U S A October 7, 2014;111(40):14466–71.

[18] Krings A, Rahman S, Huang S, Lu Y, Czernik PJ, Lecka-Czernik B. Bone marrow fat has brown adipose tissue characteristics, which are attenuated with aging and diabetes. Bone 2012;50(2):546–52.

[19] Ambrosi TH, Scialdone A, Graja A, Gohlke S, Jank A-M, Bocian C, et al. Adipocyte accumulation in the bone marrow during obesity and aging impairs stem cell-based hematopoietic and bone regeneration. Cell Stem Cell 2017;20(6):771–784.e6.

[20] Logan M, Martin JF, Nagy A, Lobe C, Olson EN, Tabin CJ. Expression of Cre Recombinase in the developing mouse limb bud driven by a Prxl enhancer. Genes 2002;33(2):77–80.

[21] Sanchez-Gurmaches J, Hsiao W-Y, Guertin DA. Highly selective in vivo labeling of subcutaneous white adipocyte precursors with Prx1-Cre. Stem Cell Rep 2015;4(4):541–50.

[22] Mizoguchi T, Pinho S, Ahmed J, Kunisaki Y, Hanoun M, Mendelson A, et al. Osterix marks distinct waves of primitive and definitive stromal progenitors during bone marrow development. Dev Cell 2014;29(3):340–9.

[23] Ono N, Ono W, Mizoguchi T, Nagasawa T, Frenette PS, Kronenberg HM. Vasculature-associated cells expressing nestin in developing bones encompass early cells in the osteoblast and endothelial lineage. Dev Cell 2014;29(3):330–9.

[24] Zhou BO, Yue R, Murphy MM, Peyer JG, Morrison SJ. Leptin-receptor-expressing mesenchymal stromal cells represent the main source of bone formed by adult bone marrow. Cell Stem Cell 2014;15(2):154–68.

[25] Pinho S, Lacombe J, Hanoun M, Mizoguchi T, Bruns I, Kunisaki Y, et al. PDGFRα and CD51 mark human nestin+ sphere-forming mesenchymal stem cells capable of hematopoietic progenitor cell expansion. J Exp Med 2013;210(7):1351–67.

[26] Yue R, Zhou BO, Shimada IS, Zhao Z, Morrison SJ. Leptin receptor promotes adipogenesis and reduces osteogenesis by regulating mesenchymal stromal cells in adult bone marrow. Cell Stem Cell 2016;18(6):782–96.

[27] Worthley DL, Churchill M, Compton JT, Tailor Y, Rao M, Si Y, et al. Gremlin 1 identifies a skeletal stem cell with bone, cartilage, and reticular stromal potential. Cell 2015;160(1–2):269–84.

[28] Liu Y, Strecker S, Wang L, Kronenberg MS, Wang W, Rowe DW, et al. Osterix-cre labeled progenitor cells contribute to the formation and maintenance of the bone marrow stroma. PLoS One 2013;8(8):e71318.

[29] Hardouin P, Rharass T, Lucas S. Bone marrow adipose tissue: to Be or not to Be a typical adipose tissue? Front Endocrinol 2016;7:85.

[30] Suchacki KJ, Cawthorn WP, Rosen CJ. Bone marrow adipose tissue: formation, function and regulation. Curr Opin Pharmacol 2016;28:50–6.

[31] Suchacki KJ, Tavares AAS, Mattiucci D, Scheller EL, Papanastasiou G, Gray C, et al. Bone marrow adipose tissue is a unique adipose subtype with distinct roles in glucose homeostasis. Nat Commun 2020;11(1):3097.

[32] Pansini V, Monnet A, Salleron J, Hardouin P, Cortet B, Cotten A. 3 Tesla (1) H MR spectroscopy of hip bone marrow in a healthy population, assessment of normal fat content values and influence of age and sex. J Magn Reson Imag 2014;39(2):369–76.

[33] Kugel H, Jung C, Schulte O, Heindel W. Age- and sex-specific differences in the 1H-spectrum of vertebral bone marrow. J Magn Reson Imag 2001;13(2):263–8.

[34] Hartsock RJ, Smith EB, Petty CS. Normal variations with aging of the amount of hematopoietic tissue in bone marrow from the anterior iliac crest. A study made from 177 cases of sudden death examined by necropsy. Am J Clin Pathol 1965;43:326–31.

[35] Hardouin P, Pansini V, Cortet B. Bone marrow fat. Joint Bone Spine 2014;81(4):313–9.

[36] Devlin MJ, Cloutier AM, Thomas NA, Panus DA, Lotinun S, Pinz I, et al. Caloric restriction leads to high marrow adiposity and low bone mass in growing mice. J Bone Miner Res Off J Am Soc Bone Miner Res 2010;25(9):2078–88.

[37] Liney GP, Bernard CP, Manton DJ, Turnbull LW, Langton CM. Age, gender, and skeletal variation in bone marrow composition: a preliminary study at 3.0Tesla. J Magn Reson Imag 2007;26(3):787–93.

[38] Griffith JF, Yeung DKW, Ma HT, Leung JCS, Kwok TCY, Leung PC. Bone marrow fat content in the elderly: a reversal of sex difference seen in younger subjects. J Magn Reson Imag 2012;36(1):225–30.

[39] Veldhuis-Vlug AG, Rosen CJ. Mechanisms of marrow adiposity and its implications for skeletal health. Metabolism 2017;67:106–14.

[40] Baum T, Rohrmeier A, Syväri J, Diefenbach MN, Franz D, Dieckmeyer M, et al. Anatomical variation of age-related changes in vertebral bone marrow composition using chemical shift encoding-based water-fat magnetic resonance imaging. Front Endocrinol 2018;9:141.

[41] Tavassoli M. Marrow adipose cells. Histochemical identification of labile and stable components. Arch Pathol Lab Med 1976;100(1):16–8.

[42] Scheller EL, Doucette CR, Learman BS, Cawthorn WP, Khandaker S, Schell B, et al. Region-specific variation in the properties of skeletal adipocytes reveals regulated and constitutive marrow adipose tissues. Nat Commun 2015;6:7808.

[43] Little-Letsinger SE, Pagnotti GM, McGrath C, Styner M. Exercise and diet: uncovering prospective mediators of skeletal fragility in bone and marrow adipose tissue. Curr Osteoporos Rep 2020;18(6):774–89.

[44] Styner M, Thompson WR, Galior K, Uzer G, Wu X, Kadari S, et al. Bone marrow fat accumulation accelerated by high fat diet is suppressed by exercise. Bone 2014;64:39–46.

[45] Liu S-Y, He Y-B, Deng S-Y, Zhu W-T, Xu S-Y, Ni G-X. Exercise affects biological characteristics of mesenchymal stromal cells derived from bone marrow and adipose tissue. Int Orthop 2017;41(6):1199–209.

[46] Menuki K, Mori T, Sakai A, Sakuma M, Okimoto N, Shimizu Y, et al. Climbing exercise enhances osteoblast differentiation and inhibits adipogenic differentiation with high expression of PTH/PTHrP receptor in bone marrow cells. Bone 2008;43(3):613–20.

[47] David V, Martin A, Lafage-Proust M-H, Malaval L, Peyroche S, Jones DB, et al. Mechanical loading down-regulates peroxisome proliferator-activated receptor gamma in bone marrow stromal cells and favors osteoblastogenesis at the expense of adipogenesis. Endocrinology 2007;148(5):2553–62.

[48] Pagnotti GM, Styner M. Exercise regulation of marrow adipose tissue. Front Endocrinol 2016;7:94.

[49] Bertheau RC, Lorbeer R, Nattenmüller J, Wintermeyer E, Machann J, Linkohr B, et al. Bone marrow fat fraction assessment in regard to physical activity: KORA FF4-3-T MR imaging in a population-based cohort. Eur Radiol 2020;30(6):3417–28.

[50] Hu M, Sheng J, Kang Z, Zou L, Guo J, Sun P. Magnetic resonance imaging and dual energy X-ray absorptiometry of the lumbar spine in professional wrestlers and untrained men. J Sports Med Phys Fitness 2014;54(4):505–10.

[51] Attané C, Estève D, Chaoui K, Iacovoni JS, Corre J, Moutahir M, et al. Human bone marrow is comprised of adipocytes with specific lipid metabolism. Cell Rep 2020;30(4):949–958.e6.

[52] Cawthorn WP, Scheller EL, Learman BS, Parlee SD, Simon BR, Mori H, et al. Bone marrow adipose tissue is an endocrine organ that contributes to increased circulating adiponectin during caloric restriction. Cell Metab 2014;20(2):368–75.

[53] Bathija A, Davis S, Trubowitz S. Bone marrow adipose tissue: response to acute starvation. Am J Hematol 1979;6(3):191–8.

[54] Tavassoli M. Differential response of bone marrow and extramedullary adipose cells to starvation. Experientia 1974;30(4):424–5.

[55] Abella E, Feliu E, Granada I, Millá F, Oriol A, Ribera JM, et al. Bone marrow changes in anorexia nervosa are correlated with the amount of weight loss and not with other clinical findings. Am J Clin Pathol 2002;118(4):582–8.

[56] Bredella MA, Torriani M, Ghomi RH, Thomas BJ, Brick DJ, Gerweck AV, et al. Vertebral bone marrow fat is positively associated with visceral fat and inversely associated with IGF-1 in obese women. Obes Silver Spring 2011;19(1):49–53.

[57] Cawthorn WP, Scheller EL, Parlee SD, Pham HA, Learman BS, Redshaw CMH, et al. Expansion of bone marrow adipose tissue during caloric restriction is associated with increased circulating glucocorticoids and not with hypoleptinemia. Endocrinology 2016;157(2):508–21.

[58] Ghali O, Al Rassy N, Hardouin P, Chauveau C. Increased bone marrow adiposity in a context of energy deficit: the tip of the iceberg? Front Endocrinol 2016;7:125.

[59] Trudel G, Payne M, Mädler B, Ramachandran N, Lecompte M, Wade C, et al. Bone marrow fat accumulation after 60 days of bed rest persisted 1 year after activities were resumed along with hemopoietic stimulation: the Women International Space Simulation for Exploration study. J Appl Physiol Bethesda 2009;107(2):540–8.

[60] Wronski TJ, Morey ER. Skeletal abnormalities in rats induced by simulated weightlessness. Metab Bone Dis Relat Res 1982;4(1):69–75.

[61] Jee WS, Wronski TJ, Morey ER, Kimmel DB. Effects of spaceflight on trabecular bone in rats. Am J Physiol 1983;244(3):R310–4.

[62] Farrell M, Fairfield H, Costa S, D'Amico A, Falank C, Brooks DJ, et al. Sclerostin-neutralizing antibody treatment rescues negative effects of rosiglitazone on mouse bone parameters. J Bone Miner Res 2021;36(1):158–69.

[63] Allen JE, Henshaw DL, Keitch PA, Fews AP, Eatough JP. Fat cells in red bone marrow of human rib: their size and spatial distribution with respect to the radon-derived dose to the haemopoietic tissue. Int J Radiat Biol 1995;68(6):669–78.

[64] Rozman C, Feliu E, Berga L, Reverter JC, Climent C, Ferrán MJ. Age-related variations of fat tissue fraction in normal human bone marrow depend both on size and number of adipocytes: a stereological study. Exp Hematol 1989;17(1):34–7.

[65] Coutel X, Olejnik C, Marchandise P, Delattre J, Béhal H, Kerckhofs G, et al. A novel microCT method for bone and marrow adipose tissue alignment identifies key differences between mandible and tibia in rats. Calcif Tissue Int 2018;103(2):189−97.

[66] Sebo ZL, Rendina-Ruedy E, Ables GP, Lindskog DM, Rodeheffer MS, Fazeli PK, et al. Bone marrow adiposity: basic and clinical implications. Endocr Rev October 1, 2019;40(5):1187−206.

[67] Bravenboer N, Bredella MA, Chauveau C, Corsi A, Douni E, Ferris WF, et al. Standardised nomenclature, abbreviations, and units for the study of bone marrow adiposity: report of the nomenclature working Group of the international bone marrow adiposity society. Front Endocrinol 2019;10:923.

[68] Karampinos DC, Ruschke S, Dieckmeyer M, Diefenbach M, Franz D, Gersing AS, et al. Quantitative MRI and spectroscopy of bone marrow. J Magn Reson Imag 2018;47(2):332−53.

[69] Goldman LW. Principles of CT and CT technology. J Nucl Med Technol 2007;35(3):115−28. quiz 129−30.

[70] Jarraya M, Bredella MA. Clinical imaging of marrow adiposity. Best Pract Res Clin Endocrinol Metabol 20 févr 2021:101511.

[71] Laval-Jeantet AM, Roger B, Bouysee S, Bergot C, Mazess RB. Influence of vertebral fat content on quantitative CT density. Radiology 1986;159(2):463−6.

[72] Di Iorgi N, Mittelman SD, Gilsanz V. Differential effect of marrow adiposity and visceral and subcutaneous fat on cardiovascular risk in young, healthy adults. Int J Obes 2008;32(12):1854−60.

[73] Di Iorgi N, Mo AO, Grimm K, Wren TAL, Dorey F, Gilsanz V. Bone acquisition in healthy young females is reciprocally related to marrow adiposity. J Clin Endocrinol Metab 2010;95(6):2977−82.

[74] Di Iorgi N, Rosol M, Mittelman SD, Gilsanz V. Reciprocal relation between marrow adiposity and the amount of bone in the axial and appendicular skeleton of young adults. J Clin Endocrinol Metab 2008;93(6):2281−6.

[75] Johnson TRC, Krauss B, Sedlmair M, Grasruck M, Bruder H, Morhard D, et al. Material differentiation by dual energy CT: initial experience. Eur Radiol 2007;17(6):1510−7.

[76] Bredella MA, Daley SM, Kalra MK, Brown JK, Miller KK, Torriani M. Marrow adipose tissue quantification of the lumbar spine by using dual-energy CT and single-voxel (1)H MR spectroscopy: a feasibility study. Radiology 2015;277(1):230−5.

[77] Arentsen L, Hansen KE, Yagi M, Takahashi Y, Shanley R, McArthur A, et al. Use of dual-energy computed tomography to measure skeletal-wide marrow composition and cancellous bone mineral density. J Bone Miner Metab 2017;35(4):428−36.

[78] Molwitz I, Leiderer M, Özden C, Yamamura J. Dual-energy computed tomography for fat quantification in the liver and bone marrow: a literature review. ROFO Fortschr Geb Rontgenstr Nuklearmed 2020;192(12):1137−53.

[79] Porter BA, Shields AF, Olson DO. Magnetic resonance imaging of bone marrow disorders. Radiol Clin North Am 1986;24(2):269−89.

[80] Delikatny EJ, Chawla S, Leung D-J, Poptani H. MR-visible lipids and the tumor microenvironment. NMR Biomed 2011;24(6):592−611.

[81] Shen W, Chen J, Gantz M, Punyanitya M, Heymsfield SB, Gallagher D, et al. MRI-measured pelvic bone marrow adipose tissue is inversely related to DXA-measured bone mineral in younger and older adults. Eur J Clin Nutr 2012;66(9):983−8.

[82] Shen W, Gong X, Weiss J, Jin Y. Comparison among T1-weighted magnetic resonance imaging, modified dixon method, and magnetic resonance spectroscopy in measuring bone marrow fat. J Obes 2013;2013:298675.

[83] Cordes C, Baum T, Dieckmeyer M, Ruschke S, Diefenbach MN, Hauner H, et al. MR-based assessment of bone marrow fat in osteoporosis, diabetes, and obesity. Front Endocrinol 2016;7:74.

[84] Zhang C, Slade JM, Miller F, Modlesky CM. Quantifying bone marrow fat using standard T1-weighted magnetic resonance images in children with typical development and in children with cerebral palsy. Sci Rep 2020;10(1):4284.

[85] Reeder SB, Hu HH, Sirlin CB. Proton density fat-fraction: a standardized MR-based biomarker of tissue fat concentration. J Magn Reson Imag 2012;36(5):1011−4.

[86] Aoki T, Yamaguchi S, Kinoshita S, Hayashida Y, Korogi Y. Quantification of bone marrow fat content using iterative decomposition of water and fat with echo asymmetry and least-squares estimation (IDEAL): reproducibility, site variation and correlation with age and menopause. Br J Radiol 2016;89(1065):20150538.

[87] Karampinos DC, Ruschke S, Dieckmeyer M, Eggers H, Kooijman H, Rummeny EJ, et al. Modeling of T2* decay in vertebral bone marrow fat quantification. NMR Biomed 2015;28(11):1535−42.

[88] Karampinos DC, Melkus G, Baum T, Bauer JS, Rummeny EJ, Krug R. Bone marrow fat quantification in the presence of trabecular bone: initial comparison between water-fat imaging and single-voxel MRS. Magn Reson Med 2014;71(3):1158−65.

[89] Gee CS, Nguyen JTK, Marquez CJ, Heunis J, Lai A, Wyatt C, et al. Validation of bone marrow fat quantification in the presence of trabecular bone using MRI. J Magn Reson Imag 2015;42(2):539−44.

[90] Arentsen L, Yagi M, Takahashi Y, Bolan PJ, White M, Yee D, et al. Validation of marrow fat assessment using noninvasive imaging with histologic examination of human bone samples. Bone 2015;72:118−22.

[91] MacEwan IJ, Glembotski NE, D'Lima D, Bae W, Masuda K, Rashidi HH, et al. Proton density water fraction as a biomarker of bone marrow cellularity: validation in ex vivo spine specimens. Magn Reson Imag 2014;32(9):1097−101.

[92] Lundbom J, Bierwagen A, Bodis K, Apostolopoulou M, Szendroedi J, Müssig K, et al. 1H-MRS of femoral red and yellow bone marrow fat composition and water content in healthy young men and women at 3 T. Magma October, 2019;32(5):591−7.

[93] Maurice F, Dutour A, Vincentelli C, Abdesselam I, Bernard M, Dufour H, et al. Active cushing syndrome patients have increased ectopic fat deposition and bone marrow fat content compared to cured patients and healthy subjects: a pilot 1H-MRS study. Eur J Endocrinol October 12, 2018;179(5):307−17.

[94] Cohen A, Shen W, Dempster DW, Zhou H, Recker RR, Lappe JM, et al. Marrow adiposity assessed on transiliac crest biopsy samples correlates with noninvasive measurement of marrow adiposity by proton magnetic resonance spectroscopy ((1)H-MRS) at the spine but not the femur. Osteoporos Int J Establ Result Coop Eur Found Osteoporos Natl Osteoporos Found USA October, 2015;26(10):2471−8.

[95] Singhal V, Miller KK, Torriani M, Bredella MA. Short- and long-term reproducibility of marrow adipose tissue quantification by 1H-MR spectroscopy. Skeletal Radiol 2016;45(2):221−5.

[96] Ren J, Dimitrov I, Sherry AD, Malloy CR. Composition of adipose tissue and marrow fat in humans by 1H NMR at 7 Tesla. J Lipid Res 2008;49(9):2055−62.

[97] Patsch JM, Li X, Baum T, Yap SP, Karampinos DC, Schwartz AV, et al. Bone marrow fat composition as a novel imaging biomarker in postmenopausal women with prevalent fragility fractures. J Bone Miner Res Off J Am Soc Bone Miner Res 2013;28(8):1721−8.

[98] Yeung DKW, Griffith JF, Antonio GE, Lee FKH, Woo J, Leung PC. Osteoporosis is associated with increased marrow fat content and decreased marrow fat unsaturation: a proton MR spectroscopy study. J Magn Reson Imag 2005;22(2):279−85.

[99] Li Z, Hardij J, Bagchi DP, Scheller EL, MacDougald OA. Development, regulation, metabolism and function of bone marrow adipose tissues. Bone 2018;110:134−40.

[100] Herrmann M. Marrow fat-secreted factors as biomarkers for osteoporosis. Curr Osteoporos Rep 2019;17(6):429−37.

[101] Laharrague P, Larrouy D, Fontanilles AM, Truel N, Campfield A, Tenenbaum R, et al. High expression of leptin by human bone marrow adipocytes in primary culture. FASEB J Off Publ Fed Am Soc Exp Biol 1998;12(9):747−52.

[102] Poloni A, Maurizi G, Serrani F, Mancini S, Zingaretti MC, Frontini A, et al. Molecular and functional characterization of human bone marrow adipocytes. Exp Hematol 2013;41(6):558−566.e2.

[103] Liu L-F, Shen W-J, Ueno M, Patel S, Kraemer FB. Characterization of age-related gene expression profiling in bone marrow and epididymal adipocytes. BMC Genomics 2011;12:212.

[104] Aaron N, Kraakman MJ, Zhou Q, Liu Q, Costa S, Yang J, et al. Adipsin promotes bone marrow adiposity by priming mesenchymal stem cells. eLife 2021;10:e69209.

[105] Scheller EL, Cawthorn WP, Burr AA, Horowitz MC, MacDougald OA. Marrow adipose tissue: trimming the fat. Trend Endocrinol Metab 2016;27(6):392−403.

[106] Corre J, Barreau C, Cousin B, Chavoin J-P, Caton D, Fournial G, et al. Human subcutaneous adipose cells support complete differentiation but not self-renewal of hematopoietic progenitors. J Cell Physiol 2006;208(2):282−8.

[107] Laharrague P, Fontanilles AM, Tkaczuk J, Corberand JX, Pénicaud L, Casteilla L. Inflammatory/haematopoietic cytokine production by human bone marrow adipocytes. Eur Cytokine Netw 2000;11(4):634−9.

[108] Hardaway AL, Herroon MK, Rajagurubandara E, Podgorski I. Marrow adipocyte-derived CXCL1 and CXCL2 contribute to osteolysis in metastatic prostate cancer. Clin Exp Metastasis 2015;32(4):353−68.

[109] Laharrague P, Truel N, Fontanilles AM, Corberand JX, Pénicaud L, Casteilla L. Regulation by cytokines of leptin expression in human bone marrow adipocytes. Horm Metab Res Horm Stoffwechselforschung Horm Metab October, 2000;32(10):381−5.

[110] Beekman KM, Zwaagstra M, Veldhuis-Vlug AG, van Essen HW, den Heijer M, Maas M, et al. Ovariectomy increases RANKL protein expression in bone marrow adipocytes of C3H/HeJ mice. Am J Physiol Endocrinol Metab. 1 déc 2019;317(6):E1050−4.

[111] Yu W, Zhong L, Yao L, Wei Y, Gui T, Li Z, et al. Bone marrow adipogenic lineage precursors promote osteoclastogenesis in bone remodeling and pathologic bone loss. J Clin Invest 2021;131(2):140214.

[112] Martin PJ, Haren N, Ghali O, Clabaut A, Chauveau C, Hardouin P, et al. Adipogenic RNAs are transferred in osteoblasts via bone marrow adipocytes-derived extracellular vesicles (EVs). BMC Cell Biol 2015;16:10.

[113] Pham TT, Ivaska KK, Hannukainen JC, Virtanen KA, Lidell ME, Enerbäck S, et al. Human bone marrow adipose tissue is a metabolically active and insulin-sensitive distinct fat depot. J Clin Endocrinol Metab 2020;105(7):dgaa216.

[114] Martin RB, Zissimos SL. Relationships between marrow fat and bone turnover in ovariectomized and intact rats. Bone 1991;12(2):123−31.

[115] Limonard EJ, Veldhuis-Vlug AG, van Dussen L, Runge JH, Tanck MW, Endert E, et al. Short-term effect of estrogen on human bone marrow fat. J Bone Miner Res Off J Am Soc Bone Miner Res 2015;30(11):2058−66.

[116] Syed FA, Oursler MJ, Hefferanm TE, Peterson JM, Riggs BL, Khosla S. Effects of estrogen therapy on bone marrow adipocytes in postmenopausal osteoporotic women. Osteoporos Int J Establ Result Coop Eur Found Osteoporos Natl Osteoporos Found USA 2008;19(9):1323−30.

[117] Sato C, Miyakoshi N, Kasukawa Y, Nozaka K, Tsuchie H, Nagahata I, et al. Teriparatide and exercise improve bone, skeletal muscle, and fat parameters in ovariectomized and tail-suspended rats. J Bone Miner Metab 2021;39(3):385−95.

[118] Yang Y, Luo X, Xie X, Yan F, Chen G, Zhao W, et al. Influences of teriparatide administration on marrow fat content in postmenopausal osteopenic women using MR spectroscopy. Climacteric J Int Menopause Soc 2016;19(3):285−91.

[119] Fan Y, Hanai J-I, Le PT, Bi R, Maridas D, DeMambro V, et al. Parathyroid hormone directs bone marrow mesenchymal cell fate. Cell Metab 2017;25(3):661−72.

[120] Shen W, Chen J, Punyanitya M, Shapses S, Heshka S, Heymsfield SB. MRI-measured bone marrow adipose tissue is inversely related to DXA-measured bone mineral in Caucasian women. Osteoporos Int J Establ Result Coop Eur Found Osteoporos Natl Osteoporos Found USA 2007;18(5):641−7.

[121] Shen W, Scherzer R, Gantz M, Chen J, Punyanitya M, Lewis CE, et al. Relationship between MRI-measured bone marrow adipose tissue and hip and spine bone mineral density in African-American and Caucasian participants: the CARDIA study. J Clin Endocrinol Metab 2012;97(4):1337−46.

[122] Meunier P, Aaron J, Edouard C, Vignon G. Osteoporosis and the replacement of cell populations of the marrow by adipose tissue. A quantitative study of 84 iliac bone biopsies. Clin Orthop 1971;80:147−54.

[123] Verma S, Rajaratnam JH, Denton J, Hoyland JA, Byers RJ. Adipocytic proportion of bone marrow is inversely related to bone formation in osteoporosis. J Clin Pathol 2002;55(9):693−8.

[124] Justesen J, Stenderup K, Ebbesen EN, Mosekilde L, Steiniche T, Kassem M. Adipocyte tissue volume in bone marrow is increased with aging and in patients with osteoporosis. Biogerontology 2001;2(3):165−71.

[125] Schwartz AV, Sigurdsson S, Hue TF, Lang TF, Harris TB, Rosen CJ, et al. Vertebral bone marrow fat associated with lower trabecular BMD and prevalent vertebral fracture in older adults. J Clin Endocrinol Metab 2013;98(6):2294−300.

[126] Griffith JF, Yeung DKW, Antonio GE, Lee FKH, Hong AWL, Wong SYS, et al. Vertebral bone mineral density, marrow perfusion, and fat content in healthy men and men with osteoporosis: dynamic contrast-enhanced MR imaging and MR spectroscopy. Radiology 2005;236(3):945−51.

[127] Pino AM, Miranda M, Figueroa C, Rodríguez JP, Rosen CJ. Qualitative aspects of bone marrow adiposity in osteoporosis. Front Endocrinol October 25, 2016;7:139.

[128] Casado-Díaz A, Santiago-Mora R, Dorado G, Quesada-Gómez JM. The omega-6 arachidonic fatty acid, but not the omega-3 fatty acids, inhibits osteoblastogenesis and induces adipogenesis of human mesenchymal stem cells: potential implication in osteoporosis. Osteoporos Int J Establ Result Coop Eur Found Osteoporos Natl Osteoporos Found U S A 2013;24(5):1647−61.

[129] Fillmore N, Huqi A, Jaswal JS, Mori J, Paulin R, Haromy A, et al. Effect of fatty acids on human bone marrow mesenchymal stem cell energy metabolism and survival. PLOS ONE 2015;10(3):e0120257.

[130] Yu A, Carballido-Gamio J, Wang L, Lang TF, Su Y, Wu X, et al. Spatial differences in the distribution of bone between femoral neck and trochanteric fractures. J Bone Miner Res Off J Am Soc Bone Miner Res 2017;32(8):1672−80.

[131] Beamer WG, Donahue LR, Rosen CJ, Baylink DJ. Genetic variability in adult bone density among inbred strains of mice. Bone 1996;18(5):397−403.

[132] Lecka-Czernik B, Moerman EJ, Grant DF, Lehmann JM, Manolagas SC, Jilka RL. Divergent effects of selective peroxisome proliferator-activated receptor-γ2 ligands on adipocyte versus osteoblast differentiation. Endocrinology 2002;143(6):2376−84.

[133] Ackert-Bicknell CL, Shockley KR, Horton LG, Lecka-Czernik B, Churchill GA, Rosen CJ. Strain-specific effects of rosiglitazone on bone mass, body composition, and serum insulin-like growth factor-I. Endocrinology 2009;150(3):1330−40.

[134] Botolin S, McCabe LR. Bone loss and increased bone adiposity in spontaneous and pharmacologically induced diabetic mice. Endocrinology 2007;148(1):198−205.

[135] Styner M, Pagnotti GM, McGrath C, Wu X, Sen B, Uzer G, et al. Exercise decreases marrow adipose tissue through ß-oxidation in obese running mice. J Bone Miner Res Off J Am Soc Bone Miner Res 2017;32(8):1692−702.

[136] Scheller EL, Khoury B, Moller KL, Wee NKY, Khandaker S, Kozloff KM, et al. Changes in skeletal integrity and marrow adiposity during high-fat diet and after weight loss. Front Endocrinol 2016;7:102.

[137] Fujita Y, Watanabe K, Maki K. Serum leptin levels negatively correlate with trabecular bone mineral density in high-fat diet-induced obesity mice. J Musculoskelet Neuronal Interact 2012;12(2):84−94.

[138] Bonnet N, Somm E, Rosen CJ. Diet and gene interactions influence the skeletal response to polyunsaturated fatty acids. Bone 2014;68:100−7.

[139] Devlin MJ, Robbins A, Cosman MN, Moursi CA, Cloutier AM, Louis L, et al. Differential effects of high fat diet and diet-induced obesity on skeletal acquisition in female C57BL/6J vs. FVB/NJ Mice. Bone Rep 2018;8:204−14.

[140] Tencerova M, Figeac F, Ditzel N, Taipaleenmäki H, Nielsen TK, Kassem M. High-fat diet-induced obesity promotes expansion of bone marrow adipose tissue and impairs skeletal stem cell functions in mice. J Bone Miner Res Off J Am Soc Bone Miner Res 2018;33(6):1154−65.

[141] Lecka-Czernik B, Stechschulte LA, Czernik PJ, Dowling AR. High bone mass in adult mice with diet-induced obesity results from a combination of initial increase in bone mass followed by attenuation in bone formation; implications for high bone mass and decreased bone quality in obesity. Mol Cell Endocrinol 2015;410:35−41.

[142] Halade GV, Rahman MM, Williams PJ, Fernandes G. Combination of conjugated linoleic acid with fish oil prevents age-associated bone marrow adiposity in C57Bl/6J mice. J Nutr Biochem 2011;22(5):459−69.

[143] Doucette CR, Horowitz MC, Berry R, MacDougald OA, Anunciado-Koza R, Koza RA, et al. A high fat diet increases bone marrow adipose tissue (MAT) but does not alter trabecular or cortical bone mass in C57BL/6J mice. J Cell Physiol 2015;230(9):2032−7.

[144] Motyl KJ, Bishop KA, DeMambro VE, Bornstein SA, Le P, Kawai M, et al. Altered thermogenesis and impaired bone remodeling in Misty mice. J Bone Miner Res 2013;28(9):1885−97.

[145] Bornstein S, Brown SA, Le PT, Wang X, DeMambro V, Horowitz MC, et al. FGF-21 and skeletal remodeling during and after lactation in C57BL/6J mice. Endocrinology 2014;155(9):3516−26.

[146] Justesen J, Mosekilde L, Holmes M, Stenderup K, Gasser J, Mullins JJ, et al. Mice deficient in 11beta-hydroxysteroid dehydrogenase type 1 lack bone marrow adipocytes, but maintain normal bone formation. Endocrinology 2004;145(4):1916−25.

[147] Iwaniec UT, Turner RT. Failure to generate bone marrow adipocytes does not protect mice from ovariectomy-induced osteopenia. Bone 2013;53(1):145−53.

[148] Hamrick MW, Della-Fera MA, Choi Y-H, Pennington C, Hartzell D, Baile CA. Leptin treatment induces loss of bone marrow adipocytes and increases bone formation in leptin-deficient ob/ob mice. J Bone Miner Res Off J Am Soc Bone Miner Res 2005;20(6):994−1001.

[149] Turner RT, Kalra SP, Wong CP, Philbrick KA, Lindenmaier LB, Boghossian S, et al. Peripheral leptin regulates bone formation. J Bone Miner Res Off J Am Soc Bone Miner Res 2013;28(1):22−34.

[150] Maurin AC, Chavassieux PM, Frappart L, Delmas PD, Serre CM, Meunier PJ. Influence of mature adipocytes on osteoblast proliferation in human primary cocultures. Bone 2000;26(5):485−9.

[151] Elbaz A, Wu X, Rivas D, Gimble JM, Duque G. Inhibition of fatty acid biosynthesis prevents adipocyte lipotoxicity on human osteoblasts in vitro. J Cell Mol Med 2010;14(4):982−91.

[152] Wang D, Haile A, Jones LC. Dexamethasone-induced lipolysis increases the adverse effect of adipocytes on osteoblasts using cells derived from human mesenchymal stem cells. Bone 2013;53(2):520−30.

[153] Kelly KA, Tanaka S, Baron R, Gimble JM. Murine bone marrow stromally derived BMS2 adipocytes support differentiation and function of osteoclast-like cells in vitro. Endocrinology 1998;139(4):2092−101.

[154] Robles H, Park S, Joens MS, Fitzpatrick JAJ, Craft CS, Scheller EL. Characterization of the bone marrow adipocyte niche with three-dimensional electron microscopy. Bone 2019;118:89−98.

[155] Naveiras O, Nardi V, Wenzel PL, Hauschka PV, Fahey F, Daley GQ. Bone-marrow adipocytes as negative regulators of the haematopoietic microenvironment. Nature 2009;460(7252):259−63.

[156] Zhu R-J, Wu M-Q, Li Z-J, Zhang Y, Liu K-Y. Hematopoietic recovery following chemotherapy is improved by BADGE-induced inhibition of adipogenesis. Int J Hematol 2013;97(1):58−72.

[157] Patel VS, Ete Chan M, Rubin J, Rubin CT. Marrow adiposity and hematopoiesis in aging and obesity: exercise as an intervention. Curr Osteoporos Rep 2018;16(2):105−15.

[158] Lamers D, Famulla S, Wronkowitz N, Hartwig S, Lehr S, Ouwens DM, et al. Dipeptidyl peptidase 4 is a novel adipokine potentially linking obesity to the metabolic syndrome. Diabetes 2011;60(7):1917−25.

[159] Marguet D, Baggio L, Kobayashi T, Bernard AM, Pierres M, Nielsen PF, et al. Enhanced insulin secretion and improved glucose tolerance in mice lacking CD26. Proc Natl Acad Sci U S A 2000;97(12):6874−9.

[160] Wilson A, Fu H, Schiffrin M, Winkler C, Koufany M, Jouzeau J-Y, et al. Lack of adipocytes alters hematopoiesis in lipodystrophic mice. Front Immunol 2018;9:2573.

[161] Spindler TJ, Tseng AW, Zhou X, Adams GB. Adipocytic cells augment the support of primitive hematopoietic cells in vitro but have no effect in the bone marrow niche under homeostatic conditions. Stem Cells Dev 2014;23(4):434−41.

[162] Zhou BO, Yu H, Yue R, Zhao Z, Rios JJ, Naveiras O, et al. Bone marrow adipocytes promote the regeneration of stem cells and haematopoiesis by secreting SCF. Nat Cell Biol 2017;19(8):891−903.

[163] Zhang Z, Huang Z, Ong B, Sahu C, Zeng H, Ruan H-B. Bone marrow adipose tissue-derived stem cell factor mediates metabolic regulation of hematopoiesis. Haematologica 2019;104(9):1731−43.

[164] Mattiucci D, Maurizi G, Izzi V, Cenci L, Ciarlantini M, Mancini S, et al. Bone marrow adipocytes support hematopoietic stem cell survival. J Cell Physiol 2018;233(2):1500−11.

[165] Bilwani FA, Knight KL. Adipocyte-derived soluble factor(s) inhibits early stages of B lymphopoiesis. J Immunol Baltim November 1 , 2012;189(9):4379−86.

[166] Kennedy DE, Knight KL. Bone marrow fat induces inflammation that inhibits B lymphopoiesis. J Immunol 2016;196(1 Suppl. ment). 122.11-122.11.

[167] Kennedy DE, Knight KL. Inhibition of B Lymphopoiesis by adipocytes and IL-1-producing myeloid-derived suppressor cells. J Immunol Baltim September 15, 2015;195(6):2666−74.

[168] Scheller EL, Burr AA, MacDougald OA, Cawthorn WP. Inside out: bone marrow adipose tissue as a source of circulating adiponectin. Adipocyte 2016;5(3):251−69.

[169] Yokota T, Meka CSR, Kouro T, Medina KL, Igarashi H, Takahashi M, et al. Adiponectin, a fat cell product, influences the earliest lymphocyte precursors in bone marrow cultures by activation of the cyclooxygenase-prostaglandin pathway in stromal cells. J Immunol Baltim November 15, 2003;171(10):5091−9.

[170] Adler BJ, Green DE, Pagnotti GM, Chan ME, Rubin CT. High fat diet rapidly suppresses B lymphopoiesis by disrupting the supportive capacity of the bone marrow niche. PLOS ONE 2014;9(3):e90639.

[171] Singer K, DelProposto J, Morris DL, Zamarron B, Mergian T, Maley N, et al. Diet-induced obesity promotes myelopoiesis in hematopoietic stem cells. Mol Metab 2014;3(6):664.

[172] Luo Y, Chen G-L, Hannemann N, Ipseiz N, Krönke G, Bäuerle T, et al. Microbiota from obese mice regulate hematopoietic stem cell differentiation by altering the bone niche. Cell Metab 2015;22(5):886−94.

[173] Trottier MD, Naaz A, Li Y, Fraker PJ. Enhancement of hematopoiesis and lymphopoiesis in diet-induced obese mice. Proc Natl Acad Sci U S A 2012;109(20):7622−9.

[174] Valet C, Batut A, Vauclard A, Dortignac A, Bellio M, Payrastre B, et al. Adipocyte fatty acid transfer supports megakaryocyte maturation. Cell Rep 2020;32(1):107875. https://doi.org/10.1016/j.celrep.2020.107875. [cité 23 juin 2021];32(1). Disponible sur: https://www.cell.com/cell-reports/abstract/S2211-1247(20)30856-1.

[175] Prost S, Relouzat F, Spentchian M, Ouzegdouh Y, Saliba J, Massonnet G, et al. Erosion of the chronic myeloid leukaemia stem cell pool by PPARγ agonists. Nature September 17, 2015;525(7569):380−3.

[176] Boyd AL, Reid JC, Salci KR, Aslostovar L, Benoit YD, Shapovalova Z, et al. Acute myeloid leukaemia disrupts endogenous myelo-erythropoiesis by compromising the adipocyte bone marrow niche. Nat Cell Biol 2017;19(11):1336−47.

[177] Larsson SC, Wolk A. Overweight and obesity and incidence of leukemia: a meta-analysis of cohort studies. Int J Canc 2008;122(6):1418−21.

[178] Castillo JJ, Reagan JL, Ingham RR, Furman M, Dalia S, Merhi B, et al. Obesity but not overweight increases the incidence and mortality of leukemia in adults: a meta-analysis of prospective cohort studies. Leuk Res 2012;36(7):868–75.

[179] Shafat MS, Oellerich T, Mohr S, Robinson SD, Edwards DR, Marlein CR, et al. Leukemic blasts program bone marrow adipocytes to generate a protumoral microenvironment. Blood 2017;129(10):1320–32.

[180] Lu W, Weng W, Zhu Q, Zhai Y, Wan Y, Liu H, et al. Small bone marrow adipocytes predict poor prognosis in acute myeloid leukemia. Haematologica 2018;103(1):e21-4.

[181] Liu H, Zhai Y, Zhao W, Wan Y, Lu W, Yang S, et al. Consolidation chemotherapy prevents relapse by indirectly regulating bone marrow adipogenesis in patients with acute myeloid leukemia. Cell Physiol Biochem Int J Exp Cell Physiol Biochem Pharmacol 2018;45(6):2389–400.

[182] Cahu X, Calvo J, Poglio S, Prade N, Colsch B, Arcangeli M-L, et al. Bone marrow sites differently imprint dormancy and chemoresistance to T-cell acute lymphoblastic leukemia. Blood Adv September 12, 2017;1(20):1760–72.

[183] Behan JW, Yun JP, Proektor MP, Ehsanipour EA, Arutyunyan A, Moses AS, et al. Adipocytes impair leukemia treatment in mice. Cancer Res October 1, 2009;69(19):7867–74.

[184] Lu Z, Xie J, Wu G, Shen J, Collins R, Chen W, et al. Fasting selectively blocks development of acute lymphoblastic leukemia via leptin-receptor upregulation. Nat Med 2017;23(1):79–90.

[185] Caers J, Deleu S, Belaid Z, De Raeve H, Van Valckenborgh E, De Bruyne E, et al. Neighboring adipocytes participate in the bone marrow microenvironment of multiple myeloma cells. Leukemia 2007;21(7):1580–4.

[186] Liu Z, Xu J, He J, Liu H, Lin P, Wan X, et al. Mature adipocytes in bone marrow protect myeloma cells against chemotherapy through autophagy activation. Oncotarget October 27, 2015;6(33):34329–41.

[187] Falank C, Fairfield H, Reagan MR. Signaling interplay between bone marrow adipose tissue and multiple myeloma cells. Front Endocrinol 2016;7:67. https://doi.org/10.3389/fendo.2016.00067. eCollection 2016.

[188] Tabe Y, Yamamoto S, Saitoh K, Sekihara K, Monma N, Ikeo K, et al. Bone marrow adipocytes facilitate fatty acid oxidation activating AMPK and a transcriptional network supporting survival of acute monocytic leukemia cells. Cancer Res 2017;77(6):1453–64.

[189] Herroon MK, Rajagurubandara E, Hardaway AL, Powell K, Turchick A, Feldmann D, et al. Bone marrow adipocytes promote tumor growth in bone via FABP4-dependent mechanisms. Oncotarget 2013;4(11):2108–23.

[190] Templeton ZS, Lie W-R, Wang W, Rosenberg-Hasson Y, Alluri RV, Tamaresis JS, et al. Breast cancer cell colonization of the human bone marrow adipose tissue niche. Neoplasia 2015;17(12):849.

[191] van der Eerden B, van Wijnen A. Meeting report of the 2016 bone marrow adiposity meeting. Adipocyte October 2, 2017;6(4):304–13.

[192] Diedrich JD, Rajagurubandara E, Herroon MK, Mahapatra G, Hüttemann M, Podgorski I. Bone marrow adipocytes promote the Warburg phenotype in metastatic prostate tumors via HIF-1α activation. Oncotarget October 4, 2016;7(40):64854–77.

[193] Guérard A, Laurent V, Fromont G, Estève D, Gilhodes J, Bonnelye E, et al. The chemokine receptor CCR3 is potentially involved in the homing of prostate cancer cells to bone: implication of bone-marrow adipocytes. Int J Mol Sci 2021;22(4):1994.

[194] Bredella MA, Fazeli PK, Miller KK, Misra M, Torriani M, Thomas BJ, et al. Increased bone marrow fat in anorexia nervosa. J Clin Endocrinol Metab 2009;94(6):2129–36.

[195] Suchacki KJ, Cawthorn WP. Molecular interaction of bone marrow adipose tissue with energy metabolism. Curr Mol Biol Rep 2018;4(2):41–9.

[196] Fazeli PK, Bredella MA, Freedman L, Thomas BJ, Breggia A, Meenaghan E, et al. Marrow fat and preadipocyte factor-1 levels decrease with recovery in women with anorexia nervosa. J Bone Miner Res Off J Am Soc Bone Miner Res 2012;27(9):1864–71.

[197] Hamrick MW, Ding K-H, Ponnala S, Ferrari SL, Isales CM. Caloric restriction decreases cortical bone mass but spares trabecular bone in the mouse skeleton: implications for the regulation of bone mass by body weight. J Bone Miner Res Off J Am Soc Bone Miner Res 2008;23(6):870–8.

[198] Benova A, Tencerova M. Obesity-induced changes in bone marrow homeostasis. Front Endocrinol 2020;11:294.

[199] de Araújo IM, Salmon CEG, Nahas AK, Nogueira-Barbosa MH, Elias J, de Paula FJA. Marrow adipose tissue spectrum in obesity and type 2 diabetes mellitus. Eur J Endocrinol 2017;176(1):21–30.

[200] Cohen A, Dempster DW, Recker RR, Lappe JM, Zhou H, Zwahlen A, et al. Abdominal fat is associated with lower bone formation and inferior bone quality in healthy premenopausal women: a transiliac bone biopsy study. J Clin Endocrinol Metab 2013;98(6):2562–72.

[201] Bredella MA, Gill CM, Gerweck AV, Landa MG, Kumar V, Daley SM, et al. Ectopic and serum lipid levels are positively associated with bone marrow fat in obesity. Radiology 2013;269(2):534–41.

[202] Blom-Høgestøl IK, Mala T, Kristinsson JA, Hauge E-M, Brunborg C, Gulseth HL, et al. Changes in bone marrow adipose tissue one year after roux-en-Y gastric bypass: a prospective cohort study. J Bone Miner Res Off J Am Soc Bone Miner Res 2019;34(10):1815–23.

[203] Piotrowska K, Tarnowski M. Bone marrow adipocytes-role in physiology and various nutritional conditions in human and animal models. Nutrients 2021;13(5):1412.

[204] Bredella MA, Greenblatt LB, Eajazi A, Torriani M, Yu EW. Effects of Roux-en-Y gastric bypass and sleeve gastrectomy on bone mineral density and marrow adipose tissue. Bone 2017;95:85–90.

[205] Bredella MA, Singhal V, Hazhir Karzar N, Animashaun A, Bose A, Stanford FC, et al. Effects of sleeve gastrectomy on bone marrow adipose tissue in adolescents and young adults with obesity. J Clin Endocrinol Metab November 1, 2020;105(11):dgaa581.

[206] Schafer AL, Li X, Schwartz AV, Tufts LS, Wheeler AL, Grunfeld C, et al. Changes in vertebral bone marrow fat and bone mass after gastric bypass surgery: a pilot study. Bone 2015;74:140–5.

[207] Kim TY, Schwartz AV, Li X, Xu K, Black DM, Petrenko DM, et al. Bone marrow fat changes after gastric bypass surgery are associated with loss of bone mass. J Bone Miner Res Off J Am Soc Bone Miner Res 2017;32(11):2239–47.

[208] Scheller EL, Khoury B, Moller KL, Wee NKY, Khandaker S, Kozloff KM, et al. Changes in skeletal integrity and marrow adiposity during high-fat diet and after weight loss. Front Endocrinol 2016;7:102. https://doi.org/10.3389/fendo.2016.00102. eCollection 2016.

[209] Corsa CAS, Walsh CM, Bagchi DP, Foss Freitas MC, Li Z, Hardij J, et al. Adipocyte-specific deletion of lamin A/C largely models human familial partial lipodystrophy type 2. Diabetes 2021;70(9):1970−84. https://doi.org/10.2337/db20-1001. Epub 2021 Jun 4.

[210] Napoli N, Chandran M, Pierroz DD, Abrahamsen B, Schwartz AV, Ferrari SL, et al. Mechanisms of diabetes mellitus-induced bone fragility. Nat Rev Endocrinol 2017;13(4):208−19.

[211] Botolin S, McCabe LR. Inhibition of PPARgamma prevents type I diabetic bone marrow adiposity but not bone loss. J Cell Physiol 2006;209(3):967−76.

[212] Carvalho AL, Massaro B, Silva LTPE, Salmon CEG, Fukada SY, Nogueira-Barbosa MH, et al. Emerging aspects of the body composition, bone marrow adipose tissue and skeletal phenotypes in type 1 diabetes mellitus. J Clin Densitom Off J Int Soc Clin Densitom 2019;22(3):420−8.

[213] Abdalrahaman N, McComb C, Foster JE, Lindsay RS, Drummond R, McKay GA, et al. The relationship between adiposity, bone density and microarchitecture is maintained in young women irrespective of diabetes status. Clin Endocrinol 2017;87(4):327−35.

[214] Sheu Y, Amati F, Schwartz AV, Danielson ME, Li X, Boudreau R, et al. Vertebral bone marrow fat, bone mineral density and diabetes: the osteoporotic fractures in men (MrOS) study. Bone 2017;97:299−305.

[215] Santopaolo M, Gu Y, Spinetti G, Madeddu P. Bone marrow fat: friend or foe in people with diabetes mellitus? Clin Sci 1979;134(8):1031−48. 30 avr 2020.

[216] Baum T, Yap SP, Karampinos DC, Nardo L, Kuo D, Burghardt AJ, et al. Does vertebral bone marrow fat content correlate with abdominal adipose tissue, lumbar spine bone mineral density, and blood biomarkers in women with type 2 diabetes mellitus? J Magn Reson Imag 2012;35(1):117−24.

[217] Devlin MJ, Van Vliet M, Motyl K, Karim L, Brooks DJ, Louis L, et al. Early-onset type 2 diabetes impairs skeletal acquisition in the male TALLYHO/JngJ mouse. Endocrinology 2014;155(10):3806−16.

Ectopic lipid deposition in skeletal muscle, liver, and myocardium strongly depends on circulating substrate concentrations. In the insulin-resistant state, the interorgan cross-talk between insulin-dependent organs is disturbed. This results in increased glucose, insulin, and NEFA levels, which majorly contribute to TAG accumulation in ectopic tissues. Other hormones might exert their impact on fat stores indirectly by modulating substrate concentrations by interfering with the action of insulin.

Thyroid hormone

Thyroid hormones are important determinants of whole-body energy metabolism. Thyroxine (T4) is the major secretory product of the thyroid gland. Its secretion is controlled by the thyroid-stimulating hormone (TSH), which is secreted from the anterior pituitary gland. As a prohormone, T4 must be converted to triiodothyronine (T3) by the deiodinase D1, D2, and D3 to acquire full biological activity, which controls the local, tissue-specific amount. T3 acts through the nuclear thyroid receptors TRα and TRβ [25].

Hypothyroidism constitutes one of the most common endocrine diseases. It is linked to a variety of changes in lipid metabolism and characterized as a hypometabolic state. Compared to euthyroid controls, hypothyroid patients exhibit markedly decreased lipid oxidation rates and low NEFA levels in combination with unchanged whole-body lipolysis, which suggests an increased synthesis of TAG [26]. Other alterations of circulating lipids include a rise in total cholesterol and low-density lipoprotein levels, which can be reversed by levothyroxine replacement therapy [27].

With regard to ectopic fat stores, hypothyroidism has been linked with TAG accumulation in the liver and the myocardium, but not in skeletal muscle.

There is a strong, inverse association between the concentration of free thyroxine (fT4) and HCL with decreased fT4 levels contributing to hepatic lipid accumulation in general population [28]. This association can be observed in subclinical and overt hypothyroidism and is independent of differences in the BMI [29]. However, we previously failed to demonstrate a significant reduction in HCL following the initiation of levothyroxine replacement therapy in a group of overtly hypothyroid patients [30]. This might most likely be explained by the short period of hypothyroidism before study inclusion, since patients were investigated 4–5 weeks after the stop of levothyroxine substitution in preparation for radioiodine therapy. On the other hand, local organ-specific thyroid hormone receptor activation in the liver prevents the development of hepatic steatosis in animal studies [31] and is currently tested in clinical trials for its therapeutic use in the treatment of nonalcoholic fatty liver disease (NAFLD) in humans [32].

The effects of thyroid hormones on hepatic lipid metabolism are complex. De novo lipogenesis is stimulated by thyroid hormones because of increased hepatic NEFA uptake, but also lipogenic gene expression. However, there is no net retention of HCL in euthyroidism and even a reduction of HCL in hyperthyroidism since fatty acid metabolism occurs at a higher rate than fatty acid synthesis. These catabolic effects of thyroid hormones on TAG stores in the liver include its impact on lipolysis, the regulation of autophagy of TAGs in lysosomes, and the stimulation of mitochondrial fatty acid oxidation [33].

In the myocardium TAG stores decrease following the initiation of a treatment by levothyroxine independent of changes in body weight [30]. This might also be explained by changes in mitochondrial lipid oxidation within the myocardium, which is enhanced by thyroid hormones [34]. Furthermore, alterations in lipoprotein lipase activity modify NEFA uptake within the heart [35]. The reduction in MYCL following treatment of hypothyroidism was associated with significant improvements in systolic left ventricular heart function, suggesting that there might be a form of cardiomyopathy due to cardiac steatosis, similar to that observed in patients with type 2 diabetes mellitus [30]. Granted that, there are also direct effects of thyroid hormones on cardiomyocytes that could explain the improvement in cardiac function [36].

In WAT thyroid hormones play a major role in the regulation of adipogenesis. T3 modulates the proliferation and differentiation of adipocytes. It is important for the development of brown adipose tissue and might stimulate a transdifferentiation from white to beige adipocytes. Furthermore, thyroid hormones regulate gene expression for lipogenesis and lipolysis in WAT, and thermogenesis in brown adipose tissue [37].

The regulation of thermogenesis and resting energy expenditure by thyroid hormones might be among the most important factors for its control of energy metabolism. Thermogenesis is mainly controlled by the mitochondrial uncoupling protein (UCP) 1, which is directly controlled by T3 and indirectly by increased sensitivity for adrenergic stimulation [38]. In hyperthyroidism, increased energy expenditure is paralleled by higher rates of lipid oxidation, which are both strongly associated with thyroid hormone concentrations [39]. In skeletal muscle, short-term treatment by T3 for 3 days markedly increased tricarboxylic acid flux without changes in ATP synthesis, highlighting the distinct promotion of thermogenesis by mitochondrial uncoupling due to UCP1 expression [40]. This also applies to the liver, where TRβ agonists have been shown to stimulate lipid oxidation and mitochondrial respiration rates [31] and have been shown to substantially reduce HCL in patients with NAFLD [41].

On the other hand, not only thyroid function exerts effects on WAT and ectopic fat stores; obesity also interferes with the hypothalamus-pituitary-thyroid axis. In patients with severe obesity, we previously observed a higher prevalence of subclinical hypothyroidism compared to general population. Furthermore, there was an association between the BMI and TSH levels, which was normalized by weight loss after bariatric surgery [42]. Several underlying mechanisms addressing the increase in TSH concentrations in obesity have been hypothesized. These include a stimulatory effect of leptin secreted in adipocytes on the hypothalamus-pituitary-thyroid axis, but also an impact of accelerated turnover of thyroid hormones resulting from increased thyroid hormone disposal due to the larger body size in obesity has been proposed [43]. However, the observation that TSH concentrations normalize after weight loss following bariatric surgery strongly suggests that the rise in TSH is more an adaptive response than a causally contributing factor.

The effects of thyroid hormones on fat stores are illustrated in Fig. 13.2.

Growth hormone

The impact of growth hormone (GH) on fat stores is unique, as it separates the otherwise tight relations between visceral and ectopic lipid deposition and insulin resistance. The secretion of GH from the somatotropic cells of the anterior pituitary is stimulated by growth hormone releasing hormone and inhibited by somatostatin from the hypothalamus. In the liver, GH stimulates the synthesis of insulin like growth factor (IGF) 1, which exerts a negative feedback on GH secretion.

GH has a central role in the regulation of whole-body lipolysis and glucose metabolism and counteracts insulin action in adipose tissue. GH is prolipolytic and thereby induces insulin resistance when secreted in excess, for example, in patients with acromegaly. In addition to these antagonistic effects of GH on insulin action GH stimulates IGF-1 secretion from the liver, a hormone that shares a structural homology with insulin and therefore also exerts insulinlike anabolic actions. However, in states of GH excess and insufficiency the direct effects of GH on lipolysis appear to largely outweigh the potential anabolic effects of IGF-1 [44,45].

Patients suffering from acromegaly, a disease characterized by excessive GH secretion due to a pituitary adenoma in almost all cases, have a markedly reduced WAT and ectopic fat mass [46]. A common metabolic consequence of acromegaly is impaired insulin sensitivity. It represents a rare exception where insulin resistance develops in the context of reduced body and liver fat [47]. This can be explained by a loss of lipid storage capacity of adipose tissue, mainly due to the lipolytic actions of GH, which has been nicely shown in mechanistic studies in healthy volunteers: Mobilization of NEFA from WAT by stimulated lipolysis in adipose tissue results in insulin resistance in skeletal muscle and the liver following GH administration. On the other hand, coadministration of Acipimox, a nicotinic acid which

FIGURE 13.2 Overview of the possible actions of thyroid hormones on the regulation of fat storage in white adipose tissue and ectopic lipid stores.

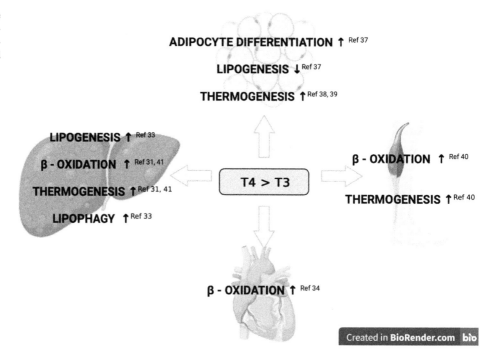

Part III

Regulation of fat stores

Chapter 13

Regulation of fat stores—endocrinological pathways

Peter Wolf, Thomas Scherer and Michael Krebs

Division of Endocrinology and Metabolism, Department of Internal Medicine III, Medical University of Vienna, Austria

Insulin

Insulin, a hormone that is secreted by beta cells in the pancreas, plays a major role in the regulation of energy metabolism and enables a balanced nutrient availability in accordance with the fluctuating demands during feeding and fasting. Under physiological conditions in the fed state insulin is a strong inhibitor of lipolysis and promoter of de novo lipogenesis in WAT acting as an anabolic hormone for lipid storage. During the transition from feeding to fasting in a metabolically flexible organism insulin levels rapidly fall and adapt to allow for lipid and energy mobilization from the fat storage compartments. Insulin's action in this complex regulation of energy homeostasis is mediated by both direct and indirect effects. It is well known that insulin binds directly to insulin receptors expressed on peripheral organs such as white adipose tissue (WAT), skeletal muscle, and the liver to regulate energy homeostasis. However, as an additional layer of complexity it also has become clear that insulin crosses the blood—brain barrier binding to insulin receptors in the brain to indirectly modulate peripheral organ function via the autonomic nervous system [1]. Brain insulin action in an acute setting is less prominent and often complementary to insulin's peripheral effects, but there is an extensive body of literature that brain insulin resistance significantly contributes to the development of whole-body insulin resistance, the metabolic syndrome, type 2 diabetes, and fatty liver disease (i.e., ectopic triacylglycerol (TAG) deposition). The role of brain insulin action in animal and human studies is extensively reviewed in Ref. [2].

In skeletal muscle insulin promotes glucose uptake, utilization, and storage under physiological conditions. In the liver, insulin lowers glucose output by activating glycogen synthesis and inhibiting gluconeogenesis, and increases lipogenic gene expression [3]. All these pathways are impaired in states of insulin resistance such as obesity and type 2 diabetes.

In obesity with adipocyte hypertrophy, inadequate vascularization and local inflammation, due to macrophage infiltration, results in insulin resistance in WAT [4]. This is followed by unrestrained lipolysis combined with impaired lipogenesis and leads to an increased release of nonesterified fatty acids (NEFA) into systemic circulation [5]. This surplus of NEFAs caused by insulin resistance, chronic overnutrition, and WAT dysfunction is compensated by an increased ectopic lipid uptake into nonadipose tissue organs where the ectopic TAGs cause lipotoxicity and further promote insulin resistance [6].

This concept of lipid-induced insulin resistance is emphasized by cross-sectional studies demonstrating higher NEFA levels in patients suffering from type 2 diabetes mellitus, but also in insulin-resistant offspring [7,8]. In metabolically healthy individuals, short time elevation of circulating NEFA by a continuous lipid infusion and heparin to activate lipoprotein lipase resulted in a marked reduction of insulin-stimulated glucose uptake in skeletal muscle and whole-body glucose oxidation [9].

These findings clearly emphasize the importance of circulating NEFAs on the development of insulin resistance. However, ectopic TAG storage in skeletal muscle is even a more sensitive predictor for impaired glucose tolerance. Intramyocellular lipid content (IMCL) is increased in the insulin resistant state [10], and was shown to be even closer associated with insulin sensitivity than NEFA levels [11]. In lean insulin resistant offspring of patients with type 2 diabetes IMCL is markedly elevated and precedes other metabolic complications [12]. Insulin resistance due to increased IMCL is mainly mediated by the accumulation of metabolically toxic intermediates of lipid metabolism, i.e., diacylglycerols and ceramides, which impair insulin signaling and decrease glucose disposal and glycogen synthesis in skeletal muscle [13].

The association between ectopic TAG accumulation and impaired insulin signaling is not restricted to skeletal muscle. In the liver, increased hepatic lipid content (HCL) is strongly associated with impaired whole-body insulin sensitivity [14].

Visceral and Ectopic Fat. https://doi.org/10.1016/B978-0-12-822186-0.00018-3

The liver is an important player in the regulation of energy homeostasis, by being the main source of endogenous glucose production and important for fatty acid disposal, as well as de novo lipogenesis. In the insulin-resistant state, glucor-egulatory effects of insulin in the liver are impaired, whereas prolipogenic effects remain preserved. This has been described as the hepatic insulin paradox and promotes a vicious circle of enhanced HCL accumulation, increased release of lipids and a further worsening of glucose tolerance [15]. Other evidence supports a more insulin-independent regulation of hepatic TAG storage, which is mainly driven by reesterification of NEFA from circulation [16]. This suggests unrestrained lipolysis in WAT as the most important factor for the increase in HCL deposition in insulin resistance. However, with regards to metabolic complications of obesity, strong evidence suggests that accumulation of TAG as ectopic fat plays a much more important role than in WAT. Elegant studies combining tracer techniques with 1H MR spectroscopy in a cohort of obese subjects directly compared the impact of HCL and WAT on metabolic abnormalities. They demonstrated that insulin sensitivity was markedly impaired in subjects with a higher than normal amount of HCL matched for WAT volume, whereas no differences were observed between subjects with different WAT volumes matched on HCL [17].

In contrast to ectopic lipid deposition in the liver and in skeletal muscle, insulin resistance as such is not associated with increased TAG accumulation in the myocardium (intramyocardial lipid content, MYCL). Intracellular TAG overload and cardiac steatosis in patients with type 2 diabetes mellitus are independent risk factors for the development of heart failure. However, insulin resistance might not be causal for ectopic fat accumulation in the heart, but cardiac steatosis rather represents a final stage after long-standing derangement of glucose and lipid metabolism [18]. Uptake of lipids by the heart is primarily determined by circulating levels of NEFA that enter the myocardium passively by diffusion or actively by transport proteins. In the resting state, approximately 70%−90% of FA entering cardiomyocytes are rapidly used for ATP synthesis, whereas only the minority is stored [19]. Oversupply with circulating NEFA results in excessive intracellular TAG accumulation, wherefore MYCL strongly depends on the regulation of lipolysis in WAT by insulin [20−22]. But even in the absence of circulating NEFA, an increase in insulin levels secondary to hyperglycemia significantly increased MYCL in healthy subjects, probably because of a local switch in substrate utilization from lipids to glucose [23].

Finally, it is important to emphasize that MYCL is highly flexible and does not inevitably relate to impaired energy metabolism, as it can be also used as a readily available source of energy in situations of increased demands [24].

An overview on the effects of insulin resistance on WAT and ectopic fat stores is shown in Fig. 13.1.

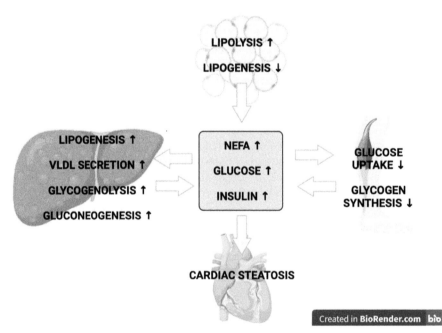

FIGURE 13.1 Overview of the consequences of insulin resistance on glucose and lipid metabolism in white adipose tissue and ectopic fat stores: in the insulin-resistant state the inhibition of lipolysis and the stimulation of lipogenesis in white adipose tissue is impaired resulting in increased concentrations of nonesterified fatty acids (NEFA); increased ectopic lipid deposition in skeletal muscle and increased circulating NEFAs impair glucose disposal and glycogen synthesis in skeletal muscle, worsening hyperglycemia. Increased ectopic lipid deposition in the liver, as well as substrate delivery by increased NEFA and glucose concentration, impairs glycogen synthesis and stimulates gluconeogenesis, lipogenesis, and VLDL secretion, worsening hypergly-cemia and dyslipidemia; increased circulating concentrations of NEFA, glucose, and insulin stimulate ectopic lipid deposition in the myocardium, resulting in cardiac steatosis (reviewed in 6,12, 24).

pharmacologically inhibits lipolysis in WAT and thereby lowers circulating NEFA concentration, mitigates these anti-insulinogenic effects of GH [48].

Visceral and subcutaneous WAT are about 70% and 80% lower in patients with active acromegaly compared to that observed in a healthy population, respectively. A significant association between disease severity and WAT distribution was observed [49]. Following pituitary surgery and disease remission, WAT increases substantially and tends to normalize compared to the control cohort [50]. Furthermore, ectopic fat stores in the liver and skeletal muscle are also lower in patients with active acromegaly [51], whereas no differences in MYCL were observed [52].

On the other hand, patients suffering from GH deficiency have a higher WAT mass, which improves following the initiation of GH substitution therapy [53,54]. Furthermore, this is associated with an increase in lipid oxidation and a decrease in protein catabolism [55]. Similar effects could be found in abdominally obese volunteers without GH deficiency, but IGF-1 in the lower normal range, in which initiation of a low dose GH substitution therapy resulted in an improved body composition, characterized by a loss of visceral fat mass and HCL [56].

Besides its impact of adipose tissue lipolysis, another factor by which GH modulates ectopic fat stores is the stimulation of beta oxidation and mitochondrial activity. In patients with active acromegaly low HCL was associated with an about 50% increase in hepatic ATP turnover compared to a group of healthy controls well matched for sex, age, BMI, and body composition [51]. Stimulated mitochondrial activity by GH might therefore prevent the liver from ectopic TAG deposition, despite elevated circulating NEFA levels and insulin resistance in acromegaly.

Other mechanisms by which GH affects HCL storage might include the inhibition of de novo lipogenesis and increased hepatic VLDL export. Data of animal models show that liver-specific GH receptor knockdown results in the early development of advanced stages of NAFLD after 7 days, independently of changes in systemic insulin sensitivity or white adipose tissue lipolysis. The observed increase in HCL was attributable to an augmented glycolysis-mediated de novo lipogenesis in the liver [57,58]. The effects of GH on hepatic lipid metabolism could be dissected from those of IGF-1, since restoration of IGF-1 improved systemic insulin sensitivity and lipid profile, but failed to protect against hepatic steatosis and inflammation in GH resistant mice [59]. However, studies confirming these effects of GH on hepatic de novo lipogenesis in humans are missing. With regards to VLDL secretion, in vivo studies in isolated perfused rat liver showed an increase following GH stimulation [60]. In humans, a study investigating the effects of 3 months of GH replacement therapy in patients with GH deficiency reported a significantly increased rate of VLDL apolipoprotein B secretion [61], whereas other studies in healthy volunteers did not show changes in VLDL kinetics following 8 days of GH administration [62].

The effects of GH on fat stores are illustrated in Fig. 13.3.

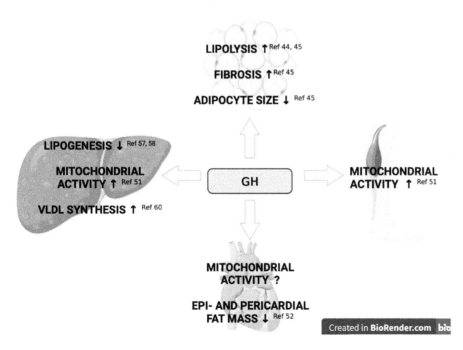

FIGURE 13.3 Overview of the possible actions of growth hormone on the regulation of fat storage in white adipose tissue and ectopic lipid stores.

Cortisol

Cortisol, a stress hormone secreted by the adrenal glands, is a major player in the regulation of energy metabolism, and disorders in cortisol secretion are strongly related with alterations in TAG storage. Cushing syndrome, resulting from endogenous hypercortisolism or chronic overexposure to exogenous glucocorticoids, is archetypical of the metabolic syndrome and clinically characterized by the accumulation of WAT in most of the patients [63]. Hypercortisolism is associated with an increase in abdominal visceral obesity and a loss of subcutaneous fat depots of the extremities. However, the underlying mechanisms are complex and only partly understood. Cortisol plays a crucial role for adipocyte differentiation by inducing key transcriptional factors. With regards to lipogenesis, cortisol has both stimulating and inhibiting effects in WAT, which also depend on the presence of insulin and the extent and duration of glucocorticoid exposure [64,65]. Furthermore, cortisol stimulates adipose tissue lipolysis directly as well as indirectly by enhancing the sensitivity to catecholamines [66]. However, abdominal WAT might have a lower lipolytic activity compared to other tissues, due to differences in glucocorticoid receptor expression [67,68]. This might explain the typical phenotype of WAT distribution in patients with Cushing syndrome [69].

Important factors for the regulation of the effects of glucocorticoids in WAT include the local activation of cortisol by conversion from cortisone by the 11b-hydroxysteroiddehydrogenase I (11bHSD1). The importance of this enzyme for the development of typical metabolic features of Cushing syndrome is highlighted by a case report of a patient with a partial defect of 11bHSD1 activity, who did not show any clinical signs despite severe hypercortisolism in biochemical analysis [70]. Animal models emphasize the impact of local 11bHSD1 on fat stores [64]. In humans, glucocorticoids were shown to stimulate 11bHSD1 expression and activity in a dose-dependent manner on short term [71]. However, in patients with Cushing syndrome, a lack of increase in 11bHSD1 expression in visceral WAT was reported, which might reflect a downregulation following prolonged exposure to high doses of glucocorticoids [72].

Another central role in the regulation of the effects of cortisol on WAT was reported for the AMP-activated protein kinase (AMPK). AMPK is a key metabolic regulator and a sensor of cellular energy status. Activation of AMPK in the fasting state results in a shift from anabolic to catabolic pathways of energy metabolism. Especially in WAT, exposure to glucocorticoids inhibited AMPK activation in animal models [73]. In line with this observation, in patients with Cushing syndrome a 70% reduction in AMPK in WAT was reported, which inversely correlated with the degree of hypercortisolism [74].

With regards to ectopic fat stores, only limited knowledge exists on the effects of hypercortisolism on IMCL, HCL, and MYCL accumulation.

In line with increased concentrations of circulating NEFAs and insulin resistance in Cushing syndrome, one might assume augmented IMCL levels in skeletal muscle. However, studies in humans showing these effects are missing.

In the liver, a relation between hypercortisolism and the development of NAFLD was suggested [75]. Elevated HCL is associated with inadequate suppression of cortisol following the overnight administration of dexamethasone [76]. Furthermore an increased prevalence of NAFLD in patients with Cushing syndrome was reported [77]. However, up to now measurements of HCL by 1H magnetic resonance spectroscopy, the gold standard method to noninvasively investigate HCL in vivo, have not been performed in patients with hypercortisolism.

With regards to the heart, an increase in pericardial fat mass was reported in patients with Cushing syndrome [78]. Pericardial fat is considered as visceral thoracic WAT, which directly surrounds the myocardium and therefore also might exert paracrine effects by adipocytokine secretion [79]. It might therefore play an important role in the development of heart disease in hypercortisolism. Biochemical disease remission decreased pericardial fat after a median follow-up of 6 months, which highlights the important impact of cortisol. On the other hand, no differences in MYCL could be observed in patients with Cushing syndrome. This is probably explained by higher rates of beta oxidation within the myocardium stimulated by cortisol excess, which prevents the heart from cardiac steatosis [80].

In patients suffering from primary adrenal insufficiency, a disease characterized by the deficiency of glucocorticoids, no differences in visceral WAT mass could be found under state-of-the-art hormone substitution therapy compared to a healthy control group in a cross-sectional study [81]. Furthermore, ectopic lipid storage in the liver and myocardium was also similar [82].

The effects of cortisol on fat stores are illustrated in Fig. 13.4.

Sex hormones

Sex hormones play a well-known role in body composition, glucose and lipid metabolism [83]. Especially androgens are characterized by sexual dimorphism [84]. In men reduced testosterone concentrations are associated with obesity, insulin resistance, and hypertension. Hypogonadism due to therapy with GnRH agonists in men suffering from prostate cancer is

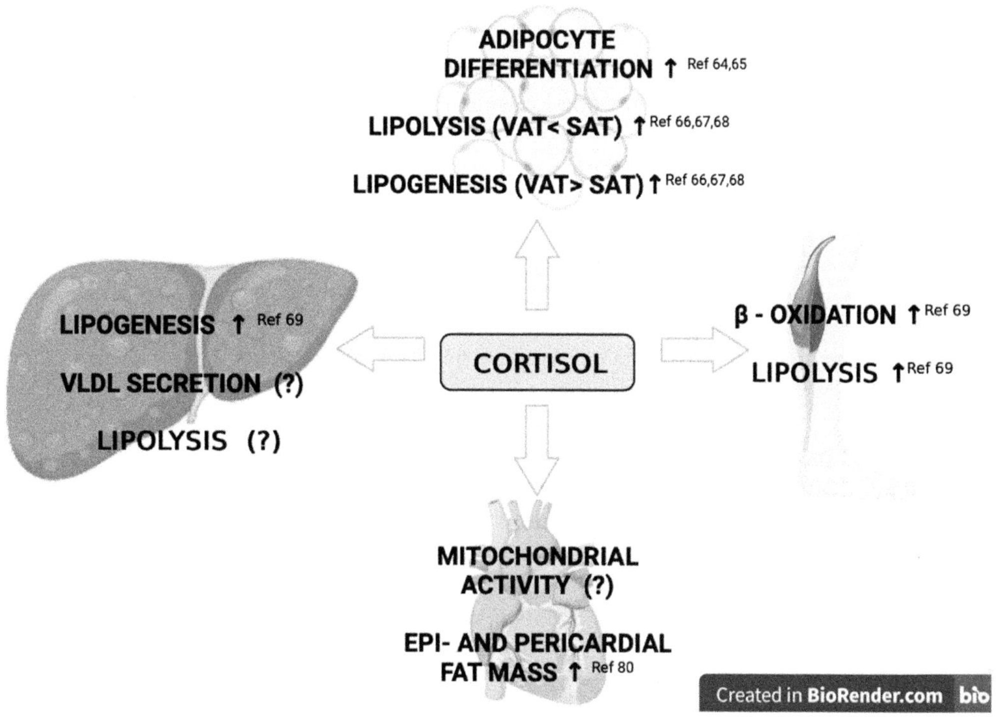

FIGURE 13.4 Overview of the possible actions of cortisol on the regulation of fat storage in white adipose tissue and ectopic lipid stores.

associated with increased fat mass [85], whereas testosterone treatment in hypogonadism improved insulin sensitivity and reduced fat mass in patients with type 2 diabetes mellitus [86].

In contrast to the favorable impact of testosterone in men, women with hyperandrogenemia have an increased risk for obesity and the metabolic syndrome [84]. The most common cause of androgen excess in women is polycystic ovary syndrome (PCOS), which is closely linked to insulin resistance, obesity, and has an unfavorable influence on women's quality of life [87].

With regards to ectopic fat stores, retrospective studies reported an increased prevalence of hypogonadism in male patients suffering from NAFLD [88]. However, testosterone replacement therapy in patients with type 2 diabetes mellitus and testosterone levels below the limit of normal, as well as in elderly men with abdominal obesity, had no effects on HCL [89,90].

With regards to skeletal muscle, no differences in IMCL and insulin sensitivity could be found 4 weeks after biochemical castration in a group of healthy volunteers [91]. Of note, the effects of testosterone replacement on changes in body composition might strongly depend on the aromatase activity and circulating estrogen concentrations [92,93]. This could in parts explain the heterogeneous findings of the effects of testosterone on lipid deposition observed in previous studies.

In women with hyperandrogenemia diagnosed with PCOS, an increased prevalence of NAFLD was reported in studies using ultrasound criteria for the definition of increased HCL [94,95], whereas recent studies using 1H MRS could not find significant differences [96]. This might be explained by the heterogeneity of patients diagnosed with PCOS, as especially those with a severe insulin resistance are at the highest risk to develop metabolic complications.

In general, men and postmenopausal women have a greater risk for the development of NAFLD than premenopausal women, highlighting the protective role of estrogen. Estrogen was shown to attenuate lipolysis in subcutaneous WAT, but not in visceral WAT [97]. These changes in regional lipid metabolism and WAT distribution—with a gynoid gluteofemoral subcutaneous WAT mass and lower android visceral adiposity— are associated with lower levels of circulating NEFAs and lower the risk for ectopic lipid accumulation [98].

On the other hand, obesity as such also has marked effects on sex hormone concentrations in a sex-specific manner. Whereas there is a high prevalence of hypogonadism in men suffering from severe obesity, androgen excess is frequently observed in women. However, weight loss following bariatric surgery significantly improved the sex hormone profile in both sexes [99].

Mechanisms that explain these differences in men are reduced levels of SHBG in adiposity, as well as the suppressive effects estrogen, which is converted from testosterone by the aromatase in adipose tissue, on the secretion of gonado-tropins. Central resistance to insulin and leptin might also play a role in the impaired stimulation of GHRH signaling mediated by proinflammatory cytokines [100]. In women, insulin resistance appears to be most important, as it stimulates androgen excess indirectly by modulating SHBG, as well as by direct promotion of androgen secretion [101].

Summary

The regulation of fat stores is tightly controlled by an interplay of different metabolically relevant hormones. Hormonal excess, as well as deficiency in various endocrine diseases, is closely linked to alterations in fat storage capacity in WAT, as well as ectopic lipid uptake into nonadipose tissue organs.

These alterations in ectopic lipid deposition can be explained by direct organ-specific hormonal effects, which stimulate local energy metabolism, as well as indirectly by modulation of lipid metabolism in WAT and circulating NEFA concentrations (see Fig. 13.5).

Treatment of endocrine diseases strongly impacts fat storage in WAT, but also in ectopic lipid depots. On the other hand, organ-specific modulation of hormone action might offer novel therapeutic targets for obesity-related disorders, as shown by the promising results of thyroid hormone receptor agonists for the reduction of HCL in nonalcoholic fatty liver disease.

For further investigating endocrinological pathways in the regulation of fat stores, rare endocrine diseases serve as ideal pathophysiological models to examine hormone-specific actions on lipid metabolism, which might help to identify and improve future treatment strategies for the obese population in general.

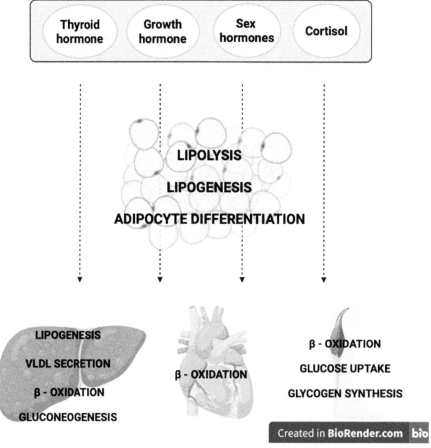

FIGURE 13.5 Overview of endocrine pathways on the hormonal regulation of fat storage in white adipose tissue and ectopic lipid stores. Thyroid hormone, growth hormone, sex hormones, and cortisol all exert effects on white adipose tissue and thereby impact glucose and lipid metabolism; this modifies ectopic fat stores indirectly by changes in circulating substrate concentrations; in addition, there are direct organ-specific effects on local energy metabolism, which modulate ectopic lipid depots.

Acknowledgments

The figures were created by using biorender.com.

References

[1] Neeland IJ, Ross R, Després JP, Matsuzawa Y, Yamashita S, Shai I, Seidell J, Magni P, Santos RD, Arsenault B, Cuevas A, Hu FB, Griffin B, Zambon A, Barter P, Fruchart JC, Eckel RH. Visceral and ectopic fat, atherosclerosis, and cardiometabolic disease: a position statement. Lancet Diabetes Endocrinol 2019;7(9):715−25.

[2] Scherer T, Sakamoto K, Buettner C. Brain insulin signalling in metabolic homeostasis and disease. Nat Rev Endocrinol 2021;17:468−83. https://doi.org/10.1038/s41574-021-00498-x. 0123456789.

[3] Petersen MC, Shulman GI. Mechanisms of insulin action and insulin resistance. Physiol Rev 2018;98(4):2133−223.

[4] Morigny P, Boucher J, Arner P, Langin D. Lipid and glucose metabolism in white adipocytes: pathways, dysfunction and therapeutics. Nat Rev Endocrinol 2021;17. https://doi.org/10.1038/s41574-021-00471-8. May.

[5] Zechner R, Zimmermann R, Eichmann T, Kohlwein S, Haemmerle G, Lass A, Madeo F. Fat signals - lipases and lipolysis in lipid metabolism and signaling. Cell Metabol 2012. https://doi.org/10.1016/j.cmet.2011.12.018.

[6] Samuel VT, Shulman GI. Mechanisms for insulin resistance: common threads and missing links. Cell 2012;148(5):852−71.

[7] Reaven GM, Hollenbeck C, Jeng CY, Wu MS, Chen YD. Measurement of plasma glucose, free fatty acid, lactate, and insulin for 24 h in patients with NIDDM. Diabetes 1988;37(8):1020−4.

[8] Perseghin G, Scifo P, De Cobelli F, Pagliato E, Battezzati A, Arcelloni C, Vanzulli A, Testolin G, Pozza G, Del Maschio A, Luzi L. Intramyocellular triglyceride content is a determinant of in vivo insulin resistance in humans: a 1H-13C nuclear magnetic resonance spectroscopy assessment in offspring of type 2 diabetic parents. Diabetes 1999;48(8):1600−6.

[9] Roden M, Price TB, Perseghin G, Petersen KF, Rothman DL, Cline GW, Shulman GI. Mechanism of free fatty acid-induced insulin resistance in humans. J Clin Invest 1996;97(12):2859−65.

[10] Pan DA, Lillioja S, Kriketos AD, Milner MR, Baur LA, Bogardus C, Jenkins AB, Storlien LH. Skeletal muscle triglyceride levels are inversely related to insulin action. Diabetes 1997;46(6):983−8.

[11] Krssak M, Falk Petersen K, Dresner A, DiPietro L, Vogel SM, Rothman DL, Roden M, Shulman GI. Intramyocellular lipid concentrations are correlated with insulin sensitivity in humans: a 1H NMR spectroscopy study. Diabetologia 1999;42(1):113−6.

[12] Petersen KF, Dufour S, Befroy D, Garcia R, Shulman GI. Impaired mitochondrial activity in the insulin-resistant offspring of patients with type 2 diabetes. N Engl J Med 2004;350(7):664−71.

[13] Roden M, Shulman GI. The integrative biology of type 2 diabetes. Nature 2019;576(7785):51−60.

[14] Angulo P. Nonalcoholic fatty liver disease. N Engl J Med 2002;346(16):1221−31.

[15] Brown MS, Goldstein JL. Selective versus total insulin resistance: a pathogenic paradox. Cell Metabol 2008;7(2):95−6.

[16] Vatner DF, Majumdar SK, Kumashiro N, Petersen MC, Rahimi Y, Gattu AK, Bears M, Camporez JPG, Cline GW, Jurczak MJ, Samuel VT, Shulman GI. Insulin-independent regulation of hepatic triglyceride synthesis by fatty acids. Proc Natl Acad Sci USA 2015;112(4):1143−8.

[17] Fabbrini E, Mohammed BS, Magkos F, Korenblat KM, Patterson BW, Klein S. Alterations in adipose tissue and hepatic lipid kinetics in obese men and women with nonalcoholic fatty liver disease. Gastroenterology 2008;134(2):424−31.

[18] Krššák M, Winhofer Y, Göbl C, Bischof M, Reiter G, Kautzky-Willer A, Luger A, Krebs M, Anderwald C. Insulin resistance is not associated with myocardial steatosis in women. Diabetologia 2011;54(7):1871−8.

[19] Stanley WC, Recchia FA, Lopaschuk GD. Myocardial substrate metabolism in the normal and failing heart. Physiol Rev 2005;85(3):1093−129.

[20] van der Meer RW, Hammer S, Lamb HJ, Frölich M, Diamant M, Rijzewijk LJ, de Roos A, Romijn JA, Smit JWA. Effects of short-term high-fat, high-energy diet on hepatic and myocardial triglyceride content in healthy men. J Clin Endocrinol Metab 2008;93(7):2702−8.

[21] Winhofer Y, Krššák M, Wolf P, Anderwald C-H, Geroldinger A, Heinze G, Baumgartner-Parzer S, Marculescu R, Stulnig T, Wolzt M, Trattnig S, Luger A, Krebs M. Free fatty acid availability is closely related to myocardial lipid storage and cardiac function in hypoglycemia counterregulation. Am J Physiol Metab 2015;308(8):E631−40.

[22] Wolf P, Winhofer Y, Krssak M, Smajis S, Harreiter J, Kosi-Trebotic L, Fürnsinn C, Anderwald CH, Baumgartner-Parzer S, Trattnig S, Luger A, Krebs M. Suppression of plasma free fatty acids reduces myocardial lipid content and systolic function in type 2 diabetes. Nutr Metabol Cardiovasc Dis 2016;26(5):387−92.

[23] Winhofer Y, Krššák M, Jankovic D, Anderwald C-H, Reiter G, Hofer A, Trattnig S, Luger A, Krebs M. Short-term hyperinsulinemia and hyperglycemia increase myocardial lipid content in normal subjects. Diabetes 2012;61(5):1210−6.

[24] Wolf P, Winhofer Y, Krššák M, Krebs M. Heart, lipids and hormones. Endocr Connect 2017;6(4):R59−69.

[25] Braverman LE, Ingbar SH, Sterling K. Conversion of thyroxine (T4) to triiodothyronine (T3) in athyreotic human subjects. J Clin Invest 1970;49(5):855−64.

[26] Gjedde S, Gormsen LC, Rungby J, Nielsen S, Jørgensen JOL, Pedersen SB, Riis AL, Weeke J, Møller N. Decreased lipid intermediate levels and lipid oxidation rates despite normal lipolysis in patients with hypothyroidism. Thyroid 2010;20(8):843−9.

[27] Kuusi T, Taskinen MR, Nikkilä EA. Lipoproteins, lipolytic enzymes, and hormonal status in hypothyroid women at different levels of substitution. J Clin Endocrinol Metab 1988;66(1):51−6.

[28] Bano A, Chaker L, Plompen EPC, Hofman A, Dehghan A, Franco OH, Janssen HLA, Darwish Murad S, Peeters RP. Thyroid function and the risk of nonalcoholic fatty liver disease: the Rotterdam study. J Clin Endocrinol Metab 2016;101(8):3204−11.

[29] Chung GE, Kim D, Kim W, Yim JY, Park MJ, Kim YJ, Yoon JH, Lee HS. Non-alcoholic fatty liver disease across the spectrum of hypothyroidism. J Hepatol 2012;57(1):150–6.

[30] Scherer T, Wolf P, Winhofer Y, Duan H, Einwallner E, Gessl A, Luger A, Trattnig S, Hoffmann M, Niessner A, Baumgartner-Parzer S, Krššák M, Krebs M. Levothyroxine replacement in hypothyroid humans reduces myocardial lipid load and improves cardiac function. J Clin Endocrinol Metab 2014;99(11):E2341–6.

[31] Vatner DF, Weismann D, Beddow SA, Kumashiro N, Erion DM, Liao X-H, Grover GJ, Webb P, Phillips KJ, Weiss RE, Bogan JS, Baxter J, Shulman GI, Samuel VT. Thyroid hormone receptor-β agonists prevent hepatic steatosis in fat-fed rats but impair insulin sensitivity via discrete pathways. Am J Physiol Endocrinol Metab 2013;305(1):E89–100.

[32] Ritter MJ, Amano I, Hollenberg AN. Thyroid hormone signaling and the liver. Hepatology 2020;72(2):742–52.

[33] Sinha RA, Singh BK, Yen PM. Direct effects of thyroid hormones on hepatic lipid metabolism. Nat Rev Endocrinol 2018;14(5):259–69.

[34] Hyyti OM, Ning X-H, Buroker NE, Ge M, Portman MA. Thyroid hormone controls myocardial substrate metabolism through nuclear receptor-mediated and rapid posttranscriptional mechanisms. Am J Physiol Endocrinol Metab 2006;290(2):E372–9.

[35] Ong JM, Simsolo RB, Saghizadeh M, Pauer A, Kern PA. Expression of lipoprotein lipase in rat muscle: regulation by feeding and hypothyroidism. J Lipid Res 1994;35(9):1542–51.

[36] Ripoli A, Pingitore A, Favilli B, Bottoni A, Turchi S, Osman NF, De Marchi D, Lombardi M, L'Abbate A, Iervasi G. Does subclinical hypothyroidism affect cardiac pump performance? Evidence from a magnetic resonance imaging study. J Am Coll Cardiol 2005;45(3):439–45.

[37] Obregon M-J. Thyroid hormone and adipocyte differentiation. Thyroid 2008;18(2):185–95.

[38] Obregon MJ. Adipose tissues and thyroid hormones. Front Physiol 2014;5:1–12. Nov.

[39] Lahesmaa M, Orava J, Schalin-Jäntti C, Soinio M, Hannukainen JC, Noponen T, Kirjavainen A, Iida H, Kudomi N, Enerbäck S, Virtanen KA, Nuutila P. Hyperthyroidism increases brown fat metabolism in humans. J Clin Endocrinol Metab 2014;99(1):28–35.

[40] Lebon V, Dufour S, Petersen KF, Ren J, Jucker BM, Slezak LA, Cline GW, Rothman DL, Shulman GI. Effect of triiodothyronine on mitochondrial energy coupling in human skeletal muscle. J Clin Invest 2001;108(5):733–7.

[41] Harrison SA, Bashir MR, Guy CD, Zhou R, Moylan CA, Frias JP, Alkhouri N, Bansal MB, Baum S, Neuschwander-Tetri BA, Taub R, Moussa SE. Resmetirom (MGL-3196) for the treatment of non-alcoholic steatohepatitis: a multicentre, randomised, double-blind, placebo-controlled, phase 2 trial. Lancet 2019;394(10213):2012–24.

[42] Janković D, Wolf P, Anderwald CH, Winhofer Y, Promintzer-Schifferl M, Hofer A, Langer F, Prager G, Ludvik B, Gessl A, Luger A, Krebs M. Prevalence of endocrine disorders in morbidly obese patients and the effects of bariatric surgery on endocrine and metabolic parameters. Obes Surg 2012;22(1):62–9.

[43] Santini F, Marzullo P, Rotondi M, Ceccarini G, Pagano L, Ippolito S, Chiovato L, Biondi B. Mechanisms in endocrinology: the crosstalk between thyroid gland and adipose tissue: signal integration in health and disease. Eur J Endocrinol 2014;171(4):R137–52.

[44] Møller N, Jørgensen JOL. Effects of growth hormone on glucose, lipid, and protein metabolism in human subjects. Endocr Rev 2009;30(2):152–77.

[45] Kopchick JJ, Berryman DE, Puri V, Lee KY, Jorgensen JOL. The effects of growth hormone on adipose tissue: old observations, new mechanisms. Nat Rev Endocrinol 2020;16(3):135–46.

[46] Melmed S, Bronstein MD, Chanson P, Klibanski A, Casanueva FF, Wass JAH, Strasburger CJ, Luger A, Clemmons DR, Giustina A. A Consensus Statement on acromegaly therapeutic outcomes. Nat Rev Endocrinol 2018;14(9):552–61.

[47] Vila G, Jørgensen JOL, Luger A, Stalla GK. Insulin resistance in patients with acromegaly. Front Endocrinol 2019;10. https://doi.org/10.3389/fendo.2019.00509. July.

[48] Nielsen S, Møller N, Christiansen JS, Jørgensen JOL. Pharmacological antilipolysis restores insulin sensitivity during growth hormone exposure. Diabetes 2001;50(10):2301–8.

[49] Freda PU, Shen W, Heymsfield SB, Reyes-Vidal CM, Geer EB, Bruce JN, Gallagher D. Lower visceral and subcutaneous but higher intermuscular adipose tissue depots in patients with growth hormone and insulin-like growth factor I excess due to acromegaly. J Clin Endocrinol Metab 2008;93(6):2334–43.

[50] Reyes-Vidal CM, Mojahed H, Shen W, Jin Z, Arias-Mendoza F, Fernandez JC, Gallagher D, Bruce JN, Post KD, Freda PU. Adipose tissue redistribution and ectopic lipid deposition in active acromegaly and effects of surgical treatment. J Clin Endocrinol Metab 2015;100(8):2946–55.

[51] Fellinger P, Wolf P, Pfleger L, Krumpolec P, Krssak M, Klavins K, Wolfsberger S, Micko A, Carey P, Gürtl B, Vila G, Raber W, Fürnsinn C, Scherer T, Trattnig S, Kautzky-Willer A, Krebs M, Winhofer Y. Increased ATP synthesis might counteract hepatic lipid accumulation in acromegaly. JCI Insight 2020;5(5):1–11.

[52] Winhofer Y, Wolf P, Krššák M, Wolfsberger S, Tura A, Pacini G, Gessl A, Raber W, Kukurova IJ, Kautzky-Willer A, Knosp E, Trattnig S, Krebs M, Luger A. No evidence of ectopic lipid accumulation in the pathophysiology of the acromegalic cardiomyopathy. J Clin Endocrinol Metab 2014;99(11):4299–306.

[53] Baum HB, Biller BM, Finkelstein JS, Cannistraro KB, Oppenhein DS, Schoenfeld DA, Michel TH, Wittink H, Klibanski A. Effects of physiologic growth hormone therapy on bone density and body composition in patients with adult-onset growth hormone deficiency. A randomized, placebo-controlled trial. Ann Intern Med 1996;125(11):883–90.

[54] Jørgensen JO, Vahl N, Hansen TB, Thuesen L, Hagen C, Christiansen JS. Growth hormone versus placebo treatment for one year in growth hormone deficient adults: increase in exercise capacity and normalization of body composition. Clin Endocrinol (Oxf) 1996;45(6):681–8.

[55] Nørrelund H, Djurhuus C, Jørgensen JOL, Nielsen S, Nair KS, Schmitz O, Christiansen JS, Møller N. Effects of GH on urea, glucose and lipid metabolism, and insulin sensitivity during fasting in GH-deficient patients. Am J Physiol Endocrinol Metab 2003;285(4):E737–43.

[56] Bredella MA, Gerweck AV, Lin E, Melissa MG, Torriani M, Schoenfeld DA, Hemphill LC, Miller KK. Effects of GH on body composition and cardiovascular risk markers in young men with abdominal obesity. J Clin Endocrinol Metab 2013;98(9):3864—72.

[57] Cordoba-Chacon J, Majumdar N, List EO, Diaz-Ruiz A, Frank SJ, Manzano A, Bartrons R, Puchowicz M, Kopchick JJ, Kineman RD. Growth hormone inhibits hepatic de novo lipogenesis in adult mice. Diabetes 2015;64(9):3093—103.

[58] Cordoba-Chacon J, Sarmento-Cabral A, Del Rio-Moreno M, Diaz-Ruiz A, Subbaiah PV, Kineman RD. Adult-Onset hepatocyte GH resistance promotes NASH in male mice, without severe systemic metabolic dysfunction. Endocrinology 2019;159(11):3761—74.

[59] Liu Z, Cordoba-Chacon J, Kineman RD, Cronstein BN, Muzumdar R, Gong Z, Werner H, Yakar S. Growth hormone control of hepatic lipid metabolism. Diabetes 2016;65(12):3598—609.

[60] Elam MB, Wilcox HG, Solomon SS, Heimberg M. In vivo growth hormone treatment stimulates secretion of very low density lipoprotein by the isolated perfused rat liver. Endocrinology 1992;131(6):2717—22.

[61] Christ ER, Cummings MH, Jackson N, Stolinski M, Lumb PJ, Wierzbicki AS, Sönksen PH, Russell-Jones DL, Umpleby AM. Effects of growth hormone (GH) replacement therapy on low-density lipoprotein apolipoprotein B100 kinetics in adult patients with GH deficiency: a stable isotope study. J Clin Endocrinol Metab 2004;89(4):1801—7.

[62] Krag MB, Gormsen LC, Guo ZK, Christiansen JS, Jensen MD, Nielsen S, Jørgensen JOL. Growth hormone-induced insulin resistance is associated with increased intramyocellular triglyceride content but unaltered VLDL-triglyceride kinetics. Am J Physiol Endocrinol Metab 2007;292(3):920—7.

[63] Chanson P, Salenave S. Metabolic syndrome in Cushing's syndrome. Neuroendocrinology 2010;92(Suppl. 1):96—101.

[64] Ferraù F, Korbonits M. Metabolic comorbidities in Cushing's syndrome. Eur J Endocrinol 2015;173(4):M133—57.

[65] Geisler CE, Renquist BJ. Hepatic lipid accumulation: cause and consequence of dysregulated glucoregulatory hormones. J Endocrinol 2017;234(1):R1—21.

[66] Mueller KM, Hartmann K, Kaltenecker D, Vettorazzi S, Bauer M, Mauser L, Amann S, Jall S, Fischer K, Esterbauer H, Müller TD, Tschöp MH, Magnes C, Haybaeck J, Scherer T, Bordag N, Tuckermann JP, Moriggl R. Adipocyte glucocorticoid receptor deficiency attenuates aging- and HFD-induced obesity and impairs the feeding-fasting transition. Diabetes 2017;66(2):272—86.

[67] Lee M-J, Fried SK, Mundt SS, Wang Y, Sullivan S, Stefanni A, Daugherty BL, Hermanowski-Vosatka A. Depot-specific regulation of the conversion of cortisone to cortisol in human adipose tissue. Obesity 2008;16(6):1178—85.

[68] Veilleux A, Rhéaume C, Daris M, Luu-The V, Tchernof A. Omental adipose tissue type 1 11 beta-hydroxysteroid dehydrogenase oxoreductase activity, body fat distribution, and metabolic alterations in women. J Clin Endocrinol Metab 2009;94(9):3550—7.

[69] Geer EB, Islam J, Buettner C. Mechanisms of glucocorticoid-induced insulin resistance. Endocrinol Metab Clin N Am 2014;43(1):75—102.

[70] Tomlinson JW, Draper N, Mackie J, Johnson AP, Holder G, Wood P, Stewart PM. Absence of cushingoid phenotype in a patient with Cushing's disease due to defective cortisone to cortisol conversion. J Clin Endocrinol Metab 2002;87(1):57—62.

[71] Morgan SA, Hassan-Smith ZK, Lavery GG. Mechanisms in endocrinology: tissue-specific activation of cortisol in Cushing's syndrome. Eur J Endocrinol 2016;175(2):R81—7.

[72] Mariniello B, Ronconi V, Rilli S, Bernante P, Boscaro M, Mantero F, Giacchetti G. Adipose tissue 11 β-hydroxysteroid dehydrogenase type 1 expression in obesity and Cushing's syndrome. Eur J Endocrinol 2006;155(3):435—41.

[73] Christ-Crain M, Kola B, Lolli F, Fekete C, Seboek D, Wittmann G, Feltrin D, Igreja SC, Ajodha S, Harvey-White J, Kunos G, Müller B, Pralong F, Aubert G, Arnaldi G, Giacchetti G, Boscaro M, Grossman AB, Korbonits M. AMP-activated protein kinase mediates glucocorticoid-induced metabolic changes: a novel mechanism in Cushing's syndrome. FASEB J Off Publ Fed Am Soc Exp Biol 2008;22(6):1672—83.

[74] Kola B, Christ-Crain M, Lolli F, Arnaldi G, Giacchetti G, Boscaro M, Grossman AB, Korbonits M. Changes in adenosine 5′-monophosphate-activated protein kinase as a mechanism of visceral obesity in Cushing's syndrome. J Clin Endocrinol Metab 2008;93(12):4969—73.

[75] Pivonello R, Isidori AM, De Martino MC, Newell-Price J, Biller BMK, Colao A. Complications of Cushing's syndrome: state of the art. Lancet Diabetes Endocrinol 2016;4(7):611—29.

[76] Zoppini G, Targher G, Venturi C, Zamboni C, Muggeo M. Relationship of nonalcoholic hepatic steatosis to overnight low-dose dexamethasone suppression test in obese individuals. Clin Endocrinol (Oxf) 2004;61(6):711—5.

[77] Rockall AG, Sohaib SA, Evans D, Kaltsas G, Isidori AM, Monson JP, Besser GM, Grossman AB, Reznek RH. Hepatic steatosis in Cushing's syndrome: a radiological assessment using computed tomography. Eur J Endocrinol 2003;149(6):543—8.

[78] Maurice F, Gaborit B, Vincentelli C, Abdesselam I, Bernard M, Graillon T, Kober F, Brue T, Castinetti F, Dutour A. Cushing syndrome is associated with subclinical LV dysfunction and increased epicardial adipose tissue. J Am Coll Cardiol 2018;72(18):2276—7.

[79] Packer M. Epicardial adipose tissue may mediate deleterious effects of obesity and inflammation on the myocardium. J Am Coll Cardiol 2018;71(20):2360—72.

[80] Wolf P, Marty B, Bouazizi B, Kachenoura N, Piedvache C, Blanchard A, Salenave S, Prigent M, Jublanc C, Ajzenberg C, Droumaguet C, Young J, Lecoq A, Kuhn E, Agostini H, Trabado S, Carlier P, Fève B, Redheuil A, Chanson P, Kamenický P. Epicardial and pericardial adiposity without myocardial steatosis in Cushing's syndrome. J Clin Endocrinol Metab 2021;106:3505—14.

[81] Bergthorsdottir R, Ragnarsson O, Skrtic S, Glad CAM, Nilsson S, Ross IL, Leonsson-Zachrisson M, Johannsson G. Visceral fat and novel biomarkers of cardiovascular disease in patients with addison's disease: a case-control study. J Clin Endocrinol Metab 2017;102(11):4264—72.

[82] Wolf P, Beiglböck H, Fellinger P, Pfleger L, Aschauer S, Gessl A, Marculescu R, Trattnig S, Kautzky-Willer A, Luger A, Winhofer Y, Krssak M, Krebs M. Plasma renin levels are associated with cardiac function in primary adrenal insufficiency. Endocrine 2019;65:399—407.

[83] Dandona P, Dhindsa S, Ghanim H, Saad F. Mechanisms underlying the metabolic actions of testosterone in humans: a narrative review. Diabetes Obes Metabol 2021;23(1):18—28.

[84] Schiffer L, Kempegowda P, Arlt W, O'Reilly MW. Mechanisms in endocrinology: the sexually dimorphic role of androgens in human metabolic disease. Eur J Endocrinol 2017;177(3):R125—43.

[85] Smith MR, Finkelstein JS, McGovern FJ, Zietman AL, Fallon MA, Schoenfeld DA, Kantoff PW. Changes in body composition during androgen deprivation therapy for prostate cancer. J Clin Endocrinol Metab 2002;87(2):599—603.

[86] Dhindsa S, Ghanim H, Batra M, Kuhadiya ND, Abuaysheh S, Sandhu S, Green K, Makdissi A, Hejna J, Chaudhuri A, Punyanitya M, Dandona P. Insulin resistance and inflammation in hypogonadotropic hypogonadism and their reduction after testosterone replacement in men with type 2 diabetes. Diabetes Care 2016;39(1):82—91.

[87] Alvarez-Blasco F, Botella-Carretero JI, San Millán JL, Escobar-Morreale HF. Prevalence and characteristics of the polycystic ovary syndrome in overweight and obese women. Arch Intern Med 2006;166(19):2081—6.

[88] Hazlehurst JM, Tomlinson JW. Non-alcoholic fatty liver disease in common endocrine disorders. Eur J Endocrinol 2013;169(2):27—37.

[89] Magnussen LV, Andersen PE, Diaz A, Ostojic J, Højlund K, Hougaard DM, Christensen AN, Nielsen TL, Andersen M. MR spectroscopy of hepatic fat and adiponectin and leptin levels during testosterone therapy in type 2 diabetes: a randomized, double-blinded, placebo-controlled trial. Eur J Endocrinol 2017;177(2):157—68.

[90] Sattler F, He J, Chukwuneke J, Kim H, Stewart Y, Colletti P, Yarasheski K, Buchanan T. Testosterone supplementation improves carbohydrate and lipid metabolism in some older men with abdominal obesity. J Gerontol Geriatr Res 2014;3(3):1000159.

[91] Rabiee A, Dwyer AA, Caronia LM, Hayes FJ, Yialamas MA, Andersen DK, Thomas B, Torriani M, Elahi D. Impact of acute biochemical castration on insulin sensitivity in healthy adult men. Endocr Res 2010;35(2):71—84.

[92] Finkelstein JS, Lee H, Burnett-Bowie S-AM, Pallais JC, Yu EW, Borges LF, Jones BF, Barry CV, Wulczyn KE, Thomas BJ, Leder BZ. Gonadal steroids and body composition, strength, and sexual function in men. N Engl J Med 2013;369(11):1011—22.

[93] Chao J, Rubinow KB, Kratz M, Amory JK, Matsumoto AM, Page ST. Short-term estrogen withdrawal increases adiposity in healthy men. J Clin Endocrinol Metab 2016;101(10):3724—31.

[94] Cerda C, Pérez-Ayuso RM, Riquelme A, Soza A, Villaseca P, Sir-Petermann T, Espinoza M, Pizarro M, Solis N, Miquel JF, Arrese M. Nonalcoholic fatty liver disease in women with polycystic ovary syndrome. J Hepatol 2007;47(3):412—7.

[95] Brzozowska MM, Ostapowicz G, Weltman MD. An association between non-alcoholic fatty liver disease and polycystic ovarian syndrome. J Gastroenterol Hepatol 2009;24(2):243—7.

[96] Leutner M, Göbl C, Wolf P, Maruszczak K, Bozkurt L, Steinbrecher H, Just-Kukurova I, Ott J, Egarter C, Trattnig S, Kautzky-Willer A. Pericardial fat relates to disturbances of glucose metabolism in women with the polycystic ovary syndrome, but not in healthy control subjects. Internet J Endocrinol 2018. https://doi.org/10.1155/2018/5406128. 2018.

[97] Pedersen SB, Kristensen K, Hermann PA, Katzenellenbogen JA, Richelsen B. Estrogen controls lipolysis by up-regulating alpha2A-adrenergic receptors directly in human adipose tissue through the estrogen receptor alpha. Implications for the female fat distribution. J Clin Endocrinol Metab 2004;89(4):1869—78.

[98] Lonardo A, Nascimbeni F, Ballestri S, Fairweather DL, Win S, Than TA, Abdelmalek MF, Suzuki A. Sex differences in nonalcoholic fatty liver disease: state of the art and identification of research gaps. Hepatology 2019;70(4):1457—69.

[99] Beiglböck H, Fellinger P, Ranzenberger-Haider T, Itariu B, Prager G, Kautzky-Willer A, Krebs M, Wolf P. Pre-operative obesity-associated hyperandrogenemia in women and hypogonadism in men have No impact on weight loss following bariatric surgery. Obes Surg 2020. https://doi.org/10.1007/s11695-020-04761-4.

[100] Grossmann M. Hypogonadism and male obesity: focus on unresolved questions. Clin Endocrinol (Oxf) 2018;89(1):11—21.

[101] McCartney CR, Marshall JC. CLINICAL PRACTICE. Polycystic ovary syndrome. N Engl J Med 2016;375(1):54—64.

Chapter 14

Inflammation of the adipose tissue: metabolic consequences during weight (re)gain and loss

Mandala Ajie[1] and Rinke Stienstra[1,2]

[1]Department of Internal Medicine, Radboud University Medical Center, Nijmegen, the Netherlands; [2]Division of Human Nutrition and Health, Wageningen University, Wageningen, the Netherlands

Introduction

Global obesity prevalence has been increasing exponentially over the past decades. Current estimates reveal that around 20% of the adult population is obese with a BMI above $30 \, kg/m^2$.[1] The presence of obesity is associated with an increased risk for the development of metabolic complications including type 2 diabetes and cardiovascular disease. Weight loss is one of the most effective ways to reduce or prevent metabolic complications associated with obesity [1−3]. However, from daily practice, it is known that nearly all individuals experience weight regain after initial weight loss [4] known as weight cycling or the yoyo effect. Weight regain causes a robust reversal of the metabolic benefits of initial weight loss and has even been suggested to promote an increased risk for the development of metabolic complications and cardiovascular disease [5−7].

The development of obesity is known to be accompanied not only by an increase in fat mass, but also impacts on the composition of the adipose tissue [8−10]. It has been well established that various types of immune cells infiltrate the adipose tissue and together drive a chronic state of inflammation (Table 14.1). Adipose tissue inflammation has been identified as one of the key contributors to the development of metabolic complications associated with obesity including insulin resistance.

In this chapter, we will zoom in on the determinants of adipose tissue inflammation during weight gain, weight loss, and regain (Fig. 14.1). We will focus on the molecular pathways underlying the development of adipose tissue inflammation and describe the effects of bodyweight loss and regain on the inflammatory status of the adipose tissue. By understanding the mechanisms underlying inflammatory responses of the adipose tissue, we could ultimately develop approaches to reverse the risk for metabolic complications associated with obesity and bodyweight cycling.

Chronic low-grade inflammation of the adipose tissue

Obesity is characterized by the excessive accumulation of lipids leading to an increase in fat mass [11]. This increase is accommodated by enlargement of adipocytes that is paralleled by changes in the immune cell composition of the adipose tissue. Various types of innate and adaptive immune cells define adipose tissue inflammation during obesity. However, it is important to emphasize that immune cells are also part of adipose tissue during lean conditions (see Table 14.1 for an overview). In fact, lean adipose tissue contains various immune cell subsets ranging from macrophages to T lymphocytes promoting tissue homeostasis [12]. However, during weight gain, an enhanced number of immune cells populate the adipose tissue [13−15]. In addition to absolute numbers, obese adipose tissue also promotes polarization of resident immune cells toward a more proinflammatory phenotype [16−18].

Visceral and Ectopic Fat. https://doi.org/10.1016/B978-0-12-822186-0.00022-5

TABLE 14.1 Characteristics of immune cell subsets residing in adipose tissue.

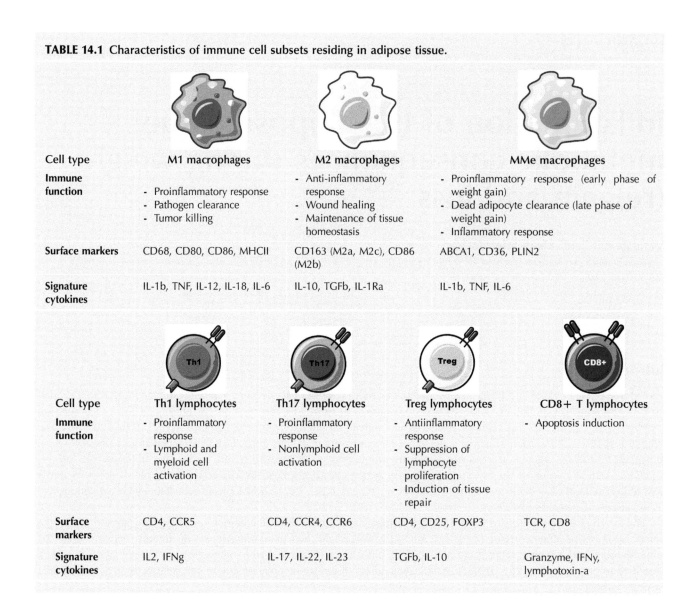

Cell type	M1 macrophages	M2 macrophages	MMe macrophages
Immune function	- Proinflammatory response - Pathogen clearance - Tumor killing	- Anti-inflammatory response - Wound healing - Maintenance of tissue homeostasis	- Proinflammatory response (early phase of weight gain) - Dead adipocyte clearance (late phase of weight gain) - Inflammatory response
Surface markers	CD68, CD80, CD86, MHCII	CD163 (M2a, M2c), CD86 (M2b)	ABCA1, CD36, PLIN2
Signature cytokines	IL-1b, TNF, IL-12, IL-18, IL-6	IL-10, TGFb, IL-1Ra	IL-1b, TNF, IL-6

Cell type	Th1 lymphocytes	Th17 lymphocytes	Treg lymphocytes	CD8+ T lymphocytes
Immune function	- Proinflammatory response - Lymphoid and myeloid cell activation	- Proinflammatory response - Nonlymphoid cell activation	- Antiinflammatory response - Suppression of lymphocyte proliferation - Induction of tissue repair	- Apoptosis induction
Surface markers	CD4, CCR5	CD4, CCR4, CCR6	CD4, CD25, FOXP3	TCR, CD8
Signature cytokines	IL2, IFNg	IL-17, IL-22, IL-23	TGFb, IL-10	Granzyme, IFNy, lymphotoxin-a

Weight gain

Although adipocytes are known for their ability to quickly change in size, the excessive and prolonged enlargement of the adipocytes during obesity leads to an increase in adipocyte death. Cell death generates a proinflammatory response involving macrophages aiming to clear the cell corpses and preventing any unwanted effects of the cellular content released into the extracellular environment [19—21]. This response is also observed in obese adipose tissue with macrophages surrounding necrotic adipocytes in an attempt to clear the dead cells. These typical structures are referred to as "crown-like structures" (CLS) and are known to promote adipose tissue inflammation [22,23].

In addition to dying cells leading to CLS formation, adipocytes are also known to contribute to the infiltration of circulating monocytes, serving as precursors cells of macrophages, even in an earlier stage (Fig. 14.2). During the development of adipocyte hypertrophy, the cells start to secrete several chemokines and cytokines initiating the recruitment of circulating monocytes into adipose tissue [23,24]. The chemokine monocyte chemoattractant protein 1 (MCP-1) is recognized by the CCR2 receptor on the surface of circulating monocytes, resulting in their migration toward obese adipose tissue [23,25]. Aside from MCP-1, other signaling molecules are released from the adipose tissue, which together impact on the number of immune cells residing in adipose tissue [26]. The effects even go beyond direct recruitment, since

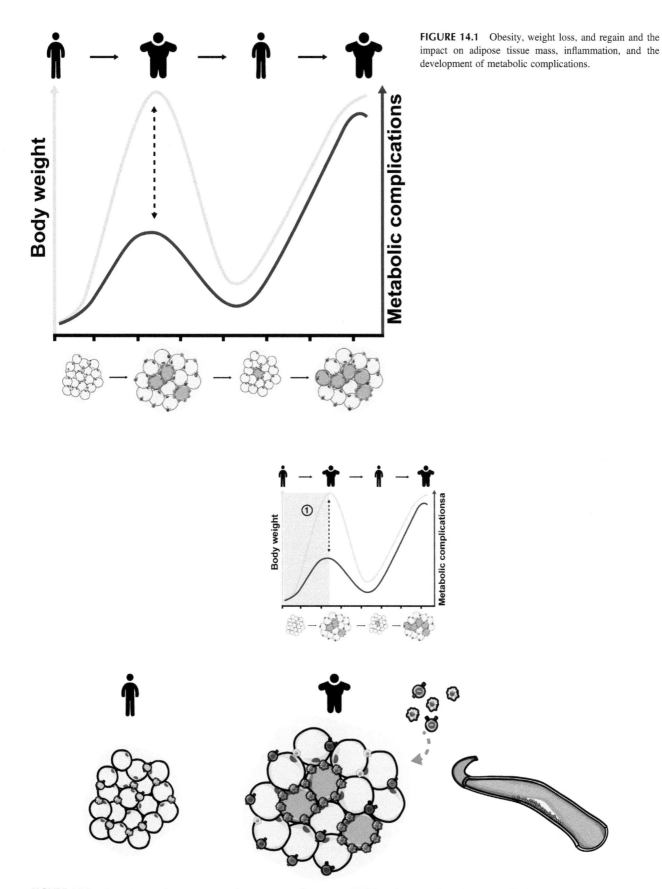

FIGURE 14.1 Obesity, weight loss, and regain and the impact on adipose tissue mass, inflammation, and the development of metabolic complications.

FIGURE 14.2 *Excessive weight gain causes adipose tissue inflammation.* Weight gain causes the enlargement of adipocytes and secretion of proinflammatory signals, hypoxic condition, and adipocyte death. This results in the recruitment of immune cells such as CD8+ T lymphocytes, CD4 T lymphocytes, and macrophages and induces their activation and differentiation into their proinflammatory subsets.

obese adipose tissue also affects myelopoiesis in the bone marrow serving to increase the number of circulating monocytes functioning as precursor cells of ATMs [27]. Other mechanisms in addition to recruitment may also contribute to increasing macrophage numbers in adipose tissue. The abundance of macrophages in obese adipose tissue has also been suggested to result from increased local proliferation of ATMs [28,29]. Additionally, studies have shown that adipose tissue macrophages exhibit reduced migratory capacity trapping cells in obese adipose tissue [30].

In addition to absolute numbers, the phenotype of a macrophage is an important determinant of its inflammatory potential. Classical phenotyping of macrophages divides them into two phenotypic groups, M1 or classical macrophages and M2 or alternative macrophages. M1 macrophages display a proinflammatory response, while M2 macrophages have an opposite phenotype. In lean individuals, ATMs display a more antiinflammatory or alternative phenotype, contributing to maintaining tissue homeostasis [23,31]. On the contrary, ATMs of obese individuals display a more M1-like phenotype [16]. However, various studies have revealed that ATMs originating from obese adipose tissue are phenotypically distinct from classical macrophages [16,32,33]. The unique trait of ATMs is being defined as metabolically activated (MMe) macrophages. This proinflammatory phenotype is driven by high levels of insulin, glucose, and palmitate, factors relevant during obesity [16,32]. In vivo, MMe macrophages form CLS around dying adipocytes and display a proinflammatory phenotype.

Interestingly, recent technical advances have revealed that the diversity of adipose tissue macrophage phenotypes even goes beyond MMe macrophages. Single cell RNAseq studies have uncovered the existence of a wide variety of different macrophage phenotypes residing in obese adipose tissue [34−37]. Single-cell RNAseq approaches in both animal and human studies have corroborated the presence of pro- and antiinflammatory macrophages in the adipose tissue of obese individuals [37]. However, immunological phenotypes of these cells are highly distinct, implying important roles of macrophage subsets other than the M1/M2/MMe phenotypes in obesity [34,38]. Identifying both the existence and function of different macrophage phenotypes in modulating inflammatory responses in the adipose tissue would be crucial for our understanding of the pathogenesis of low-grade chronic inflammation and can ultimately lead to the identification of novel targets to modulate adipose tissue inflammation.

Aside from innate immune cells, it is important to emphasize that adaptive immune cells also contribute to exacerbating adipose tissue inflammation in obesity. Studies have shown enrichment of CD4+ and CD8+ T cells in adipose tissue of obese individuals as opposed to healthy controls [39]. Moreover, the increase in proinflammatory T cell numbers in adipose tissue has been associated with chronic grade inflammation [40]. In an animal model, accumulation of CD4+ and CD8+ cells in the adipose tissue was shown to precede macrophage infiltration [41]. Moreover, the rate of macrophage infiltration was also reduced when CD8+ cells were depleted from the adipose tissue. Thus, adipose tissue inflammatory status is the net result of an interaction between various types of cells residing in adipose tissue including hypertrophic adipocytes, innate, and adaptive immune cells (see Fig. 14.2).

Altogether, these mechanisms result in an increased inflammatory state of obese adipose tissue. By producing various proinflammatory mediators that interfere with insulin signaling pathways, this will promote the development of insulin resistance and type 2 diabetes. In addition, other complications associated with obesity, including cardiovascular diseases, are also known to be driven by proinflammatory activation partly originating from obese adipose tissue [42,43].

Weight loss

Weight loss is an effective way to reverse many metabolic complications associated with obesity. Weight loss not only leads to a reduction in adipose mass but also leads to specific immune responses within the tissue. Different weight loss methods, i.e. calorie restriction, bariatric surgery, and exercise, will cause differential changes in immune response dynamics within adipose tissue [44,45]. Here, we will focus on immune responses occurring after caloric restriction, as this is the most widely used approach to lose body weight (see Fig. 14.3).

Weight loss has been associated with a reduction in the chronic inflammatory state both locally in adipose tissue [46] and systemically based on circulation markers [47]. In adipose tissue, this process is driven by dynamic interactions between adipocytes and ATMs, in which adipose tissue inflammation is exacerbated during the early phase of weight loss, but resolved at a later stage.

Immune cell responses during weight loss can therefore be divided into two distinct phases: (1) an early phase and (2) a late phase [48]. During the early phase of weight loss, an inflammatory response accommodates adipose tissue remodeling [49,50]. Caloric restriction causes the activation of lipolysis and adipokine production of the adipocytes [50]. The subsequent release of free fatty acids and adipokines induces recruitment of macrophages, which partly serve to buffer the high concentrations of free fatty acids [50]. At the later stage of weight loss, the recruitment of macrophages into the adipose tissue is reduced, stabilizing the numbers of ATMs [48].

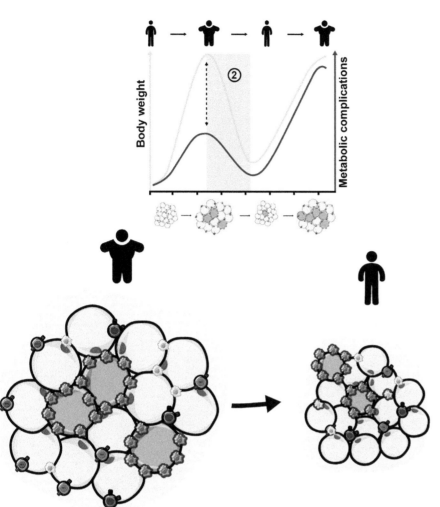

FIGURE 14.3 *Adipose tissue inflammation persists after weight loss.* Weight loss results in the normalization of adipocyte size and reduction in inflammation. However, a proinflammatory state persists even after weight loss.

Systemically, weight loss results in decreased levels of circulating inflammatory markers such as IL-6, IL-18, and C-reactive protein (CRP), while at the same time elevates circulating adiponectin levels known to promote insulin sensitivity [51–53].

However, despite the fact that adipose tissue mass is reduced upon weight loss, several studies have shown that a chronic low-grade level of inflammation persists in adipose tissue following weight loss [54–56] with circulating inflammatory markers that remain elevated [57,58]. The persistence of low-grade inflammation despite weight loss is illustrated by an elevated expression of inflammatory markers in adipose tissue paralleled by increased numbers of CLS [52,53]. Although the persistency of adipose tissue inflammation after weight loss is likely affected by various factors, such as age, time to achieve weight loss (rapid vs. gradual), and timing of the inflammatory measurements (directly after weight loss vs. after a weight stable period) [46,55,59,60], these results suggest a certain level of irreversibility of adipose tissue inflammation and the presence of a memory toward a previous period of obesity [54,55,61].

Weight regain

Although weight loss is a very effective way to reduce obesity-associated metabolic complications, the majority of individuals regain their lost weight within 5 years after initial weight loss, thereby reversing many metabolic benefits [4].

From an inflammatory perspective, it has been shown that even partial weight regain in individuals with a history of obesity induces inflammation of the adipose tissue (see Fig. 14.4) [61]. The level of inflammation is similar to, or even higher than, the levels observed during the initial period of obesity [8,54,56,62,63]. These findings may partly be explained by the presence of an obesogenic memory triggering elevated immune responses upon weight regain. The existence of a

FIGURE 14.4 *Weight regain exacerbates adipose tissue inflammation.* Weight regain causes adipocyte hypertrophy and recruitment of immune cells into the adipose tissue, leading to a worsening of the inflammatory response of the tissue as compared with the initial weight gain period.

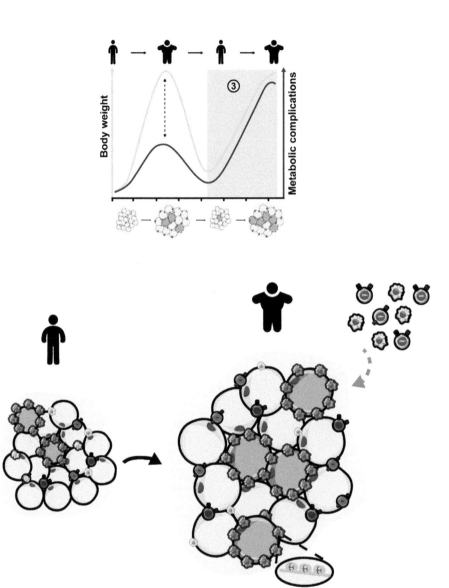

memory toward a previous period of obesity may subsequently result in an increased risk for the development of obesity-induced metabolic complications [54].

From a mechanistic point of view, several explanations may exist for the development of an obesogenic memory of the adipose tissue. A number of human studies have linked obesity to long-term epigenetic reprogramming of the adipose tissue in genes directly responsible for adipokine production including leptin and adiponectin [64–66]. Upon weight regain, this may lead to dysregulation of adipokines that may ultimately result in alterations of lipid metabolism and insulin sensitivity [66]. Obesity has also been shown to cause epigenetic changes of the immune cells in adipose tissue involving activation of proinflammatory genes in the macrophages, while suppressing antiinflammatory genes in different animal models [67–70]. Since epigenetic reprogramming can persist long after the environmental stimuli have disappeared, epigenetic remodeling of adipocytes and immune cells may play a significant role in maintaining the inflammatory trait after weight loss. These changes may even go beyond the adipose tissue itself and involve more systemic effects. A recent in vivo study showed that a western diet induces enhanced inflammatory response of the innate immune cells that persist after the dietary intake is normalized [71]. These changes are partly mediated by epigenetic reprogramming of the progenitor myeloid cells residing in the bone marrow. This phenomenon is called trained immunity and describes the enhanced inflammatory response of primed immune cells upon exposure to nonrelated stimuli [72–74]. Epigenetic changes on both immune progenitor cells and adipocytes may explain obesogenic memory and the subsequent enhanced inflammatory response of ATMs upon weight regain (see Fig. 14.4), ultimately leading to worsening of metabolic complications. However, future studies are needed to identify potential mechanisms underlying the obesogenic memory response.

Adipose tissue inflammation during obesity: how does it lead to complications?

Although obesity and weight cycling result in exacerbated inflammation locally, the inflammatory response may lead to systemic effects due to the endocrine role of the adipose tissue. Adipose tissue releases adipokines allowing for cross-talk with other cells and distant organs. Inflamed adipose tissue releases proinflammatory mediators that can impact on other distant tissues and cells leading to metabolic complications.

Insulin resistance

Adipocytes along with the proinflammatory immune cells in the adipose tissue secrete a number of proinflammatory cytokines and chemokines. Proinflammatory cytokines such as IL-6, TNFα, IL-1β and others are known to negatively impact on the insulin signaling cascade driving resistance [75]. Due to the endocrine nature of the adipose tissue, the enhanced release of these cytokines may not only lead to local effects, yet may also promote insulin resistance in more distant tissues. IL-6 produced from the adipose tissue, for example, is linked to the development of insulin resistance in the liver [15]. Metabolic dysfunction and insulin resistance of the adipose tissue also promote other metabolic complications. For example, the increased efflux of free fatty acids from the adipocytes results in the excessive accumulation of fat in the liver, as well as dyslipidemia causing metabolic complications [43].

Atherosclerosis

Proinflammatory cytokines such as IL-6, TNFα, and IL-1β also induce the secretion of adhesion molecules from endothelial cells, promoting immune cell adhesion and local inflammation [43,76]. Moreover, these inflammatory cytokines also induce immune cell activation and differentiation, making them more proinflammatory. Chemokines such as MCP-1 promote immune cell recruitment into the vasculature, initiating a cascade of events that lead to atherosclerosis [43]. A number of observational studies have linked adipose tissue enlargement and inflammation to atherosclerosis [77−79].

Hence, reducing adipose tissue inflammation during obesity should be considered as a therapeutic approach to lower the risk for developing metabolic complications.

Determining adipose tissue inflammation

Since adipose tissue inflammation is an important driver of metabolic complications during obesity, accurate assessment of the inflammatory status of the adipose tissue may prove useful to design specific and personalized interventions. Conventional assessment of adipose tissue inflammation is done through histological analyses such as crown-like structure staining and adipocyte size measurements. These methods require an invasive tissue biopsy and are less suitable to easily screen adipose tissue inflammatory status.

In recent years, a number of noninvasive imaging techniques have been tested to determine adipose tissue inflammation. Imaging techniques such as PET scan and MRI can be used as a proxy to determine adipose tissue inflammation and are based upon physiological and metabolic changes in the adipose tissue. For example, the higher metabolic rate of inflamed adipose tissue makes it possible to utilize 18-F FDG/PET techniques to determine adipose tissue inflammation due to the higher consumption rate of glucose [80]. MRI-based methods have also been utilized to measure adipose tissue enlargement and/or inflammation [79,81−83]. For example, certain MRI measurements including the T1 relaxation time may be used as surrogate makers to determine the inflammatory status of the adipose tissue including the presence of crown-like structure formation and a shift in triglyceride composition [83]. Adipose tissue inflammation can also lead to tissue scarring and fibrosis [84]. The changes in tissue elasticity due to fibrosis can be detected using AdipoScan, an ultrasound-based tool for detecting fibrosis in subcutaneous AT [85].

These and other imaging techniques may prove useful to determine the degree of adipose tissue inflammation allowing for the identification of those individuals that would benefit most from therapeutic approaches to reverse the inflammatory state.

A number of studies have been exploring the possibility of reversing the metabolic complications of obesity through controlling or reducing adipose tissue inflammation [86−88]. One approach would be to use pharmacology and specifically block those pathways driving the chronic state of inflammation. Colchicine, an antiinflammatory drug used to treat rheumatoid arthritis has been shown to ameliorate inflammation in obese individuals [88]. Type 2 diabetes individuals treated with anakinra, a receptor antagonist of IL-1 receptor, showed sustained improvement in glycemic control [89]. Obese individuals treated with salsalate also showed improvement in glycemia [90,91], although this was not accompanied by a reduction in adipose tissue inflammation [91,92].

Alternatively, a dietary or lifestyle approach could be used to modulate adipose tissue inflammatory status [93,94]. A Mediterranean style diet that is rich in legumes, vegetables, and olive oil consumption is linked with reduced adipose tissue inflammation and decreased cardiometabolic disease risk [93,94]. Exercise also ameliorates adipose tissue inflammation although to a lesser degree compared with dietary intervention [95].

By using these approaches in those individuals with high levels of adipose tissue inflammation, we might be able to reverse metabolic complications during obesity.

Conclusion

The development of obesity leads to a chronic inflammatory state of the adipose tissue driven by adipocyte hypertrophy and increased numbers of innate and adaptive immune cells. Chronic inflammation is an important driver of the development of various complications associated with obesity including insulin resistance and cardiovascular disease. Although weight loss is an effective way to reduce inflammation of the adipose tissue, this is often followed by weight regain. This process of weight loss followed by weight regain is known as the yoyo effect or weight cycling and appears to exacerbate adipose tissue inflammation, which has systemic effects on metabolic complications.

By using noninvasive tools to assess adipose tissue inflammation, personalized treatment targeting obese individuals with a high degree of inflammation may potentially lead to a reduction of metabolic complications.

References

[1] Bray GA, et al. The science of obesity management: an endocrine society scientific statement. Endocr Rev 2018;39:79—132.

[2] Delahanty LM, et al. Effects of weight loss, weight cycling, and weight loss maintenance on diabetes incidence and change in cardiometabolic traits in the Diabetes Prevention Program. Diabetes Care 2014;37:2738—45.

[3] Ryan DH, Yockey SR. Weight loss and improvement in comorbidity: differences at 5%, 10%, 15%, and over. Curr Obes Rep 2017;6:187—94.

[4] van Baak MA, Mariman ECM. Mechanisms of weight regain after weight loss - the role of adipose tissue. Nat Rev Endocrinol 2019;15:274—87.

[5] Zou J, et al. CD4+ T cells memorize obesity and promote weight regain. Cell Mol Immunol 2018;15:630—9.

[6] Rhee EJ, et al. Increased risk of diabetes development in individuals with weight cycling over 4 years: the Kangbuk Samsung Health study. Diabetes Res Clin Pract 2018;139:230—8.

[7] Kakinami L, Knaüper B, Brunet J. Weight cycling is associated with adverse cardiometabolic markers in a cross-sectional representative US sample. J Epidemiol Community Health 2020;74:662.

[8] Barbosa-da-Silva S, Fraulob-Aquino JC, Lopes JR, Mandarim-de-Lacerda CA, Aguila MB. Weight cycling enhances adipose tissue inflammatory responses in male mice. PLoS One 2012;7.

[9] Bertola A, et al. Identification of adipose tissue dendritic cells correlated with obesity-associated insulin-resistance and inducing Th17 responses in mice and patients. Diabetes 2012;61:2238—47.

[10] Barra NG, Henriksbo BD, Anhê FF, Schertzer JD. The NLRP3 inflammasome regulates adipose tissue metabolism. Biochem J 2020;477:1089—107.

[11] Bluher M. Obesity: global epidemiology and pathogenesis. Nat Rev Endocrinol 2019;15:288—98.

[12] Asghar A, Sheikh N. Role of immune cells in obesity induced low grade inflammation and insulin resistance. Cell Immunol 2017;315:18—26.

[13] Monteiro R, Azevedo I. Chronic inflammation in obesity and the metabolic syndrome. Mediat Inflamm 2010. https://doi.org/10.1155/2010/289645. 2010.

[14] Ellulu MS, Patimah I, Khaza'ai H, Rahmat A, Abed Y. Obesity and inflammation: the linking mechanism and the complications. Arch Med Sci 2017;13:851.

[15] Zatterale F, et al. Chronic adipose tissue inflammation linking obesity to insulin resistance and type 2 diabetes. Front Physiol 2020;10.

[16] Kratz M, et al. Metabolic dysfunction drives a mechanistically distinct proinflammatory phenotype in adipose tissue macrophages. Cell Metabol 2014;20:614—25.

[17] Saltiel AR, Olefsky JM. Inflammatory mechanisms linking obesity and metabolic disease. J Clin Invest 2017;127:1—4.

[18] Kawai T, Autieri MV, Scalia R. Adipose tissue inflammation and metabolic dysfunction in obesity. Am J Physiol Cell Physiol 2021;320:C375—91.

[19] Cinti S, et al. Adipocyte death defines macrophage localization and function in adipose tissue of obese mice and humans. J Lipid Res 2005;46:2347—55.

[20] Nishimoto S, et al. Obesity-induced DNA released from adipocytes stimulates chronic adipose tissue inflammation and insulin resistance. Sci Adv 2016;2.

[21] Lindhorst A, et al. Adipocyte death triggers a pro-inflammatory response and induces metabolic activation of resident macrophages. Cell Death Dis 2021:1—15. 2021 126 12.

[22] Patel PS, Buras ED, Balasubramanyam A. The role of the immune system in obesity and insulin resistance. J Obes 2013. https://doi.org/10.1155/2013/616193. 2013.

[23] Bai Y, Sun Q. Macrophage recruitment in obese adipose tissue. Obes Rev 2015;16:127−36.

[24] Suganami T, Nishida J, Ogawa Y. A paracrine loop between adipocytes and macrophages aggravates inflammatory changes: role of free fatty acids and tumor necrosis factor α. Arterioscler Thromb Vasc Biol 2005;25:2062−8.

[25] Kanda H, et al. MCP-1 contributes to macrophage infiltration into adipose tissue, insulin resistance, and hepatic steatosis in obesity. J Clin Invest 2006;116:1494−505.

[26] Phillips CL, Grayson BE. The immune remodel: weight loss-mediated inflammatory changes to obesity. Exp Biol Med (Maywood, NJ, U S) 2020;245:109−21.

[27] Nagareddy PR, et al. Hyperglycemia promotes myelopoiesis and impairs the resolution of atherosclerosis. Cell Metabol 2013;17:695−708.

[28] Amano SU, et al. Local proliferation of macrophages contributes to obesity-associated adipose tissue inflammation. Cell Metabol 2014;19:162−71.

[29] Morita Y, et al. Impact of tissue macrophage proliferation on peripheral and systemic insulin resistance in obese mice with diabetes. BMJ Open Diabetes Res Care 2020;8:e001578.

[30] Ramkhelawon B, et al. Netrin-1 promotes adipose tissue macrophage retention and insulin resistance in obesity. Nat Med 2014;20:377−84.

[31] Feuerer M, et al. Lean, but not obese, fat is enriched for a unique population of regulatory T cells that affect metabolic parameters. Nat Med 2009:930−9. 2009 158 15.

[32] Coats BR, et al. Metabolically activated adipose tissue macrophages perform detrimental and beneficial functions during diet-induced obesity. Cell Rep 2017;20:3149.

[33] Tiwari P, et al. Metabolically activated adipose tissue macrophages link obesity to triple-negative breast cancer. J Exp Med 2019;216:1345−58.

[34] Jaitin DA, et al. Lipid-associated macrophages control metabolic homeostasis in a Trem2-dependent manner. Cell 2019;178:686−98. e14.

[35] Li C, et al. Single cell transcriptomics based-MacSpectrum reveals novel macrophage activation signatures in diseases. JCI insight 2019;5.

[36] A W, et al. Single-cell RNA sequencing of visceral adipose tissue leukocytes reveals that caloric restriction following obesity promotes the accumulation of a distinct macrophage population with features of phagocytic cells. Immunometabolism 2019;1.

[37] Vijay J, et al. Single-cell analysis of human adipose tissue identifies depot and disease specific cell types. Nat Metab 2020;2:97−109.

[38] Hill DA, et al. Distinct macrophage populations direct inflammatory versus physiological changes in adipose tissue. Proc Natl Acad Sci USA 2018;115:E5096−105.

[39] Herck MAV, et al. The differential roles of T cells in non-alcoholic fatty liver disease and obesity. Front Immunol 2019;10.

[40] Porsche CE, Delproposto JB, Geletka L, O'Rourke R, Lumeng CN. Obesity results in adipose tissue T cell exhaustion. JCI insight 2021;6.

[41] Nishimura S, et al. CD8+ effector T cells contribute to macrophage recruitment and adipose tissue inflammation in obesity. Nat Med 2009;15:914−20.

[42] Akoumianakis I, Antoniades C. The interplay between adipose tissue and the cardiovascular system: is fat always bad? Cardiovasc Res 2017;113:999−1008.

[43] Chait A, den Hartigh LJ. Adipose tissue distribution, inflammation and its metabolic consequences, including diabetes and cardiovascular disease. Front Cardiovasc Med 2020;7:22.

[44] Wasinski F, et al. Exercise and caloric restriction alter the immune system of mice submitted to a high-fat diet. Mediat Inflamm 2013;2013.

[45] Lips MA, et al. Weight loss induced by very low calorie diet is associated with a more beneficial systemic inflammatory profile than by Roux-en-Y gastric bypass. Metabolism 2016;65:1614−20.

[46] Alemán JO, et al. Effects of rapid weight loss on systemic and adipose tissue inflammation and metabolism in obese postmenopausal women. J Endocr Soc 2017;1:625.

[47] Bianchi VE. Weight loss is a critical factor to reduce inflammation. Clin Nutr ESPEN 2018;28:21−35.

[48] Kosteli A, et al. Weight loss and lipolysis promote a dynamic immune response in murine adipose tissue. J Clin Invest 2010;120:3466−79.

[49] Buzelle SL, MacPherson REK, Peppler WT, Castellani L, Wright DC. The contribution of IL-6 to beta 3 adrenergic receptor mediated adipose tissue remodeling. Phys Rep 2015;3.

[50] Lacerda DR, et al. Role of adipose tissue inflammation in fat pad loss induced by fasting in lean and mildly obese mice. J Nutr Biochem 2019;72.

[51] Esposito K, et al. Effect of weight loss and lifestyle changes on vascular inflammatory markers in obese women: a randomized trial. JAMA 2003;289:1799−804.

[52] Madsen EL, et al. Weight loss larger than 10% is needed for general improvement of levels of circulating adiponectin and markers of inflammation in obese subjects: a 3-year weight loss study. Eur J Endocrinol 2008;158:179−87.

[53] Van Gemert WA, et al. Effect of weight loss with or without exercise on inflammatory markers and adipokines in postmenopausal women: the SHAPE-2 trial, A randomized controlled trial. Cancer Epidemiol Biomarkers Prev 2016;25:799−806.

[54] Schmitz J, et al. Obesogenic memory can confer long-term increases in adipose tissue but not liver inflammation and insulin resistance after weight loss. Mol Metabol 2016;5:328−39.

[55] AM B, et al. Obesogenic memory maintains adipose tissue inflammation and insulin resistance. Immunometabolism 2020;2.

[56] Zamarron BF, et al. Macrophage proliferation sustains adipose tissue inflammation in formerly obese mice. Diabetes 2017;66:392−406.

[57] Salas-Salvadó J, et al. Subcutaneous adipose tissue cytokine production is not responsible for the restoration of systemic inflammation markers during weight loss. Int J Obes 2006;30:1714−20.

[58] Strączkowski M, et al. The effect of moderate weight loss, with or without (1, 3)(1, 6)-β-glucan addition, on subcutaneous adipose tissue inflammatory gene expression in young subjects with uncomplicated obesity. Endocrine 2018;61:275−84.

[59] Willemsen L, et al. Peritoneal macrophages have an impaired immune response in obesity which can be reversed by subsequent weight loss. BMJ open diabetes Res care 2019;7.

[60] Rodrigues MOM, et al. Caloric restriction-induced weight loss with a high-fat diet does not fully recover visceral adipose tissue inflammation in previously obese C57BL/6 mice. Appl Physiol Nutr Metabol 2020;45:1353—9.

[61] Roumans NJT, Vink RG, Fazelzadeh P, Van Baak MA, Mariman ECM. A role for leukocyte integrins and extracellular matrix remodeling of adipose tissue in the risk of weight regain after weight loss. Am J Clin Nutr 2017;105:1054—62.

[62] Blomain ES, Dirhan DA, Valentino MA, Kim GW, Waldman SA. Mechanisms of weight regain following weight loss. ISRN Obes 2013:210524. 2013.

[63] Sougiannis AT, et al. Impact of weight loss and partial weight regain on immune cell and inflammatory markers in adipose tissue in male mice. J Appl Physiol 2020;129:909—19.

[64] Herrera BM, Keildson S, Lindgren CM. Genetics and epigenetics of obesity. Maturitas 2011;69:41—9.

[65] Lopomo A, Burgio E, Migliore L. Epigenetics of obesity. Prog Mol Biol Transl Sci 2016;140:151—84.

[66] Ling C, Rönn T. Epigenetics in human obesity and type 2 diabetes. Cell Metabol 2019;29:1028—44.

[67] Brasacchio D, et al. Hyperglycemia induces a dynamic cooperativity of histone methylase and demethylase enzymes associated with gene-activating epigenetic marks that coexist on the lysine tail. Diabetes 2009;58:1229—36.

[68] Yang X, et al. Epigenetic regulation of macrophage polarization by DNA methyltransferase 3b. Mol Endocrinol 2014;28:565—74.

[69] Wang X, et al. Epigenetic regulation of macrophage polarization and inflammation by DNA methylation in obesity. JCI insight 2016;1.

[70] Ahmed M, de Winther MPJ, Van den Bossche J. Epigenetic mechanisms of macrophage activation in type 2 diabetes. Immunobiology 2017;222:937—43.

[71] Christ A, et al. Western diet triggers NLRP3-dependent innate immune reprogramming. Cell 2018;172:162—75. e14.

[72] Kleinnijenhuis J, et al. Long-lasting effects of BCG vaccination on both heterologous Th1/Th17 responses and innate trained immunity. J Innate Immun 2014;6:152—8.

[73] Arts RJW, et al. Immunometabolic pathways in BCG-induced trained immunity. Cell Rep 2016;17:2562—71.

[74] Netea MG, et al. Trained immunity: a program of innate immune memory in health and disease. Science 2016;352:aaf1098.

[75] Zand H, Morshedzadeh N, Naghashian F. Signaling pathways linking inflammation to insulin resistance. Diabetes Metabol Syndr 2017;11(Suppl. 1):S307—9.

[76] Rana MN, Neeland IJ. Adipose tissue inflammation and cardiovascular disease: an update. Curr Diabetes Rep 2022;22.

[77] Mazzotta C, et al. Perivascular adipose tissue inflammation in ischemic heart disease. Arterioscler Thromb Vasc Biol 2021;41:1239—50.

[78] Reijrink M, et al. Visceral adipose tissue volume is associated with premature atherosclerosis in early type 2 diabetes mellitus independent of traditional risk factors. Atherosclerosis 2019;290:87—93.

[79] Gast KB, et al. Individual contributions of visceral fat and total body fat to subclinical atherosclerosis: the NEO study. Atherosclerosis 2015;241:547—54.

[80] Bucerius J, et al. Arterial and fat tissue inflammation are highly correlated: a prospective 18F-FDG PET/CT study. Eur J Nucl Med Mol Imag 2014;41:934—45.

[81] Ong HH, et al. Fat-water MRI is sensitive to local adipose tissue inflammatory changes in a diet-induced obesity mouse model at 15T. In: Medical Imaging 2015: Biomedical Applications in Molecular, Structural, and Functional Imaging. 9417; 2015. 94170C.

[82] Ong HH, et al. Fat-water MRI of a diet-induced obesity mouse model at 15.2T. J Med Imaging 2016;3:026002.

[83] Garnov N, et al. Comparison of T1 relaxation times in adipose tissue of severely obese patients and healthy lean subjects measured by 1.5 T MRI. NMR Biomed 2014;27:1123—8.

[84] Debari MK, Abbott RD. Adipose tissue fibrosis: mechanisms, models, and importance. Int J Mol Sci 2020;21:1—24.

[85] Sasso M, et al. AdipoScan: a novel transient elastography-based tool used to non-invasively assess subcutaneous adipose tissue shear wave speed in obesity. Ultrasound Med Biol 2016;42:2401—13.

[86] Wang Y, et al. Improvement of obesity-associated disorders by a small-molecule drug targeting mitochondria of adipose tissue macrophages. Nat Commun 2021:1—16. 2021 121 12.

[87] Alsaggar M, et al. Silibinin attenuates adipose tissue inflammation and reverses obesity and its complications in diet-induced obesity model in mice. BMC Pharmacol Toxicol 2020;21.

[88] Demidowich AP, et al. Effects of colchicine in adults with metabolic syndrome: a pilot randomized controlled trial. Diabetes Obes Metabol 2019;21:1642—51.

[89] van Asseldonk EJP, et al. One week treatment with the IL-1 receptor antagonist anakinra leads to a sustained improvement in insulin sensitivity in insulin resistant patients with type 1 diabetes mellitus. Clin Immunol 2015;160:155—62.

[90] Fleischman A, Shoelson SE, Bernier R, Goldfine AB. Salsalate improves glycemia and inflammatory parameters in obese young adults. Diabetes Care 2008;31:289.

[91] Alderete TL, et al. Salsalate treatment improves glycemia without altering adipose tissue in nondiabetic obese hispanics. Obesity 2015;23:543—51.

[92] Kim MS, et al. Regulation of diet-induced adipose tissue and systemic inflammation by salicylates and pioglitazone. PLoS One 2013;8:e82847.

[93] Jovanović GK, et al. The efficacy of an energy-restricted anti-inflammatory diet for the management of obesity in younger adults. Nutrients 2020;12:1—23.

[94] Estruch R, et al. Primary prevention of cardiovascular disease with a Mediterranean diet supplemented with extra-virgin olive oil or nuts. N Engl J Med 2018;378:e34.

[95] van den Hoek AM, et al. Diet and exercise reduce pre-existing NASH and fibrosis and have additional beneficial effects on the vasculature, adipose tissue and skeletal muscle via organ-crosstalk. Metabolism 2021;124.

Part IV

Clinical aspects

Chapter 15

Role of adipose tissue remodeling in diabetic heart disease

Amanda MacCannell[1], Sam Straw[1,2] and Eylem Levelt[1,2]

[1]University of Leeds, Multidisciplinary Cardiovascular Research Centre and Biomedical Imaging Science Department, Leeds Institute of Cardiovascular and Metabolic Medicine, Leeds, United Kingdom; [2]Leeds Teaching Hospitals NHS Trust, Department of Cardiology, Leeds, United Kingdom

Adipose tissue physiology in health and the pathophysiological role of adipose tissue in transition from obesity to diabetes

Cardiovascular disease (CVD) remains a leading cause of morbidity and mortality globally despite substantial advances in prevention and treatment [1]. Obesity is a major contributor to a range of serious health complications including CVD [2]. The medical progress at tackling CVD has been counteracted by the consequences of the obesity epidemic. Driven by the obesity epidemic, the two diseases that have the largest stress on the healthcare community are hypertension and type 2 diabetes mellitus (T2DM) [3,4]. Both conditions are among the most important CVD risk factors and leading causes of mortality [5]. Hypertension is twice as common among obese adults than normal weight individuals. The prevalence of T2DM in obese adults is 11% compared with 2% in normal weight individuals [6].

The role of adipose tissue in CVD pathogenesis is more complex than simple metrics of obesity. Accumulating evidence suggests that adipose tissue distribution is an important determinant of CVD risk (Fig. 15.1) [7—14], which influences function and severity of CVD [15]. Subcutaneous white adipose tissue (sWAT) was once thought to have minimal risks for metabolic disease development; however, there is now a growing body of literature that suggests otherwise (Fig. 15.2) [16—18]. Visceral white adipose tissue (vWAT) is located within the abdominal cavity [19] and is associated with a higher risk of metabolic disease, insulin resistance, and cardiovascular disease in both men and women [20,21]. vWAT is composed of more adipocytes than sWAT, which are generally larger in size, with a higher capacity to hold lipid [22]. Venous blood from vWAT is drained into the liver through the portal vein directing free fatty acids (FFAs), secreted from visceral adipocytes, to the liver [23]. Increased liver fat accumulation can impair liver function, and continued accumulation can lead to nonalcoholic fatty liver disease (NAFLD) [23,24].

Adipose tissue is histologically classified into two types, white adipose tissue (WAT) and brown adipose tissue (BAT), which are visibly distinguishable based on tissue color (Fig. 15.2). BAT functions to generate heat through nonshivering thermogenesis in response to cold [25]. BAT converts fatty acids into measurable changes in heat production through the futile cycling of the mitochondrial electron transport chain (ETC) mediated by uncoupling protein 1 (UCP1) [26]. Evidence suggests active BAT may protect against obesity and cardiometabolic disease [27]. The aging process decreases both BAT and WAT function, causing changes to abundance, distribution, cellular composition, and endocrine signaling, which lead to increased disease burden. The functionality and volume of BAT in humans has been observed to decline with age and body mass index (BMI) [28,29]. Patients with obesity have less BAT volume but also decrease function through UCP1. Decreased UCP1, among other morphological changes, causes the BAT to begin to resemble WAT in a process termed "whitening" [30]. Whitening is observed to a greater extent in the BAT of patients with both obesity and T2DM compared with obese but nondiabetic controls [31].

Diabetes is a chronic disorder that alters the metabolism of patients and has serious long-term complications. Diabetes compromises the body's ability to store circulating glucose via malfunctioning insulin signaling, the main hormone involved in blood glucose homeostasis. In early stages of T2DM, there is a decrease in insulin secretion from pancreatic β-

Visceral and Ectopic Fat. https://doi.org/10.1016/B978-0-12-822186-0.00004-3

FIGURE 15.1 Human adipose tissue depots. When excess lipid cannot be stored in adipocytes, other cell types begin to store excess lipid.

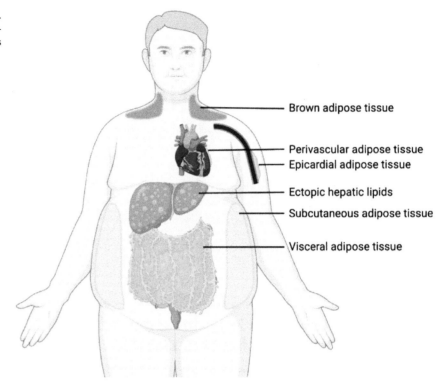

- Brown adipose tissue
- Perivascular adipose tissue
- Epicardial adipose tissue
- Ectopic hepatic lipids
- Subcutaneous adipose tissue
- Visceral adipose tissue

Langerhans islet cells, in the setting of peripheral tissue insulin resistance, in which the tissues fail to respond effectively to insulin signaling, reducing glucose uptake [32]. Through the "fat but fit theory," it is thought obesity itself does not cause adverse effects on health as long as the fat is stored effectively within adipocytes that respond to insulin [33]. The adipose tissue expandability hypothesis states that adipocytes have a maximum capacity and overexpansion of adipocytes can lead to hypoxia and inappropriate fat storage (Fig. 15.3). Hypoxia can cause insulin-resistant adipocytes by inhibiting phosphorylation of the insulin receptor tyrosine, leading to a decrease in glucose transport through inflammation within the adipocyte [34]. Failure to store fat effectively increases dyslipidemia and ectopic fat deposition in tissues such as muscle and liver, which further impairs insulin signaling [35].

Adipose tissue and signaling pathways in diabetes and heart disease

While the primary function of adipose tissue was considered to be a storage center for triacylglycerols (TAGs), recent studies have highlighted adipose tissue to be a prominent endocrine organ, able to influence almost all organs and cell types (Fig. 15.4). Adipose tissue signals can elicit a variety of responses including metabolic, immune, endocrine, and cardiovascular. Both visceral and subcutaneous adipose tissue secrete free fatty acids (FFA) and adipokines, which include leptin, adiponectin, tumor necrosis factor alpha (TNFα), Toll-like receptor (TLR) expression, and interleukin-6 (IL-6) [36]. These adipokines have the ability to act on organs both centrally and peripherally [37] to regulate food intake, energy balance, and insulin sensitivity [38].

Obesity occurs when food intake chronically exceeds energy expenditure. Energy intake consists of calories consumed, while energy expenditure includes basal metabolism, physical activity, and adaptive thermogenesis, which is considerably more difficult to measure. Energy balance, food intake and energy expenditure, is largely regulated by stimulus on the brain and central nervous system. Leptin and insulin act on the brain and are responsible for adiposity feedback signals, which influence appetite. Leptin signaling is proportional to adipose amount; increased leptin regulates adiposity by supporting energy expenditure and limiting energy intake [39]. Like insulin intolerance, patients can develop leptin intolerance, which occurs when the brain no longer responds to leptin signals, preventing limitation of food intake and reducing energy expenditure [40]. One mechanism of leptin resistance is through C-reactive protein (CRP). CRP is secreted by adipocytes and is a known marker of systemic inflammation, which increases with obesity [41]. CRP inhibits leptin signaling by preventing leptin from binding its receptor, impairing the ability of leptin to prevent food intake and energy expenditure

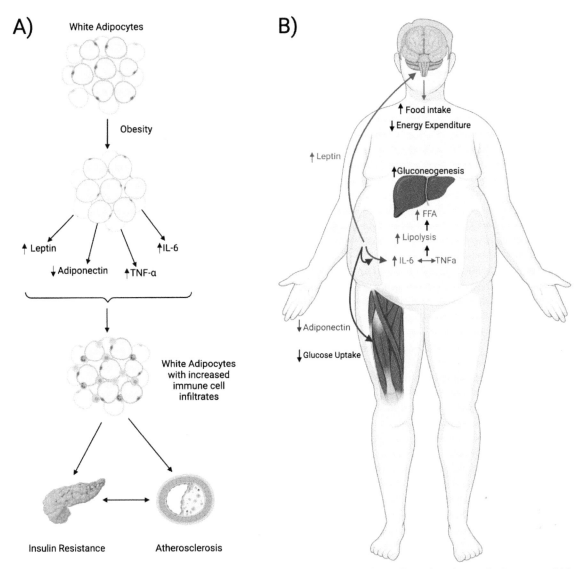

FIGURE 15.2 Histological classification of adipose tissue and adipose tissue secretory function. Adipose tissue is an endocrine organ, which secretes adipokines to regulate other organs. (A) When adipocytes expand in obesity, the levels of secreted adipokines change, leading to insulin resistance and atherosclerosis at a whole-body level. (B) Pathway-specific changes caused by changes to circulating adipokines.

[42]. Leptin is involved in not only energy balance but glucose and insulin homeostasis [43]. Leptin influences glucose—insulin metabolism by decreasing glycemia, insulinemia, and insulin resistance. Leptin increases insulin sensitivity by decreasing adiposity and lipotoxicity alongside decreasing hepatic production of glucose to reduce plasma glucose levels [44]. In addition to leptin regulating insulin and glucose metabolism, leptin secondarily stimulates vascular inflammation, oxidative stress, and vascular smooth muscle hypertrophy, which may contribute to pathogenesis of T2DM, hypertension, atherosclerosis, and coronary heart disease [45—47].

Adipose tissue cytokines have both autocrine and paracrine affects. Adipose tissue produces over 100 proinflammatory, anti-inflammatory, and immunomodulating proteins and peptides. Adipose tissue inflammation is considered a crucial event, leading to metabolic syndrome, T2DM, and atherosclerotic cardiovascular diseases. Chronic inflammation and activation of the immune system can lead to obesity-related insulin resistance and T2DM. TNFα plays a direct role in decreasing insulin signaling and subsequently glucose uptake within adipocytes [48,49]. Improvement in insulin sensitivity induced by weight loss is accompanied by a decrease in the expression of proinflammatory genes [50]. TNFα is not solely responsible for causing T2DM; acute elevations of FFA levels that usually stimulate insulin secretion but chronic elevation of FFA concentrations impair β-cell function [51]. Increased BMI has been associated with increased risk of CVD and mortality of humans across both sexes [7,52].

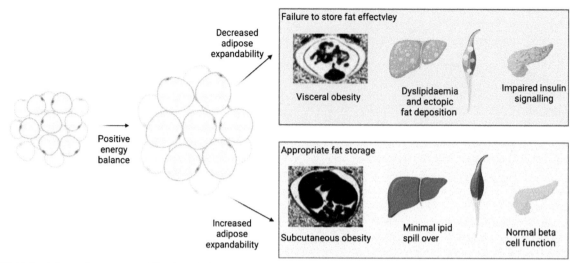

FIGURE 15.3 Adipose tissue expandability hypothesis proposes that during positive energy balance, adipocytes have a maximum capacity and overexpansion of adipocytes can lead to hypoxia and inappropriate fat storage. Excess lipid accumulated as visceral adipose tissue, ectopic fat deposition causing impair insulin signaling in peripheral tissues, leading to β-cell failure and type 2 diabetes mellitus.

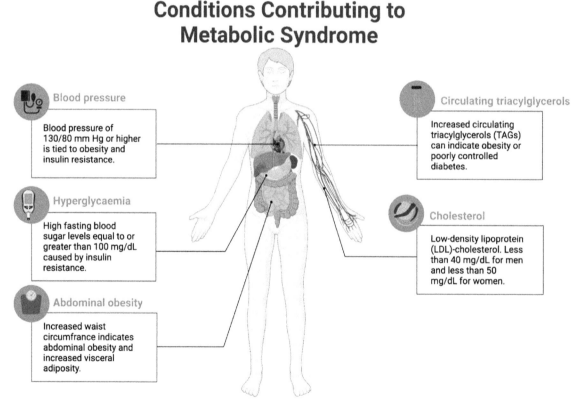

FIGURE 15.4 Metabolic syndrome (MetS) is a cluster of conditions that occur together, increasing your risk of heart disease, stroke, and type 2 diabetes. Metabolic syndrome is a combination of high waist circumference, circulating levels of triacylglycerols (TAGs), and low-density lipoprotein (LDL) cholesterol, fasting hyperglycemia and high blood pressure.

Adipokines are not only altered by changes to energy intake but also influenced by circadian rhythm disruptions. Circadian clocks exist to control daily physiological events through the suprachiasmatic nucleus (SCN), which coordinates with peripheral organs through CLOCK (circadian locomotor output cycles kaput) and BMAL1 genes. Our bodies operate on a 24-h clock, which includes a circadian rhythm of food intake governed by predictable daily mealtimes. Due to the anticipatory nature of food intake, our bodies anticipate the need for insulin and increase plasma insulin levels prior to food intake [53]. Altered timing of food intake and changes to food composition can cause desynchronization of the central pacemaker and peripheral clocks, which can lead to the development of metabolic disorders [54]. Alterations to both adipose tissue and liver peripheral clocks have shown to directly contribute to metabolic disease. BMAL1 and CLOCK control expression of cytokines involved in glucose and lipid homeostasis [55]. Adiponectin, which is involved in regulating glucose concentrations and fatty acid breakdown, has shown to have a delay in expression caused by obesity due to alterations in BMAL1 signaling [56,57]. Alterations to adiponectin signaling reduced the positive response of adiponectin increasing susceptibility to steatosis and T2DM [58,59].

Sex differences in adipose tissue remodeling effects on cardiovascular disease

Sexual dimorphism of both adipose tissue distribution and overall adiposity translates to sex differences in the prevalence of metabolic syndrome and T2DM [60,61]. Obesity perturbs numerous metabolic pathways [62] and increases the risk for metabolic syndrome (MetS), a combination of high waist circumference, circulating levels of triacylglycerols (TAGs), and low-density lipoprotein (LDL) cholesterol, fasting hyperglycemia and high blood pressure [63]. In turn, MetS increases the risk of developing T2DM and cardiovascular disease [64]. MetS is a cluster of different conditions, and each of these conditions has difference severity and prevalence among men and women (Fig. 15.4).

Premenopausal women have fewer incidents of obesity-related metabolic disorders than age-matched men, although women have ~10% higher body fat compared with men (Fig. 15.5) [65]. Premenopausal women accrue more sWAT, which is associated with relatively less adverse consequences of obesity and MetS compared with vWAT. The sexual dimorphism of systemic metabolic characteristics has been linked to higher proportions of sWAT and lower proportions of vWAT in women compared with men. Even lean men carry a greater proportion of their body fat as vWAT compared with lean women. After menopause, adipose tissue distribution in women shifts to favor deposition in vWAT, which correlates with a shift in metabolic disease risk, closely resembling the same risk as seen in age-matched men [66]. Sex differences in adipose tissue distribution are caused by sex differences in determinates of fat uptake and storage. The rate-limiting step in accumulation of fat derived from circulating fatty acids and TAGs is through lipoprotein lipase. Lipoprotein lipase activity is higher in sWAT compared with vWAT in women, which is the opposite to men [67]. The sex differences in adipose tissue distribution are determined through lipoprotein lipase activity suppression by testosterone in femoral subcutaneous

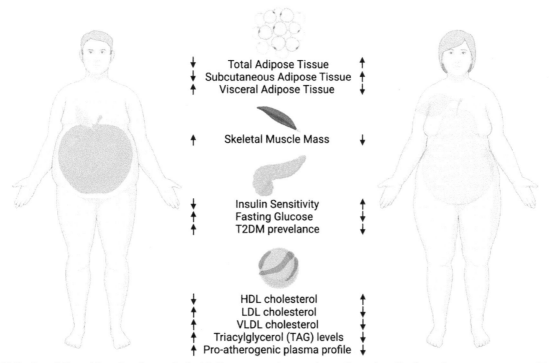

FIGURE 15.5 Sexual dimorphism of cardiovascular health. Premenopausal women have a "pear-shaped" adipose tissue storage pattern, with increased subcutaneous adipose tissue. Men have an "apple-shaped" adipose tissue storage pattern with increased visceral adipose storage. ↑, increased; ↓, decreased.

adipose in men [68]. Women have higher HDL cholesterol levels and lower LDL cholesterol, VLDL cholesterol, and triacylglycerol (TAG) levels, reflecting a less proatherogenic plasma lipid profile than men matched for age and BMI [69].

The postmenopausal hormone shift is a key contributor to increase incidents of CVD. Women that begin estrogen treatment during the perimenopausal period have reduced CVD disease risk compared with postmenopausal women [70]. The timing of hormonal treatment has proven to be very important, and delayed start of hormonal treatment does not have the same effect on reducing CVD risk [70]. Taken together, sex hormones contribute to sex differences in substrate metabolism and cardiometabolic disease susceptibility. The cardiovascular advantage women have disappeared after menopause, but also with the development of T2DM. Alongside premenopausal women having decreased incident of CVD, women also have lower risk of insulin resistance and T2DM than age-matched men and reduced fasting glucose levels [71,72], showing a link between glucose homeostasis and CVD. Women have higher whole-body insulin sensitivity in women than in men when expressed per unit of fat-free mass rather than in terms of body weight [69].

Adiponectin, proinflammatory adipocytokines, and cardiovascular disease in diabetes

Adiponectin is an important adipokine with direct anti-inflammatory and antioxidant effects on the vasculature and the heart. Adiponectin is secreted solely by adipose tissue, is abundant in human plasma, and is a protective factor with anti-inflammatory, antiatherogenic, and insulin-sensitizing effects [73]. Adiponectin is normally found in circulation as one of the most abundant plasma proteins and circulating adiponectin levels generally decrease in individuals with obesity and diabetes [74]. Adiponectin knockout (Ad-KO) mice have been particularly informative in terms of elucidating the regulation of cardiac function and remodeling events such as apoptosis and fibrosis by adiponectin [75]. Despite adiponectin being associated with a favorable risk profile in healthy individuals, higher levels have been associated with worse outcomes in people with existing heart failure—a so-called "adiponectin paradox" where excess secretion serves as a protective mechanism or a compensatory response to advanced cardiovascular disease [76]. Similarly in diabetes mellitus, the protective effects of high circulating adiponectin are lost, or even reversed [77]. Adiponectin exerts a direct protective effect, and in humans, adiponectin is accumulated in myocardial tissue damaged by ischemia and exerts protective effects inhibiting inducible nitric oxide synthase and expression and thereby oxidative stress [78,79].

Inflammation is a key feature of atherogenesis, preceding the development of atherosclerotic plaques while also predisposing to plaque destabilization and rupture [80]. Adiponectin exerts endocrine and paracrine effects on the vascular wall [81], suppressing the TNFα-induced expression of adhesion molecules in vascular endothelial cells, as well as inhibiting macrophage release of cytokines and transformation into foam cells, key components in the development of atherosclerosis [82,83]. Adiponectin also increases insulin sensitivity by stimulating tissue fat oxidation, resulting in reduced circulating FFA concentrations and reduced hepatic and skeletal muscle triglyceride concentrations [84]. Furthermore, adiponectin induces endothelial nitric oxide synthase in endothelial cell cultures, increasing nitric oxide concentrations that might explain the vasoprotective effects of adiponectin in T2DM [85].

In metabolic disease states such as T2DM, a shift between anti-inflammatory and proinflammatory adipocytokines occurs, with this imbalance predisposing to chronic, low-grade inflammation that contributes to the development of CVD. As well as the CVD, low-grade adipose tissue inflammation is also thought to play an adverse prognostic role in the severe acute respiratory syndrome coronavirus 2 (SARS-CoV-2) infection-related morbidity and mortality. The severity of coronavirus disease 2019 (COVID-19) is associated with the presence of comorbidities; while obesity alone is responsible for 20% of COVID-19 hospitalizations, obesity in combination with T2DM and hypertension accounts for 58% [86]. A recent study investigating the ultrastructural features of vWAT among individuals with COVID-19 showed the presence of higher local vWAT inflammation and higher prevalence of pulmonary fat embolism of subjects who died due to COVID-19 [87]. TNFα, a proinflammatory cytokine, is associated with insulin resistance and obesity [88] as well as being upregulated following myocardial infarction and in heart failure [89]. TNFα induces the expression of proinflammatory genes and, in vascular smooth muscle cells, induces migration, proliferation, and apoptosis as well as increasing expression of adhesion molecules within endothelial cells [90]. Leptin has a broader biological role than merely influencing adipose stores and promotes atherogenesis by increasing oxidative stress within endothelial cells [91] and promoting the release of proinflammatory cytokines.

Imaging ectopic adiposity in patients with type 2 diabetes mellitus

Computed tomography (CT), magnetic resonance imaging (MRI), ultrasonography, and proton (^{1}H)-MR spectroscopy (MRS) have all been used to quantify adipose tissue amount or lipid content within an organ and to examine the association of various fat depots with both systemic and local manifestations of disease [92−97]. Recently, using these techniques, it was demonstrated that, irrespective of body mass index, diabetes is related to significant abnormalities in cardiac function, energetics, and cardiac and hepatic steatosis [24]. However, obese patients with T2DM showed a greater propensity for ectopic fat deposition that is associated with cardiac contractile dysfunction and fibroinflammatory liver disease than lean T2DM patients [24]. Moreover, an inverse correlation of epicardial adipose tissue volumes with cardiac systolic strain was demonstrated [24]. Similarly, excess liver fat, which is a form of ectopic fat, has been shown to be accompanied by cardiac structural and functional changes [98].

The most exciting recent development in adipose tissue imaging is the demonstration of the ability of CT angiography methodology to quantify the phenotypic changes in perivascular adipose tissue (PVAT) induced by vascular inflammation. Vascular inflammation is a key feature of vascular atherosclerotic disease pathogenesis and leads to the release of inflammatory signals that disseminate into local fat, inducing local lipolysis and inhibiting adipogenesis [99]. The study by Charalambos et al. demonstrated that vascular inflammation induces a shift of PVAT's composition from lipid to aqueous phase, which results into increased CT attenuation around the inflamed artery, forming a gradient with increasing attenuation closer to the inflamed coronary artery wall. This ability of PVAT to sense inflammatory signals from the vascular wall was used as a "thermometer" of the vascular wall, allowing for noninvasive detection of coronary inflammation [99]. These spatial changes in PVAT's attenuation were shown to be detected with high sensitivity around culprit lesions during acute coronary syndromes. A new biomarker designed to capture these spatial changes in PVAT's attenuation around the human coronary arteries, the Fat Attenuation Index (FAI), was shown to have additional predictive value in stable patients for cardiac mortality and nonfatal heart attacks, above the prediction provided by the current state-of-the-art diagnostic approach that includes risk factors, calcium score, and presence of high-risk plaque features. This new diagnostic test was therefore able to identify the those patients most at risk enabling application of targeted treatments in primary or secondary prevention, to prevent the development of clinical cardiovascular disease. The use of perivascular FAI in clinical practice may change the way cardiovascular CT angiography is interpreted, as it is applicable to any coronary CT angiogram, and it offers dynamic information about the inflammatory burden of the coronary arteries, providing potential guidance for preventive measures and invasive treatments.

Conclusions

Adipose tissue produces a wide range of adipocytokines with a diverse range of metabolic functions. In metabolic disease states, a shift between anti-inflammatory and proinflammatory adipocytokines occurs, with this imbalance predisposing to chronic, low-grade inflammation that contributes to the development of cardiovascular disease.

References

[1] Virani SS, Alonso A, Benjamin EJ, Bittencourt MS, Callaway CW, Carson AP, et al. Heart disease and stroke statistics-2020 update: a report from the American heart association. Circulation 2020;141:e139—596. https://doi.org/10.1161/CIR.0000000000000757.

[2] Poirier P, Giles TD, Bray GA, Hong Y, Stern JS, Pi-Sunyer FX, et al. Obesity and cardiovascular disease: pathophysiology, evaluation, and effect of weight loss: an update of the 1997 American heart association scientific statement on obesity and heart disease from the obesity committee of the council on nutrition, physical activity, and metabolism. Circulation 2006;113:898—918. https://doi.org/10.1161/CIRCULATIONAHA.106.171016.

[3] Emerging Risk Factors Collaboration, Sarwar N, Gao P, Seshasai SRK, Gobin R, Kaptoge S, et al. Diabetes mellitus, fasting blood glucose concentration, and risk of vascular disease: a collaborative meta-analysis of 102 prospective studies. Lancet 2010;375:2215—22. https://doi.org/10.1016/S0140-6736(10)60484-9.

[4] Khurram M, Paracha SJ, Hamama-tul-Bushra Khar ZH. Obesity related complications in 100 obese subjects and their age matched controls. JPMA 2006;56.

[5] Organization WH. Global report on diabetes. World Health Organization; 2016.

[6] Gatineau M, Hancock C, Holman N, Outhwaite H, Oldridge L, Christie A, et al. Adult obesity and type 2 diabetes. Oxford: Public Health England; 2014.

[7] Kenchaiah S, Evans JC, Levy D, Wilson PWF, Benjamin EJ, Larson MG, et al. Obesity and the risk of heart failure. N Engl J Med 2002;347:305—13. https://doi.org/10.1056/NEJMoa020245.

[8] Després J-P. The insulin resistance—dyslipidemic syndrome of visceral obesity: effect on patients' risk. Obes Res 1998;6:8S—17S. https://doi.org/10.1002/j.1550-8528.1998.tb00683.x.

[9] Van Gaal LF, Mertens IL, De Block CE. Mechanisms linking obesity with cardiovascular disease. Nature 2006;444:875—80. https://doi.org/10.1038/nature05487.

[10] Giamila F, Theodore M. Adipose tissue and atherosclerosis. Arterioscler Thromb Vasc Biol 2007;27:996—1003. https://doi.org/10.1161/ATVBAHA.106.131755.

[11] Bowden DW, Cox AJ. Diabetes: unravelling the enigma of T2DM and cardiovascular disease. Nat Rev Endocrinol 2013;9:632—3. https://doi.org/10.1038/nrendo.2013.192.

[12] Okura T, Nakata Y, Yamabuki K, Tanaka K. Regional body composition changes exhibit opposing effects on coronary heart disease risk factors. Arterioscler Thromb Vasc Biol 2004;24:923−9. https://doi.org/10.1161/01.ATV.0000125702.26272.f6.

[13] Pou KM, Massaro JM, Hoffmann U, Vasan RS, Maurovich-Horvat P, Larson MG, et al. Visceral and subcutaneous adipose tissue volumes are cross-sectionally related to markers of inflammation and oxidative stress: the Framingham Heart Study. Circulation 2007;116:1234−41. https://doi.org/10.1161/CIRCULATIONAHA.107.710509.

[14] Schmidt MI, Duncan BB, Sharrett AR, Lindberg G, Savage PJ, Offenbacher S, et al. Markers of inflammation and prediction of diabetes mellitus in adults (atherosclerosis risk in communities study): a cohort study. Lancet 1999;353:1649−52. https://doi.org/10.1016/s0140-6736(99)01046-6.

[15] Tchernof A, Després J-P. Pathophysiology of human visceral obesity: an update. Physiol Rev 2013;93:359−404. https://doi.org/10.1152/physrev.00033.2011.

[16] Grundy SM. Adipose tissue and metabolic syndrome: too much, too little or neither. Eur J Clin Invest 2015;45:1209−17. https://doi.org/10.1111/eci.12519.

[17] Yang X, Smith U. Adipose tissue distribution and risk of metabolic disease: does thiazolidinedione-induced adipose tissue redistribution provide a clue to the answer? Diabetologia 2007;50:1127−39. https://doi.org/10.1007/s00125-007-0640-1.

[18] Wajchenberg BL. Subcutaneous and visceral adipose tissue: their relation to the metabolic syndrome. Endocr Rev 2000;21:697−738. https://doi.org/10.1210/edrv.21.6.0415.

[19] Wronska A, Kmiec Z. Structural and biochemical characteristics of various white adipose tissue depots. Acta Physiol 2012;205:194−208.

[20] Ross R, Aru J, Freeman J, Hudson R, Janssen I. Abdominal adiposity and insulin resistance in obese men. Am J Physiol-Endocrinol Metabol 2002;282:E657−63. https://doi.org/10.1152/ajpendo.00469.2001.

[21] Ross R, Freeman J, Hudson R, Janssen I. Abdominal obesity, muscle composition, and insulin resistance in premenopausal women. J Clin Endocrinol Metab 2002;87:5044−51. https://doi.org/10.1210/jc.2002-020570.

[22] Verboven K, Wouters K, Gaens K, Hansen D, Bijnen M, Wetzels S, et al. Abdominal subcutaneous and visceral adipocyte size, lipolysis and inflammation relate to insulin resistance in male obese humans. Sci Rep 2018;8:4677. https://doi.org/10.1038/s41598-018-22962-x.

[23] Heilbronn L, Smith SR, Ravussin E. Failure of fat cell proliferation, mitochondrial function and fat oxidation results in ectopic fat storage, insulin resistance and type II diabetes mellitus. Int J Obes Relat Metab Disord 2004;28(Suppl. 4):S12−21. https://doi.org/10.1038/sj.ijo.0802853.

[24] Levelt E, Pavlides M, Banerjee R, Mahmod M, Kelly C, Sellwood J, et al. Ectopic and visceral fat deposition in lean and obese patients with type 2 diabetes. J Am Coll Cardiol 2016;68:53−63. https://doi.org/10.1016/j.jacc.2016.03.597.

[25] Frontini A, Cinti S. Distribution and development of Brown adipocytes in the murine and human adipose organ. Cell Metabol 2010;11:253−6. https://doi.org/10.1016/j.cmet.2010.03.004.

[26] Golozoubova V, Cannon B, Nedergaard J. UCP1 is essential for adaptive adrenergic nonshivering thermogenesis. Am J Physiol-Endocrinol Metabol 2006;291:E350−7. https://doi.org/10.1152/ajpendo.00387.2005.

[27] Betz MJ, Enerbäck S. Human brown adipose tissue: what we have learned so far. Diabetes 2015;64:2352−60. https://doi.org/10.2337/db15-0146.

[28] Palmer AK, Kirkland JL. Aging and adipose tissue: potential interventions for diabetes and regenerative medicine. Exp Gerontol 2016;86:97−105. https://doi.org/10.1016/j.exger.2016.02.013.

[29] Saito M, Okamatsu-Ogura Y, Matsushita M, Watanabe K, Yoneshiro T, Nio-Kobayashi J, et al. High incidence of metabolically active brown adipose tissue in healthy adult humans: effects of cold exposure and adiposity. Diabetes 2009;58:1526−31. https://doi.org/10.2337/db09-0530.

[30] Shimizu I, Aprahamian T, Kikuchi R, Shimizu A, Papanicolaou KN, MacLauchlan S, et al. Vascular rarefaction mediates whitening of brown fat in obesity. J Clin Invest 2014;124:2099−112. https://doi.org/10.1172/JCI71643.

[31] Timmons JA, Pedersen BK. The importance of brown adipose tissue. N Engl J Med 2009;361:415−6. https://doi.org/10.1056/NEJMc091009. author reply 418-421.

[32] Cerf ME. Beta cell dysfunction and insulin resistance. Front Endocrinol 2013;4. https://doi.org/10.3389/fendo.2013.00037.

[33] Røder ME, Porte D, Schwartz RS, Kahn SE. Disproportionately elevated proinsulin levels reflect the degree of impaired B cell secretory capacity in patients with noninsulin-dependent diabetes mellitus. J Clin Endocrinol Metab 1998;83:604−8. https://doi.org/10.1210/jcem.83.2.4544.

[34] Trayhurn P, Wang B, Wood IS. Hypoxia in adipose tissue: a basis for the dysregulation of tissue function in obesity? Br J Nutr 2008;100:227−35. https://doi.org/10.1017/S0007114508971282.

[35] Virtue S, Vidal-Puig A. Adipose tissue expandability, lipotoxicity and the metabolic syndrome — an allostatic perspective. Biochim Biophys Acta Mol Cell Biol Lipids 2010;1801:338−49. https://doi.org/10.1016/j.bbalip.2009.12.006.

[36] Vázquez-Vela MEF, Torres N, Tovar AR. White adipose tissue as endocrine organ and its role in obesity. Arch Med Res 2008;39:715−28. https://doi.org/10.1016/j.arcmed.2008.09.005.

[37] Friedman JM, Halaas JL. Leptin and the regulation of body weight in mammals. Nature 1998;395:763−70. https://doi.org/10.1038/27376.

[38] Rosen E, Spiegelman BM. Adipocytes as regulators of energy balance and glucose homeostasis. Nature 2006;444:847−53.

[39] Denroche HC, Huynh FK, Kieffer TJ. The role of leptin in glucose homeostasis. J Diabetes Investig 2012;3:115−29. https://doi.org/10.1111/j.2040-1124.2012.00203.x. 2012.

[40] Gruzdeva O, Borodkina D, Uchasova E, Dyleva Y, Barbarash O. Leptin resistance: underlying mechanisms and diagnosis. Diab Metab Syndr Obes 2019;12:191−8. https://doi.org/10.2147/DMSO.S182406.

[41] Festa A, Williams K, D'Agostino R, Wagenknecht LE, Haffner SM. The natural course of beta-cell function in nondiabetic and diabetic individuals: the insulin resistance atherosclerosis study. Diabetes 2006;55:1114−20. https://doi.org/10.2337/diabetes.55.04.06.db05-1100.

[42] Chen K, Li F, Li J, Cai H, Strom S, Bisello A, et al. Induction of leptin resistance through direct interaction of C-reactive protein with leptin. Nat Med 2006;12:425−32. https://doi.org/10.1038/nm1372.

[43] Schwartz MW, Porte D. Diabetes, obesity, and the brain. Science 2005;307:375−9. https://doi.org/10.1126/science.1104344.

[44] Paz-Filho G, Mastronardi C, Wong M-L, Licinio J. Leptin therapy, insulin sensitivity, and glucose homeostasis. Indian J Endocrinol Metab 2012;16:S549−55. https://doi.org/10.4103/2230-8210.105571.

[45] Seufert J. Leptin effects on pancreatic beta-cell gene expression and function. Diabetes 2004;53(Suppl. 1):S152−8. https://doi.org/10.2337/diabetes.53.2007.s152.

[46] Bełtowski J. Role of leptin in blood pressure regulation and arterial hypertension. J Hypertens 2006;24:789−801. https://doi.org/10.1097/01.hjh.0000222743.06584.66.

[47] Beltowski J. Leptin and atherosclerosis. Atherosclerosis 2006;189:47−60. https://doi.org/10.1016/j.atherosclerosis.2006.03.003.

[48] Hotamisligil GS, Spiegelman BM. Tumor necrosis factor α: a key component of the obesity-diabetes link. Diabetes 1994;43:1271−8. https://doi.org/10.2337/diab.43.11.1271.

[49] Engelman JA, Berg AH, Lewis RY, Lisanti MP, Scherer PE. Tumor necrosis factor alpha-mediated insulin resistance, but not dedifferentiation, is abrogated by MEK1/2 inhibitors in 3T3-L1 adipocytes. Mol Endocrinol 2000;14:1557−69. https://doi.org/10.1210/mend.14.10.0542.

[50] Hotamisligil GS, Arner P, Caro JF, Atkinson RL, Spiegelman BM. Increased adipose tissue expression of tumor necrosis factor-alpha in human obesity and insulin resistance. J Clin Invest 1995;95:2409−15. https://doi.org/10.1172/JCI117936.

[51] McGarry JD, Dobbins R. Fatty acids, lipotoxicity and insulin secretion. Diabetologia 1999;42:128−38. https://doi.org/10.1007/s001250051130.

[52] Manson JE, Willett WC, Stampfer MJ, Colditz GA, Hunter DJ, Hankinson SE, et al. Body weight and mortality among women. N Engl J Med 1995;333:677−85.

[53] Tahara Y, Shibata S. Chronobiology and nutrition. Neuroscience 2013;253:78−88. https://doi.org/10.1016/j.neuroscience.2013.08.049.

[54] Barclay JL, Husse J, Bode B, Naujokat N, Meyer-Kovac J, Schmid SM, et al. Circadian desynchrony promotes metabolic disruption in a mouse model of shiftwork. PLoS One 2012;7. https://doi.org/10.1371/journal.pone.0037150.

[55] Maury E, Ramsey KM, Bass J. Circadian rhythms and metabolic syndrome. Circ Res 2010;106:447−62. https://doi.org/10.1161/CIRCRESAHA.109.208355.

[56] Lamia KA, Storch K-F, Weitz CJ. Physiological significance of a peripheral tissue circadian clock. Proc Natl Acad Sci U S A 2008;105:15172−7. https://doi.org/10.1073/pnas.0806717105.

[57] Shimba S, Ishii N, Ohta Y, Ohno T, Watabe Y, Hayashi M, et al. Brain and muscle Arnt-like protein-1 (BMAL1), a component of the molecular clock, regulates adipogenesis. Proc Natl Acad Sci USA 2005;102:12071−6. https://doi.org/10.1073/pnas.0502383102.

[58] Barnea M, Madar Z, Froy O. High-fat diet delays and fasting advances the circadian expression of adiponectin signaling components in mouse liver. Endocrinology 2009;150:161−8. https://doi.org/10.1210/en.2008-0944.

[59] Kamada Y, Takehara T, Hayashi N. Adipocytokines and liver disease. J Gastroenterol 2008;43:811−22. https://doi.org/10.1007/s00535-008-2213-6.

[60] Power ML, Schulkin J. Sex differences in fat storage, fat metabolism, and the health risks from obesity: possible evolutionary origins. Br J Nutr 2008;99:931−40. https://doi.org/10.1017/S0007114507853347.

[61] Shi H, Seeley RJ, Clegg DJ. Sexual differences in the control of energy homeostasis. Front Neuroendocrin 2009;30:396−404. https://doi.org/10.1016/j.yfrne.2009.03.004.

[62] Grundy SM. Obesity, metabolic syndrome, and cardiovascular disease. J Clin Endocrinol Metab 2004;89:2595−600. https://doi.org/10.1210/jc.2004-0372.

[63] Huang PL. A comprehensive definition for metabolic syndrome. Dis Model Mech 2009;2:231−7. https://doi.org/10.1242/dmm.001180.

[64] Galassi A, Reynolds K, He J. Metabolic syndrome and risk of cardiovascular disease: a meta-analysis. Am J Med 2006;119:812−9. https://doi.org/10.1016/j.amjmed.2006.02.031.

[65] Jackson AS, Stanforth PR, Gagnon J, Rankinen T, Leon AS, Rao DC, et al. The effect of sex, age and race on estimating percentage body fat from body mass index: the heritage family study. Int J Obes 2002;26:789−96. https://doi.org/10.1038/sj.ijo.0802006.

[66] Colditz GA, Willett WC, Stampfer MJ, Rosner B, Speizer FE, Hennekens CH. Menopause and the risk of coronary heart disease in women. N Engl J Med 1987;316:1105−10. https://doi.org/10.1056/NEJM198704303161801.

[67] Arner P, Lithell H, Wahrenberg H, Brönnegard M. Expression of lipoprotein lipase in different human subcutaneous adipose tissue regions. J Lipid Res 1991;32:423−9. https://doi.org/10.1016/S0022-2275(20)42065-6.

[68] Ramirez ME, McMurry MP, Wiebke GA, Felten KJ, Ren K, Meikle AW, et al. Evidence for sex steroid inhibition of lipoprotein lipase in men: comparison of abdominal and femoral adipose tissue. Metabolism 1997;46:179−85. https://doi.org/10.1016/S0026-0495(97)90299-7.

[69] Goossens GH, Jocken JWE, Blaak EE. Sexual dimorphism in cardiometabolic health: the role of adipose tissue, muscle and liver. Nat Rev Endocrinol 2021;17:47−66. https://doi.org/10.1038/s41574-020-00431-8.

[70] Reslan OM, Khalil RA. Vascular effects of estrogenic menopausal hormone therapy. Rev Rec Clin Trials 2012;7:47−70.

[71] Kuhl J, Hilding A, Ostenson CG, Grill V, Efendic S, Båvenholm P. Characterisation of subjects with early abnormalities of glucose tolerance in the stockholm diabetes prevention programme: the impact of sex and type 2 diabetes heredity. Diabetologia 2005;48:35−40. https://doi.org/10.1007/s00125-004-1614-1.

[72] Peters SAE, Muntner P, Woodward M. Sex differences in the prevalence of, and trends in, cardiovascular risk factors, treatment, and control in the United States, 2001 to 2016. Circulation 2019;139:1025−35. https://doi.org/10.1161/CIRCULATIONAHA.118.035550.

[73] Golia E, Limongelli G, Natale F, Fimiani F, Maddaloni V, Russo PE, Riegler L, Bianchi R, Crisci M, Palma GD, et al. Adipose tissue and vascular inflammation in coronary artery disease. World J Cardiol 2014;6:539−54. https://doi.org/10.4330/wjc.v6.i7.539.

[74] Liu Y, Retnakaran R, Fau - Hanley A, Hanley A, Fau - Tungtrongchitr R, Tungtrongchitr R, Fau - Shaw C, Shaw C, Fau - Sweeney G, Sweeney G. Total and high molecular weight but not trimeric or hexameric forms of adiponectin correlate with markers of the metabolic syndrome and liver injury in Thai subjects. 2007.

[75] Yamauchi T, Kadowaki T. Physiological and pathophysiological roles of adiponectin and adiponectin receptors in the integrated regulation of metabolic and cardiovascular diseases. Int J Obes 2008;32:S13—8. https://doi.org/10.1038/ijo.2008.233.

[76] Wannamethee SG, Whincup PH, Lennon L, Sattar N. Circulating adiponectin levels and mortality in elderly men with and without cardiovascular disease and heart failure. Arch Intern Med 2007;167:1510—7. https://doi.org/10.1001/archinte.167.14.1510.

[77] Beatty AL, Zhang MH, Ku IA, Na B, Schiller NB, Whooley MA. Adiponectin is associated with increased mortality and heart failure in patients with stable ischemic heart disease: data from the Heart and Soul Study. Atherosclerosis 2012;220:587—92. https://doi.org/10.1016/j.atherosclerosis.2011.11.038.

[78] Tao L, Gao E, Jiao X, Yuan Y, Li S, Christopher TA, Lopez BL, Koch W, Chan L, Goldstein BJ, et al. Adiponectin cardioprotection after myocardial ischemia/reperfusion involves the reduction of oxidative/nitrative stress. Circulation 2007;115:1408—16. https://doi.org/10.1161/CIRCULATIONAHA.106.666941.

[79] Shibata R, Izumiya Y, Sato K, Papanicolaou K, Kihara S, Colucci WS, Sam F, Ouchi N, Walsh K. Adiponectin protects against the development of systolic dysfunction following myocardial infarction. J Mol Cell Cardiol 2007;42:1065—74. https://doi.org/10.1016/j.yjmcc.2007.03.808.

[80] Ross R. Atherosclerosis–an inflammatory disease. N Engl J Med 1999;340:115—26. https://doi.org/10.1056/NEJM199901143400207.

[81] Antoniades C, Antonopoulos AS, Tousoulis D, Stefanadis C. Adiponectin: from obesity to cardiovascular disease. Obes Rev 2009;10:269—79. https://doi.org/10.1111/j.1467-789X.2009.00571.x.

[82] Ouchi N, Kihara S, Arita Y, Okamoto Y, Maeda K, Kuriyama H, Hotta K, Nishida M, Takahashi M, Muraguchi M, et al. Adiponectin, an adipocyte-derived plasma protein, inhibits endothelial NF-kappaB signaling through a cAMP-dependent pathway. Circulation 2000;102:1296—301. https://doi.org/10.1161/01.cir.102.11.1296.

[83] Ouchi N, Kihara S, Arita Y, Maeda K, Kuriyama H, Okamoto Y, Hotta K, Nishida M, Takahashi M, Nakamura T, et al. Novel modulator for endothelial adhesion molecules: adipocyte-derived plasma protein adiponectin. Circulation 1999;100:2473—6. https://doi.org/10.1161/01.cir.100.25.2473.

[84] Yamauchi T, Kamon J, Waki H, Terauchi Y, Kubota N, Hara K, Mori Y, Ide T, Murakami K, Tsuboyama-Kasaoka N, et al. The fat-derived hormone adiponectin reverses insulin resistance associated with both lipoatrophy and obesity. Nat Med 2001;7:941—6. https://doi.org/10.1038/90984.

[85] Hattori Y, Suzuki M, Hattori S, Kasai K. Globular adiponectin upregulates nitric oxide production in vascular endothelial cells. Diabetologia 2003;46:1543—9. https://doi.org/10.1007/s00125-003-1224-3.

[86] Stefan N, Birkenfeld AL, Schulze MB. Global pandemics interconnected — obesity, impaired metabolic health and COVID-19. Nat Rev Endocrinol 2021;17:135—49. https://doi.org/10.1038/s41574-020-00462-1.

[87] Colleluori G, Graciotti L, Pesaresi M, Di Vincenzo A, Perugini J, Di Mercurio E, Caucci S, Bagnarelli P, Zingaretti CM, Nisoli E, et al. Visceral fat inflammation and fat embolism are associated with lung's lipidic hyaline membranes in subjects with COVID-19. Int J Obes 2022. https://doi.org/10.1038/s41366-022-01071-w.

[88] Ziccardi P, Nappo F, Giugliano G, Esposito K, Marfella R, Cioffi M, D'Andrea F, Molinari AM, Giugliano D. Reduction of inflammatory cytokine concentrations and improvement of endothelial functions in obese women after weight loss over one year. Circulation 2002;105:804—9. https://doi.org/10.1161/hc0702.104279.

[89] Kleinbongard P, Heusch G, Schulz R. TNFalpha in atherosclerosis, myocardial ischemia/reperfusion and heart failure. Pharmacol Ther 2010;127:295—314. https://doi.org/10.1016/j.pharmthera.2010.05.002.

[90] Slowik MR, De Luca LG, Fiers W, Pober JS. Tumor necrosis factor activates human endothelial cells through the p55 tumor necrosis factor receptor but the p75 receptor contributes to activation at low tumor necrosis factor concentration. Am J Pathol 1993;143:1724—30.

[91] Bouloumie A, Marumo T, Lafontan M, Busse R. Leptin induces oxidative stress in human endothelial cells. FASEB J 1999;13:1231—8.

[92] Fox CS, Massaro JM, Hoffmann U, Pou KM, Maurovich-Horvat P, Liu C-Y, Vasan RS, Murabito JM, Meigs JB, Cupples LA, et al. Abdominal visceral and subcutaneous adipose tissue compartments: association with metabolic risk factors in the framingham heart study. Circulation 2007;116:39—48. https://doi.org/10.1161/circulationaha.106.675355.

[93] Fox CS, Gona P, Hoffmann U, Porter SA, Salton CJ, Massaro JM, Levy D, Larson MG, D'Agostino RB, O'Donnell CJ, et al. Pericardial fat, intrathoracic fat, and measures of left ventricular structure and function: the framingham heart study. Circulation 2009;119:1586—91. https://doi.org/10.1161/circulationaha.108.828970.

[94] Fox CS, Massaro JM, Schlett CL, Lehman SJ, Meigs JB, O'Donnell CJ, Hoffmann U, Murabito JM. Periaortic fat deposition is associated with peripheral arterial disease: the framingham heart study. Circul: Cardiovas Imag 2010;3:515—9. https://doi.org/10.1161/circimaging.110.958884.

[95] Rijzewijk LJ, van der Meer RW, Smit JWA, Diamant M, Bax JJ, Hammer S, Romijn JA, de Roos A, Lamb HJ. Myocardial steatosis is an independent predictor of diastolic dysfunction in type 2 diabetes mellitus. J Am Coll Cardiol 2008;52:1793—9. https://doi.org/10.1016/j.jacc.2008.07.062.

[96] Rijzewijk LJ, Jonker JT, van der Meer RW, Lubberink M, de Jong HW, Romijn JA, Bax JJ, de Roos A, Heine RJ, Twisk JW, et al. Effects of hepatic triglyceride content on myocardial metabolism in type 2 diabetes. J Am Coll Cardiol 2010;56:225—33. https://doi.org/10.1016/j.jacc.2010.02.049.

[97] McGavock JM, Lingvay I, Zib I, Tillery T, Salas N, Unger R, Levine BD, Raskin P, Victor RG, Szczepaniak LS. Cardiac steatosis in diabetes mellitus: a 1H-magnetic resonance spectroscopy study. Circulation 2007;116:1170—5. https://doi.org/10.1161/CIRCULATIONAHA.106.645614.

[98] Petta S, Argano C, Colomba D, Cammà C, Di Marco V, Cabibi D, Tuttolomondo A, Marchesini G, Pinto A, Licata G, et al. Epicardial fat, cardiac geometry and cardiac function in patients with non-alcoholic fatty liver disease: association with the severity of liver disease. J Hepatol 2015;62:928—33. https://doi.org/10.1016/j.jhep.2014.11.030.

[99] Antonopoulos AA-O, Sanna FA-O, Sabharwal NA-OX, Thomas SA-OX, Oikonomou EA-O, Herdman LA-O, Margaritis MA-O, Shirodaria C, Kampoli AM, Akoumianakis IA-O, et al. Detecting human coronary inflammation by imaging perivascular fat. 2017. LID - eaal2658 [pii] LID - 10.1126/scitranslmed.aal2658 [doi].

Chapter 16

Cardiovascular disease

Michiel Sala[1], Albert de Roos[1] and Hildo J. Lamb[2]

[1]Leiden University Medical Center, Radiology Department, Leiden, the Netherlands; [2]Department of Radiology, Cardio Vascular Imaging Group (CVIG), Leiden University Medical Center, Leiden, the Netherlands

Introduction

Individuals with similar measures of overall adiposity such as body mass index may have distinct metabolic cardiovascular risk profiles. This may be explained by individual differences in regional body fat distribution (e.g., high-risk obesities) and the ability of subcutaneous adipose tissue to expand (e.g., dysfunctional adipose tissue). The majority of the association between adiposity and cardiovascular disease appears to be explained by altered cardiometabolic risk factors and comorbidities. High-risk obesities are the main drivers of altered cardiometabolic risk mediators including type 2 diabetes, increased blood pressure, abnormal lipid metabolism, inflammation, and endothelial dysfunction. In this chapter we will discuss the association between obesity and cardiovascular disease outcomes including obesity hypertension, coronary artery disease, arrhythmias, and heart failure. Specifically, different imaging techniques including computed tomography and magnetic resonance imaging are reviewed in relation to obesity and cardiovascular disease.

Obesity hypertension: role of magnetic resonance imaging

Obesity is associated with many adverse metabolic and cardiovascular outcomes, increasingly concerning among them is obesity hypertension. Obesity is one of the strongest predictors of hypertension, but how obesity increases blood pressure is currently unknown. Obesity affects the function of kidney, liver, adipose tissues, heart, brain, and blood vessels, and a clearly defined mechanism would aid in the development of better antihypertensive medications for obese subjects. However, the pathophysiology of obesity hypertension is very complex and is mediated by various interconnected organ systems. Impaired renal pressure—natriuresis, autonomic dysfunction, leptin, and vascular dysfunction are implicated in the development of obesity hypertension [1]. Neurohumoral mechanisms via stimulation of the renal-angiotensin system, leptin activity, sympathetic overdrive, and proinflammatory processes that potentiate vascular remodeling result in a higher incidence of the progression of many known cardiovascular complications. Endothelial dysfunction in obesity occurs from inflammation, oxidative and mechanical stress. These mechanisms perpetuate vascular stiffening and atherosclerosis. Leptin may also cause endothelial dysfunction by oxidatively damaging endogenous nitric oxide synthase [1]. In addition, emerging evidence suggests that changes in the gut bacterial microbiome, associated with genetic and dietary factors, can lead to metabolic disorders that result in obesity, insulin resistance, type 2 diabetes mellitus, and hypertension.

Imaging may play an important role to assess several contributing factors to the occurrence of hypertension in obesity, notably by imaging the various fat deposits throughout the body and by imaging the various organ manifestations and cardiovascular interactions. Retroperitoneal and visceral adiposity are better predictors of increased blood pressure than subcutaneous fat deposits in obesity hypertension emphasizing the potential role of assessing various deep lying fat depots as early markers of disease. Visceral adiposity, in fact, plays a central role in blood pressure increase, through a greater release of free fatty acids in the systemic circulation and a consequent increase in insulin resistance and hyperinsulinemia. These changes are firmly related to augmented arterial stiffness and a decrease in vasodilation (Fig. 16.1). Perivascular adipose tissue represents adipose tissue that surrounds blood vessels. Its main function is to provide mechanical support to vessels and regulate vascular homeostasis. Obesity leads to a dysfunction of perivascular fat which releases elevated levels of proinflammatory factors adipokines such as leptin, cytokines, and chemokines directly to the vascular wall, contributing to

Visceral and Ectopic Fat. https://doi.org/10.1016/B978-0-12-822186-0.00002-X

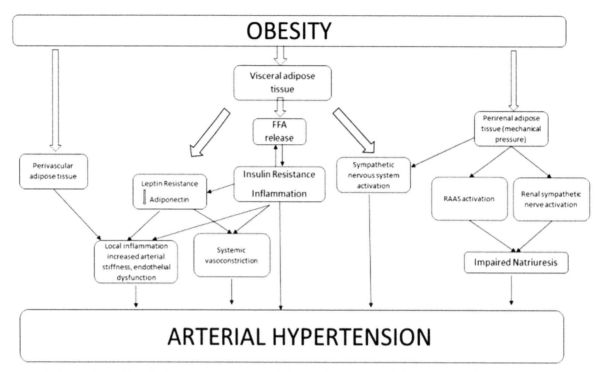

FIGURE 16.1 Mechanisms linking obesity to hypertension. Visceral adiposity plays a central role in blood pressure increase, through a greater release of free fatty acids in the systemic circulation and a consequent increase in insulin resistance and hyperinsulinemia. These changes are related to augmented arterial stiffness and a decrease in vasodilation. Perivascular adipose tissue provides mechanical support to vessels and regulates vascular homeostasis. Obesity can lead to a dysfunction of perivascular fat, which releases elevated levels of proinflammatory factors adipokines such as leptin, cytokines, and chemokines directly to the vascular wall, contributing to endothelial dysfunction and inflammation. Mechanical compression of the kidneys by fat in and around the kidneys can impair renal pressure natriuresis as a key component contributing to the occurrence of hypertension. *Adapted from Fantin et al. (2019).*

endothelial dysfunction and inflammation (Fig. 16.1). Mechanical compression of the kidneys by fat in and around the kidneys may impair renal-pressure natriuresis as a key component contributing to the occurrence of hypertension (Fig. 16.1).

Modern imaging technology such as magnetic resonance imaging (MRI) and computed tomography (CT) can visualize and quantify these various fat depots which may play a role in causing obesity hypertension and may help to understand their biological contribution to cardiometabolic disease (Figs. 16.2–16.4). In this chapter specifically the potential role of MRI applications is reviewed that may help to understand the contribution of fat depots and hemodynamic interaction between the heart and vascular system in causing obesity hypertension.

Fat deposits in obesity hypertension

In men with essential hypertension, fat is selectively accumulated in the visceral abdominal and intrathoracic region. This visceral adiposity appears to be an inherent feature of the hypertensive phenotype because it was found in newly diagnosed, untreated cases. It is quantitatively related to both height of blood pressure and degree of insulin resistance [2]. A study from India showed that body visceral fat percentage was significantly associated with hypertension, dyslipidemia, and type 2 diabetes among a local indigenous ethnic population [3]. A cross-sectional epidemiological study in African American and Hispanic American families suggests that visceral fat, independent of total body adiposity, is associated with prevalent hypertension [4]. These results are consistent with previous studies, and suggest that visceral fat may be particularly associated with hypertension among women. The results also suggest that behaviors that reduce visceral fat, such as regular physical activity and healthy dietary patterns, will have a beneficial effect upon blood pressure. Fig. 16.2 illustrates possible pathophysiological mechanisms assessable by MRI, related to various fat depots in obesity that may lead to cardiovascular atherosclerosis and vascular stiffening, contributing to the occurrence of obesity hypertension. The stiffness and distensibility of the arterial system are commonly used markers of atherosclerosis. Besides atherogenic dyslipidemia, most of the other factors that define metabolic syndrome (directly or indirectly) influence vascular wall properties, leading to increased arterial wall stiffness. In hypertension, vascular tone is increased, and hypertension leads to

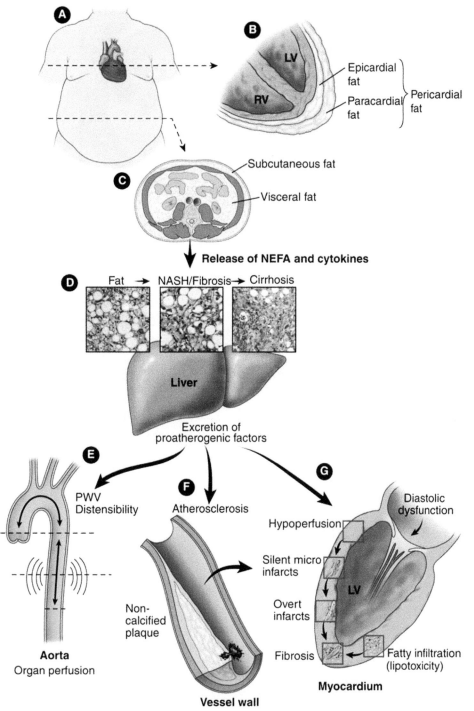

FIGURE 16.2 Schematic of possible mechanisms for cardiovascular disease in obesity assessed by MRI. (A) Imaging of heart and abdomen (dashed lines) in an obese person. (B) Adipose tissue expands and accumulates around heart and coronary vessels. Pericardial fat can be divided into epicardial and paracardial layers. Epicardial fat is a source of several inflammatory mediators and may be a cause of cardiac dysfunction and coronary artery disease. (C) Distribution of visceral and subcutaneous fat depots in obesity. Increased lipolysis in the excessive amount of visceral fat leads to increased amounts of nonesterified fatty acid (NEFA) and inflammatory cytokines in blood pool. Excessive NEFAs are taken up by nonadipose organs such as, (D), liver and, (G), heart. When uptake exceeds oxidative capacities, steatosis occurs. Liver is both target (mediated by NEFAs and cytokines) and amplifier of proatherogenic factors. (D) In liver, uncomplicated steatosis may develop into nonalcoholic steatohepatitis (NASH) and fibrosis and eventually result in cirrhosis, which predisposes to hepatocellular carcinoma. Fatty liver excretes increased amounts of proatherogenic factors that may contribute to, (E–G), development of cardiovascular disease. (F), Atherosclerotic coronary plaques develop that may result in plaque rupture and occlusion of the artery leading to ischemic heart disease. (G), Myocardial hypoperfusion, silent microinfarcts, overt myocardial infarction, myocardial fibrosis, and cardiac lipotoxicity are putative mechanisms of LV diastolic dysfunction and heart failure. Atherosclerosis causes endothelial dysfunction and vascular stiffening, which can be assessed with pulse-wave velocity (PWV) and distensibility measurements in aorta and other vascular beds (E). Aortic stiffening is an independent predictor of cardiovascular disease and plays a central role in organ perfusion, leading to hypoperfusion of heart and other organs. *Adapted from van der Meer RW, Lamb, HJ, Smit JWA, de Roos A. MR imaging evaluation of cardiovascular risk in metabolic syndrome. Radiology 2012;264(1):21–37. https://doi.org/10.1148/radiol.12110772.*

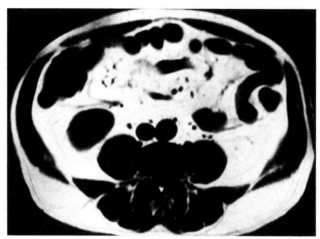

FIGURE 16.3 MRI of visceral and subcutaneous fat. A transverse section at the level of the L5 vertebra is acquired with fat-selective imaging. (A) Fat signal is of high intensity, all other tissue is nulled. (B) By using dedicated software, visceral (red) and subcutaneous (green) fat compartments can be differentiated easily. *Adapted from van der Meer RW, Lamb, HJ, Smit JWA, de Roos A. MR imaging evaluation of cardiovascular risk in metabolic syndrome. Radiology 2012;264(1):21—37. https://doi.org/10.1148/radiol.12110772.*

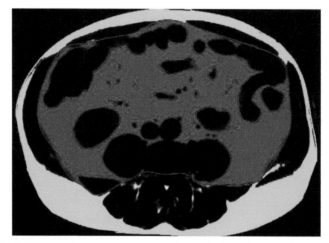

FIGURE 16.4 MRI of visceral and subcutaneous fat. A transverse section at the level of the L5 vertebra is acquired with fat-selective imaging. (A) Fat signal is of high intensity, all other tissue is nulled. (B) By using dedicated software, visceral (red) and subcutaneous (green) fat compartments can be differentiated easily. *Adapted from van der Meer RW, Lamb, HJ, Smit JWA, de Roos A. MR imaging evaluation of cardiovascular risk in metabolic syndrome. Radiology 2012;264(1):21—37. https://doi.org/10.1148/radiol.12110772.*

arterial wall thickening to restore wall stress to normal levels. Impaired glucose tolerance enhances nonenzymatic glycation of proteins with covalent cross-linking of collagen (advanced glycation end products), thereby altering the mechanical properties of interstitial tissue of the arterial wall [5].

An example of MRI assessment of subcutaneous and visceral fat is shown in Figs. 16.3 and 16.4. There is growing interest in CT-based opportunistic screening, whereby these additional imaging data can be used for assessment of abdominal fat distribution and prediction of future adverse clinical events [6] as illustrated in Fig. 16.5.

Cardiovascular structure and function in obesity hypertension

The relationship between hypertension and obesity is multifaceted, including vascular changes assessable by imaging such as MRI. Alterations in the vasculature including structural changes, endothelial dysfunction, enhanced contractile response, and altered stiffness are hallmarks of obesity. These vascular abnormalities are thought to contribute and even predict the development of hypertension and other cardiovascular complications. Consistent with the notion that in obesity vascular alterations precede hypertension, experimental research demonstrated that diet-induced obese mice develop arterial

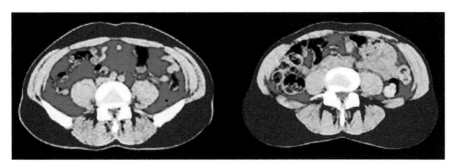

FIGURE 16.5 CT assessment of abdominal fat. Abdominal computed tomography images at the level of the fifth lumbar vertebra, 8.0 mm slice thickness. Area in red represents visceral fat and the blue areas represent subcutaneous fat. Left panel: 49-year-old male, BMI of 26, the visceral fat area measured 119.6 cm^2 and the subcutaneous fat area 156.8 cm^2. Right panel: 50-year-old female, BMI of 20.1, the visceral fat area measured 39.6 cm^2 and the subcutaneous fat area 150.2 cm^2. These findings illustrate the difference between so-called apple- and pear-shaped body habitus, respectively. This difference can be quantified by using the visceral-to-subcutaneous fat ratio. Increased visceral-to-subcutaneous fat ratio for the individual on the left portends a higher cardiovascular risk. *Adapted from Sala et al. (2015).*

stiffness and endothelial dysfunction before the onset of hypertension [7]. Endothelial dysfunction and arterial stiffness are thought to be the earliest manifestations of vascular dysfunction in obesity and precede the development of pre-hypertension and hypertension. Increased arterial stiffness is seen in patients who are normotensive but have obesity and who are predisposed to develop hypertension; moreover, incident hypertension is more robustly predicted in patients who are in the highest quartile of arterial stiffness. Changes in the extracellular matrix and vascular smooth muscle dysfunction contribute to arterial stiffness; however, accumulating evidence suggests that endothelial dysfunction also contributes to vascular stiffness, which is in turn strongly associated with insulin resistance [7].

Obesity is associated with hemodynamic overload. The increased metabolic demand imposed by the expanded adipose tissue and augmented fat-free mass in obesity results in a hyperdynamic circulation with increased blood volume. In addition to the increased preload, left ventricular afterload is also elevated in obese individuals due to both increased peripheral resistance and greater conduit artery stiffness. Cardiac output is often higher in obesity, due to an augmented stroke volume and an increase in heart rate. Ventricular systolic function as assessed by ejection fraction is usually normal in obesity [8]. Recent studies suggest that high left ventricle ejection force is responsible for hypertension. High ejection force in stage 1 hypertension is due to high acceleration (i.e., aortic flow values), high peak systolic velocity and short acceleration time associated with increased basal sympathetic activity. Highest ejection force in stage 2 hypertension is due to high acceleration, i.e., high stroke volume delivered during acceleration phase associated with normal baseline sympathetic activity. The possible mechanism of hypertension is supposed to start from increase in baseline sympathetic activity. This results in increased left ventricular ejection force, without significantly changing stroke volume, and this increased ejection force leads to stage 1 hypertension. Accordingly, it has been suggested that hypertension is caused by increased cardiac output and/or increased peripheral resistance. Blood pressure is defined as the product of cardiac output and peripheral resistance. Hypertension is, therefore, said to be caused by increased cardiac output and/or increased peripheral resistance. Cardiac output is determined by stroke volume and heart rate; stroke volume is related to myocardial contractility and to the size of the vascular compartment. Peripheral resistance is determined by functional and anatomic changes in small arteries and arterioles [9].

Applanation tonometry has revealed that pulsatile components of blood pressure may be more relevant for prognosis than traditional estimates of mean arterial blood pressure, which is a common target for antihypertensive therapy. The Framingham Heart Study has shown that higher forward pressure wave amplitude, as a measure of proximal aortic geometry and stiffness, is associated with increased risk for incident cardiovascular disease, whereas mean arterial pressure and relative wave reflection, as measured by applanation tonometry, were not related to events. It is important to note that these observations may be relevant to understand the potential adverse effect of vasodilatation in antihypertensive therapy, by which increased cardiac output and peak flow may inadvertently increase forward pressure wave amplitude and also increase penetration of excessive pressure and flow pulsatility into the microcirculation. Furthermore, recently it was shown that in healthy and relatively young adults, increased arterial stiffness assessed by applanation tonometry is superior to blood pressure in predicting cognitive decline in all domains, underscoring the relevance of arterial stiffness as a potential target for therapy [9].

Hemodynamic interaction between the heart and proximal aorta are also implicated in causing obesity hypertension. The proximal aorta acts as a buffer and cushion for left ventricular systolic load, by which ventricular-aortic coupling between the left ventricle and the elastic proximal aorta is modulated. Aortic stiffness in combination with stroke volume and ejection velocity is a determinant of arterial pressure wave amplitude, influencing systolic and diastolic blood pressure and pulse pressure. Left ventricular ejection pattern, aortic wall stiffness, and aortic lumen diameter are interrelated and interact, resulting in altered hemodynamics and hypertension. For example, systolic blood pressure could be normal in the presence of a stiffened aortic wall if mean arterial pressure is normal or left ventricular peak ejection rate and aortic lumen area are optimized to maintain a low pulse pressure. Conversely, higher mean arterial pressure may increase aortic stiffness in the presence of mid-life hypertension because of the effects of distending pressure alone without necessary intrinsic aortic wall abnormalities. A mismatch between increasing stroke volume and relative small aortic diameter enhances aortic stiffness, thereby increasing pulse pressure, which will result in systolic hypertension [10].

MRI is well suited to assess the interaction and hemodynamics between the heart and proximal aorta (Fig. 16.6). Cardiac MRI, which provides accurate and highly reproducible measurement of left ventricular mass, volumes, and systolic function, is not limited by acoustic windows as is echocardiography; it does not rely on geometric assumptions about the shape of the ventricle, and does not require exposure to ionizing radiation. Thus, MRI is an appropriate noninvasive imaging technology for investigating alterations in heart function. Furthermore, MRI also allows unhampered imaging of aortic size, function, and flow in conjunction with heart evaluation. The hemodynamic coupling between the function of the left ventricle and proximal aorta as assessed by MRI may provide a number of key parameters that contribute to the development of obesity hypertension, including left ventricular end-systolic volume, end-diastolic volume, stroke volume, cardiac output, ejection fraction, and (indexed) left ventricular mass and hypertrophy. MRI also provides a number of key components of proximal aortic anatomy and function that may be implicated in obesity hypertension, including aortic size, wall thickness/plaques, aortic root motion (i.e., circumferential strain, longitudinal strain), distensibility, aortic flow quantification (stroke volume, cardiac output, flow velocity, flow volume), and regional pulse wave velocity as a marker of vascular stiffness.

Many obese subjects with heart failure have nonischemic dilated cardiomyopathy. Additionally, isolated diastolic dysfunction is common in obese subjects, and systolic dysfunction is typically a late finding, or not seen at all. An elevated circulating blood volume in obese subjects leads to larger stroke volumes and subsequent left ventricular dilatation. To compensate for the higher wall stress, eccentric hypertrophy develops. This hypertrophy may cause impaired diastolic relaxation and diastolic heart failure, or combined systolic and diastolic failure if the hypertrophy cannot match the output demands [10]. Numerous epidemiological investigations have illustrated the relationship between hypertension and obesity and increased risk for incident heart failure. The effect of hypertension may be attenuated by antihypertensive medication, consistent with SPRINT (Systolic Blood Pressure Intervention Trial), a randomized controlled trial that showed aggressive blood pressure treatment substantially reduced heart failure risks in patients with hypertension. Prevention of hypertension, obesity, and diabetes by ages 45 and 55 years may substantially prolong heart failure-free survival, decrease heart failure-related morbidity, and reduce the public health impact of heart failure [11].

Coronary artery disease in obesity

Individuals with obesity are at increased risk for coronary artery disease (CAD). It has been shown that excess adiposity, visceral adipose tissue in particular, accelerates progression of atherosclerosis many years before the clinical manifestation of CAD [12]. Longer duration of overall and abdominal adiposity has been associated with coronary artery calcification, a marker of subclinical coronary artery assessed by CT, and its progression, independent of the degree of adiposity [13]. Autopsy studies have shown that vulnerable coronary artery lesions were frequently present in association with abdominal obesity [12]. These findings were independent of other cardiovascular risk factors, indicating the importance of abdominal adiposity in the pathogenesis of atherosclerotic disease.

Epicardial adipose tissue (EAT), which is of similar embryological origin as abdominal mesenteric and omental visceral fat, also relates to CAD. By using CT, epicardial adipose tissue is visualized as a tissue with attenuation ranging from -190 to -30 Hounsfield Units (HU). Within this attenuation range, fat voxels inside the visceral pericardium are classified as epicardial fat [14]. In the multiethnic study of atherosclerosis, epicardial fat accumulation assessed by CT was associated with coronary events and atherosclerosis burden in the general population, independently of other cardiovascular risk factors [15]. In addition, excess epicardial fat deposition has been related to coronary plaque vulnerability and severity of CAD [16]. Focal obstructive coronary lesions occur in these segments that are immediately adjacent to areas of epicardial fat with the greatest thickness [17]. The mechanisms linking obesity to CAD are complex. Altered lipid-lipoprotein metabolism leads to increased plasma total cholesterol and LDL levels, as well as decreased HDL levels, which may accelerate the development of atherosclerosis and CAD [14]. In addition, CAD development in obesity, especially in visceral adiposity including EAT, appears to be mediated by the production of various cytokines causing chronic low-

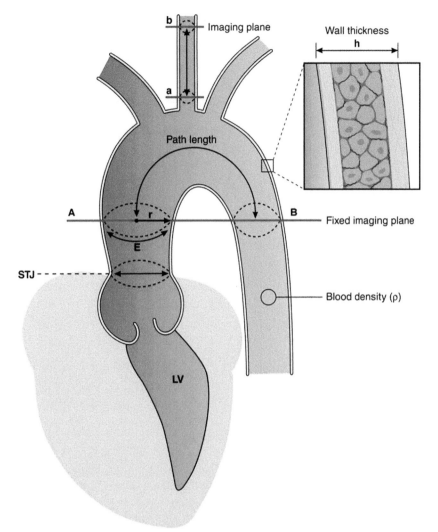

FIGURE 16.6 Proposed mechanism of interaction between left ventricular and proximal aortic function in obesity hypertension. Distensibility and pulse wave velocity (PWV) in proximal aorta and carotid vessels estimated by magnetic resonance imaging. The luminal area change or diameter change of the aorta at the sinotubular junction (STJ) determines local distensibility according to the formula: distensibility = (Amax − Amin)/(Amin × PP) (in mmHg−1), where PP is central pulse pressure and Amax and Amin the maximal and minimal cross-sectional area, respectively. A fixed magnetic resonance imaging plane at the level of the ascending aorta (A) and transecting also the proximal descending aorta (B) is used to estimate aortic arch PWV. The path length Δx (in meters) between levels A and B is divided by the difference in arrival time Δt (in seconds) between flow curves measured by velocity-encoded magnetic resonance imaging at levels A and B simultaneously to calculate PWV (expressed in meters/second). Vascular PWV is determined by: E (circumferential Young's modulus, representing material rigidity), h (vessel wall thickness), r (luminal aortic radius), and rho ρ (blood density). The relation among these parameters is represented in the Moens−Korteweg equation according to the formula: PWV = √(E × h/2r × ρ). PWV and distensibility are inversely related to one another as defined by the Bramwell−Hill equation: PWV = √(1/(ρ × distensibility)). These factors interact with left ventricular (LV) function (e.g., increased cardiac output in obesity) resulting in a stiffer proximal aorta (PWV>) as a consequence of more collagen and less elastin in aortic wall (E>), increased wall thickness (h>), and change in aortic radius (>decreases PWV, <increases PWV). When aortic diameter is relatively small compared with LV function with increased aortic flow and cardiac output, aortic flow and increased aortic stiffness cause increased forward pressure wave amplitude, resulting in increased pulse pressure and systolic hypertension. Similarly to aortic arch stiffness, carotid artery stiffness can be estimated from two imaging levels (a and b) using velocity-encoded magnetic resonance imaging to measure the path length between a and b as well as the difference in arrival time between flow curves. *Adapted from de Roos A, van der Grond J, Mitchell G, Westenberg J. Magnetic resonance imaging of cardiovascular function and the brain: is dementia a cardiovascular-driven disease? Circulation 2017;135(22):2178−2195. https://doi.org/ 10.1161/CIRCULATIONAHA.116.021978.*

grade inflammation [16]. Normal EAT contributes to maintaining vascular homeostasis through production of antiinflammatory substances. In the presence of excess energy supply, insulin resistance, and diabetes, the EAT becomes hypertrophic and dysfunctional (Fig. 16.7). Adipose tissue−derived adipocytokines, inflammation and systemic mediators including reactive oxygen species favor development of a local proatherogenic environment [14].

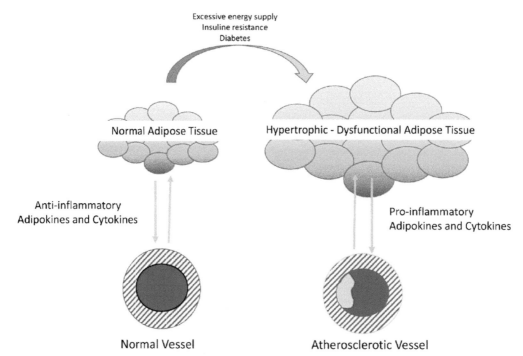

FIGURE 16.7 Relation between EAT and atherosclerosis. Normal EAT/PCAT contributes to maintaining vascular homeostasis through the production of substances with an antiinflammatory effect. In the presence of stressful conditions, the EAT may become hypertrophic and dysfunctional, releasing detrimental adipokines related to atherosclerosis formation and progression. *EAT*, epicardial adipose tissue; *PCAT*, pericoronary adipose tissue. *Adapted from Guglielmo M, Lin A, Dey D, Baggiano A, Fusini L, Muscogiuri G, Pontone G. Epicardial fat and coronary artery disease: role of cardiac imaging. Atherosclerosis 2021;321:30−38. https://doi.org/10.1016/j.atherosclerosis.2021.02.008.*

Pericoronary adipose tissue (PCAT), the portion of epicardial fat directly surrounding the coronary arteries, may have a local effect in atherosclerosis development due to its close anatomical location to the coronary artery wall. Inflammatory pathways have been suggested via local paracrine and vasocrine effects in relation to CAD development. Indeed, inflammation of PCAT has been shown in patients with advanced CAD undergoing elective surgery for coronary artery bypass grafting [18] where tissue sampling has been performed. In addition, by using 18F-FDG PET-CT, higher standardized uptake values were found in PCAT in patients with CAD compared to controls, indicating inflammation. On the other hand, while results from many studies indicate that inflammation of PCAT has detrimental effect on coronary arteries in terms of atherogenesis and CAD development, recently it has been suggested that changes in PCAT that can be detected by CT imaging may be a biomarker of coronary inflammation rather than a driver of vascular inflammation [17]. Inflamed coronary arteries release cytokines that prevent lipid accumulation in PCAT-derived preadipocytes. In the presence of inflammation, smaller preadipocytes with less intracellular lipid and higher aqueous content cause an increase in PCAT attenuation values [17] as assessed by CT imaging. These increased PCAT attenuation values (up to −30 HU), also referred to as fat attenuation index (FAI), are assessed by CT in a cylindrical layer of fat tissue within a radial distance from the outer coronary artery wall equal to the average diameter of the corresponding vessel (Fig. 16.8). It has been shown that FAI was higher in CAD patients as compared to individuals without CAD [17]. Furthermore, in patients with acute coronary syndrome, PCAT attenuation values were increased around culprit coronary lesions compared to nonculprit lesions and compared with high-grade coronary stenosis lesions in patients with stable CAD [17]. Moreover, increased FAI values have been found to predict all-cause and cardiac mortality, and provide incremental prognostic value over and above high-risk plaques (e.g., positive remodeling, low-attenuation plaque, spotty calcification or napkin-ring sign on coronary CT angiography) [17].

Radiomics has emerged as a promising clinical research application in cardiovascular imaging. It allows for extraction of more information than what can be obtained by visual image assessment alone. In short, quantitative image features based on texture, shape, or transformation (e.g., utilize spatial information to create new data from images) can produce a more specific phenotype than traditional first-order statistics (e.g., histogram-based distribution of Hounsfield units in a region of interest) [19]. One recent study used cardiac CT radiomics to evaluate patients with acute myocardial infarction [20]. They compared radiomics parameters of PCAT in patients with acute myocardial infarction and patients with stable or

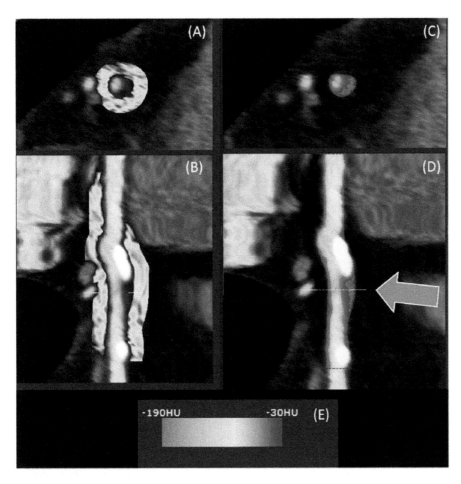

FIGURE 16.8 PCAT and plaque CT attenuation quantification in a lesion in the proximal LAD. (A) Cross-section and (B) straightened view illustrating PCAT assessment. (C) Cross-section and (D) straightened view with plaque attenuation assessment. There is a lipid core and positive remodeling (orange overlay, orange arrow). (E) Range of Hounsfield units (HU) to detect adipose tissue. *PCAT*, pericoronary adipose tissue; *LAD*, left anterior descending artery. *Adapted from Guglielmo M, Lin A, Dey D, Baggiano A, Fusini L, Muscogiuri G, Pontone G. Epicardial fat and coronary artery disease: role of cardiac imaging. Atherosclerosis 2021;321:30−38. https://doi.org/10.1016/j.atherosclerosis.2021.02.008.*

no CAD and found that texture- and geometry-based parameters were the most important radiomics parameters for distinguishing patients with or without myocardial infarction. This information was not provided by PCAT in this study. These results suggest that data from CT-based radiomics can detect biomarkers that may identify vulnerable patients.

In addition to changes in macrovasculature related to obesity (e.g., coronary atherosclerosis), obesity has been related to coronary microvascular dysfunction, assessed by stress positron emission computed tomography [21]. Microvascular dysfunction is defined as impaired coronary flow reserve in the absence of flow-limiting CAD [22]. Coronary microvascular dysfunction may be due to endothelial dysfunction and small vessel remodeling and provides prognostic information regarding cardiovascular risk in obesity. It has been shown that the severity of coronary microvascular dysfunction relates to the amount of abdominal visceral fat [23]. Importantly, surgical weight-loss procedures have shown improvement in coronary microvascular function after treatment [24].

Arrhythmias

Atrial fibrillation (AF) is the most common sustained cardiac arrhythmia and has a significant impact on heart failure progression and an increased risk of thromboembolism, resulting in increased mortality and morbidity [25]. Many studies have shown an increased prevalence of atrial fibrillation in obesity, which is multifactorial in cause, and might be attributable to increased prevalence of systemic hypertension, as well as to increased left atrial size and volume [26].

In addition to overall adiposity, the amount of epicardial fat as assessed by CT and MRI has been independently associated with the presence, severity (e.g., symptom burden, chronicity, and subtype), and recurrence of atrial fibrillation [14,27]. There is an increasing interest in the identification of epicardial fat around the left atrium, which shows a nonuniform spatial distribution [25]. Tsao et al. found that left atrial epicardial fat volume as assessed by CT was significantly increased in patients with AF compared to controls. Abundance of epicardial fat was independently related to AF recurrence after ablation [28]. Most periatrial fat was located adjacent to the anterior roof, left atrial appendage, and lateral mitral isthmus. These findings illustrate the importance of volumetric assessment using 3-dimensional imaging (e.g., in contrast to single-slice epicardial fat area or epicardial fat thickness [27] for accurate assessment of left atrial epicardial fat volume). While CT-imaging provides volumetric quantification of epicardial fat with high spatial resolution and high reproducibility, MRI can also be used to quantify fat around heart. This imaging modality is not limited by radiation exposure or need for an iodinated contrast agent. While conventional cine magnetic resonance images do not allow for reliable quantification of adipose tissue, fat—water separation sequences such as Dixon technique can be used for this purpose (Fig. 16.9). By using 3-dimensional Dixon MRI, Nakamori et al. showed that left atrium epicardial fat volume is significantly increased in atrial fibrillation patients [25]. They also found that the integration of LA-epicardial fat and LA volume provides greater discriminatory performance for identifying atrial fibrillation patients than LA volume alone.

It has been suggested that proinflammatory and profibrotic cytokines may diffuse from epicardial fat into the adjacent myocardium and promote fibrosis and an arrhythmogenic substrate leading to increased risk for atrial fibrillation [26]. Furthermore, increased sympathetic or parasympathetic tone related to dense innervation of fat depots may play a role in AF development [26]. MRI can be used for combined assessment of atrial and ventricular volumes, myocardial (e.g., ventricular) fibrosis, and myocardial perfusion, all of which may provide additional insights into AF pathogenesis.

Increasing evidence support a close relation between epicardial fat and inflammation [29]. By using CT imaging, density of epicardial fat can be measured, where higher density reflects the presence of inflammation [30]. By using this measure, it has been shown that increased epicardial fat density was significantly associated with the presence of atrial fibrillation after adjusting for other risk factors [30]. Inflammatory activity of epicardial fat in patients with atrial fibrillation has also been shown by using 18-fluorodeoxyglucose positron emission tomography [31], where increased maximal standardized uptake values indicating inflammation have been found in atrial fibrillation patients compared to controls.

Heart failure

Many studies have shown that body composition plays an important role in the development of heart failure. Obesity has a negative impact on many of the established cardiovascular risk factors. Indeed, obesity-related metabolic, inflammatory, and hormonal changes lead to an increased risk for CAD and hypertension, which in turn are major risk factors for development of heart failure. In addition, the relationship between obesity and heart failure has been shown to involve adverse hemodynamic and anatomic changes including left ventricular hypertrophy (especially in the presence of hypertension) and diastolic dysfunction [14].

Obese individuals have increased blood volume to meet the increased metabolic demand of the extra body weight related to a greater perfusion of adipose tissue and an increase in lean body weight. This requires increased cardiac output via increasing stroke volume, which results in a greater cardiac workload. These hemodynamic changes are associated with increased left ventricular size, wall stress, and left ventricular hypertrophy, which predispose to development of left

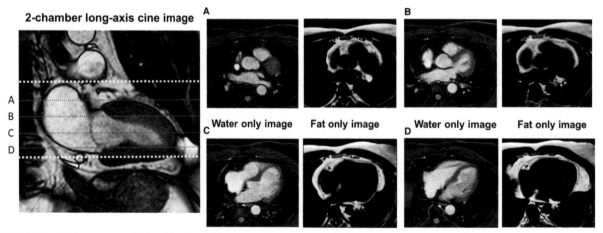

FIGURE 16.9 MRI assessment of left atrial epicardial fat volume. Dixon image analysis for assessment of left atrial epicardial fat volume (LA epicardial fat) at high level (A), high-middle level (B), low-middle level (C), and low level (D) in the LA. The dotted yellow lines indicate the caudal and cranial limits for the measurement of LA-epicardial fat and the arrows point at the counter of the pericardial outline. A region of interest was placed on high signal intensity area inside pericardial outline around LA (C) for each image. Total LA-epicardial fat was calculated as the sum of epicardial fat multiplied by the slice thickness of 5 mm. *Adapted from Nakamori S, Nezafat M, Ngo LH, Manning WJ, Nezafat R. Left atrial epicardial fat volume is associated with atrial fibrillation: a prospective cardiovascular magnetic resonance 3D dixon study J Am Heart Assoc 2018;7(6). https://doi.org/10.1161/JAHA.117.008232.*

ventricular failure [32]. In addition, in the presence of left ventricular failure, pulmonary venous pressure increases which leads to right ventricular hypertrophy and subsequent pulmonary hypertension. Furthermore, obstructive sleep apnea is frequently present in obesity, which results in hypoxia and acidosis, further increasing the aforementioned changes.

Alterations in cardiac energy metabolism may also contribute to heart failure pathophysiology. Advanced imaging modalities enable in vivo assessment of myocardial energetics. Proton magnetic resonance spectroscopy (^{1}H-MRS) can be used to quantify myocardial steatosis (Fig. 16.10) [33]. Increased myocardial storage of triglycerides reflects abundance of toxic lipids that may impair cardiomyocyte integrity and function. It has been shown that myocardial steatosis is an independent predictor of diastolic dysfunction in obesity. Importantly, these changes are reversible. In addition to excess myocardial fat content, impaired myocardial energetics has also been shown to be an important contributor to impaired cardiac function in obesity. The human heart requires large amounts of adenosine triphosphate (ATP) as a primary carrier of chemical energy. By using phosphorus magnetic resonance spectroscopy (^{31}P-MRS), the phosphocreatine (PCr)/ATP ratio can be quantified (Fig. 16.11) [33], which has been used as an indicator of cardiac energy reserve and metabolic efficiency. A decreased ratio is associated with diastolic and systolic dysfunction, and predicts mortality. In heart failure patients, PCr/ATP ratio relates to left ventricular systolic function and has greater prognostic value than left ventricular ejection fraction [34]. A significant decrease in PCr/ATP ratio was found with increasing BMI, indicating impaired myocardial energetics in obesity. In addition, visceral fat was found to be associated with decreased PCr/ATP ratio in obese diabetic men without other cardiovascular risk factors [14].

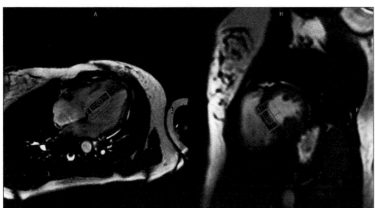

FIGURE 16.10 Proton magnetic resonance spectroscopy to quantify myocardial steatosis. 1H-MRS is subject to motion artifacts owing to contraction and breathing. To overcome these issues, cardiac 1H-MRS is usually performed with electrocardiographic gating and either breath-holding or free breathing with respiratory motion triggering/compensation. To prevent contamination of pericardial fat, the voxel of interest (VOI) is placed in the interventricular septum (upper panel). The water-suppressed spectrum displayed in the lower panel shows signals from creatine (Cr), triglycerides (TG), and trimethyl ammonium (TMA). *Adapted from Bizino MB, Sala ML, de Heer P, van der Tol P, Smit JWA, Webb AG, de Roos A, Lamb HJ. MR of multi-organ involvement in the metabolic syndrome. Magn Reson Imag Clin N Am 2015;23(1):41–58. https://doi.org/10.1016/j.mric.2014.09.010.*

FIGURE 16.11 Phosphorus magnetic resonance spectroscopy (31P-MRS) to assess high-energy phosphates. Imaging is performed by positioning a volume of interest (square box) over almost the entire heart (A, B); eliminating signal contamination from skeletal muscle is essential. The PCr/ATP ratio, which has been used as an indicator of cardiac energy reserve and metabolic efficiency, can be calculated from the spectrum (C). *ATP*, adenosine triphosphate; *2,3 DPG*, 2,3-diphosphoglycerate; *PCr*, phosphocreatine; *PDE*, phosphodiesters; *ppm*, parts per million. *Adapted from Bizino MB, Sala ML, de Heer P, van der Tol P, Smit JWA, Webb AG, de Roos A, Lamb HJ. MR of multi-organ involvement in the metabolic syndrome. Magn Reson Imag Clin N Am 2015;23(1):41−58. https://doi.org/10.1016/j.mric.2014.09.010.*

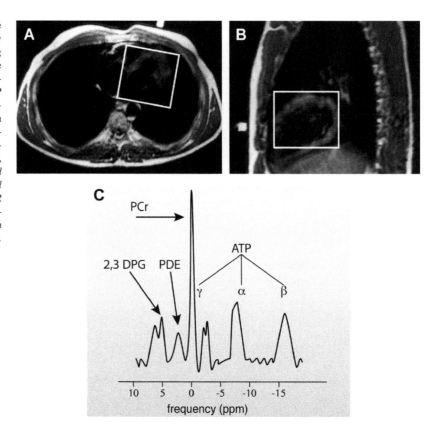

Abnormal fat accumulation in specific body compartments may lead to cardiac changes that relate to development of heart failure. Previous CT studies have shown that visceral fat is of particular importance regarding the risk of heart failure, especially heart failure with preserved ejection fraction, and subsequent prognosis in patients with heart failure. Many individuals with obesity develop heart failure with preserved ejection fraction. These cases can be challenging to diagnose in clinical practice because the left ventricular ejection fraction (a conventional clinical parameter for systolic function) is normal [14]. Previous studies have shown that by using MRI, imaging evidence of subclinical myocardial dysfunction as indicated by abnormal myocardial strain is present in up to 54% of obese individuals [14]. One recent study investigated the effect of increased epicardial fat volume on left ventricular myocardial fat content and burden of interstitial myocardial fibrosis, and their subsequent effects on myocardial contractile function [35]. Myocardial fat content was assessed by ^{1}H-MRS and MOLLI T1 mapping was used to quantify left ventricular extracellular volume, which is a measure of interstitial fibrosis. It was found that increased EAT volume was independently associated with increased myocardial fat content and burden of interstitial myocardial fibrosis. In addition, increased EAT volume was independently associated with reduced myocardial contractile function as indicated by left ventricular global longitudinal strain imaging. These findings indicate that the observed myocardial dysfunction in obesity may be secondary to functional (e.g., direct vasocrine and paracrine effects of adipokines secreted by EAT) and structural myocardial changes (myocardial fibrosis due to inflammation) mediated by increased EAT volume. Regarding these structural myocardial changes in obesity, while increased intracellular myocardial triglyceride is likely inert, increased shunting of free fatty acid into nonoxidative pathway can lead to accumulation of toxic fatty acid intermediates that disrupt normal cellular signaling pathways and can lead to cellular apoptosis and myocardial replacement fibrosis [35].

It has been shown that bariatric surgery prevents development of heart failure and improves heart failure symptoms including heart failure with preserved ejection fraction. Identification of individuals with high-risk obesities and subclinical cardiac changes related to heart failure is of importance as early treatment may prevent progression of heart failure and improve clinical outcome.

Conclusion

Cardiovascular risk may vary between individuals with similar measures of overall adiposity. This seems to be explained by the presence of high-risk obesities and dysfunctional adipose tissue. The majority of the association between adiposity and cardiovascular disease may be explained by altered cardiometabolic risk factors and comorbidities. High-risk obesities are the main drivers of altered cardiometabolic risk mediators including type 2 diabetes, increased blood pressure, abnormal lipid metabolism, inflammation, and endothelial dysfunction. Cardiovascular disease outcomes include hypertension, coronary artery disease, arrhythmias, and heart failure. Different imaging techniques including computed tomography and magnetic resonance imaging can be used to assess imaging markers related to these disease outcomes.

Individuals with similar measures of overall adiposity such as body mass index may have distinct metabolic cardiovascular risk profiles. This may be explained by individual differences in regional body fat distribution (e.g., high-risk obesities) and the ability of subcutaneous adipose tissue to expand (e.g., dysfunctional adipose tissue). The majority of the association between adiposity and cardiovascular disease appears to be explained by altered cardiometabolic risk factors and comorbidities. High-risk obesities are the main drivers of altered cardiometabolic risk mediators including type 2 diabetes, increased blood pressure, abnormal lipid metabolism, inflammation, and endothelial dysfunction. In this chapter we will discuss the association between obesity and cardiovascular disease outcomes including obesity, hypertension, coronary artery disease, arrhythmias, and heart failure. Specifically, different imaging techniques including computed tomography and magnetic resonance imaging are reviewed in relation to obesity and cardiovascular disease.

References

[1] Mendoza MF, Kachur SM, Lavie CJ. Hypertension in obesity. Curr Opin Cardiol 2020;35(4):389−96. https://doi.org/10.1097/HCO.0000000000000749.

[2] Sironi AM, Gastaldelli A, Mari A, Ciociaro D, Positano V, Postano V, Buzzigoli E, Ghione S, Turchi S, Lombardi M, Ferrannini E. Visceral fat in hypertension: influence on insulin resistance and beta-cell function. Hypertension 2004;44(2):127−33.

[3] Goswami B, Reang T, Sarkar S, Sengupta S, Bhattacharjee B. Role of body visceral fat in hypertension and dyslipidemia among the diabetic and nondiabetic ethnic population of Tripura-A comparative study. J Fam Med Prim Care 2020;9(6):2885−90. https://doi.org/10.4103/jfmpc.jfmpc_187_20.

[4] Foy CG, Hsu F-C, Haffner SM, Norris JM, Rotter JI, Henkin LF, Bryer-Ash M, Chen Y-DI, Wagenknecht LE. Visceral fat and prevalence of hypertension among African Americans and Hispanic Americans: findings from the IRAS family study. Am J Hypertens 2008;21(8):910−6. https://doi.org/10.1038/ajh.2008.213.

[5] van der Meer RW, Lamb HJ, Smit JWA, de Roos A. MR imaging evaluation of cardiovascular risk in metabolic syndrome. Radiology 2012;264(1):21−37. https://doi.org/10.1148/radiol.12110772.

[6] Pickhardt PJ, Graffy PM, Perez AA, Lubner MG, Elton DC, Summers RM. Opportunistic screening at abdominal CT: use of automated body composition biomarkers for added cardiometabolic value. Radiograph: Rev Publicat Radiol Soci North Am 2021;41(2):524−42. https://doi.org/10.1148/rg.2021200056.

[7] Rahmouni K. Obesity-associated hypertension: recent progress in deciphering the pathogenesis. Hypertension 2014;64(2):215−21. https://doi.org/10.1161/HYPERTENSIONAHA.114.00920.

[8] Vasan RS. Cardiac function and obesity. Heart 2003;89(10):1127−9.

[9] Saxena T, Ali AO, Saxena M. Pathophysiology of essential hypertension: an update. Expet Rev Cardiovasc Ther 2018;16(12):879−87. https://doi.org/10.1080/14779072.2018.1540301.

[10] de Roos A, van der Grond J, Mitchell G, Westenberg J. Magnetic resonance imaging of cardiovascular function and the brain: is dementia a cardiovascular-driven disease? Circulation 2017;135(22):2178−95. https://doi.org/10.1161/CIRCULATIONAHA.116.021978.

[11] Sack MN. Obesity and cardiac function - the role of caloric excess and its reversal. Drug discovery today. Dis Mech 2013;10(1−2):e41−6.

[12] McGill HC, McMahan CA, Malcom GT, Oalmann MC, Strong JP. Relation of glycohemoglobin and adiposity to atherosclerosis in youth. Pathobiological determinants of atherosclerosis in youth (PDAY) research group. Arterioscler Thromb Vasc Biol 1995;15(4):431−40.

[13] Reis JP, Loria CM, Lewis CE, Powell-Wiley TM, Wei GS, Carr JJ, Terry JG, Liu K. Association between duration of overall and abdominal obesity beginning in young adulthood and coronary artery calcification in middle age. JAMA 2013;310(3):280−8. https://doi.org/10.1001/jama.2013.7833.

[14] Piché M-E, Tchernof A, Després J-P. Obesity phenotypes, diabetes, and cardiovascular diseases. Circ Res 2020;126(11):1477−500. https://doi.org/10.1161/CIRCRESAHA.120.316101.

[15] Shah RV, Anderson A, Ding J, Budoff M, Rider O, Petersen SE, Jensen MK, Koch M, Allison M, Kawel-Boehm N, Wisocky J, Jerosch-Herold M, Mukamal K, Lima JAC, Murthy VL. Pericardial, but not hepatic, fat by CT is associated with CV outcomes and structure: the multi-ethnic study of atherosclerosis. JACC. Cardiovasc Imag 2017;10(9):1016−27. https://doi.org/10.1016/j.jcmg.2016.10.024.

[16] Packer M. Epicardial adipose tissue may mediate deleterious effects of obesity and inflammation on the myocardium. J Am Coll Cardiol 2018;71(20):2360−72. https://doi.org/10.1016/j.jacc.2018.03.509.

[17] Guglielmo M, Lin A, Dey D, Baggiano A, Fusini L, Muscogiuri G, Pontone G. Epicardial fat and coronary artery disease: role of cardiac imaging. Atherosclerosis 2021;321:30−8. https://doi.org/10.1016/j.atherosclerosis.2021.02.008.

[18] Mazurek T, Zhang L, Zalewski A, Mannion JD, Diehl JT, Arafat H, Sarov-Blat L, O'Brien S, Keiper EA, Johnson AG, Martin J, Goldstein BJ, Shi Y. Human epicardial adipose tissue is a source of inflammatory mediators. Circulation 2003;108(20):2460−6.

[19] Xu P, Xue Y, Schoepf UJ, Varga-Szemes A, Griffith J, Yacoub B, Zhou F, Zhou C, Yang Y, Xing W, Zhang L. Radiomics: the next frontier of cardiac computed tomography. Circulation. Cardiovasc Imag 2021;14(3):e011747. https://doi.org/10.1161/CIRCIMAGING.120.011747.

[20] Lin A, Kolossváry M, Yuvaraj J, Cadet S, McElhinney PA, Jiang C, Nerlekar N, Nicholls SJ, Slomka PJ, Maurovich-Horvat P, Wong DTL, Dey D. Myocardial infarction associates with a distinct pericoronary adipose tissue radiomic phenotype: a prospective case-control study. jacc. Cardiovasc Imag 2020;13(11):2371−83. https://doi.org/10.1016/j.jcmg.2020.06.033.

[21] Bajaj NS, Osborne MT, Gupta A, Tavakkoli A, Bravo PE, Vita T, Bibbo CF, Hainer J, Dorbala S, Blankstein R, Bhatt DL, Di Carli MF, Taqueti VR. Coronary microvascular dysfunction and cardiovascular risk in obese patients. J Am Coll Cardiol 2018;72(7):707−17. https://doi.org/10.1016/j.jacc.2018.05.049.

[22] Taqueti VR, Di Carli MF. Coronary microvascular disease pathogenic mechanisms and therapeutic options: JACC state-of-the-art review. J Am Coll Cardiol 2018;72(21):2625−41. https://doi.org/10.1016/j.jacc.2018.09.042.

[23] Sorop O, Olver TD, van de Wouw J, Heinonen I, van Duin RW, Duncker DJ, Merkus D. The microcirculation: a key player in obesity-associated cardiovascular disease. Cardiovasc Res 2017;113(9):1035−45. https://doi.org/10.1093/cvr/cvx093.

[24] Quercioli A, Montecucco F, Pataky Z, Thomas A, Ambrosio G, Staub C, Di Marzo V, Ratib O, Mach F, Golay A, Schindler TH. Improvement in coronary circulatory function in morbidly obese individuals after gastric bypass-induced weight loss: relation to alterations in endocannabinoids and adipocytokines. Eur Heart J 2013;34(27):2063−73. https://doi.org/10.1093/eurheartj/eht085.

[25] Nakamori S, Nezafat M, Ngo LH, Manning WJ, Nezafat R. Left atrial epicardial fat volume is associated with atrial fibrillation: a prospective cardiovascular magnetic resonance 3D Dixon study. J Am Heart Assoc 2018;7(6). https://doi.org/10.1161/JAHA.117.008232.

[26] Neeland IJ, Poirier P, Després J-P. Cardiovascular and metabolic heterogeneity of obesity: clinical challenges and implications for management. Circulation 2018;137(13):1391−406. https://doi.org/10.1161/CIRCULATIONAHA.117.029617.

[27] Wong CX, Ganesan AN, Selvanayagam JB. Epicardial fat and atrial fibrillation: current evidence, potential mechanisms, clinical implications, and future directions. Eur Heart J 2017;38(17):1294−302. https://doi.org/10.1093/eurheartj/ehw045.

[28] Tsao H-M, Hu W-C, Wu M-H, Tai C-T, Lin Y-J, Chang S-L, Lo L-W, Hu Y-F, Tuan T-C, Wu T-J, Sheu M-H, Chang C-Y, Chen S-A. Quantitative analysis of quantity and distribution of epicardial adipose tissue surrounding the left atrium in patients with atrial fibrillation and effect of recurrence after ablation. Am J Cardiol 2011;107(10):1498−503. https://doi.org/10.1016/j.amjcard.2011.01.027.

[29] Bonou M, Mavrogeni S, Kapelios CJ, Markousis-Mavrogenis G, Aggeli C, Cholongitas E, Protogerou AD, Barbetseas J. Cardiac adiposity and arrhythmias: the role of imaging. Diagnostics 2021;11(2). https://doi.org/10.3390/diagnostics11020362.

[30] Kusayama T, Furusho H, Kashiwagi H, Kato T, Murai H, Usui S, Kaneko S, Takamura M. Inflammation of left atrial epicardial adipose tissue is associated with paroxysmal atrial fibrillation. J Cardiol 2016;68(5):406−11. https://doi.org/10.1016/j.jjcc.2015.11.005.

[31] Mazurek T, Kiliszek M, Kobylecka M, Skubisz-Głuchowska J, Kochman J, Filipiak K, Królicki L, Opolski G. Relation of proinflammatory activity of epicardial adipose tissue to the occurrence of atrial fibrillation. Am J Cardiol 2014;113(9):1505−8. https://doi.org/10.1016/j.amjcard.2014.02.005.

[32] Datta T, Lee AJ, Cain R, McCarey M, Whellan DJ. Weighing in on heart failure: the potential impact of bariatric surgery. Heart Fail Rev 2021. https://doi.org/10.1007/s10741-021-10078-w.

[33] Bizino MB, Sala ML, de Heer P, van der Tol P, Smit JWA, Webb AG, de Roos A, Lamb HJ. MR of multi-organ involvement in the metabolic syndrome. Magn Reson Imag Clin N Am 2015;23(1):41−58. https://doi.org/10.1016/j.mric.2014.09.010.

[34] Neubauer S. The failing heart–an engine out of fuel. N Engl J Med 2007;356(11):1140−51.

[35] Ng ACT, Strudwick M, van der Geest RJ, Ng ACC, Gillinder L, Goo SY, Cowin G, Delgado V, Wang WYS, Bax JJ. Impact of epicardial adipose tissue, left ventricular myocardial fat content, and interstitial fibrosis on myocardial contractile function. Circulat Cardiovasc Imag 2018;11(8):e007372. https://doi.org/10.1161/CIRCIMAGING.117.007372.

Chapter 17

Obesity in relation to cardiorenal function

Isabel T.N. Nguyen[1], Jaap A. Joles[1], Marianne C. Verhaar[1], Hildo J. Lamb[2] and Ilona A. Dekkers[2]

[1]*Department of Nephrology and Hypertension, University Medical Center Utrecht, Utrecht, the Netherlands;* [2]*Department of Radiology, Cardio Vascular Imaging Group (CVIG), Leiden University Medical Center, Leiden, the Netherlands*

Introduction

Obesity (defined as a Body Mass Index (BMI) $\geq 30 \, \text{kg/m}^2$) is a growing pandemic with serious impact on renal and cardiovascular function. The current rise in obesity coincides with an increase in chronic kidney disease (CKD) and cardiovascular disease (CVD) in Western societies [1]. Approximately 10% of the Western population have chronic kidney damage of which a significant number is related to obesity and obesity-associated risk factors. Additionally, type-2 diabetes is nine times more prevalent in obese individuals than in the nonoverweight population and CVD is three times more often diagnosed [2]. The association of obesity with incident heart failure is stronger than those for other CVD subtypes and was largely unexplained by adjustment for traditional CVD risk factors [3]. The two leading causes of CKD worldwide—hypertensive glomerulosclerosis and type-2 diabetic nephropathy—are both largely attributable to obesity [4]. Obesity plays a central role in the development of the metabolic syndrome, which affects approximately 25% of the adult population [5], and is also a common feature of both CKD and CVD. The complex associations between obesity and cardiorenal function involve several pathological metabolic, neurohormonal, and inflammatory processes, also referred to as obesity-related cardiorenal syndrome. An increasing number of studies have investigated the underlying processes of obesity-related cardiorenal syndrome in both animal studies as well as translational studies in humans. However, the underlying pathophysiology of obesity-related kidney disease and relation of obesity with CVD and heart failure is complex and not fully elucidated. Until now it has been challenging to determine which obese patients are at increased risk of obesity-related kidney disease. BMI has shown to be an independent risk factor for CKD and end-stage renal disease (ESRD) [6] and obesity progresses preexisting CKD irrespective of the underlying nephropathy [7]. Moreover, BMI is associated with an increased risk of heart failure [8]. The number of obese with CVD and heart failure, and obese with end-stage kidney disease on maintenance dialysis is projected to markedly increase in the future [9]. This makes obesity a rapidly emerging problem for both the cardiovascular and renal community.

Obesity-related cardiorenal dysfunction

The heart and kidneys are organs that both play a major role in hemodynamic regulation including vascular tone, end-organ perfusion, and volume status. As such, the heart and kidneys are highly interconnected and disturbance of either cardiac or renal function has via complex processes subsequent effects on the other organ. In the context of obesity and metabolic dysregulation, the physiological interdependence of the heart and kidneys can lead to dysfunction of both organs, referred to as cardiorenal syndrome (CRS).

Overview of five-part classification system for cardiorenal syndrome

The Acute Dialysis Quality Initiative classification has categorized CRS in five different subtypes based on the primary and secondary involved organ and processes, and development over time [10]. In short, in type 1 CRS (acute CRS), the primary

Classification of the cardiorenal syndrome

	Type	Name	Mechanism	Examples
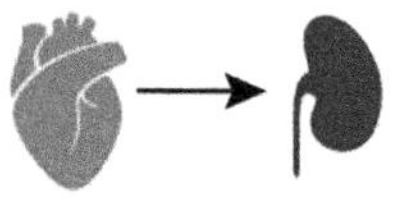	1	Acute cardiorenal syndrome	Acute impairment of the cardiac function leading to acute kidney injury	Acute myocardial infarction Cardiogenic shock
	2	Chronic cardiorenal syndrome	Chronic abnormalities in cardiac function causing progressive chronic kidney disease	Chronic congestive heart failure
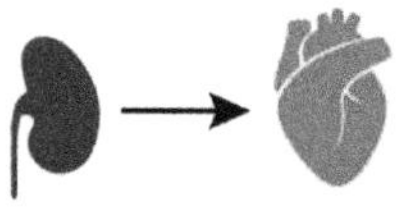	3	Acute renocardiac syndrome	Acute primary worsening of renal function that leads to cardiac dysfunction	Acute kidney injury, glomerulonephritis, hyperkalemia and uremia
	4	Chronic renocardiac syndrome	Primary chronic kidney disease contributing to decreased cardiac function	Chronic glomerular disease, uremic cardiomyopathy, anemia, hypertension
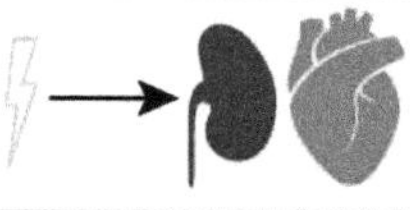	5	Secondary cardiorenal syndrome	An acute or chronic systemic condition causing both cardiac and renal dysfunction	Diabetes mellitus, amyloidosis, sepsis, cirrhosis

FIGURE 17.1 Overview of the five-part classification system for the cardiorenal syndrome.

process is acute cardiac impairment leading secondary to acute renal impairment and can be described as heart failure resulting in acute kidney injury (Fig. 17.1). Type 2 CRS (chronic CRS) is characterized by chronic cardiac dysfunction leading to chronic renal dysfunction, e.g., chronic heart failure resulting in CKD. In type 3 CRS (acute renocardiac syndrome), acute kidney injury precedes acute heart failure. CRS type 4 (chronic renocardiac syndrome) is characterized by chronic renal impairment preceding cardiac dysfunction such as CKD-associated (uremic) cardiomyopathy leading to left ventricular hypertrophy and heart failure. Finally, in type 5 CRS (secondary CRS) a systemic condition, such as amyloidosis, sepsis or cirrhosis is the primary underlying process leading secondary to cardiac and renal dysfunction. In this chapter the focus is on chronic subtypes of CRS in relation to obesity.

The pathophysiology of cardiorenal syndrome

The complex associations between obesity and cardiorenal function involve several pathological processes including: the metabolic syndrome, dyslipidemia and atherosclerosis, systemic inflammation, microvascular dysfunction and heart failure, sympathetic activation and leptin, renin-angiotensin-aldosterone system (RAAS), and hyperuricemia. A summary of the processes discussed below that are involved in cardiorenal interaction in obesity is provided in Fig. 17.2.

Metabolic syndrome

The metabolic syndrome is a constellation of hypertension, abdominal obesity, hypertriglyceridemia, hyperglycemia, and/or insulin resistance, and is a well-known risk factor for cardiovascular disease, diabetes, and diabetic nephropathy (Fig. 17.3). In addition, the metabolic syndrome may directly affect the kidney; however, the underlying etiology between metabolic syndrome and CKD risk remains unclear [11]. The shared risk factors of the metabolic syndrome and the combined negative influences on heart and kidneys have also been referred to as the metabolic CRS. These are supported by the notion that impaired insulin signaling contributes to impaired diastolic mechanics of the heart [12] and that obesity and insulin resistance are strongly correlated with impaired kidney function [13].

Dyslipidemia and atherosclerosis

Obesity has been associated with an abnormal lipid profile consisting of increased serum triglycerides and free fatty acids, decreased high-density lipoprotein (HDL) with HDL dysfunction, and normal or slightly elevated levels of low-density lipoprotein (LDL) with increased levels of small, dense LDL [14]. Lipid abnormalities associated with obesity and a

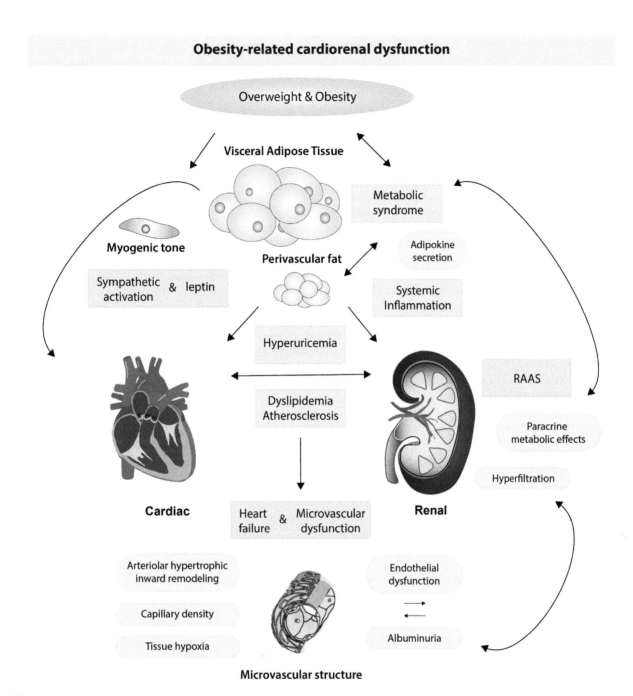

FIGURE 17.2 Overview of interacting pathways in obesity that are associated with maladaptive changes in the heart and kidney that contribute to the development of CRS. RAAS, renin-angiotensin-aldosterone system. The pathophysiological processes involved discussed above are visualized in the *orange* rectangular text boxes, and in the *blue* oval text boxes the subsequent affected functional and morphological changes.

typical feature of the metabolic syndrome are small, dense LDL, accumulation of atherogenic remnants during postprandial hyperlipidemia as well as lipoproteins containing apolipoprotein B that are produced in excess by the liver [15]. These lipid abnormalities are associated with proinflammatory changes which may be produced by adipose tissue and have been linked to endothelial dysfunction, subendothelial macrophage uptake of LDL leading to foam cell and atherosclerotic plaque formation [16]. In relation to CRS, renal atherosclerosis is of particular relevance considering the development of renal artery stenosis is an independent risk factor for adverse coronary events and contributes to renovascular hypertension and ischemic nephropathy [17].

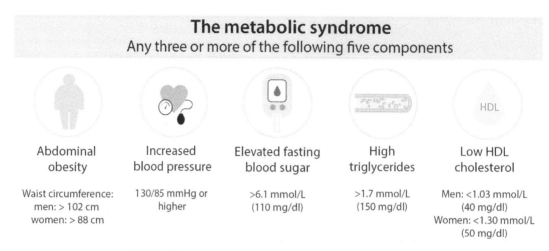

The metabolic syndrome

Any three or more of the following five components

Abdominal obesity	Increased blood pressure	Elevated fasting blood sugar	High triglycerides	Low HDL cholesterol
Waist circumference: men: > 102 cm women: > 88 cm	130/85 mmHg or higher	>6.1 mmol/L (110 mg/dl)	>1.7 mmol/L (150 mg/dl)	Men: <1.03 mmol/L (40 mg/dl) Women: <1.30 mmol/L (50 mg/dl)

FIGURE 17.3 An overview of the criteria for the metabolic syndrome.

Systemic inflammation, microvascular dysfunction, and heart failure

Obesity has been linked to a low-grade systemic inflammation which contributes to the excretion of inflammatory cytokine profile [18]. These systemic inflammatory effects negatively influence vascular reactivity and endothelial function, promote atherosclerosis, and have been suggested to contribute to renocardiovascular and cerebrovascular disease [19,20]. In addition to obstructive atherosclerosis, the regulation of microvascular function might have a more important role in the development of CRS than previously recognized. In patients without obstructive coronary artery disease, coronary microvascular dysfunction (CMD) has been linked to impaired renal function, cardiovascular events [21], and severity of CKD stage [22,23]. Additionally, CMD has been linked to conventional CVD and CKD risk factors including obesity, dyslipidemia, and hypertension [24]. The central pathophysiological mechanism in the association between CMD and CKD is endothelial dysfunction, which has been linked to vascular rarefaction in glomerular capillaries and subsequent tissue hypoxia and kidney damage, see also Fig. 17.2 [25]. In addition, in CKD patients the presence of uremia-related risk factors, RAAS-activation, oxidative stress, and low-grade inflammation have been associated with microvascular rarefaction and myocardial fibrosis [26−28]. Recently, it was proposed that the combined burden of systemic comorbidities contributes to a proinflammatory state that negatively affects the coronary endothelium and activates the perivascular environment which ultimately leads to stiffening of the ventricle and diastolic dysfunction [29,30]. This comorbidity-associated CMD has been proposed as the main driver of myocardial dysfunction and remodeling in heart failure with preserved ejection fraction (HFpEF) [29]. This is in contrast to heart failure with reduced ejection fraction (HFrEF), characterized by a lack of contractility, in which remodeling is caused by an insult leading to cardiomyocyte loss and functional impairment [31]. HFpEF accounts for over 50% of all heart failure cases, yet currently no effective treatment is available for this specific form of heart failure while these do exist for HFrEF. To address this unmet need, an increasing number of (pre-)clinical studies focus on further understanding the mechanisms involved in HFpEF.

Sympathetic activation and leptin

Chronic cardiac sympathetic overstimulation in obesity has been linked to increased catecholamine levels and obesity-related hypertension [32]. The increase in sympathetic nervous system activity in response to weight gain is believed to be an adaptive mechanism to increase energy expenditure and promote restoration of the previous weight [33]. The rise in central sympathetic outflow combined with elevated levels of circulating fatty acids, insulin, leptin, and angiotensin II contribute to an increase in arterial stiffness, affecting the cardiovascular system and renal vasculature [34,35]. Leptin is an adipocyte-secreted hormone that is a key regulator of appetite and energy homeostasis. In physiological conditions, a minor increase in leptin concentrations reduces appetite, food intake, and body weight [36]. However, in obesity it has been found that despite increased leptin concentrations, its appetite reducing effects are decreased. This ultimately leads to the development of leptin resistance due to a defect in the intracellular signaling associated with the leptin receptor [37]. Several rodent models for obesity research originated from leptin deficiency with either nonfunctional leptin or leptin receptors.

Renin-angiotensin-aldosterone system (RAAS)

The renin-angiotensin-aldosterone system (RAAS) plays an important role in the regulation of both cardiovascular function and renal function. As such, the RAAS is considered to play a central role in the CRS. Translational studies in pigs and humans have shown that renin is exclusively derived from the kidney, and disappears from the circulation after bilateral nephrectomy [38]. In obese individuals, it has been shown that plasma renin activity is reduced and that plasma aldosterone levels are elevated and positively associated with blood pressure, waist circumference, and insulin resistance. These changes promote renal sodium and water retention and aldosterone production, which subsequently contributes to vascular inflammation and oxidative stress [39]. Finally, overactivation of the RAAS has been linked to adverse cardiorenal changes such as cardiac fibrosis and hypertrophy, and at a renal level with tubulointerstitial inflammation, glomerulosclerosis, mesangial proliferation, and podocyte dysfunction [39].

Hyperuricemia

Previously, the relationship between serum uric acid levels and cardiometabolic disease was considered to be merely a simple epiphenomenon. However, increasing evidence indicates that hyperuricemia is an independent risk factor for metabolic syndrome, supporting the complex role of serum uric acid levels as a consequence of both hypertension and metabolic syndrome [40]. Hyperuricemia contributes to various negative effects on the cardiovascular and renal system via different processes leading to oxidative stress [41], inhibition of endothelial NO synthase [42], vascular adaptations due to stimulation of smooth muscle cell proliferation [43] and RAAS activation [44]. As such, hyperuricemia is increasingly recognized as an important obesity-related risk factor for several renocardiovascular conditions, such as atherosclerosis [45], endothelial dysfunction [46], and heart failure [47]. A recent metaanalysis found that hyperuricemia is associated with worsening estimated glomerular filtration rate (GFR), albuminuria, CKD, and renal failure [48]. Moreover, long-term urate-lowering therapies were found to have a positive effect on renal function and reducing proteinuria [48].

Preclinical studies

Obese animal models of cardiorenal syndrome

The important connection between cardiac and renal pathophysiology is demonstrated by the high prevalence of CKD in patients with heart failure and vice versa, where dysfunction of one organ leads to progressive dysfunction of the other organ, eventually resulting in the failure of both organs [49]. Although studies have been performed on the association between CKD and HFrEF, less is known about the link between CKD and HFpEF. There is a strong relationship between CRS and metabolic risk factors that include obesity, dyslipidemia, high blood pressure, and hyperglycemia. While several of these links are understood, some of the mechanisms for the cardiorenal interaction remain incompletely explained. The availability of animal models of the metabolic CRS allows us to further explore these mechanisms, and more importantly, potential therapeutic strategies. As the CRS is a complex disorder, it is not possible to reproduce all the disease components in one single animal model. Nevertheless, animal models have provided valuable insights in the pathogenesis of the metabolic CRS [50].

The interaction of cardiac and renal dysfunction in obesity has been investigated in a wide range of species, from rodent to swine models. The acute types of the CRS are typically investigated in nonobese animal models; therefore, these types will not be discussed in this chapter. An overview of studies performed in the most commonly used obese animal models of CRS is given in Table 17.1. Efforts to incorporate obesity in animal models have been performed through Western diets high in fat, fructose, or salt, either alone or in combination with additional stressors, as well as models predisposed to exhibit metabolic syndrome [64]. Mutations in the gene responsible for the production of leptin (Lep) or its receptor (Lepr), which are important in the control of appetite, lead to excessive eating and eventually obesity at a young age in rodent models. Mice homozygous for the spontaneous mutation Lep^{ob}, the ob/ob mice, develop hyperphagia, obesity, hyperglycemia, and hyperinsulinemia as a result of the inability of leptin to bind to its receptor [65,66]. Their obesity is characterized by a growth in the number and size of adipocytes and they will develop cardiac and renal dysfunction with microvascular complications [67].

The db/db mouse is another mouse model in which the spontaneous leptin receptor mutation *db* leads to the development of morbid obesity, dyslipidemia, and diabetes [68]. The defective leptin receptor leads to the overproduction of extracellular leptin, but lacks the intracellular leptin action through the receptor [65]. Mice homozygous for this mutation exhibit albuminuria, glomerulopathy, and left ventricular diastolic dysfunction as indicated by increased left ventricular mass and E/e' ratio [51,52]. Homozygous ob/ob and db/db mice have severe, rapid, spontaneous and early onset obesity that is already apparent at 4 weeks of age [69].

TABLE 17.1 Overview of obese animal models exhibiting cardiorenal syndrome (compared to lean controls).

Model	M/F	Age	Systemic features	Cardiac function	Renal function	Cardiac morphology	Renal morphology	Refs.
db/db mice	M + F	26W	Hyperglycemia, hypertension	↑ LV mass, EDV ↔ EF ↑ E/e', ↑ LVDEP (females)	ND	↑ Cardiomyocyte size ↑ Interstitial fibrosis Capillary rarefaction (males)	ND	[51]
db/db mice	M	20W	Hyperglycemia	ND	↑ Albuminuria	ND	↑ Hypertrophy of glomeruli and proximal tubular cells ↑ Glomerular inflammation	[52]
db/db mice	M	28W	Hyperglycemia	ND	↑ Albuminuria ↑ GFR (inulin)	ND	ND	[53]
ob/ob mice	F	11W	Hyperglycemia, dyslipidemia	↑ LV mass ↓ E/A	ND	↑ Lipid accumulation	ND	[54]
Zucker rat	M	14W	Hyperglycemia hypertension	↔ LVPWd ↔ EF ↔ LVEDP, ↔ tau	↑ BUN	↔ Fibrosis ↔ Cardiomyocyte size	↔ Fibrosis	[55]
ZDF rat	M	36W	Hyperglycemia	↓ LV mass, ↑ EDV, ↑ESV ↑ LVDEP	↑ Albuminuria	ND	Hydronephrosis	[56]
ZDF rat	F	20W	Hyperglycemia, dyslipidemia	↑ LVPWd, ↑ LV mass ↑ E/e'	ND	↑ Fibrosis	ND	[57]
ZSF1 rat	M+F	26W	Hyperglycemia (males), dyslipidemia	↔ EF ↑ E/e'	ND	↑ Fibrosis	ND	[58]
ZSF1 rat	M	32W	Hyperglycemia, dyslipidemia	ND	↔ GFR (inulin) ↑ Proteinuria ↑ Albuminuria	↑ Lipid deposition	↑ Lipid deposition ↑ Glomerulosclerosis ↑ Inflammation	[59]
ZSF1 rat	M	25W	Hyperglycemia	↑ LVPWd, ↑ LV mass ↔ EF ↓ E/A, ↑ E/e'	↑ Proteinuria ↑ TBARS	↑ Fibrosis ↑ Inflammation	↑Tubulointerstitial damage ↑ Glomerulosclerosis Vascular rarefaction	[60]

Model	M/F	W	Comorbidities	Cardiac function	Renal function	Cardiac histology	Renal histology	Ref
Obese Dahl-SS rat	F	15W	Hyperglycemia, dyslipidemia, hypertension	↑LVPWd, ↑ LV mass ↔ EF ↓ E/A	↑ BUN, proteinuria ↓ Creatinine clearance	↑ Cardiomyocyte size ↑ Fibrosis ↑ Inflammation	ND	[61]
Obese Dahl-SS rat	M	18W	Hypertension	ND	↑ Proteinuria	ND	↑ Glomerulosclerosis ↑ Glomerular lipid deposition	[62]
DM+HC+HT swine	F	26W	Hyperglycemia hypertension	↓ LVEDV, ↓ SV, ↔ EF ↓ E/A	↓ GFR ↑ Cystatin C	↑ Collagen deposition ↓ Capillary/fiber ratio	↑ Tubulointerstitial damage	[63]
Göttingen mini-swine	F	20W	Dyslipidemia, hypertension, IR	↑ LV mass, ↑ LVPWd ↔ EF ↑ E/e', ↑ LVEDP	ND	↑ LV fibrosis	↑ Renal fibrosis	[64]

BUN, blood urea nitrogen; *EDV*, end-diastolic volume; *EF*, ejection fraction; *GFR*, glomerular filtration rate; *IR*, insulin resistance; *LV*, left ventricle; *LVEDP*, left ventricular end-diastolic pressure; *LVPWd*, left ventricular posterior wall thickness in diastole; *M/F*, male/female; *ND*, not determined; *W*, weeks.

Many of the available rat models of obesity are derived from the selective crossing between rats comprising one of the two most significant mutations in the leptin receptor, *fa* and *cp* [60]. A missense mutation in the leptin receptor gene (*fa*) leads to the production of nonfunctional leptin receptors [65]. The Zucker rat and its substrain, the Zucker Diabetic rat (ZDF), are both homozygous for the spontaneous Lepr^{fa} mutation. The corpulent (*cp*) phenotype, resulting from an autosomal recessive mutation on the Lepr gene was first found in spontaneously hypertensive obese rats (SHROB or Koletsky rat) [70]. Rats homozygous for this mutation completely lack functional leptin receptors and are leptin-resistant with high levels of circulating leptin. Several substrains have been bred from the SHROB rat since the discovery of the *cp* mutation. Recently, the obese diabetic Zucker Fatty/spontaneously hypertensive heart failure F1 hybrid (ZSF1) rat, which contains both the *fa* and the *cp* mutation, has been proposed as a relevant model for the metabolic CRS [58,60].

In addition to the rodent models, obesity or metabolic syndrome—induced CRS has been studied in larger animal models. Often several comorbidities are induced in these models via a combination of a high caloric diet and chemical and surgical interventions to mimic human disease progression as close as possible. Recently, a female swine model was developed with multiple common comorbidities that ultimately leads to left ventricular dysfunction [63]. The combination of obesity induced by a high diet, diabetes induced by streptozotocin, and hypertension resulting from renal artery embolization leads to the development of renal dysfunction, impaired coronary microvascular function, and myocardial stiffening. Another model that has been recently developed is the Göttingen mini swine model with multiple comorbidities that develops HFpEF. Obesity induced via a diet containing high levels of fat, fructose, cholesterol, and salt on top of the administration of the aldosterone agonist deoxycorticosterone acetate leads to the development of metabolic syndrome and consequently heart failure [64].

The Zucker rat and substrains as proposed models of the metabolic cardiorenal syndrome

The obese Zucker rat and its substrains (Fig. 17.4) have been widely used as a research model for obesity-related cardiac and renal dysfunction. In addition to obesity and dyslipidemia, they exhibit mild glucose intolerance and peripheral insulin resistance. These abnormalities precede the development of albuminuria and glomerular injury with a parallel deterioration in cardiac output and renal function [50].

A substrain of Zucker rats, the ZDF rat, was selectively inbred for hyperglycemia. They were derived by selective inbreeding of the hyperglycemic rats containing both the recessive Lepr mutation and autosomal recessive defect in β-cell transcription. This defect in itself is not sufficient to initiate diabetes development, only in combination with the Lepr mutation does it lead to hyperglycemia [71]. ZDF rats have a decrease in β-cell mass which results in an inability to compensate for severe insulin resistance. Their hyperphagia leads to hyperinsulinemia, which upregulates transcription factors that stimulate lipogenesis. This results in the ectopic deposition of triacylglycerol in nonadipocytes, thereby providing a fatty acid substrate for pathological nonoxidative metabolism, such as ceramide synthesis [72].

A new rat model of the metabolic syndrome, the obese Dahl salt-sensitive (SS) leptin receptor mutant rat (SS^{LepR-}mutant), was derived from crossing the Dahl-SS rat with the Zucker rat. The obese Dahl-SS rat develops salt-induced hypertension and subsequently goes from cardiac hypertrophy to heart failure [73]. The early development of progressive proteinuria is associated with renal hyperfiltration followed by a decline in renal function in obese rats. These rats exhibit more glomerulosclerosis and glomerular lipid accumulation compared to control rats [62].

The ZSF1 rat is derived by crossing a lean female ZDF rat (*fa*) with a lean male spontaneously hypertensive heart failure rat (SHHF, *cp*) (see Fig. 17.2) [74]. Homozygous rats develop obesity, severe dyslipidemia, mild hypertension, hyperglycemia and insulin resistance. Heterozygous rats are used as control as they do not develop obesity. Both obese and lean ZSF1 rats exhibit elevated blood pressure, as they inherit the hypertensive gene from the SHHF strain [75]. Obese ZSF1 rats develop metabolic syndrome as early as 8 weeks of age. The obese rats die (at age ±12 months) with symptoms of end-stage renal failure accompanied by marked cardiac hypertrophy [76].

Abnormalities in cardiac function in obesity

Obesity is associated with both pressure overload and volume overload [77]. The increased metabolic demand imposed by the expanded adipose tissue and augmented fat-free mass in obesity results in a hyperdynamic circulation with increased blood volume [78]. Arterial and ventricular remodeling in response to the increased load involves changes in the cardiomyocytes and extracellular matrix. Initially, cardiac remodeling is activated as an adaptive response to normalize wall stress and results in both concentric and eccentric changes in the left ventricle [77]. Pressure overload causes concentric hypertrophy associated with increased extracellular matrix synthesis by fibroblasts and diastolic dysfunction, whereas volume overload induces dilation accompanied by matrix degradation [79]. Additionally, ectopic fat storage might

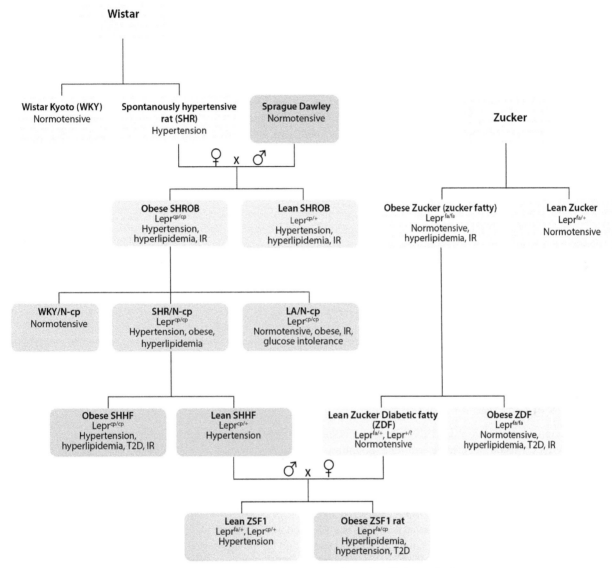

FIGURE 17.4 Schematic overview of the obese Zucker rat family.

contribute to the development of cardiac dysfunction. Obesity is associated with the intramyocardial deposition of lipids [80]. The accumulation of large amounts of triglycerides may trigger a pathological signaling cascade resulting in apoptosis and systolic dysfunction [80]. Indeed, cardiac lipid accumulation has been observed in obese rat models. Twenty-weeks-old male ZDF rats showed elevated myocardial triglyceride and ceramide content, with increased apoptosis and mild contractile dysfunction [81]. ZDF rats at 30 weeks of age showed a marked accumulation of neutral lipid droplets within cardiomyocytes [82]. This was accompanied with increased apoptosis, fibrosis, hypertrophy, and diastolic dysfunction while ejection fraction was preserved.

It has been demonstrated that patients with HFpEF, especially women, had significantly more intramyocardial fat than HFrEF patients or nonheart failure controls and that the amount of intramyocardial fat assessed by proton magnetic resonance spectroscopy (^{1}H-MRS) correlated with left ventricular diastolic dysfunction parameters [83]. Additionally, healthy individuals with obesity and normal ejection fraction who have elevated myocardial triglyceride levels develop left ventricular concentric hypertrophy [84]. Similarly, in 32-weeks-old female obese ZSF1 rats a high degree of intramyocardial fat deposition was found, especially at the mitral valve annulus, in parallel with diastolic dysfunction and left ventricular hypertrophy [85].

Adipose tissue can be broadly classified into two types: white or brown adipose tissue [86]. White fat stores a large amount of energy in the form of triglycerides in big droplets and also serves as an important endocrine organ. In contrast, brown fat contains smaller droplets and a high amount of mitochondria and is a key player in energy expenditure by converting large amounts of energy to heat (thermogenesis) [87]. In obesity, white adipocyte dysfunction is associated with the release of proinflammatory adipokines and chemokines. Cardiac visceral adipose tissue (CVAT) of obese ZSF1 rats revealed a white adipose tissuelike phenotype accompanied by adipocyte hypertrophy and further analysis showed enrichment of proteins involved in triglyceride metabolic processes [88]. In contrast, mitochondrial proteins were prominent in CVAT obtained from lean ZSF1 rats, suggesting a more brown adipose tissuelike phenotype. Incubation of myocardial organocultures with cultured media obtained from CVAT of obese ZSF1 rats significantly reduced cell viability, induced cardiomyocyte hypertrophy and fibrosis [88]. High resolution ^{1}H-MRS was applied to study adipose tissue in lean and obese Zucker rats [89]. Adipose tissue in obese rats was qualitative different from lean rats, with the indication that adipose tissue in obese rats was more active compared to lean controls. White adipose tissue was characterized by lower unsaturation and polyunsaturation indexes in obese versus lean rats, suggesting abnormal lipid metabolism in obese Zucker rats.

Excessive weight gain, especially when associated with increased visceral or retroperitoneal adiposity, is a well-established cause of hypertension [90]. The hemodynamic changes imposed by hypertension can induce cardiac remodeling involving cardiomyocyte hypertrophy, interstitial inflammation, fibrosis, and microvascular rarefaction [91]. Extracellular matrix composition is primarily controlled by matrix metalloproteinase and tissue inhibitors of metalloproteinases. An increase in the activity of matrix metalloproteinase-2, a gelatinase involved in the process of myocardial remodeling, was observed in obese female ZSF1 rats compared to lean controls [85]. Perivascular fibrosis was enhanced in obese rats, with increased expression of collagen type I and III in left ventricular tissue. Additionally, increased cardiac deposition of collagen and cardiomyocyte hypertrophy was observed in both male and female obese ZSF1 rats [58].

The combination of a mild increase in blood pressure, increase in cardiac output, ectopic fat storage within and around the heart, could have additive effects resulting in systolic and diastolic dysfunction in obesity, which in the long term promotes heart failure.

Abnormalities in renal function in obesity

Excess fat accumulation in and around the kidneys is associated with increased intrarenal pressures, impaired pressure natriuresis and hypertension [90]. Increased renal sodium reabsorption plays a major role in initiating the rise in blood pressure that is associated with obesity and obese individuals have been found to require higher than normal pressure to maintain sodium balance, indicating impaired renal pressure natriuresis [92]. Many mechanisms have been suggested to explain the abnormal sodium handling including increased renal nerve sympathetic activity and activation of the RAAS including the activation of mineralocorticoid receptors independent of aldosterone. Additionally, the accumulation of fat within the renal sinus, also referred to as renal sinus fat, is associated with the increased intraabdominal pressure of visceral obesity and may physically compress the renal papilla, renal vein, and lymphatic vessels, altering intrarenal physical forces that favor sodium reabsorption and arterial hypertension [80]. Also, CKD may over a much longer time amplify the effects of these mechanisms, making obesity-associated hypertension more difficult to control and less easily reversed by weight loss.

Over time functional changes in renal function in obesity involve glomerular hyperfiltration in the early phase, followed by normal filtration and eventually a gradual decline in GFR because of renal injury and loss of nephrons [93]. Nephron loss, which is often masked by hyperfiltration, is believed to start in the early phases. In the early phases, urinary albumin excretion becomes evident and progressively increases until so many nephrons are lost that in the final stages urinary albumin excretion starts to fall [90]. GFR was significantly elevated two–threefold in 10-weeks-old male obese ZSF1 rats compared to lean age-matched controls, indicating glomerular hyperfiltration at early time points [94]. The GFR subsequently declined over time in parallel with worsening dyslipidemia in obese ZSF1 rats, with similar GFR found between obese and lean ZSF1 rats at 32 weeks of age. At this time point, renal fibrosis and glomerulosclerosis score were elevated in obese ZSF1 rats compared to lean rats. Obese ZSF1 rats showed regression of the peritubular and glomerular microvasculature, accompanied by proteinuria, tubulointerstitial damage, and glomerulosclerosis [60].

CKD as a risk factor for HFpEF in obese animals

The coexistence of CKD and HFpEF is partially due to common underlying comorbidities, such as obesity, hypertension, and diabetes. Renal dysfunction, even in mild stages, can cause metabolic and systemic derangements in circulating factors that introduce a systemic proinflammatory state [29]. The proinflammatory state further impairs microvascular function, evidenced by endothelial oxidative stress, impaired nitric oxide availability, reduced endothelial cell survival and regeneration, and pericyte loss. This eventually leads to cardiomyocyte stiffening, myocardial fibrosis, diastolic dysfunction, and HFpEF. Microvascular inflammatory endothelial activation, oxidative stress, endothelial nitric oxide synthase uncoupling, and impaired cGMP-PKG signaling were found in the left ventricle of 20-weeks-old obese male ZSF1 rats and HFpEF patients [95].

Conversely, HFpEF is able to further worsen CKD. Increased filling pressures found in HFpEF cause a decreased cardiac output, especially in situations of high demand, and increase central venous pressure. This potentially causes a reduction in renal blood flow and renal perfusion pressure, activating the RAAS and the sympathetic nervous system, leading to a reduction in GFR [96]. Additionally, the higher central and venous pressure raises intrarenal interstitial pressure, leading to renal fibrosis and increased tubular pressure, thereby further reducing GFR and ultimately resulting in renal dysfunction [97].

Sex differences in the cardiorenal interaction

Obesity is highly prevalent in patients with CKD and HFpEF, more specifically in older women [98]. Obesity in women in particular harbors greater risk of HFpEF versus HFrEF, whereas this difference is less pronounced in men. However, when looking at preclinical rodent studies, female sex is often underrepresented. Nonobese male rats are more susceptible to developing heart failure compared to females and often the phenotype in female rats is milder compared to their male counterparts [99,100]. As a result, female animals are often not included in experimental studies.

The major advantage of the spontaneous obese animal models is that there is no need for invasive procedures or timeconsuming feeding schemes to induce the disease [65]. However, in some of these models certain characteristics of the metabolic syndrome do not develop in female rats and dietary manipulations are necessary. In obese ZDF and ZSF1 rats, only the male rats develop hyperglycemia from early age on. The female rats do not become diabetic without providing them a specific diet, such as the Purina 5008 diet or Research Diets 12,468 [57,101,102]. The dyslipidemia in female obese rats seems to be more severe compared to males, with higher plasma triglyceride and cholesterol levels observed in obese female ZSF1 rats [58]. Even though the female rats did not develop hyperglycemia, the severity of diastolic dysfunction and cardiac hypertrophy and fibrosis was similar to the obese males. In addition, female obese ZSF1 rats showed delayed proteinuria and less renal fibrosis compared to obese male rats [94]. Even though cardiac phenotype was similar between male and female rats, females exhibit milder renal dysfunction.

Epidemiological and translational studies in humans

Estimating obesity's risk for renal and cardiac dysfunction

Currently, BMI is used to classify overweight ($>25 \text{ kg/m}^2$) and obese ($>30 \text{ kg/m}^2$) individuals. However, BMI differentiates poorly between body fat, muscle mass, and water, whereas there is a wide range of body fat distribution in both lean and obese adults [103]. Several studies have shown that abdominal or central obesity, reflected as waist circumference (WC) or waist-to-hip ratio (WHR), is a better marker of cardiometabolic risk and mortality than overall obesity measured with BMI; and is also associated with renal impairment [104,105]. However, WHR and WC discriminate suboptimal between abdominal subcutaneous (aSAT) and visceral adipose tissue (VAT). This distinction is important since both compartments convey different cardiovascular risk factors that cluster together in the metabolic syndrome [106−108]. VAT is a better predictor of type-2 diabetes and risk factors for CVD compared to aSAT and anthropometric measures such as BMI and WC [109]. Importantly, the risk of CKD increases with the number of cardiovascular risk factors of the metabolic syndrome [110], and as such VAT might be a better predictor of CKD than conventional measures of obesity. Studies investigating the effect of aSAT/VAT on prevalent CKD are limited, and neither VAT nor SAT assessed by computed tomography (CT) was independently associated with CKD in the combined Framingham Offspring and MDCT cohort [109]. On the other hand, VAT was associated with (micro)albuminuria in men, whereas aSAT was more associated with (micro)albuminuria in women using partly the same cohorts [107]. A diminished adipose tissue expandability in CKD might be a possible explanation for the lack of association of aSAT/VAT with CKD, however it remains unclear whether aSAT/VAT can improve on predicting CKD compared to traditional anthropometric measures. In addition, increased VAT is also indicative of an increased risk of CVD. With regard to cardiac function, population-based imaging studies such as the Framingham Heart Study and the UK Biobank study have showed that VAT is associated with left ventricular remodeling and systolic and diastolic dysfunction [111,112]. A recent large Mendelian Randomization study in the UK

Biobank showed that VAT is a causal risk factor for hypertension, heart attack/angina, type 2 diabetes and hyperlipidemia [113], making VAT an important indicator for obesity's risk of both renal and cardiac dysfunction, as well as CRS.

The interplay between adipose tissue and the cardiovascular system can be considered bidirectional, with vascular and cardiac signals directly affecting adipose tissue biology, and vice versa [114]. This is supported by increasing evidence indicating that fat accumulation around blood vessels also referred to as perivascular adipose tissue (PVAT) plays an important role in the cross-talk between adipose tissue and the renocardiovascular system [114]. Regional phenotypic and functional differences exist among PVAT depots (depending on the specific location of the involved vascular bed), leading to specific endocrine and paracrine effects and related disease states, such as endothelial dysfunction, atherosclerosis, or insulin resistance [115]. In the context of CRS, in particular, visceral fat surrounding the epi- and pericardium and renal sinus is of interest. Cardiac visceral fat has shown to be independently and positively associated with coronary stenosis, myocardial ischemia, major adverse cardiac events [116], and incidence of atrial fibrillation [117]. Renal sinus fat is a PVAT compartment surrounding the vasculature of the hilum of the kidney [118], and has shown to contain dormant brown fat [119]. Renal sinus fat has been associated with exercise-induced albuminuria in nondiabetic individuals at increased risk of type-2 diabetes independent of VAT [120], supporting the pathophysiologic link between renal sinus fat and microalbuminuria. Magnetic resonance imaging (MRI) studies in individuals with prediabetes, diabetes, and normal glucose tolerance have showed that renal volume and in particular renal sinus fat volume increases in (pre)diabetes and is associated with VAT [121,122]. Decreased renal sinus fat after dietary intervention, however, has been associated with improved hepatic parameters rather than renal function [123]. In addition, renal sinus fat indexed for VAT is an independent risk indicator of coronary artery calcium in patients with suspected coronary artery disease [124]. These findings suggest that renal sinus fat is a potential link between metabolic syndrome and CRS, making renal sinus fat a potential imaging biomarker for obesity-related CRS (see Fig. 17.5).

Metabolic imaging studies of ectopic fat storage in heart and kidney

Another way to look at obesity's risk for cardiorenal dysfunction is to look at ectopic fat storage. Diminished expandability of aSAT and VAT may lead to an overflow of lipids resulting in an accumulation of lipids in nonadipose tissue such as liver, skeletal muscle, and heart [127]. Consequently, this ectopic lipid may be a better biomarker for cardiometabolic risk of obesity. The archetypical example of ectopic lipid accumulation in metabolic unhealthy obesity is nonalcoholic fatty liver disease (NAFLD). Fatty liver may contribute to hepatic insulin resistance, gluconeogenesis, and systemic levels of inflammatory adipokines and cytokines that may influence both obesity-related kidney disease and CVD. A large meta-analysis showed that NAFLD is independently associated with CKD [128], albeit none of the included studies adjusted for VAT and used either echography or CT for the assessment of liver fat rather than MRI or related techniques such as ^{1}H-MRS. Notably, a Chinese study in 400 individuals showed that NAFLD measured using ^{1}H-MRS was indeed independently associated with CKD after adjustment for VAT [129]. However, recent Mendelian Randomization studies in

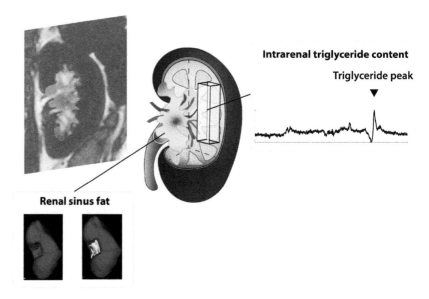

FIGURE 17.5 Schematic drawing of renal sinus fat in yellow (=perivascular fat around the kidney hilum) assessed on an isotropic fat only DIXON scan (left) versus the spectral peak of intrarenal triglyceride content (=fat accumulating inside the kidney) (right) assessed using ^{1}H-MRS at 3T [122,125,126].

Intrarenal triglyceride content

Triglyceride peak

Renal sinus fat

community dwelling Caucasian populations suggest that VAT was more important compared to liver fat (measured by ^{1}H-MRS) in the etiology microalbuminuria (which is an established surrogate marker of early diabetic nephropathy and glomerular microangiopathy) [130] and eGFR [131].

Similar to ectopic lipid accumulation in the liver, the accumulation of lipids in renal parenchyma (referred to as fatty kidney) occurs in obesity and has been hypothesized to contribute to obesity-related CKD leading to specific obesity-related changes in the kidney (Fig. 17.6) [132]. This hypothesis is supported by the positive association between BMI and triglycerides in human kidney cortex samples from nephrectomy samples [133]. Translational studies in humans on ectopic lipid accumulation in obesity-related CKD are scarce as biopsies are considered unethical. ^{1}H-MRS is a valid noninvasive in vivo metabolic imaging technique to study lipid content in tissues such as liver, muscle, and heart [134,135]. MR spectroscopy of the heart and kidney is considered one of the most technically challenging techniques, since it requires the highest level of technical knowledge on MR system hardware and software, as well as development of spectral analysis tools [136]. Automated respiratory motion corrected ^{1}H-MRS of the human heart enabled measurement of intramyocardial and intrarenal triglyceride depositions [137,138]. ^{1}H-MRS is the most powerful method for assessing energy metabolism in heart failure, since it entails in vivo assessment of turnover rates of glucose and fatty acids, rates of oxidative phosphorylation and ATP transfer providing the foundation for the fuel depletion hypothesis in heart failure [139]. The application of ^{1}H-MRS for measuring renal triglyceride content in the kidney is a unique and novel way to study renal lipid metabolism noninvasively.

Dietary effects on ectopic fat storage in heart and kidney

The concept of fatty kidney has been studied in animal models investigating the effects of a 6-month fast food cafeteria diet and standard diet in obese type-2 diabetes minipigs compared with nonobese, nondiabetic minipigs. Type-2 diabetes was induced by combining low-dose streptozotocin (STZ) to cause beta cell damage and frank hyperglycemia in the presence of normal insulin concentrations (noninsulin dependent) in nongenetic outbred pigs [140]. This study showed a close correlation between ectopic lipid in liver and kidney suggesting that NAFLD might constitute a proxy of fatty kidney (Fig. 17.7A). The type-2 diabetes arm had a significantly higher renal cortex triglyceride quantity compared to the fast food and standard diet arm only (Fig. 17.7B), supporting the hypothesis that high caloric intake, obesity, and type-2 diabetes are associated with fatty kidney.

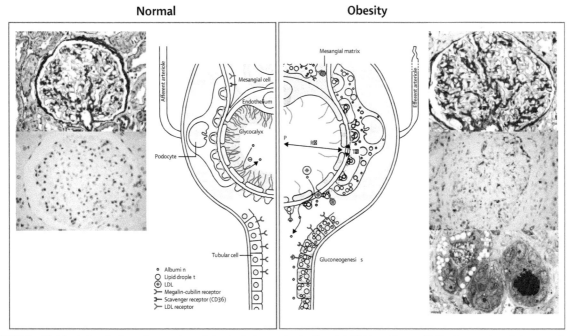

FIGURE 17.6 Histological and schematic overview of structural changes in obesity-related kidney disease. Light microscopic and electron microscopic findings in a healthy individual (left) and in obesity-related nephropathy and diabetic nephropathy (right). Pathological obesity-related changes in the kidney include glomerulomegaly (upper row, right column), lipid droplets in the glomeruli (middle row, right column), and lipid-laden degenerating epithelial cells (bottom row, right column). *Figure adapted from de Vries, A.P. et al. Fatty kidney: emerging role of ectopic lipid in obesity-related renal disease. Lancet Diabetes Endocrinol 2014;2(5):417−426.*

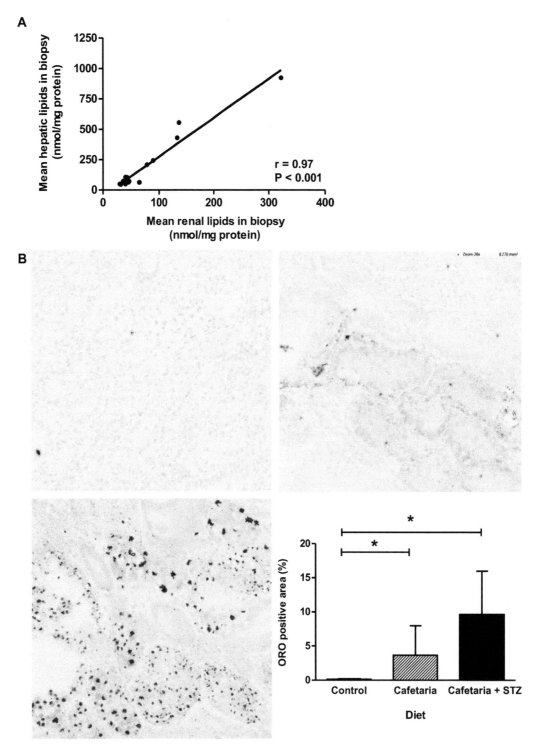

FIGURE 17.7 (A) Correlation between renal and hepatic lipid content after 9 months of diet (n = 14), measured by enzymatic essay. (B) Three representative examples of Oil Red O staining for lipids in kidney biopsies from minipigs on a 9-months control, cafeteria or cafeteria with streptozocin diet. Percentage of Oil Red O stained renal section in the three diet groups (mean ± SEM, N = 5/group). *P < .05 between groups. *Adapted from Jonker, J.T., et al. Metabolic imaging of fatty kidney in diabesity: validation and dietary intervention. Nephrol Dial Transplant 2018;33(2):224−230.*

Technical advances of MR spectroscopy over the last decade have opened a window of opportunity to also explore physiologic processes in the kidney (Fig. 17.8). In addition, it was shown that it is feasible to measure intrarenal triglyceride content of human kidney in vivo using ^{1}H-MRS on 1.5T MRI [138] and 3T MRI [141], and showed good

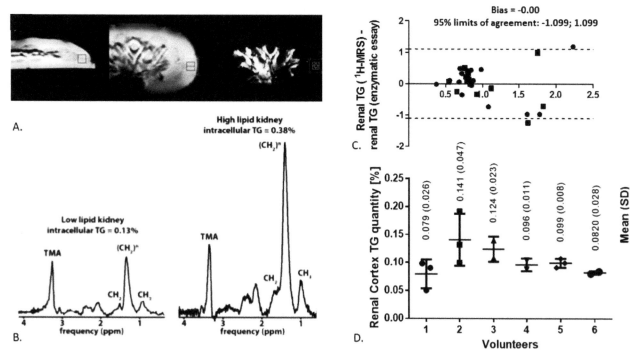

FIGURE 17.8 (A) Placement of the voxel (red box) in the kidney cortex of a porcine kidney on a transverse and coronal survey and Dixon fat image showing renal sinus fat as hyperintense signal. (B) The two kidney MR spectra with a large difference in measured triglyceride quantity. The spectra are scaled to water spectra to allow direct comparison. (C) Bland-Altman plot showing good comparison between renal triglyceride content measured using ^{1}H-MRS and enzymatic assay (unpublished data). (D) Reproducibility of triglyceride quantity (%) in six human volunteers using respiratory motion correction on 3T (unpublished data). *(A, B) Adapted from Jonker, J.T. et al. Metabolic imaging of fatty kidney in diabesity: validation and dietary intervention. Nephrol Dial Transplant 2018;33(2):224–230.*

agreement with gold-standard enzymatic assay [140]. The increased amount of intrarenal triglyceride content relates to dysfunctional adipose tissue expandability [127], where the excess of fat leads to ectopic lipid accumulation in nonadipose tissue, such as the kidney parenchyma, and impairs organ function. The total cortical triglyceride content was measured around 0.12% in healthy, young volunteers and was similar to older studies quantifying the overall lipid content of normal human kidneys [142]. At this moment no studies have been performed that investigate the dietary effects on ectopic lipid in the kidney in humans.

One of the landmark studies by Hall et al. in dogs showed that obesity induced by a beef fat supplement is associated with hypertension and increased GFR and filtration fraction even under conditions of standardized salt intake [143]. Studies on short-term caloric reduction in severely obese type-2 diabetics with stage two CKD and advanced diabetic nephropathy showed that caloric restriction also influenced GFR [144–146], but it remains unknown whether these changes relate to ectopic lipid accumulation in the kidney. For the heart, it was shown that a 3-day (short-term) very low caloric diet induces accumulation of myocardial triglycerides and decreases left ventricular diastolic function, without alterations in myocardial high-energy phosphate metabolism [147]. Moreover, progressive caloric restriction induces a dose-dependent increase in myocardial triglyceride content and hepatic triglyceride content shows a differential response to progressive caloric restriction [148]. This indicates that redistribution of endogenous triglyceride stores is tissue specific, at least in lean healthy men. Another study showed that short-term, high-fat, high-energy diet in healthy men results in major increases in hepatic fat content, whereas it did not influence myocardial triglyceride content or myocardial function [149]. This suggests a differential tissue-specific partitioning of either triglyceride or fatty acids or both between nonadipose organs such as the human heart and liver during different physiological conditions, and possibly also the kidney. Additionally, this study found that high fat intake results in increased intracellular fat in the liver, but not in the heart. No studies in humans thus far have evaluated the physiological variation of intrarenal triglyceride content following dietary intervention.

Effects of glycemic control on ectopic fat storage in heart and kidney

The UKPDS [150] and ADVANCE [151] studies have demonstrated that improved glycemic control reduces microvascular disease and end-stage renal disease. Additionally, treatment of hypertension and proteinuria, in particular using RAAS inhibitors, conveyed a 30% risk reduction for end-stage renal disease [152,153]. However, the incidence of end-stage renal disease by diabetic kidney disease continues to rise despite of these cornerstone therapies, indicating possible involvement of other (nonproteinuric) pathways related to metabolic regulation and hyperfiltration [154]. Novel antihyperglycemic medications, including glucagon-like peptide 1 (GLP1) agonists liraglutide [155], and sodium–glucose transporter 2 (SGLT2) inhibitors canagliflozin [156], dapagliflozin [157], and empagliflozin [158] have demonstrated significant benefits on major renocardiovascular endpoints in diabetic patients. Moreover, preclinical studies have suggested that inflammatory impairment of cardiac microvascular endothelium can be restored by empagliflozin [159]. Furthermore, it has been suggested that single dose treatment with dapagliflozin improves renal cortical oxygenation which might indicate reduced proximal tubule transport workload [160]. Possible explanations for improved renocardiovascular endpoints are improved glycemia, amended blood pressure regulation and reduction of weight, and/or ectopic fat depots such as liver fat [161–163] and cardiac visceral fat [164]. Several studies have investigated whether these novel antihyperglycemic medications affected the metabolic myocardial expenditure in humans in vivo using ^{1}H-MRS. Interestingly, albeit significant reductions were found for liver fat no significant changes were found for epicardial, myocardial fat or myocardial energetics, challenging the thrifty substrate hypothesis [165] for cardiovascular protection by empagliflozin [166,167] and liraglutide [168,169]. Human studies evaluating the effects of these drugs on lipid metabolism in the kidney remain scarce. A recent secondary end-point study of the MAGNA VICTORIA trial showed that 26 weeks of glycemic control resulted in lower levels of renal triglyceride content, in particular for liraglutide [125]. However larger clinical studies are needed to assess whether these changes reflect a true effect of glycemic control on renal steatosis.

Future outlook

Novel developments in preclinical studies

Recent technological advances have provided high-throughput detection of genes (genomics), mRNA (transcriptomics), proteins (proteomics), and metabolites (metabolomics) in a biological sample in a nontargeted and nonbiased way [170]. This provides us with a comprehensive overview of biological processes such as interactions in and between signal transduction pathways leading to a better understanding of the CRS. The multiomics approach in the setting of cardiorenal disease may improve disease management by identifying molecular abnormalities that could help with disease detection and diagnosis, suggesting a link between genotype and phenotype and new therapeutic strategies [171]. Multiomics approach may represent the basis for precision medicine, providing personalized health care. Additionally, the molecular technology known as clustered regularly interspaced palindromic repeats (CRISPR)-associated protein (Cas) could become a promising therapeutic gene-editing tool in the treatment of obesity and diabetes in the far future. The attraction of CRISPR/Cas9 lies in its ability to efficiently edit DNA or modulate gene expression in living eukaryotic cells and organisms. Recently, Wang et al. used the CRISPR-Cas9 gene-editing technology to engineer human white fat so that it displays the properties of brown fat. These brown-fat engineered cells were then transplanted into obese mice. Obese mice receiving the engineered cells showed a sustained improvement in glucose tolerance and insulin sensitivity, as well as increased energy expenditure compared to mice receiving white control fat cells [172]. These data demonstrate the utility of using CRISPR-Cas9 to engineer human white adipocytes to display brown-fat-like phenotype providing a cell-based opportunity to treat obesity and diabetes.

Multiorgan imaging in the management of CRS in obese individuals

Understanding of the pathophysiologic mechanisms involved in CRS is direly needed for diagnosis, prevention, and intervention of obesity-related kidney damage and cardiac dysfunction [173]. Imaging provides the opportunity to capture personalized information on adipose tissue distribution and organ function throughout the human body. Different imaging modalities exist, with specific advantages and disadvantages. Echography is widely available, noninvasive, and enables measurement of thickness of superficial adipose tissue layers (e.g., abdominal, subcutaneous, epicardial, and perirenal), while assessing cardiac function and kidney structure. Limitations of echography are its user-dependency and lack of information on VAT depots as well as limited functional renal parameters. MRI is one of the most versatile in-vivo imaging modalities today that allows for detailed assessment of both cardiac and kidney structures, functions, and metabolism while avoiding the need for ionizing radiation. With regard to fat imaging, MRI combined with ^{1}H-MRS enables assessment of whole body fat distribution and quantification of ectopic fat. Extension with dedicated functional cardiac and renal imaging protocols provides the opportunity for deep phenotyping of cardiometabolic abnormalities [174,175]. For example, the recent cardiorenal MRI study by Breidthardt et al. showed that renal dysfunction in patients with chronic heart failure was not primarily mediated by decreased renal perfusion, but rather by chronic renoparenchymal damage underlying chronic CRS [176]. This study illustrates the use of MRI to study the consequences of metabolic derangements in obesity on various endorgans including heart and kidney in a single scan session [177]. Limitations of MRI are high costs related to scanner infrastructure and lack of standardization. CT enables highly detailed and accurate assessment of fat depots and vascular calcifications, but requires ionizing radiation [178,179]. In addition, the use of iodinated contrast media compromises the application of CT angiography and CT perfusion (including GFR measurement) in CRS patients with eGFR <30 mL/min/1.73 m^2. Metabolic imaging using nuclear medicine techniques such as positron-emission tomography (PET) can be combined with either CT or MRI, and depending on the user tracer-specific metabolic or functional properties can be quantified. Potentially relevant examples of PET in CRS include evaluation of CMD in obesity using radioactive flow tracers [180] or brown adipose tissue localization using radioactive sugar [181]; however, the application of PET for functional and metabolic evaluation of the kidney is still in its infancy. PET is limited by high costs related to the need for dedicated infrastructure (both scanner and radiopharmaceutical related), radiation exposure, and poor resolution.

Personalized approach in the management of obesity-related CRS

Imaging biomarkers can offer a noninvasive approach to more precisely estimate an individual's risk for cardiac and renal dysfunction in obesity. As such, imaging strategies providing detailed structural and functional information of the heart and kidneys can be used for a personalized approach in the management of obesity-related CRS. Implementation of such a multiorgan imaging approach in combination with novel insights from multiomics data could aid in tailoring clinical decisions, for example, living-kidney donation from obese donors, guiding bariatric surgery in high-risk individuals or assessing an obese person's risk for CKD after (oncologic) nephrectomy. Furthermore, it will be necessary to use such novel techniques in designated centers to create therapeutic breakthroughs in obesity-related kidney disease that may have worldwide impact, such as in the evaluation of new pharmacologic agents that may positively affect both the heart and kidneys. In addition, novel methods have been developed to predict total body VAT, without the need for MRI, using individual-specific data such as age, sex, and anthropometric measurements [182]. Such prediction equations might facilitate a wider application of VAT instead of BMI, and as such contribute to the identification of individuals at increased risk of CRS.

Conclusion

Obesity, particularly in the context of metabolic syndrome, plays an important role for the development and progression of the cardiorenal syndrome. Ectopic lipid deposition, reflecting diminished adipose tissue expandability, is suggested to be a better biomarker of obesity-related endorgan dysfunction compared to traditional measures of obesity such as BMI and waist circumference. The interplay of fat compartments and ectopic lipid deposition on renal and cardiac function have been explored in both animal models and humans, evaluating dietary effects and the effects of glycemic control using novel antihyperglycemic medications. For the future, the implementation of novel imaging strategies in combination with insights from multiomics data might contribute to the identification of individuals at increased risk of CRS and a more personalized medicine-based approach in the management of obesity-related chronic kidney disease and cardiovascular disease.

Funding

This study was supported by a grant from the Netherlands CardioVascular Research Initiative: an initiative with support of the Dutch Heart Foundation [CVON2014-11 (RECONNECT, RECONNEXT)].

References

[1] Meguid El Nahas A, Bello AK. Chronic kidney disease: the global challenge. Lancet 2005;365(9456):331−40.

[2] Collaboration NCDRF. Worldwide trends in body-mass index, underweight, overweight, and obesity from 1975 to 2016: a pooled analysis of 2416 population-based measurement studies in 128.9 million children, adolescents, and adults. Lancet 2017;390(10113):2627−42.

[3] Ndumele CE, et al. Obesity and subtypes of incident cardiovascular disease. J Am Heart Assoc 2016;5(8).

[4] Webster AC, et al. Chronic kidney disease. Lancet 2017;389(10075):1238–52.

[5] Neeland IJ, et al. Visceral and ectopic fat, atherosclerosis, and cardiometabolic disease: a position statement. Lancet Diab Endocrinol 2019;7(9):715–25.

[6] Ejerblad E, et al. Obesity and risk for chronic renal failure. J Am Soc Nephrol 2006;17(6):1695–702.

[7] Praga M, Morales E. Obesity, proteinuria and progression of renal failure. Curr Opin Nephrol Hypertens 2006;15(5):481–6.

[8] Kenchaiah S, et al. Obesity and the risk of heart failure. N Engl J Med 2002;347(5):305–13.

[9] Stenvinkel P, Zoccali C, Ikizler TA. Obesity in CKD–what should nephrologists know? J Am Soc Nephrol 2013;24(11):1727–36.

[10] Ronco C, et al. Cardiorenal syndromes: an executive summary from the consensus conference of the Acute Dialysis Quality Initiative (ADQI). Contrib Nephrol 2010;165:54–67.

[11] Prasad GV. Metabolic syndrome and chronic kidney disease: current status and future directions. World J Nephrol 2014;3(4):210–9.

[12] Mentz RJ, et al. Noncardiac comorbidities in heart failure with reduced versus preserved ejection fraction. J Am Coll Cardiol 2014;64(21):2281–93.

[13] Chen J, et al. The metabolic syndrome and chronic kidney disease in U.S. adults. Ann Intern Med 2004;140(3):167–74.

[14] Klop B, Elte JW, Cabezas MC. Dyslipidemia in obesity: mechanisms and potential targets. Nutrients 2013;5(4):1218–40.

[15] Wang H, Peng DQ. New insights into the mechanism of low high-density lipoprotein cholesterol in obesity. Lipids Health Dis 2011;10:176.

[16] Chapman MJ, Sposito AC. Hypertension and dyslipidaemia in obesity and insulin resistance: pathophysiology, impact on atherosclerotic disease and pharmacotherapy. Pharmacol Ther 2008;117(3):354–73.

[17] Edwards MS, et al. Renovascular disease and the risk of adverse coronary events in the elderly: a prospective, population-based study. Arch Intern Med 2005;165(2):207–13.

[18] Trayhurn P, Wang B, Wood IS. Hypoxia and the endocrine and signalling role of white adipose tissue. Arch Physiol Biochem 2008;114(4):267–76.

[19] Vila E, Salaices M. Cytokines and vascular reactivity in resistance arteries. Am J Physiol Heart Circ Physiol 2005;288(3):H1016–21.

[20] Virdis A, Schiffrin EL. Vascular inflammation: a role in vascular disease in hypertension? Curr Opin Nephrol Hypertens 2003;12(2):181–7.

[21] Bajaj NS, et al. Coronary microvascular dysfunction, left ventricular remodeling, and clinical outcomes in patients with chronic kidney impairment. Circulation 2020;141(1):21–33.

[22] Nelson AJ, et al. End-stage renal failure is associated with impaired coronary microvascular function. Coron Artery Dis 2019;30(7):520–7.

[23] Charytan DM, et al. Coronary flow reserve is predictive of the risk of cardiovascular death regardless of chronic kidney disease stage. Kidney Int 2018;93(2):501–9.

[24] Camici PG, et al. Coronary microvascular dysfunction in hypertrophy and heart failure. Cardiovasc Res 2020;116(4):806–16.

[25] Fliser D, et al. The dysfunctional endothelium in CKD and in cardiovascular disease: mapping the origin(s) of cardiovascular problems in CKD and of kidney disease in cardiovascular conditions for a research agenda. Kidney Int Suppl 2011;1(1):6–9. 2011.

[26] Prommer HU, et al. Chronic kidney disease induces a systemic microangiopathy, tissue hypoxia and dysfunctional angiogenesis. Sci Rep 2018;8(1):5317.

[27] Charytan DM, et al. Increased concentration of circulating angiogenesis and nitric oxide inhibitors induces endothelial to mesenchymal transition and myocardial fibrosis in patients with chronic kidney disease. Int J Cardiol 2014;176(1):99–109.

[28] Cachofeiro V, et al. Oxidative stress and inflammation, a link between chronic kidney disease and cardiovascular disease. Kidney Int Suppl 2008;(111):S4–9.

[29] Paulus WJ, Tschope C. A novel paradigm for heart failure with preserved ejection fraction: comorbidities drive myocardial dysfunction and remodeling through coronary microvascular endothelial inflammation. J Am Coll Cardiol 2013;62(4):263–71.

[30] Ohanyan V, et al. A chicken and egg conundrum: coronary microvascular dysfunction and heart failure with preserved ejection fraction. Am J Physiol Heart Circ Physiol 2018;314(6):H1262–3.

[31] Borlaug BA, Paulus WJ. Heart failure with preserved ejection fraction: pathophysiology, diagnosis, and treatment. Eur Heart J 2011;32(6):670–9.

[32] Esler M, et al. Mechanisms of sympathetic activation in obesity-related hypertension. Hypertension 2006;48(5):787–96.

[33] Guarino D, et al. The role of the autonomic nervous system in the pathophysiology of obesity. Front Physiol 2017;8:665.

[34] Grassi G, et al. Sympathetic activation in obese normotensive subjects. Hypertension 1995;25(4 Pt 1):560–3.

[35] Kotsis VT, et al. Impact of obesity in intima media thickness of carotid arteries. Obesity 2006;14(10):1708–15.

[36] Izquierdo AG, et al. Leptin, obesity, and leptin resistance: where are we 25 Years later? Nutrients 2019;11(11).

[37] Farr OM, Gavrieli A, Mantzoros CS. Leptin applications in 2015: what have we learned about leptin and obesity? Curr Opin Endocrinol Diabetes Obes 2015;22(5):353–9.

[38] Krop M, et al. Renin and prorenin disappearance in humans post-nephrectomy: evidence for binding? Front Biosci 2008;13:3931–9.

[39] Briet M, Schiffrin EL. Aldosterone: effects on the kidney and cardiovascular system. Nat Rev Nephrol 2010;6(5):261–73.

[40] Nakagawa T, et al. A causal role for uric acid in fructose-induced metabolic syndrome. Am J Physiol Ren Physiol 2006;290(3):F625–31.

[41] Lanaspa MA, et al. Uric acid induces hepatic steatosis by generation of mitochondrial oxidative stress: potential role in fructose-dependent and -independent fatty liver. J Biol Chem 2012;287(48):40732–44.

[42] Khosla UM, et al. Hyperuricemia induces endothelial dysfunction. Kidney Int 2005;67(5):1739–42.

[43] Johnson RJ, et al. Is there a pathogenetic role for uric acid in hypertension and cardiovascular and renal disease? Hypertension 2003;41(6):1183–90.

[44] Mazzali M, et al. Elevated uric acid increases blood pressure in the rat by a novel crystal-independent mechanism. Hypertension 2001;38(5):1101−6.

[45] Kanbay M, et al. Uric acid and pentraxin-3 levels are independently associated with coronary artery disease risk in patients with stage 2 and 3 kidney disease. Am J Nephrol 2011;33(4):325−31.

[46] Kanbay M, et al. Serum uric acid level and endothelial dysfunction in patients with nondiabetic chronic kidney disease. Am J Nephrol 2011;33(4):298−304.

[47] Anker SD, et al. Uric acid and survival in chronic heart failure: validation and application in metabolic, functional, and hemodynamic staging. Circulation 2003;107(15):1991−7.

[48] Sharma G, et al. Hyperuricemia, urate-lowering therapy, and kidney outcomes: a systematic review and meta-analysis. Ther Adv Musculoskelet Dis 2021;13. 1759720X211016661.

[49] Rubattu S, et al. Pathogenesis of chronic cardiorenal syndrome: is there a role for oxidative stress? Int J Mol Sci 2013;14(11):23011−32.

[50] Hewitson TD, Holt SG, Smith ER. Animal models to study links between cardiovascular disease and renal failure and their relevance to human pathology. Front Immunol 2015;6:465.

[51] Alex L, et al. Characterization of a mouse model of obesity-related fibrotic cardiomyopathy that recapitulates features of human heart failure with preserved ejection fraction. Am J Physiol Heart Circ Physiol 2018;315(4):H934−49.

[52] Brezniceanu ML, et al. Attenuation of interstitial fibrosis and tubular apoptosis in db/db transgenic mice overexpressing catalase in renal proximal tubular cells. Diabetes 2008;57(2):451−9.

[53] Bivona BJ, Park S, Harrison-Bernard LM. Glomerular filtration rate determinations in conscious type II diabetic mice. Am J Physiol Ren Physiol 2011;300(3):F618−25.

[54] Christoffersen C, et al. Cardiac lipid accumulation associated with diastolic dysfunction in obese mice. Endocrinology 2003;144(8):3483−90.

[55] Marsh SA, et al. Cardiovascular dysfunction in Zucker obese and Zucker diabetic fatty rats: role of hydronephrosis. Am J Physiol Heart Circ Physiol 2007;293(1):H292−8.

[56] Baynes J, Murray DB. Cardiac and renal function are progressively impaired with aging in Zucker diabetic fatty type II diabetic rats. Oxid Med Cell Longev 2009;2(5):328−34.

[57] Lum-Naihe K, et al. Cardiovascular disease progression in female Zucker Diabetic Fatty rats occurs via unique mechanisms compared to males. Sci Rep 2017;7(1):17823.

[58] Nguyen ITN, et al. Both male and female obese ZSF1 rats develop cardiac dysfunction in obesity-induced heart failure with preserved ejection fraction. PLoS One 2020;15(5):e0232399.

[59] Bilan VP, et al. Diabetic nephropathy and long-term treatment effects of rosiglitazone and enalapril in obese ZSF1 rats. J Endocrinol 2011;210(3):293−308.

[60] van Dijk CG, et al. Distinct endothelial cell responses in the heart and kidney microvasculature characterize the progression of heart failure with preserved ejection fraction in the obese ZSF1 rat with cardiorenal metabolic syndrome. Circ Heart Fail 2016;9(4):e002760.

[61] Murase T, et al. Cardiac remodeling and diastolic dysfunction in DahlS.Z-Lepr(fa)/Lepr(fa) rats: a new animal model of metabolic syndrome. Hypertens Res 2012;35(2):186−93.

[62] McPherson KC, et al. Altered renal hemodynamics is associated with glomerular lipid accumulation in obese Dahl salt-sensitive leptin receptor mutant rats. Am J Physiol Ren Physiol 2020;318(4):F911−21.

[63] Sorop O, et al. Multiple common comorbidities produce left ventricular diastolic dysfunction associated with coronary microvascular dysfunction, oxidative stress, and myocardial stiffening. Cardiovasc Res 2018;114(7):954−64.

[64] Sharp 3rd TE, et al. Novel gottingen miniswine model of heart failure with preserved ejection fraction integrating multiple comorbidities. JACC Basic Transl Sci 2021;6(2):154−70.

[65] Wang B, Chandrasekera PC, Pippin JJ. Leptin- and leptin receptor-deficient rodent models: relevance for human type 2 diabetes. Curr Diabetes Rev 2014;10(2):131−45.

[66] Lindstrom P. The physiology of obese-hyperglycemic mice [ob/ob mice]. Sci World J 2007;7:666−85.

[67] Westergren HU, et al. Impaired coronary and renal vascular function in spontaneously type 2 diabetic leptin-deficient mice. PLoS One 2015;10(6):e0130648.

[68] Sharma K, McCue P, Dunn SR. Diabetic kidney disease in the db/db mouse. Am J Physiol Ren Physiol 2003;284(6):F1138−44.

[69] Della-Fera MA, et al. Sensitivity of ob/ob mice to leptin-induced adipose tissue apoptosis. Obes Res 2005;13(9):1540−7.

[70] Koletsky S. Animal model: obese hypertensive rat. Am J Pathol 1975;81(2):463−6.

[71] Griffen SC, Wang J, German MS. A genetic defect in beta-cell gene expression segregates independently from the fa locus in the ZDF rat. Diabetes 2001;50(1):63−8.

[72] Unger RH, Orci L. Diseases of liporegulation: new perspective on obesity and related disorders. Faseb J 2001;15(2):312−21.

[73] Hattori T, et al. Characterization of a new animal model of metabolic syndrome: the DahlS.Z-Lepr(fa)/Lepr(fa) rat. Nutr Diabetes 2011;1:e1.

[74] Tofovic SP, Jackson EK. Rat models of the metabolic syndrome. Methods Mol Med 2003;86:29−46.

[75] Tofovic SP, et al. Renal function and structure in diabetic, hypertensive, obese ZDFxSHHF-hybrid rats. Ren Fail 2000;22(4):387−406.

[76] Valero-Munoz M, Backman W, Sam F. Murine models of heart failure with preserved ejection fraction: a "fishing expedition". JACC Basic Transl Sci 2017;2(6):770−89.

[77] Carroll JF, Tyagi SC. Extracellular matrix remodeling in the heart of the homocysteinemic obese rabbit. Am J Hypertens 2005;18(5 Pt 1):692−8.

[78] Vasan RS. Cardiac function and obesity. Heart 2003;89(10):1127−9.

[79] Cavalera M, Wang J, Frangogiannis NG. Obesity, metabolic dysfunction, and cardiac fibrosis: pathophysiological pathways, molecular mechanisms, and therapeutic opportunities. Transl Res 2014;164(4):323−35.

[80] Montani JP, et al. Ectopic fat storage in heart, blood vessels and kidneys in the pathogenesis of cardiovascular diseases. Int J Obes Relat Metab Disord 2004;28(Suppl. 4):S58−65.

[81] Zhou YT, et al. Lipotoxic heart disease in obese rats: implications for human obesity. Proc Natl Acad Sci U S A 2000;97(4):1784−9.

[82] Ramirez E, et al. Eplerenone attenuated cardiac steatosis, apoptosis and diastolic dysfunction in experimental type-II diabetes. Cardiovasc Diabetol 2013;12:172.

[83] Wu CK, et al. Myocardial adipose deposition and the development of heart failure with preserved ejection fraction. Eur J Heart Fail 2020;22(3):445−54.

[84] Szczepaniak LS, et al. Myocardial triglycerides and systolic function in humans: in vivo evaluation by localized proton spectroscopy and cardiac imaging. Magn Reson Med 2003;49(3):417−23.

[85] Schauer A, et al. Sacubitril/valsartan improves diastolic function but not skeletal muscle function in a rat model of HFpEF. Int J Mol Sci 2021;22(7).

[86] Zhang T, et al. Interaction between adipocytes and high-density lipoprotein:new insights into the mechanism of obesity-induced dyslipidemia and atherosclerosis. Lipids Health Dis 2019;18(1):223.

[87] Fenzl A, Kiefer FW. Brown adipose tissue and thermogenesis. Horm Mol Biol Clin Invest 2014;19(1):25−37.

[88] Conceicao G, et al. Fat quality matters: distinct proteomic signatures between lean and obese cardiac visceral adipose tissue underlie its differential myocardial impact. Cell Physiol Biochem 2020;54(3):384−400.

[89] Mosconi E, et al. Investigation of adipose tissues in Zucker rats using in vivo and ex vivo magnetic resonance spectroscopy. J Lipid Res 2011;52(2):330−6.

[90] Hall JE, et al. Obesity-induced hypertension: interaction of neurohumoral and renal mechanisms. Circ Res 2015;116(6):991−1006.

[91] Drazner MH. The progression of hypertensive heart disease. Circulation 2011;123(3):327−34.

[92] Hirohama D, Fujita T. Evaluation of the pathophysiological mechanisms of salt-sensitive hypertension. Hypertens Res 2019;42(12):1848−57.

[93] Mascali A, et al. Obesity and kidney disease: beyond the hyperfiltration. Int J Immunopathol Pharmacol 2016;29(3):354−63.

[94] Su Z, et al. Longitudinal changes in measured glomerular filtration rate, renal fibrosis and biomarkers in a rat model of type 2 diabetic nephropathy. Am J Nephrol 2016;44(5):339−53.

[95] Franssen C, et al. Myocardial microvascular inflammatory endothelial activation in heart failure with preserved ejection fraction. JACC Heart Fail 2016;4(4):312−24.

[96] Ter Maaten JM, et al. Connecting heart failure with preserved ejection fraction and renal dysfunction: the role of endothelial dysfunction and inflammation. Eur J Heart Fail 2016;18(6):588−98.

[97] Damman K, Testani JM. The kidney in heart failure: an update. Eur Heart J 2015;36(23):1437−44.

[98] Beale AL, et al. Sex differences in cardiovascular pathophysiology: why women are overrepresented in heart failure with preserved ejection fraction. Circulation 2018;138(2):198−205.

[99] Chan V, et al. Cardiovascular changes during maturation and ageing in male and female spontaneously hypertensive rats. J Cardiovasc Pharmacol 2011;57(4):469−78.

[100] Litwin SE, et al. Gender differences in postinfarction left ventricular remodeling. Cardiology 1999;91(3):173−83.

[101] Corsetti JP, et al. Effect of dietary fat on the development of non-insulin dependent diabetes mellitus in obese Zucker diabetic fatty male and female rats. Atherosclerosis 2000;148(2):231−41.

[102] Gustavsson C, et al. Sex-dependent hepatic transcripts and metabolites in the development of glucose intolerance and insulin resistance in Zucker diabetic fatty rats. J Mol Endocrinol 2011;47(2):129−43.

[103] Rothman KJ. BMI-related errors in the measurement of obesity. Int J Obes 2008;32(Suppl. 3):S56−9.

[104] Elsayed EF, et al. Waist-to-hip ratio, body mass index, and subsequent kidney disease and death. Am J Kidney Dis 2008;52(1):29−38.

[105] Pinto-Sietsma SJ, et al. A central body fat distribution is related to renal function impairment, even in lean subjects. Am J Kidney Dis 2003;41(4):733−41.

[106] Fox CS, et al. Abdominal visceral and subcutaneous adipose tissue compartments: association with metabolic risk factors in the Framingham Heart Study. Circulation 2007;116(1):39−48.

[107] Foster MC, et al. Association of subcutaneous and visceral adiposity with albuminuria: the Framingham Heart Study. Obesity 2011;19(6):1284−9.

[108] Rosenquist KJ, et al. Visceral and subcutaneous fat quality and cardiometabolic risk. JACC Cardiovasc Imag 2013;6(7):762−71.

[109] Young JA, et al. Association of visceral and subcutaneous adiposity with kidney function. Clin J Am Soc Nephrol 2008;3(6):1786−91.

[110] Kwakernaak AJ, et al. Central body fat distribution associates with unfavorable renal hemodynamics independent of body mass index. J Am Soc Nephrol 2013;24(6):987−94.

[111] Fox CS, et al. Pericardial fat, intrathoracic fat, and measures of left ventricular structure and function: the Framingham Heart Study. Circulation 2009;119(12):1586−91.

[112] van Hout MJP, et al. The impact of visceral and general obesity on vascular and left ventricular function and geometry: a cross-sectional magnetic resonance imaging study of the UK Biobank. Eur Heart J Cardiovasc Imag 2020;21(3):273−81.

[113] Karlsson T, et al. Contribution of genetics to visceral adiposity and its relation to cardiovascular and metabolic disease. Nat Med 2019;25(9):1390−5.

[114] Oikonomou EK, Antoniades C. The role of adipose tissue in cardiovascular health and disease. Nat Rev Cardiol 2019;16(2):83−99.

[115] Gil-Ortega M, et al. Regional differences in perivascular adipose tissue impacting vascular homeostasis. Trends Endocrinol Metab 2015;26(7):367–75.

[116] Mancio J, et al. Epicardial adipose tissue volume assessed by computed tomography and coronary artery disease: a systematic review and meta-analysis. Eur Heart J Cardiovasc Imag 2018;19(5):490–7.

[117] Heckbert SR, et al. Pericardial fat volume and incident atrial fibrillation in the multi-ethnic study of atherosclerosis and jackson heart study. Obesity 2017;25(6):1115–21.

[118] Siegel-Axel DI, Haring HU. Perivascular adipose tissue: an unique fat compartment relevant for the cardiometabolic syndrome. Rev Endocr Metab Disord 2016;17(1):51–60.

[119] Jespersen NZ, et al. Heterogeneity in the perirenal region of humans suggests presence of dormant brown adipose tissue that contains brown fat precursor cells. Mol Metab 2019;24:30–43.

[120] Wagner R, et al. Exercise-induced albuminuria is associated with perivascular renal sinus fat in individuals at increased risk of type 2 diabetes. Diabetologia 2012;55(7):2054–8.

[121] Notohamiprodjo M, et al. Renal and renal sinus fat volumes as quantified by magnetic resonance imaging in subjects with prediabetes, diabetes, and normal glucose tolerance. PLoS One 2020;15(2):e0216635.

[122] Lin L, et al. Renal sinus fat volume in type 2 diabetes mellitus is associated with glycated hemoglobin and metabolic risk factors. J Diabet Complicat 2021:107973.

[123] Zelicha H, et al. Changes of renal sinus fat and renal parenchymal fat during an 18-month randomized weight loss trial. Clin Nutr 2018;37(4):1145–53.

[124] Murakami Y, et al. Renal sinus fat volume on computed tomography in middle-aged patients at risk for cardiovascular disease and its association with coronary artery calcification. Atherosclerosis 2016;246:374–81.

[125] Dekkers IA, et al. The effect of glycemic control on renal triglyceride content assessed by proton spectroscopy in patients with type 2 diabetes mellitus: a single-center parallel-group trial. J Ren Nutr 2021;31(6):611–9.

[126] Dekkers IA, et al. Reproducibility of native T1 mapping for renal tissue characterization at 3T. J Magn Reson Imag 2019;49(2):588–96.

[127] Despres JP, Lemieux I. Abdominal obesity and metabolic syndrome. Nature 2006;444(7121):881–7.

[128] Mantovani A, et al. Nonalcoholic fatty liver disease increases risk of incident chronic kidney disease: a systematic review and meta-analysis. Metabolism 2018;79:64–76.

[129] Pan LL, et al. Intrahepatic triglyceride content is independently associated with chronic kidney disease in obese adults: a cross-sectional study. Metabolism 2015;64(9):1077–85.

[130] Dekkers IA, et al. The separate contributions of visceral fat and liver fat to chronic kidney disease-related renal outcomes. J Ren Nutr 2020;30(4):286–95.

[131] Park S, et al. Causal effects from non-alcoholic fatty liver disease on kidney function: a Mendelian randomization study. Liver Int 2022;42(2):412–8.

[132] de Vries AP, et al. Fatty kidney: emerging role of ectopic lipid in obesity-related renal disease. Lancet Diabetes Endocrinol 2014;2(5):417–26.

[133] Bobulescu IA, et al. Triglycerides in the human kidney cortex: relationship with body size. PLoS One 2014;9(8):e101285.

[134] Szczepaniak LS, et al. Magnetic resonance spectroscopy to measure hepatic triglyceride content: prevalence of hepatic steatosis in the general population. Am J Physiol Endocrinol Metab 2005;288(2):E462–8.

[135] Szczepaniak LS, et al. Measurement of intracellular triglyceride stores by H spectroscopy: validation in vivo. Am J Physiol 1999;276(5):E977–89.

[136] Bizino MB, Hammer S, Lamb HJ. Metabolic imaging of the human heart: clinical application of magnetic resonance spectroscopy. Heart 2014;100(11):881–90.

[137] van der Meer RW, et al. Metabolic imaging of myocardial triglyceride content: reproducibility of 1H MR spectroscopy with respiratory navigator gating in volunteers. Radiology 2007;245(1):251–7.

[138] Hammer S, et al. Metabolic imaging of human kidney triglyceride content: reproducibility of proton magnetic resonance spectroscopy. PLoS One 2013;8(4):e62209.

[139] Neubauer S. The failing heart–an engine out of fuel. N Engl J Med 2007;356(11):1140–51.

[140] Jonker JT, et al. Metabolic imaging of fatty kidney in diabesity: validation and dietary intervention. Nephrol Dial Transplant 2018;33(2):224–30.

[141] Dekkers IA, et al. (1) H-MRS for the assessment of renal triglyceride content in humans at 3T: a primer and reproducibility study. J Magn Reson Imag 2018;48(2):507–13.

[142] Bobulescu IA. Renal lipid metabolism and lipotoxicity. Curr Opin Nephrol Hypertens 2010;19(4):393–402.

[143] Hall JE, et al. Obesity-induced hypertension. Renal function and systemic hemodynamics. Hypertension 1993;22(3):292–9.

[144] Ruggenenti P, et al. Renal and systemic effects of calorie restriction in patients with type 2 diabetes with abdominal obesity: a randomized controlled trial. Diabetes 2017;66(1):75–86.

[145] Giordani I, et al. Acute caloric restriction improves glomerular filtration rate in patients with morbid obesity and type 2 diabetes. Diabetes Metab 2014;40(2):158–60.

[146] Friedman AN, et al. Short-term changes after a weight reduction intervention in advanced diabetic nephropathy. Clin J Am Soc Nephrol 2013;8(11):1892–8.

[147] van der Meer RW, et al. Short-term caloric restriction induces accumulation of myocardial triglycerides and decreases left ventricular diastolic function in healthy subjects. Diabetes 2007;56(12):2849–53.

[148] Hammer S, et al. Progressive caloric restriction induces dose-dependent changes in myocardial triglyceride content and diastolic function in healthy men. J Clin Endocrinol Metab 2008;93(2):497−503.

[149] van der Meer RW, et al. Effects of short-term high-fat, high-energy diet on hepatic and myocardial triglyceride content in healthy men. J Clin Endocrinol Metab 2008;93(7):2702−8.

[150] Holman RR, et al. 10-year follow-up of intensive glucose control in type 2 diabetes. N Engl J Med 2008;359(15):1577−89.

[151] Perkovic V, et al. Intensive glucose control improves kidney outcomes in patients with type 2 diabetes. Kidney Int 2013;83(3):517−23.

[152] Brenner BM, et al. Effects of losartan on renal and cardiovascular outcomes in patients with type 2 diabetes and nephropathy. N Engl J Med 2001;345(12):861−9.

[153] Lewis EJ, et al. Renoprotective effect of the angiotensin-receptor antagonist irbesartan in patients with nephropathy due to type 2 diabetes. N Engl J Med 2001;345(12):851−60.

[154] Porrini E, et al. Non-proteinuric pathways in loss of renal function in patients with type 2 diabetes. Lancet Diabetes Endocrinol 2015;3(5):382−91.

[155] Mann JFE, et al. Liraglutide and renal outcomes in type 2 diabetes. N Engl J Med 2017;377(9):839−48.

[156] Neal B, et al. Canagliflozin and cardiovascular and renal events in type 2 diabetes. N Engl J Med 2017;377(7):644−57.

[157] Heerspink HJL, et al. Dapagliflozin in patients with chronic kidney disease. N Engl J Med 2020;383(15):1436−46.

[158] Packer M, et al. Cardiovascular and renal outcomes with empagliflozin in heart failure. N Engl J Med 2020;383(15):1413−24.

[159] Juni RP, et al. Cardiac microvascular endothelial enhancement of cardiomyocyte function is impaired by inflammation and restored by empagliflozin. JACC Basic Transl Sci 2019;4(5):575−91.

[160] Laursen JC, et al. Acute effects of dapagliflozin on renal oxygenation and perfusion in type 1 diabetes with albuminuria: a randomised, double-blind, placebo-controlled crossover trial. EClinicalMedicine 2021;37(100895).

[161] Arase Y, et al. Effect of sodium glucose Co-transporter 2 inhibitors on liver fat mass and body composition in patients with nonalcoholic fatty liver disease and type 2 diabetes mellitus. Clin Drug Invest 2019;39(7):631−41.

[162] Cusi K, et al. Effect of canagliflozin treatment on hepatic triglyceride content and glucose metabolism in patients with type 2 diabetes. Diabetes Obes Metabol 2019;21(4):812−21.

[163] Cuthbertson DJ, et al. Improved glycaemia correlates with liver fat reduction in obese, type 2 diabetes, patients given glucagon-like peptide-1 (GLP-1) receptor agonists. PLoS One 2012;7(12):e50117.

[164] Iacobellis G, et al. Liraglutide causes large and rapid epicardial fat reduction. Obesity 2017;25(2):311−6.

[165] Ferrannini E, Mark M, Mayoux E. CV protection in the EMPA-REG outcome trial: a "thrifty substrate" hypothesis. Diabetes Care 2016;39(7):1108−14.

[166] Gaborit B, et al. Effect of empagliflozin on ectopic fat stores and myocardial energetics in type 2 diabetes: the EMPACEF study. Cardiovasc Diabetol 2021;20(1):57.

[167] Hiruma S, et al. A prospective randomized study comparing effects of empagliflozin to sitagliptin on cardiac fat accumulation, cardiac function, and cardiac metabolism in patients with early-stage type 2 diabetes: the ASSET study. Cardiovasc Diabetol 2021;20(1):32.

[168] Paiman EHM, et al. Effect of liraglutide on cardiovascular function and myocardial tissue characteristics in type 2 diabetes patients of south asian descent living in The Netherlands: a double-blind, randomized, placebo-controlled trial. J Magn Reson Imag 2020;51(6):1679−88.

[169] Bizino MB, et al. Placebo-controlled randomised trial with liraglutide on magnetic resonance endpoints in individuals with type 2 diabetes: a pre-specified secondary study on ectopic fat accumulation. Diabetologia 2020;63(1):65−74.

[170] Sun YV, Hu YJ. Integrative analysis of multi-omics data for discovery and functional studies of complex human diseases. Adv Genet 2016;93:147−90.

[171] Virzi GM, et al. Multi-omics approach: new potential key mechanisms implicated in cardiorenal syndromes. Cardiorenal Med 2019;9(4):201−11.

[172] Wang CH, et al. CRISPR-engineered human brown-like adipocytes prevent diet-induced obesity and ameliorate metabolic syndrome in mice. Sci Transl Med 2020;12(558).

[173] Lin L, Zhou X, Dekkers IA, Lamb HJ. Cardiorenal syndrome: emerging role of medical imaging for clinical diagnosis and management. J Personalized Med 2021;11(8):734.

[174] Paiman EHM, et al. Phenotyping diabetic cardiomyopathy in Europeans and south asians. Cardiovasc Diabetol 2019;18(1):133.

[175] Pursnani A, Prasad PV. Science to practice: can functional MR imaging Be useful in the evaluation of cardiorenal syndrome? Radiology 2018;286(1):1−3.

[176] Breidthardt T, et al. The pathophysiology of the chronic cardiorenal syndrome: a magnetic resonance imaging study. Eur Radiol 2015;25(6):1684−91.

[177] Bizino MB, et al. MR of multi-organ involvement in the metabolic syndrome. Magn Reson Imag Clin N Am 2015;23(1):41−58.

[178] van der Molen AJ, et al. Post-contrast acute kidney injury - Part 1: definition, clinical features, incidence, role of contrast medium and risk factors : recommendations for updated ESUR Contrast Medium Safety Committee guidelines. Eur Radiol 2018;28(7):2845−55.

[179] van der Molen AJ, et al. Post-contrast acute kidney injury. Part 2: risk stratification, role of hydration and other prophylactic measures, patients taking metformin and chronic dialysis patients : recommendations for updated ESUR Contrast Medium Safety Committee guidelines. Eur Radiol 2018;28(7):2856−69.

[180] Bajaj NS, et al. Coronary microvascular dysfunction and cardiovascular risk in obese patients. J Am Coll Cardiol 2018;72(7):707−17.

[181] Leitner BP, et al. Mapping of human brown adipose tissue in lean and obese young men. Proc Natl Acad Sci U S A 2017;114(32):8649−54.

[182] Lin L, et al. Novel artificial neural network and linear regression based equation for estimating visceral adipose tissue volume. Clin Nutr 2020;39(10):3182−8.

Chapter 18

Obesity and asthma

Daisuke Murakami, Yuichi Saito and Ryota Higuchi

Department of Otorhinolaryngology, Graduate School of Medical Sciences, Kyushu University, Fukuoka, Japan

Obesity is a major public health problem. Obesity is a state not only of having excess bodyweight but also of excessive accumulation of body fat. It is the cause of many diseases related to metabolic syndrome including lifestyle-related diseases such as diabetes, dyslipidemia, hypertension, and cardiovascular disease. Obesity is greatly involved in the pathophysiology of asthma in both children and adults. Obesity is related to an increased risk of asthma; comorbid obesity is related to worse symptom control and quality of life, and more severe disease in patients with asthma. Obesity also increases resistance to treatment. Asthma associated with obesity is considered a complex syndrome involving several different pathologies. This chapter first describes the background genetic factors related to obesity that affects bronchial asthma and how obesity affects respiratory function. Second, we describe the clinical features and findings of obesity-related asthma in epidemiological studies to date. Finally, we describe the current understanding of its pathogenesis.

Physical function: lung function and genetic factors

Physical effects and genetic background of obesity and asthma

Obesity causes significant changes in normal lung physiology and leads to airway hyperresponsiveness due to excessive accumulation of fat in the thoracic and abdominal cavities. Furthermore, both asthma and obesity have a considerable hereditary component. Therefore, it is thought that the pathophysiology of asthma and obesity changes depending on racial and genetic factors.

Obesity and respiratory function

Obesity affects respiratory function in many ways, including decreased thoracic compliance, increased strain on respiratory muscles, unequal ventilation blood flow, increased airway resistance, and increased airway hyperresponsiveness [1].

In respiratory function tests, total lung capacity (TLC), vital capacity (VC), and tidal volume (TV) decrease directly with increasing body mass index (BMI). Furthermore, within the lung volume fraction, both functional residual capacity (FRC) and expiratory reserve volume (ERV) decrease directly with increasing BMI as shown in Figs. 18.1 and 18.2. This may be due to the presence of obesity, which causes diaphragmatic elevation due to intraabdominal fat and increased chest wall mass. Furthermore, the decrease in lung compliance is caused by peripheral airway obstruction due to decreased lung

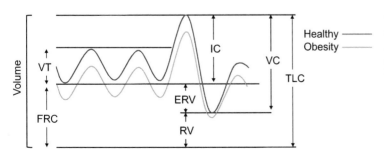

FIGURE 18.1 Mechanical effects of lung compression in obese individuals compared with normal weight individuals. *ERV*, expiratory reserve volume; *FRC*, functional residual capacity; *IC*, inspiratory capacity; *RV*, residual volume; *TLC*, total lung capacity; *VC*, vital capacity; *VT*, tidal volume.

Visceral and Ectopic Fat. https://doi.org/10.1016/B978-0-12-822186-0.00012-2

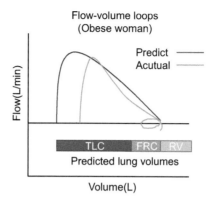

FIGURE 18.2 Expiratory flow volume curve of an obese woman. *FRC*, functional residual capacity; *RV*, residual volume; *TLC*, total lung capacity.

volume, and the pressure and volume curves of the respiratory system deviate to the lower right due to decreased thorax compliance and lung compliance. Moreover, the FRC, which is the lung capacity at the point of equilibrium between thorax elastic expansion pressure and lung elastic contraction pressure, is decreased.

Expiratory flow, forced expiratory volume in one second (FEV1), and forced vital capacity (FVC) also decrease with increasing BMI (Fig. 18.3 shows normal spirometry). Forced expiratory volume percentage in one second (FEV1%) is often maintained, but when the FVC is substantially reduced, it will typically increase. Lower FEV1 and FVC have been associated with obesity, especially abdominal obesity. Regarding ventilatory blood flow ratio, in severe obesity, the FRC falls below the closing capacity, and when bronchi become obstructed during resting expiration, an inequality in ventilatory blood flow occurs [2]. A decrease in ventilation volume causes a shortening and reduction of airway smooth muscle, and a decrease in muscle tone narrows the peripheral airway diameter and increases airway hyperresponsiveness. Furthermore, decreased physical activity, chronic inflammation, complications (sleep apnea syndrome, and gastroesophageal reflux), and abnormal secretion of adipokines have been postulated to be involved.

Airway hyperresponsiveness is also a feature of asthma, and a prospective cohort study investigating the relationship between obesity and airway hyperresponsiveness reported that the risk of airway hyperresponsiveness increased with BMI and that weight gain was a risk factor for developing airway hyperresponsiveness. Smaller studies have failed to find a relationship, which may be due to small sample size and interpatient population differences [3,4,5].

Racial differences

In the field of obesity research, the differences in the characteristics of obesity between Asian and Western populations are well known. Compared with Westerners of the same age, sex, and BMI, the percentage of body fat is higher in the Asian populations [6]. It has also been found that central obesity is more prevalent among obese Asian populations [7]. Because increased visceral fat is associated with obesity-related disease risk [8], there may be differences in the risk of developing obesity-related diseases due to differences in the amount of visceral fat among racial groups.

Genetic factors in obesity and asthma

Both obesity and asthma have a substantial genetic component. Previous studies have reported several genes associated with asthma and BMI, including *PRKCA*, *LEP*, and *ADRB3*.

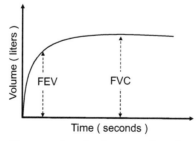

FIGURE 18.3 Normal spirometry. Spirometry is used to measure lung function, measuring volume against time. Patients are usually sitting up in a chair. They are asked to take a maximal inspiration in and are then asked to expel air for as long and as quickly as possible. Measurements are included: forced expiratory volume in one second (FEV1); forced vital capacity (FVC); the ratio of the two volumes (FEV1/FVC).

Other approaches have yielded more promising results; one study using gene-by-environment analysis found that seven single nucleotide polymorphisms in 17q21 (often referred to as the asthma-associated locus) were associated with BMI only among asthmatics among two independent cohorts [9]. A small pilot study in children reported different epigenome-wide DNA methylation patterns in children according to obesity and asthma status. Additionally, a study in mice and humans revealed that the expression of the *CHI3L1* gene is induced by a high-fat diet, and its product (chitinase 3-like 1) may contribute to both obesity and asthma symptoms [10].

Another recent study using RNA sequencing and reverse transcription polymerase chain reaction in individuals of European descent identified 34 shared loci that positively correlated with the obesity index and delayed onset asthma, defined as an age of onset of asthma >16 years. Furthermore, in experiments with obese and control mice, RNA sequencing analysis of lung samples identified *ACOXL* and *MYL6* as genes associated with both asthma and obesity [11].

Epidemiology: clinical features and findings

Epidemiological study of obesity and asthma in children and adults

The prevalence of obesity in children and adults is on the rise worldwide and has led to repeated warnings being published by the World Health Organization and other organizations [12,13,14]. Obesity is not only a risk for metabolic syndrome, which includes hypertension, secondary diabetes, and hyperlipidemia, but also involved in the onset and exacerbation of asthma. However, the association between obesity and asthma in children is not always the same as that in adults.

Epidemiological studies in children

Obesity and asthma

A metaanalysis of six studies in children younger than 18 years showed that overweight (95th > BMI ≥ 85th percentile) and obesity (BMI ≥ 95th percentile) significantly increased the risk of asthma [15]. Obesity is related to not only an increased prevalence of asthma, but it also tends to also make asthma more severe [16,17,18] and more difficult to control [19] and leads to lower quality of life [20].

Obese children with asthma receive less therapeutic effect from inhaled steroids than nonobese children with asthma [21], and once they have an asthma attack [22,23], they are more likely to experience more severe effects. Once hospitalized, the hospitalization period is typically longer, and the risk of requiring ventilatory support is higher [18]. Obese children with asthma are also prone to exacerbation due to indoor pollutants [24]. Many obese children with asthma tend to have a Th1-biased response to inflammatory stimuli caused by systemic inflammation associated with dyslipidemia and insulin resistance [25], [26], [27].

One study reported that obesity is not involved in asthma [28]. The study did not find a significant relationship between obesity and the frequency of asthma attacks requiring oral corticosteroids or the asymptomatic duration of asthma attacks, and that the dyspnea reported by obese children did not necessarily arise from asthma-related pathology.

These results show that obese children with asthma will need to be managed and evaluated based on objective indicators, as well as symptoms.

Definition of obesity in pediatric clinical studies

Most studies of the relationship between obesity and asthma use BMI as an indicator of obesity; however, some researchers have questioned whether BMI is the best indicator of obesity [29]. Abdominal circumference/buttock ratio, abdominal circumference, and abdominal circumference/height ratio, which are indicators of central obesity, have been reported to be more clearly associated with asthma than BMI [30]. Another study found that high BMI was associated with high airway resistance and a significantly higher risk of wheezing [31]. Furthermore, when the relationship with fat distribution was examined, fractional exhaled nitric oxide (FeNO) was lower when the android to gynoid fat mass ratio was higher, FeNO was higher when the preperitoneal fat mass was higher, and there was no relationship between subcutaneous fat mass and FeNO as shown in Fig. 18.4. Further studies are needed on how different distributions of fat deposits are associated with asthma, allergic inflammation, and metabolic disorders.

Relationship between weight change and asthma

Cross-sectional studies cannot explain the causal relationship between asthma and obesity, that is, whether asthma causes obesity or whether obesity induces asthma. However, many studies that have analyzed effects over time, such as

FIGURE 18.4 Body fat mass distribution and fractional exhaled nitric oxide.

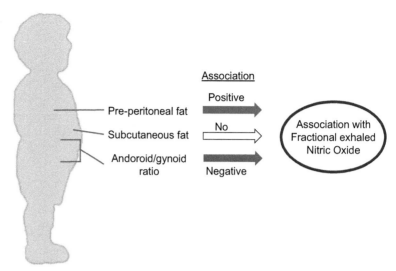

birth cohort studies, often show that obesity precedes asthma symptoms. Birth cohort studies have shown that high BMI at age 6–7 years, regardless of previous BMI, is a risk factor for dyspnea and airway hyperresponsiveness at age 8 [32]. Therefore, even if infants are obese, if the BMI is normal at the age of 6–7 years, there is no increased risk of dyspnea or increased airway hyperresponsiveness. A metaanalysis of eight birth cohort studies in Europe also showed that children with a rapid growth in BMI by 2 years of age were at increased risk of developing asthma by 6 years of age [33]. Other studies have also reported that rapid weight gain up to 3 months of age poses a risk of developing asthma up to 4 years of age, regardless of birth weight [34] and is related to asthma onset and respiratory dysfunction at 5 years of age [35].

Asthma has also been shown to increase the risk of becoming obese. It has been reported that asthma reduces the amount of exercise in daily life and that lower exercise levels tend to cause asthma in adolescence [36,37]. Furthermore, a 10-year follow-up study of children aged 5–8 years found that nonobese children with asthma at enrollment, regardless of their level of daily activity, had a 51% higher risk of subsequent obesity than nonobese nonasthmatic children [38]. Early-onset asthma and wheezing may also affect the increased risk of developing obesity in late childhood [39].

Relationship between obesity and weight gain in pregnant mothers and asthma in childhood

Studies have shown that maternal body weight is associated with wheezing and asthma in their children [40,41]. Maternal obesity early in pregnancy and significant maternal weight gain during pregnancy are associated with the development of asthma in children [42]. Although this effect diminishes with increasing age of the child, analysis of the relationship with the time of onset of asthma showed that it was most strongly associated with asthma that developed by 6 years of age, followed by asthma that developed between 6 and 12 years of age.

Sex differences in obesity and asthma in children

The prevalence of asthma in children is higher in boys before puberty and higher in girls after puberty; furthermore, the severity of asthma is higher in girls after puberty [43]. In a cohort study in the United States, girls who became obese between the ages of 6 and 11 years were more likely to have asthma at the age of 13 years than girls who did not become obese at that time; however, no such tendency was observed in boys [44]. The relationship between obesity and asthma was clear in girls who had menarche by the age of 11 years, but no effect was observed in girls who had menarche after the age of 11 years [45]. Moreover, when asthma was divided into allergic and nonallergic and the relationship with the change in body weight from birth was examined, the effect was different between boys and girls with allergic asthma; in only boys, allergic asthma was related to being underweight at birth regardless of whether they remained so or become overweight. Only girls who had been obese since birth showed an association with allergic asthma at the age of 9–11 years [46].

A cross-sectional study from New Zealand reported, however, that there is no difference between the male and female population in any generation regarding the prevalence of obesity and asthma [47].

Epidemiological studies in adults

Obesity and asthma

A prospective study of obesity and asthma has shown that obesity is a risk factor for the development of asthma [48]. A 4-year follow-up of women aged 26–46 years showed that the development of bronchial asthma was strongly associated with BMI. Since then, several studies supporting this result have been reported [49,50,51,52,53,54,55]. Furthermore, in a retrospective metaanalysis study, the odds ratio for asthma was 1.5 and that for the obese group was 1.9, relative to the lean group [56]. This result is reflected in US statistical data, with a prevalence of asthma of 7.1% among lean adults and 11.1% among obese adults. This tendency was particularly remarkable in women, with prevalence of 7.9% and 14.6%, respectively [57].

Obesity is an intractable and aggravating factor for asthma in adults as well as in children [58,59,60,61,62, 63,64,65,66,67,68]. Among asthma patients with obesity, the rate of emergency outpatient visits due to exacerbation of asthma was higher, the symptoms were more severe at the time of the emergency visit [60,61], and there was a higher possibility that mechanical ventilation management would be required [62]. Furthermore, it was shown that asthmatic patients with obesity have reduced responsiveness to corticosteroids [69,70,71]. One study has shown that in obese patients, responsiveness to leukotriene receptor antagonists remains unchanged, but responsiveness to inhaled corticosteroids is decreased [71].

Definition of obesity in adult clinical studies

Most studies define obesity in adults and children using BMI as an indicator. Obesity in adults is defined as a BMI of ≥ 30 kg/m^2; however, the physiology and metabolic health differ greatly depending on the given BMI. Metabolic alterations are more associated with visceral fat than BMI [72,73,74,75,76,77].

There are few reports on the relationship between actual fat distribution and asthma; however, there are reports that abdominal or visceral obesity is associated with the development of asthma [78]. Visceral fat accumulation (VFA) has also been found to be associated with the development of asthma in patients with type 2 diabetes in a more direct evaluation of VFA using computed tomography (CT) [79].

Phenotypes of obese patients with asthma

There are at least two phenotypes in obese asthma patients [80],61]. One is early onset, which is a phenotype with high IgE levels and severe type 2 inflammation [80]. This phenotype is the most severe seen in obese asthma patients, and weight loss is not expected to improve asthma control. This phenotype is considered to reflect a condition in which obesity is combined with allergic asthma to modify the pathological condition. Although the relationship between obesity and enhanced eosinophil inflammation has been previously reported, the detailed mechanism of asthma exacerbation has not yet been elucidated [81].

The other is a phenotype that is common in the female population and characterized by late-onset, non–type 2 inflammation, and excessive oxidative stress. In this phenotype, adipose tissue–derived cytokines and oxidative stress contribute to the exacerbation of airway inflammation, and parasympathetic tone due to obesity is involved in airway narrowing [80],82]. Furthermore, the effect of fat deposition on respiratory function is also considered to be strongly involved in the exacerbation of asthma [81], and weight loss can be expected to improve asthma control [83] as shown in Fig. 18.5. Therefore, it is presumed that the pathological condition caused by obesity causes the pathological condition of asthma. It is sometimes referred to as a phenotype associated with neutrophil inflammation [84]. In adult asthma patients with obesity, the late-onset type accounts for the majority of cases, but as described before, it should be noted that there is an early-onset type with severe type 2 inflammation.

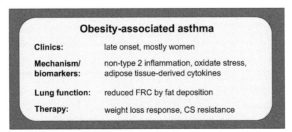

Obesity-associated asthma

Clinics:	late onset, mostly women
Mechanism/ biomarkers:	non-type 2 inflammation, oxidate stress, adipose tissue-derived cytokines
Lung function:	reduced FRC by fat deposition
Therapy:	weight loss response, CS resistance

FIGURE 18.5 Basic characteristics of obesity-associated asthma. *FRC*, functional residual capacity; CS, corticosteroids.

Sex differences in obesity and asthma in adults

As described before, the late-onset phenotype is characterized by non—type 2 inflammatory and strong oxidative stress, and cytokines derived from adipose tissue and oxidative stress contribute to the exacerbation of airway inflammation, which is a common phenotype in women. It has been reported that visceral fat is associated with asthma in women [85]. Although the amount of adipose tissue around organs in women is less than that in men, the activity of the adipose tissue is higher, which is thought to affect the pathophysiology of asthma [86].

Effect on asthma due to obesity-related complications

Among obesity-related complications, obstructive sleep apnea syndrome (OSAS) and gastroesophageal reflux disease (GERD) have received particular attention in relation to asthma control and deterioration. It has been reported that patients with severe asthma have a higher incidence of OSAS [87]. Among patients with OSAS, systemic oxidative stress is elevated due to repeated episodes of hypoxia and reoxygenation [88,89]. Furthermore, this increased oxidative stress has been reported to be ameliorated by continuous positive airway pressure (CPAP) therapy [88].

Asthma patients with GERD have more frequent asthma exacerbations than those without GERD [59]. Furthermore, patients with severe asthma and obesity have a higher frequency of GERD-related complications [90]. These findings suggest that the presence of GERD may be involved in the deterioration of asthma control in obese patients. OSAS and GERD may also be involved in the exacerbation of asthma in obese children [91]. Adolescent obese patients have other complications that may worsen bronchial asthma, such as a decreased immune response to viral infections and increased rates of depression [92].

Disease pathogenesis: immunological mechanisms

Pathogenesis of obesity and asthma

Among the various factors that have been found to be associated with the pathogenesis of asthma, obesity has been shown to be a cause of the onset of asthma and affect its severity. There are multiple pathways through which obesity affects the pathogenesis of asthma, including abnormalities in lipid metabolism, increased oxidative stress, increased inflammation in the airways and adipose tissue, abnormalities in adipokines, decreased steroid sensitivity, and insulin resistance.

Abnormal lipid metabolism

It has been suggested that lipid metabolism directly influences the pathogenesis of asthma; this is because histamine released from basophils triggered by hydrolysis of low-density lipoprotein (LDL) and very-low-density lipoprotein (VLDL) has been shown to lead to airway smooth muscle contraction [93].

In obese patients with asthma, increased nucleotide oligomerization domain-like receptor protein 3 (*NLRP3*) gene expression and elevated IL-1β protein levels in the sputum due to activation of the NLRP3 inflammasome have been shown to increase airway inflammation. It has also been shown that a high-fat diet is associated with airway inflammation because saturated fatty acid intake increases sputum neutrophils and *NLRP3* gene expression in patients with asthma [94].

Metabolic syndrome is characterized by mitochondrial dysfunction in various organs.

Studies using mouse and human specimens have shown that mitochondrial dysfunction also exists in airway epithelial cells in asthma, suggesting that metabolic syndrome associated with obesity may cause mitochondrial abnormalities in the airway epithelium that exacerbate asthma pathology [95]; [96—98,99]. In fact, compared with lean patients with asthma, the mitochondria of airway epithelial cells in obese patients have a greater maximal oxygen respiration rate and glycolytic rate and produce more oxidants. This leads to increased oxidative phosphorylation rates and enhanced production of mitochondria-derived reactive oxygen species (ROS), which may activate inflammasomes and activate downstream inflammatory pathways [100].

Increased oxidative stress

Oxidative stress occurs in obesity, and increased airway oxidative stress has been reported to occur in obese adults, especially those with late-onset asthma [101].

This is thought to be related to decreased bioavailability of arginine, a substrate for the production of nitric oxide (NO), a messenger molecule involved in a variety of pathologies including endothelial dysfunction, airway inflammation, and smooth muscle contraction. L-arginine, a semiessential amino acid, is a substrate for NO synthase (NOS), which plays an

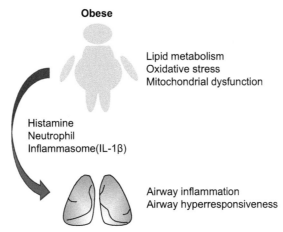

FIGURE 18.6   Metabolic abnormalities and oxidative stress due to obesity affect asthma pathology.

important role in NO homeostasis. It has been found that arginase expression and activity are increased in asthma [102,103,104]. Degradation of L-arginine, a substrate for NO production, leads to impaired NOS function. This results in NOS uncoupling, a phenomenon in which superoxide anions are preferentially produced, and oxidative stress is induced [105,106].

In obese patients with late-onset asthma, the decreased ratio of arginase activity to asymmetric dimethylarginine (ADMA), an NOS inhibitor, has been found to be associated with increased respiratory symptoms and decreased lung function [101,107]. Fig. 18.6 is a schema that summarizes these pathologies.

Increased airway inflammation

Eosinophils have been shown to influence the underlying pathogenesis of asthma, including airway goblet cell metaplasia, epithelial cell mucin accumulation, airway hyperresponsiveness, and remodeling in vivo [108].

One study reported that obese patients with asthma had higher IL-5 levels in the sputum than nonobese patients, which correlated with eosinophil levels under the airway mucosa and obesity [109].

Neutrophils have also been shown to promote asthma pathogenesis through various pathways in animal experiments and human specimens [110,111,112,113]. It has been reported that IL-17 and neutrophil levels in the sputum are significantly higher in obese asthma patients than among nonobese patients [84,114,115]. These findings suggest that airway inflammation caused by eosinophils/Th17 is enhanced in obese asthmatics.

In obese humans, the Th1/Th2 ratio of blood CD4-positive T cells is elevated [26]. In the adipose tissue, it has been reported that the proportion of Th1 and Th17 cells is higher than that of Th2 and regulatory T cells in obese patients [116]. Changes in the polarity of these T cells may affect the severity and control of asthma. It has been suggested that changes in the polarity of these T cells are associated with worsening severity and control of asthma and lung function abnormalities.

Studies using mouse models of obesity have reported that type 2 and type 3 innate lymphocytes (ILCs) exacerbate asthma pathology, and the effects of innate lymphocytes on obesity and asthma pathology have been suggested in humans [117,118]. Fig. 18.7 is a schema that summarizes these pathologies.

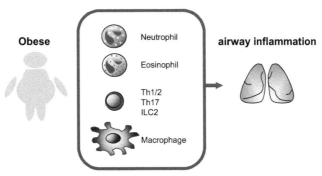

FIGURE 18.7   Obesity increases airway inflammation via various cells.

Inflammation in adipose tissue

The main immune cells in adipose tissue are adipose tissue macrophages. Obesity and adipose tissue macrophages have been found to be correlated, and most cytokines produced in adipose tissue due to obesity are produced by adipose tissue macrophages [119,120]. In adipocytes in obese patients, hypoxic stress causes cell death, and inflammatory cytokines, such as IL-6, TNF-α, and monocyte chemoattractant protein (MCP-1), are produced during processing by adipose tissue macrophages [121]. In a study of asthma patients, subjects with high blood IL-6 levels tended to have more severe obesity and a higher frequency of asthma exacerbations, severity of asthma, and blood neutrophil count, suggesting that obesity-induced increased IL-6 levels contribute to the worsening of asthma pathology [122,123].

Abnormalities in adipokines

Adipokines are produced by adipocytes, and abnormalities in their production have been shown to affect the pathogenesis of asthma [124,125,126,127,128,129,130].

Adiponectin has been shown in animal studies to inhibit the production of inflammatory cytokines, such as TNF and IL-6, from adipocytes and macrophages [131,132,133]. It has also been shown to protect against airway inflammation and oxidative stress in mouse models of asthma [134]. Although visceral adipocytes are the most important source of adiponectin, obesity decreases whole-body adiponectin levels, suggesting an adiponectin-mediated effect of obesity on the pathogenesis of asthma [135,136].

Leptin has been shown to directly activate human airway epithelial cells, increasing ICAM-1 expression; inducing CCL11, VEGF, G-CSF, and IL-6 synthesis; inducing migration; inhibiting apoptosis; and promoting cell proliferation [137]. Furthermore, leptin increases airway inflammation mediated by T cells, ILC2, and eosinophils. Leptin has also been reported to increase airway inflammation mediated via T cells, ILC2, and eosinophils [138,139]. There is a significant association between serum leptin levels and BMI in patients with asthma, suggesting an effect of obesity on asthma pathogenesis [140]. Fig. 18.8 is a schema that summarizes these pathologies.

Decreased steroid responsiveness

Steroid resistance in obese patients with asthma is clinically known, but there are various possibilities for its cause [70]. In vitro experiments using samples from obese patients with asthma have found decreased steroid sensitivity among peripheral blood mononuclear cells and cells in bronchoalveolar lavage fluid [141].

Insulin resistance

Insulin resistance, a hallmark of metabolic disorders in obese patients, leads to hyperinsulinemia. Studies of adult patients with asthma have shown that there is a positive relationship between obesity and asthma and that insulin resistance modifies this relationship [142]. Animal studies have also shown that insulin increases lung tissue remodeling, fibrosis, and airway hyperresponsiveness [143]. In the central nervous system, high insulin increases airway responsiveness through activation of cholinergic nerves [144] Experiments on human specimens have also shown that insulin causes smooth muscle cell proliferation and collagen production [143]. Fig. 18.9 is a schema that summarizes these pathologies.

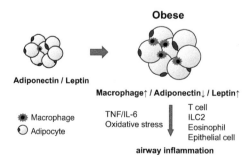

FIGURE 18.8 Obesity increases airway inflammation via adipose tissue macrophages or adipocytokines.

Metabolic disorders

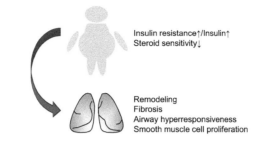

Insulin resistance↑/Insulin↑
Steroid sensitivity↓

Remodeling
Fibrosis
Airway hyperresponsiveness
Smooth muscle cell proliferation

FIGURE 18.9 Systemic changes caused by obesity exacerbates asthma.

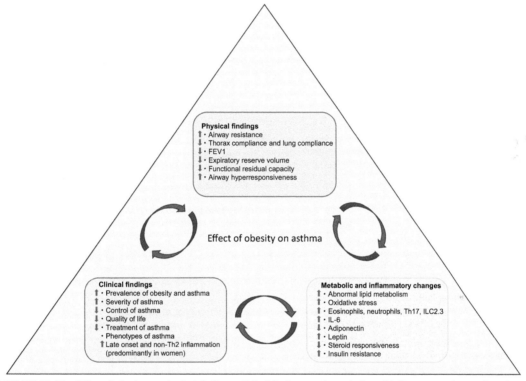

Physical findings
↑ · Airway resistance
↓ · Thorax compliance and lung compliance
↓ · FEV1
↓ · Expiratory reserve volume
↓ · Functional residual capacity
↑ · Airway hyperresponsiveness

Effect of obesity on asthma

Clinical findings
↑ · Prevalence of obesity and asthma
↑ · Severity of asthma
↓ · Control of asthma
↓ · Quality of life
↓ · Treatment of asthma
  · Phenotypes of asthma
↑ Late onset and non-Th2 inflammation
  (predominantly in women)

Metabolic and inflammatory changes
↑ · Abnormal lipid metabolism
↑ · Oxidative stress
↑ · Eosinophils, neutrophils, Th17, ILC2.3
↑ · IL-6
↓ · Adiponectin
↑ · Leptin
↓ · Steroid responsiveness
↑ · Insulin resistance

FIGURE 18.10 Effect of obesity on physical findings, clinical findings, and metabolic and inflammatory changes in asthma.

Summary

Obesity exacerbates bronchial asthma, the mechanism of which varies greatly depending on age, sex, respiratory function, type (i.e., allergic vs. nonallergic), location of fat deposition, and associated immunological changes with metabolic disorders (Fig. 18.10). The detailed molecular mechanism of how each factor is involved in the exacerbation of asthma remains unclear. In the future, the accumulation of knowledge will promote the development of more individualized treatments for obesity and severe asthma and preventive measures to reduce obesity.

Acknowledgments

We thank John Holmes, MSc., from Edanz (https://jp.edanz.com/ac), for editing a draft of this chapter.

References

[1] Dixon AE, Peters U. The effect of obesity on lung function. Expet Rev Respir Med 2018;12(9):755−67. https://doi.org/10.1080/17476348.2018.1506331.

[2] Yamane T, Date T, Tokuda M, Aramaki Y, Inada K, Matsuo S, Shibayama K, Miyanaga S, Miyazaki H, Sugimoto KI, Yoshimura M. Hypoxemia in inferior pulmonary veins in supine position is dependent on obesity. Am J Respir Crit Care Med 2008;178(3):295−9. https://doi.org/10.1164/rccm.200801-113OC.

[3] Bustos P, Amigo H, Oyarzún M, Rona RJ. Is there a causal relation between obesity and asthma? Evidence from Chile. Int J Obes 2005;29(7):804−9. https://doi.org/10.1038/sj.ijo.0802958.

[4] Litonjua AA, Sparrow D, Celedon JC, DeMolles D, Weiss ST. Association of body mass index with the development of methacholine airway hyperresponsiveness in men: the Normative Aging Study. Thorax 2002;57(7):581−5. https://doi.org/10.1136/thorax.57.7.581.

[5] Schachter LM, Salome CM, Peat JK, Woolcock AJ. Obesity is a risk for asthma and wheeze but not airway hyperresponsiveness. Thorax 2001;56(1):4−8. https://doi.org/10.1136/thorax.56.1.4.

[6] Appropriate bodymass index for Asian populations and its implications for policy and intervention strategies. In: WHO expert consultation, vol. 363; 2004. p. 157−63.

[7] McNeely MJ, Boyko EJ, Shofer JB, Newell-Morris L, Leonetti DL, Fujimoto WY. Standard definitions of overweight and central adiposity for determining diabetes risk in Japanese Americans. Am J Clin Nutr 2001;74(1):101−7. https://doi.org/10.1093/ajcn/74.1.101.

[8] Després JP. Is visceral obesity the cause of the metabolic syndrome? Ann Med 2006;38(1):52−63. https://doi.org/10.1080/07853890500383895.

[9] Wang L, Murk W, DeWan AT, Mersha TB. Genome-wide gene by environment interaction analysis identifies common SNPs at 17q21.2 that are associated with increased body mass index only among asthmatics. PLoS One 2015;10(12):e0144114. https://doi.org/10.1371/journal.pone.0144114.

[10] Ahangari F, Sood A, Ma B, Takyar S, Schuyler M, Qualls C, Dela Cruz CS, Chupp GL, Lee CG, Elias JA. Chitinase 3-like-1 regulates both visceral fat accumulation and asthma-like Th2 inflammation. Am J Respir Crit Care Med 2015;191(7):746−57. https://doi.org/10.1164/rccm.201405-0796OC.

[11] Zhu Z, Guo Y, Shi H, Liu CL, Panganiban RA, Chung W, O'Connor LJ, Himes BE, Gazal S, Hasegawa K, Camargo CA, Qi L, Moffatt MF, Hu FB, Lu Q, Cookson WOC, Liang L. Shared genetic and experimental links between obesity-related traits and asthma subtypes in UK Biobank. J Allergy Clin Immunol 2020;145(2):537−49. https://doi.org/10.1016/j.jaci.2019.09.035.

[12] The GBD 2015 Obesity Collaborators. Heath effects of overweight and obesity in 195 countries over 25 years. N Engl J Med 2015;377(1):13−27.

[13] World Health Organization. Noncommunicable diseases: childhood overweight and obesity. 2021. https://www.who.int/news-room/q-a-detail/noncommunicable-diseases-childhood-overweight-and-obesity.

[14] World Health Organization. Obesity and overweight. 2021. https://www.who.int/news-room/fact-sheets/detail/obesity-and-overweight.

[15] Egan KB, Ettinger AS, Bracken MB. Childhood body mass index and subsequent physician-diagnosed asthma: a systematic review and meta-analysis of prospective cohort studies. BMC Pediatr 2013;13(1). https://doi.org/10.1186/1471-2431-13-121.

[16] Ahmadizar F, Vijverberg SJH, Arets HGM, De Boer A, Lang JE, Kattan M, Palmer CNA, Mukhopadhyay S, Turner S, Der Zee AHMV. Childhood obesity in relation to poor asthma control and exacerbation: a meta-analysis. Eur Respir J 2016;48(4):1063−73. https://doi.org/10.1183/13993003.00766-2016.

[17] Aragona E, El-Magbri E, Wang J, Scheckelhoff T, Scheckelhoff T, Hyacinthe A, Nair S, Khan A, Nino G, Pillai DK. Impact of obesity on clinical outcomes in urban children hospitalized for status asthmaticus. Hosp Pediatr 2016;6(4):211−8. https://doi.org/10.1542/hpeds.2015-0094.

[18] Okubo Y, Nochioka K, Hataya H, Sakakibara H, Terakawa T, Testa M. Burden of obesity on pediatric inpatients with acute asthma exacerbation in the United States. J Allergy Clin Immunol Pract 2016;4(6):1227−31. https://doi.org/10.1016/j.jaip.2016.06.004.

[19] van Gent R, van der Ent CK, Rovers MM, Kimpen JLL, van Essen-Zandvliet LEM, de Meer G. Excessive body weight is associated with additional loss of quality of life in children with asthma. J Allergy Clin Immunol 2007;119(3):591−6. https://doi.org/10.1016/j.jaci.2006.11.007.

[20] Borrell LN, Nguyen EA, Roth LA, Oh SS, Tcheurekdjian H, Sen S, Davis A, Farber HJ, Avila PC, Brigino-Buenaventura E, LeNoir MA, Lurmann F, Meade K, Serebrisky D, Rodriguez-Cintron W, Kumar R, Rodriguez-Santana JR, Thyne SM, Burchard EG. Childhood obesity and asthma control in the GALA II and SAGE II studies. Am J Respir Crit Care Med 2013;187(7):697−702. https://doi.org/10.1164/rccm.201211-2116OC.

[21] Forno E, Lescher R, Strunk R, Weiss S, Fuhlbrigge A, Celedón JC. Decreased response to inhaled steroids in overweight and obese asthmatic children. J Allergy Clin Immunol 2011;127(3):741−9. https://doi.org/10.1016/j.jaci.2010.12.010.

[22] Carroll CL, Bhandari A, Zucker AR, Schramm CM. Childhood obesity increases duration of therapy during severe asthma exacerbations. Pediatr Crit Care Med 2006;7(6):527−31. https://doi.org/10.1097/01.PCC.0000243749.14555.E8.

[23] Carroll CL, Stoltz P, Raykov N, Smith SR, Zucker AR. Childhood overweight increases hospital admission rates for asthma. Pediatrics 2007;120(4):734−40. https://doi.org/10.1542/peds.2007-0409.

[24] Lu KD, Breysse PN, Diette GB, Curtin-Brosnan J, Aloe C, Williams DL, Peng RD, McCormack MC, Matsui EC. Being overweight increases susceptibility to indoor pollutants among urban children with asthma. J Allergy Clin Immunol 2013;131(4):1017−e3. https://doi.org/10.1016/j.jaci.2012.12.1570.

[25] Eising JB, Uiterwaal CSPM, Evelein AMV, Visseren FLJ, Van Der Ent CK. Relationship between leptin and lung function in young healthy children. Eur Respir J 2014;43(4):1189−92. https://doi.org/10.1183/09031936.00149613.

[26] Rastogi D, Fraser S, Oh J, Huber AM, Schulman Y, Bhagtani RH, Khan ZS, Tesfa L, Hall CB, Macian F. Inflammation, metabolic dysregulation, and pulmonary function among obese urban adolescents with asthma. Am J Respir Crit Care Med 2015a;191(2):149−60. https://doi.org/10.1164/rccm.201409-1587OC.

[27] Vinding RK, Stokholm J, Chawes BLK, Bisgaard H. Blood lipid levels associate with childhood asthma, airway obstruction, bronchial hyper-responsiveness, and aeroallergen sensitization. J Allergy Clin Immunol 2016;137(1):68−74.e4. https://doi.org/10.1016/j.jaci.2015.05.033.

[28] Mahut B, Beydon N, Delclaux C. Overweight is not a comorbidity factor during childhood asthma: the GrowthOb study. Eur Respir J 2012;39(5):1120–6. https://doi.org/10.1183/09031936.00103311.

[29] Forno E. Childhood obesity and asthma: to BMI or not to BMI? J Allergy Clin Immunol 2017;139(3):767–8. https://doi.org/10.1016/j.jaci.2016.08.020.

[30] Chen YC, Tu YK, Huang KC, Chen PC, Chu DC, Lee YL. Pathway from central obesity to childhood asthma: physical fitness and sedentary time are leading factors. Am J Respir Crit Care Med 2014;189(10):1194–203. https://doi.org/10.1164/rccm.201401-0097OC.

[31] Dekker, Jongste RK, de, Reiss J, Jaddoe I, Duijts V. Body fat mass distribution and interrupter resistance, fractional exhaled nitric oxide, and asthma at school-age. J Allergy Clin Immunol 2017;139(3):810–8.

[32] Scholtens S, Wijga AH, Seidell JC, Brunekreef B, de Jongste JC, Gehring U, Postma DS, Kerkhof M, Smit HA. Overweight and changes in weight status during childhood in relation to asthma symptoms at 8 years of age. J Allergy Clin Immunol 2009;123(6):1312–e2. https://doi.org/10.1016/j.jaci.2009.02.029.

[33] Rzehak P, Wijga, Keil T, Eller E, Bindslev-Jensen C, Smit H, et al. GA^{2}LEN-WP 1.5 Birth Cohorts. Body mass index trajectory classes and incident asthma in childhood: results from 8 European Birth Cohorts–a Global Allergy and Asthma European Network initiative. J Allergy Clin Immunol 2013;131(6):1528–36.

[34] Sonnenschein-van Der Voort AMM, Jaddoe VWV, Raat H, Moll HA, Hofman A, De Jongste JC, Duijts L. Fetal and infant growth and asthma symptoms in preschool children: the generation R study. Am J Respir Crit Care Med 2012;185(7):731–7. https://doi.org/10.1164/rccm.201107-1266OC.

[35] Van Der Gugten AC, Koopman M, Evelein AMV, Verheij TJM, Uiterwaal CSPM, Van Der Ent CK. Rapid early weight gain is associated with wheeze and reduced lung function in childhood. Eur Respir J 2012;39(2):403–10. https://doi.org/10.1183/09031936.00188310.

[36] Rasmussen F, Lambrechtsen J, Siersted HC, Hansen HS, Hansen NCG. Low physical fitness in childhood is associated with the development of asthma in young adulthood: the Odense schoolchild study. Eur Respir J 2000;16(5):866–70. https://doi.org/10.1183/09031936.00.16586600.

[37] Vahlkvist S, Pedersen S. Fitness, daily activity and body composition in children with newly diagnosed, untreated asthma. Allergy 2009;64(11):1649–55. https://doi.org/10.1111/j.1398-9995.2009.02081.x.

[38] Chen Z, Salam MT, Alderete TL, Habre R, Bastain TM, Berhane K, et al. Effects of childhood asthma on the development of obesity among school-aged children. Am J Respir Crit Care Med 2017;195(9):1181–8. https://doi.org/10.1164/rccm.201608-1691OC.

[39] Contreras ZA, Chen Z, Roumeliotaki T, Annesi-Maesano I, Baïz N, von Berg A, Bergström A, Crozier S, Duijts L, Ekström S, Eller E, Fantini MP, Kjaer HF, Forastiere F, Gerhard B, Gori D, Harskamp-Van Ginkel MW, Heinrich J, Iñiguez C, et al. Does early onset asthma increase childhood obesity risk? A pooled analysis of 16 European cohorts. Eur Respir J 2018;52(3). https://doi.org/10.1183/13993003.00504-2018.

[40] Forno E, Young OM, Kumar R, Simhan H, Celedón JC. Maternal obesity in pregnancy, gestational weight gain, and risk of childhood asthma. Pediatrics 2014;134(2):e535–46. https://doi.org/10.1542/peds.2014-0439.

[41] Rusconi F, Popovic M. Maternal obesity and childhood wheezing and asthma. Paediatr Respir Rev 2017;22:66–71. https://doi.org/10.1016/j.prrv.2016.08.009.

[42] Dumas O, Varraso R, Gillman MW, Field AE, Camargo CA. Longitudinal study of maternal body mass index, gestational weight gain, and offspring asthma. Aller: Euro J Aller Clin Immunol 2016;71(9):1295–304. https://doi.org/10.1111/all.12876.

[43] Fu L, Freishtat RJ, Gordish-Dressman H, Teach SJ, Resca L, Hoffman EP, Wang Z. Natural progression of childhood asthma symptoms and strong influence of sex and puberty. Ann Am Thor Soci 2014;11(6):898–907. https://doi.org/10.1513/AnnalsATS.201402-084OC.

[44] Castro-Rodríguez JA, Holberg CJ, Morgan WJ, Wright AL, Martinez FD. Increased incidence of asthmalike symptoms in girls who become overweight or obese during the school years. Am J Respir Crit Care Med 2001;163(6):1344–9. https://doi.org/10.1164/ajrccm.163.6.2006140.

[45] Castro-Rodriguez JA. A new childhood asthma phenotype: obese with early menarche. Paediatr Respir Rev 2016;18:85–9. https://doi.org/10.1016/j.prrv.2015.10.006.

[46] Chastang J, Baiz N, Parnet L, Cadwallader JS, De Blay F, Caillaud D, Charpin DA, Dwyer J, Lavaud F, Raherison C, Ibanez G, Annesi-Maesano I. Changes in body mass index during childhood and risk of various asthma phenotypes: a retrospective analysis. Pediatr Allergy Immunol 2017;28(3):273–9. https://doi.org/10.1111/pai.12699.

[47] Wickens K, Barry D, Friezema A, Rhodius R, Bone N, Purdie G, Crane J. Obesity and asthma in 11-12 year old New Zealand children in 1989 and 2000. Thorax 2005;60(1):7–12. https://doi.org/10.1136/thx.2002.001529.

[48] Camargo CA, Weiss ST, Zhang S, Willett WC, Speizer FE. Prospective study of body mass index, weight change, and risk of adult- onset asthma in women. Arch Intern Med 1999;159(21):2582–8. https://doi.org/10.1001/archinte.159.21.2582.

[49] Chen Y, Dales R, Tang M, Krewski D. Obesity may increase the incidence of asthma in women but not in men: longitudinal observations from the Canadian National Population Health Surveys. Am J Epidemiol 2002;155(3):191–7. https://doi.org/10.1093/aje/155.3.191.

[50] Ford ES, Mannino DM, Redd SC, Mokdad AH, Mott JA. Body mass index and asthma incidence among USA adults. Eur Respir J 2004;24(5):740–4. https://doi.org/10.1183/09031936.04.00088003.

[51] Gunnbjörnsdóttir MI, Omenaas E, Gíslason T, Norrman E, Olin AC, Jõgi R, Jensen EJ, Lindberg E, Björnsson E, Franklin K, Janson C, Gulsvik A, Laerum B, Svanes C, Torén K, Tunsäter A, Lillienberg L, Gíslason D, Blöndal T, et al. Obesity and nocturnal gastro-oesophageal reflux are related to onset of asthma and respiratory symptoms. Eur Respir J 2004;24(1):116–21. https://doi.org/10.1183/09031936.04.00042603.

[52] Hjellvik V, Tverdal A, Furu K. Body mass index as predictor for asthma: a cohort study of 118,723 males and females. Eur Respir J 2010;35(6):1235–42. https://doi.org/10.1183/09031936.00192408.

[53] Huovinen E, Kaprio J, Koskenvuo M. Factors associated to lifestyle and risk of adult onset asthma. Respir Med 2003;97(3):273–80. https://doi.org/10.1053/rmed.2003.1419.

[54] Kim S, Camargo CA. Sex-race differences in the relationship between obesity and asthma: the behavioral risk factor surveillance system, 2000. Ann Epidemiol 2003;13(10):666—73. https://doi.org/10.1016/S1047-2797(03)00054-1.

[55] Nystad W, Meyer HE, Nafstad P, Tverdal A, Engeland A. Body mass index in relation to adult asthma among 135,000 Norwegian men and women. Am J Epidemiol 2004;160(10):969—76. https://doi.org/10.1093/aje/kwh303.

[56] Beuther DA, Sutherland ER. Overweight, obesity, and incident asthma: a meta-analysis of prospective epidemiologic studies. Am J Respir Crit Care Med 2007;175(7):661—6. https://doi.org/10.1164/rccm.200611-1717OC.

[57] Akinbami L, Fryar CD. Current asthma prevalence by weight status among adults: United States. NCHS Data Brief 2001;239:1—8.

[58] Akerman MJH, Calacanis CM, Madsen MK. Relationship between asthma severity and obesity. J Asthma 2004;41(5):521—6. https://doi.org/10.1081/JAS-120037651.

[59] Gibeon D, Batuwita K, Osmond M, Heaney LG, Brightling CE, Niven R, Mansur A, Chaudhuri R, Bucknall CE, Rowe A, Guo Y, Bhavsar PK, Chung KF, Menzies-Gow A. Obesity-associated severe asthma represents a distinct clinical phenotype analysis of the british thoracic society diffi cult asthma registry patient cohort according to bmi. Chest 2013;143(2):406—14. https://doi.org/10.1378/chest.12-0872.

[60] Hasegawa K, Tsugawa Y, Lopez BL, Smithline HA, Sullivan AF, Camargo CA. Body mass index and risk of hospitalization among adults presenting with asthma exacerbation to the emergency department. Ann Am Thor Soci 2014;11(9):1439—44. https://doi.org/10.1513/AnnalsATS.201406-270BC.

[61] Holguin F, Bleecker ER, Busse WW, Calhoun WJ, Castro M, Erzurum SC, Fitzpatrick AM, Gaston B, Israel E, Jarjour NN, Moore WC, Peters SP, Yonas M, Teague WG, Wenzel SE. Obesity and asthma: an association modified by age of asthma onset. J Allergy Clin Immunol 2011;127(6):1486—e2. https://doi.org/10.1016/j.jaci.2011.03.036.

[62] Luthe SK, Hirayama A, Goto T, Faridi MK, Camargo CA, Hasegawa K. Association between obesity and acute severity among patients hospitalized for asthma exacerbation. J Allergy Clin Immunol Pract 2018;6(6):1936—1941.e4. https://doi.org/10.1016/j.jaip.2018.02.001.

[63] Mosen DM, Schatz M, Magid DJ, Camargo CA. The relationship between obesity and asthma severity and control in adults. J Allergy Clin Immunol 2008;122(3):507—e6. https://doi.org/10.1016/j.jaci.2008.06.024.

[64] Rodrigo GJ, Plaza V. Body mass index and response to emergency department treatment in adults with severe asthma exacerbations: a prospective cohort study. Chest 2007;132(5):1513—9. https://doi.org/10.1378/chest.07-0936.

[65] Saint-Pierre P, Bourdin A, Chanez P, Daures JP, Godard P. Are overweight asthmatics more difficult to control? Allergy: Europ J Aller Clin Immunol 2006;61(1):79—84. https://doi.org/10.1111/j.1398-9995.2005.00953.x.

[66] Schatz M, Zeiger RS, Zhang F, Chen W, Yang SJ, Camargo CA. Overweight/obesity and risk of seasonal asthma exacerbations. J Allergy Clin Immunol Pract 2013;1(6):618—22. https://doi.org/10.1016/j.jaip.2013.07.009.

[67] Taylor B, Mannino D, Brown C, Crocker D, Twum-Baah N, Holguin F. Body mass index and asthma severity in the National Asthma Survey. Thorax 2008;63(1):14—20. https://doi.org/10.1136/thx.2007.082784.

[68] Varraso R, Siroux V, Maccario J, Pin I, Kauffmann F. Asthma severity is associated with body mass index and early menarche in women. Am J Respir Crit Care Med 2005;171(4):334—9. https://doi.org/10.1164/rccm.200405-674OC.

[69] Anderson WJ, Lipworth BJ. Does body mass index influence responsiveness to inhaled corticosteroids in persistent asthma? Ann Allergy Asthma Immunol 2012;108(4):237—42. https://doi.org/10.1016/j.anai.2011.12.006.

[70] Boulet LP, Franssen E. Influence of obesity on response to fluticasone with or without salmeterol in moderate asthma. Respir Med 2007;101(11):2240—7. https://doi.org/10.1016/j.rmed.2007.06.031.

[71] Peters-Golden M, Swern A, Bird SS, Hustad CM, Grant E, Edelman JM. Influence of body mass index on the response to asthma controller agents. Eur Respir J 2006;27(3):495—503. https://doi.org/10.1183/09031936.06.00077205.

[72] Dandona P, Aljada A, Chaudhuri A, Mohanty P, Garg R. Metabolic syndrome: a comprehensive perspective based on interactions between obesity, diabetes, and inflammation. Circulation 2005;111(11):1448—54. https://doi.org/10.1161/01.CIR.0000158483.13093.9D.

[73] Eckel RH, Grundy SM, Zimmet PZ. The metabolic syndrome. In: Lancet, vol. 365. Elsevier Limited; 2005. p. 1415—28. https://doi.org/10.1016/S0140-6736(05)66378-7. 9468.

[74] Kahn R, Buse J, Ferrannini E, Stern M. The metabolic syndrome: time for a critical appraisal: joint statement from the American diabetes association and the European association for the study of diabetes. Diab Care 2005;48(9):2289—304. https://doi.org/10.2337/diacare.28.9.2289.

[75] Karelis AD, St-Pierre DH, Conus F, Rabasa-Lhoret R, Poehlman ET. Metabolic and body composition factors in subgroups of obesity: what do we know?. In: Journal of clinical endocrinology and metabolism, vol. 89; 2004. p. 2569—75. https://doi.org/10.1210/jc.2004-0165. 6.

[76] Larsson B. Obesity, fat distribution and cardiovascular disease. Int J Obes 1991;15:53—7.

[77] Wajchenberg BL. Subcutaneous and visceral adipose tissue: their relation to the metabolic syndrome. Endocr Rev 2000;21(6):697—738. https://doi.org/10.1210/edrv.21.6.0415.

[78] Brumpton B, Langhammer A, Romundstad P, Chen Y, Mai XM. General and abdominal obesity and incident asthma in adults: the HUNT study. Eur Respir J 2013;41(2):323—9. https://doi.org/10.1183/09031936.00012112.

[79] Murakami D, Anan F, Masaki T, Umeno Y, Shigenaga T, Eshima N, Nakagawa T. Visceral fat accumulation is associated with asthma in patients with type 2 diabetes. J Diabetes Res 2019. https://doi.org/10.1155/2019/3129286. 2019.

[80] Dixon AE, Poynter ME. Mechanisms of asthma in obesity pleiotropic aspects of obesity produce distinct asthma phenotypes. Am J Respir Cell Mol Biol 2016;54(5):601—8. https://doi.org/10.1165/rcmb.2016-0017PS.

[81] Bates JHT, Poynter ME, Frodella CM, Peters U, Dixon AE, Suratt BT. Pathophysiology to phenotype in the asthma of obesity. Ann Am Tho Soci 2017;14:S395—8. https://doi.org/10.1513/AnnalsATS.201702-122AW.

[82] Sideleva O, Suratt BT, Black KE, Tharp WG, Pratley RE, Forgione P, Dienz O, Irvin CG, Dixon AE. Obesity and asthma: an inflammatory disease of adipose tissue not the airway. Am J Respir Crit Care Med 2012;186(7):598−605. https://doi.org/10.1164/rccm.201203-0573OC.

[83] Dixon AE, Pratley RE, Forgione PM, Kaminsky DA, Whittaker-Leclair LA, Griffes LA, Garudathri J, Raymond D, Poynter ME, Bunn JY, Irvin CG. Effects of obesity and bariatric surgery on airway hyperresponsiveness, asthma control, and inflammation. J Allergy Clin Immunol 2011;128(3):508−e2. https://doi.org/10.1016/j.jaci.2011.06.009.

[84] Scott HA, Gibson PG, Garg ML, Wood LG. Airway inflammation is augmented by obesity and fatty acids in asthma. Eur Respir J 2011a;38(3):594−602. https://doi.org/10.1183/09031936.00139810.

[85] Sood A, Qualls C, Li R, Schuyler M, Beckett WS, Smith LJ, Thyagarajan B, Lewis CE, Jacobs DR. Lean mass predicts asthma better than fat mass among females. Eur Respir J 2011;37(1):65−71. https://doi.org/10.1183/09031936.00193709.

[86] Sood A. Sex differences: implications for the obesity-asthma association. Exerc Sport Sci Rev 2011;39(1):48−56. https://doi.org/10.1097/JES.0b013e318201f0c4.

[87] Julien JY, Martin JG, Ernst P, Olivenstein R, Hamid Q, Lemière C, Pepe C, Naor N, Olha A, Kimoff RJ. Prevalence of obstructive sleep apnea-hypopnea in severe versus moderate asthma. J Allergy Clin Immunol 2009;124(2):371−6. https://doi.org/10.1016/j.jaci.2009.05.016.

[88] Barceló A, Miralles C, Barbé F, Vila M, Pons S, Agustí AGN. Abnormal lipid peroxidation in patients with sleep apnoea. Eur Respir J 2000;16(4):644. https://doi.org/10.1034/j.1399-3003.2000.16d13.x.

[89] Lavie L, Vishnevsky A, Lavie P. Evidence for lipid peroxidation in obstructive sleep apnea. Sleep 2004;27(1):123−8.

[90] Denlinger LC, Phillips BR, Ramratnam S, Ross K, Bhakta NR, Cardet JC, Castro M, Peters SP, Phipatanakul W, Aujla S, Bacharier LB, Bleecker ER, Comhair SAA, Coverstone A, DeBoer M, Erzurum SC, Fain SB, Fajt M, Fitzpatrick AM, et al. Inflammatory and comorbid features of patients with severe asthma and frequent exacerbations. Am J Respir Crit Care Med 2017;195(3):302−13. https://doi.org/10.1164/rccm.201602-0419OC.

[91] Lang JE. Contribution of comorbidities to obesity-related asthma in children. Paediatr Respir Rev 2021;37:22−9. https://doi.org/10.1016/j.prrv.2020.07.006.

[92] Mannan M, Mamun A, Doi S, Clavarino A, Homberg J. Prospective associations between depression and obesity for adolescent males and females-A systematic review and meta-analysis of longitudinal studies. PLoS One 2016;11(6):e0157240. https://doi.org/10.1371/journal.pone.0157240.

[93] Gonen B, O'Donnell P, Post TJ, Quinn TJ, Schulman ES. Very low density lipoproteins (VLDL) trigger the release of histamine from human basophils. Biochim Biophys Acta Lipids Lipid Metabol 1987;917(3):418−24. https://doi.org/10.1016/0005-2760(87)90121-4.

[94] Wood LG, Li Q, Scott HA, Rutting S, Berthon BS, Gibson PG, Hansbro PM, Williams E, Horvat J, Simpson JL, Young P, Oliver BG, Baines KJ. Saturated fatty acids, obesity, and the nucleotide oligomerization domain−like receptor protein 3 (NLRP3) inflammasome in asthmatic patients. J Allergy Clin Immunol 2019;143(1):305−15. https://doi.org/10.1016/j.jaci.2018.04.037.

[95] Aguilera-Aguirre L, Bacsi A, Saavedra-Molina A, Kurosky A, Sur S, Boldogh I. Mitochondrial dysfunction increases allergic airway inflammation. J Immunol 2009;183(8):5379−87. https://doi.org/10.4049/jimmunol.0900228.

[96] Mabalirajan U, Dinda AK, Kumar S, Roshan R, Gupta P, Sharma SK, Ghosh B. Mitochondrial structural changes and dysfunction are associated with experimental allergic asthma. J Immunol 2008;181(5):3540−8. https://doi.org/10.4049/jimmunol.181.5.3540.

[97] Mabalirajan U, Rehman R, Ahmad T, Kumar S, Singh S, Leishangthem GD, Aich J, Kumar M, Khanna K, Singh VP, Dinda AK, Biswal S, Agrawal A, Ghosh B. Linoleic acid metabolite drives severe asthma by causing airway epithelial injury. Sci Rep 2013;3. https://doi.org/10.1038/srep01349.

[98] Mabalirajan U, Ghosh B. Mitochondrial dysfunction in metabolic syndrome and asthma. J Allergy 2013:1−12. https://doi.org/10.1155/2013/340476.

[99] Xu W, Comhair S, Janocha, Mavrakis L, Erzurum SC. Alteration of nitric oxide synthesis related to abnormal cellular bioenergetics in asthmatic airway epithelium. Am J Respir Crit Care Med 2010;181.

[100] Winnica D, Corey C, Mullett S, Reynolds M, Hill G, Wendell S, Que L, Holguin F, Shiva S. Bioenergetic differences in the airway epithelium of lean versus obese asthmatics are driven by nitric oxide and reflected in circulating platelets. Antioxidants Redox Signal 2019;31(10):673−86. https://doi.org/10.1089/ars.2018.7627.

[101] Holguin F, Comhair SAA, Hazen SL, Powers RW, Khatri SS, Bleecker ER, Busse WW, Calhoun WJ, Castro M, Fitzpatrick AM, Gaston B, Israel E, Jarjour NN, Moore WC, Peters SP, Teague WG, Chung KF, Erzurum SC, Wenzel SE. An association between L-arginine/asymmetric dimethyl arginine balance, obesity, and the age of asthma onset phenotype. Am J Respir Crit Care Med 2013;187(2):153−9. https://doi.org/10.1164/rccm.201207-1270OC.

[102] Morris CR, Poljakovic M, Lavrisha L, Machado L, Kuypers FA, Morris SM. Decreased arginine bioavailability and increased serum arginase activity in asthma. Am J Respir Crit Care Med 2004;170(2):148−53. https://doi.org/10.1164/rccm.200309-1304oc.

[103] North ML, Khanna N, Marsden PA, Grasemann H, Scott JA. Functionally important role for arginase 1 in the airway hyperresponsiveness of asthma. Am J Physiol Lung Cell Mol Physiol 2009;296(6):L911−20. https://doi.org/10.1152/ajplung.00025.2009.

[104] Zimmermann N, King NE, Laporte J, Yang M, Mishra A, Pope SM, Muntel EE, Witte DP, Pegg AA, Foster PS, Hamid Q, Rothenberg ME. Dissection of experimental asthma with DNA microarray analysis identifies arginase in asthma pathogenesis. J Clin Invest 2003;111(12):1863−74. https://doi.org/10.1172/JCI200317912.

[105] Antoniades, Shirodaria, Antonopoulos L, Van-Assche W, et al. Association of plasma asymmetrical dimethylarginine (ADMA) with elevated vascular superoxide production and endothelial nitric oxide synthase uncoupling: implications for endothelial function in human atherosclerosis. Am J Respir Cell Mol Biol 2007;30(9):520−8.

[106] Wells SM, Holian A. Asymmetric dimethylarginine induces oxidative and nitrosative stress in murine lung epithelial cells. Am J Respir Cell Mol Biol 2007;36(5):520−8. https://doi.org/10.1165/rcmb.2006-0302SM.

[107] Holguin F, Khatri S, Serpil, Powers R, Trudeau J, Wenzel SE. Reduced L- arginine/ADMA as a potential mechanism to explain increased symptom severity and reduced atopy in late onset obese asthmatics. Am J Respir Crit Care Med 2012;185.

[108] Ochkur SI, Doyle AD, Jacobsen EA, LeSuer WE, Li W, Protheroe CA, Zellner KR, Colbert D, Shen HHH, Irvin CG, Lee JJ, Lee NA. Frontline science: eosinophil-deficient MBP-1 and EPX double-knockout mice link pulmonary remodeling and airway dysfunction with type 2 inflammation. J Leukoc Biol 2017;102(3):589–99. https://doi.org/10.1189/jlb.3HI1116-488RR.

[109] Desai D, Newby C, Symon FA, Haldar P, Shah S, Gupta S, Bafadhel M, Singapuri A, Siddiqui S, Woods J, Herath A, Anderson IK, Bradding P, Green R, Kulkarni N, Pavord I, Marshall RP, Sousa AR, May RD, et al. Elevated sputum interleukin-5 and submucosal eosinophilia in obese individuals with severe asthma. Am J Respir Crit Care Med 2013;188(6):657–63. https://doi.org/10.1164/rccm.201208-1470oc.

[110] Hosoki K, Aguilera-Aguirre L, Brasier AR, Kurosky A, Boldogh I, Sur S. Facilitation of allergic sensitization and allergic airway inflammation by pollen-induced innate neutrophil recruitment. Am J Respir Cell Mol Biol 2016;54(1):81–90. https://doi.org/10.1165/rcmb.2015-0044OC.

[111] Pothoven KL, Norton JE, Suh LA, Carter RG, Harris KE, Biyasheva A, Welch K, Shintani-Smith S, Conley DB, Liu MC, Kato A, Avila PC, Hamid Q, Grammer LC, Peters AT, Kern RC, Tan BK, Schleimer RP. Neutrophils are a major source of the epithelial barrier disrupting cytokine oncostatin M in patients with mucosal airways disease. J Allergy Clin Immunol 2017;139(6):1966–1978.e9. https://doi.org/10.1016/j.jaci.2016.10.039.

[112] Toussaint M, Jackson DJ, Swieboda D, Guedán A, Tsourouktsoglou TD, Ching YM, Radermecker C, Makrinioti H, Aniscenko J, Edwards MR, Solari R, Farnir F, Papayannopoulos V, Bureau F, Marichal T, Johnston SL. Host DNA released by NETosis promotes rhinovirus-induced type-2 allergic asthma exacerbation. Nat Med 2017;23(6):681–91. https://doi.org/10.1038/nm.4332.

[113] Ventura I, Vega A, Chacón P, Chamorro C, Aroca R, Gómez E, Bellido V, Puente Y, Blanca M, Monteseirín J. Neutrophils from allergic asthmatic patients produce and release metalloproteinase-9 upon direct exposure to allergens. Allergy 2014;69(7):898–905. https://doi.org/10.1111/all.12414.

[114] Marijsse GS, Seys SF, Schelpe AS, Dilissen E, Goeminne P, Dupont LJ, et al. Obese individuals with asthma preferentially have a high IL-5/IL-17A/IL-25 sputum inflammatory pattern. Am J Respir Crit Care Med 2014;189(10):1284–5. https://doi.org/10.1164/rccm.201310-1841LE.

[115] Telenga ED, Tideman SW, Kerstjens HAM, Hacken NHT, Timens W, Postma DS, et al. Obesity in asthma: more neutrophilic inflammation as a possible explanation for a reduced treatment response. Allergy 2012;67(8):1060–8. https://doi.org/10.1111/j.1398-9995.2012.02855.x.

[116] McLaughlin T, Liu L-F, Lamendola C, Shen L, Morton J, Rivas H, Winer D, Tolentino L, Choi O, Zhang H, Hui Yen Chng M, Engleman E. T-cell profile in adipose tissue is associated with insulin resistance and systemic inflammation in humans. Arterioscler Thromb Vasc Biol 2014;34(12):2637–43. https://doi.org/10.1161/atvbaha.114.304636.

[117] Everaere L, Ait-Yahia S, Molendi-Coste O, Vorng H, Quemener S, Le Vu P, et al. Innate lymphoid cells contribute to allergic airway disease exacerbation by obesity. J Allergy Clin Immunol 2016;138(5):1309–18. https://doi.org/10.1016/j.jaci.2016.03.019. e11.

[118] Kim HY, Lee HY, Chang YJ, Pichavant M, Shore SA, Fitzgerald KA, et al. Interleukin-17-producing innate lymphoid cells and the NLRP3 inflammasome facilitate obesity-associated airway hyperreactivity. Nat Med 2014;20(1):54–61. https://doi.org/10.1038/nm.3423.

[119] Weisberg SP, Hunter D, Huber R, Lemieux J, Slaymaker S, Vaddi K, et al. CCR2 modulates inflammatory and metabolic effects of high-fat feeding. J Clin Invest 2006;116(1):115–24. https://doi.org/10.1172/JCI24335.

[120] Xu H, Barnes GT, Yang Q, Tan G, Yang D, Chou CJ, et al. Chronic inflammation in fat plays a crucial role in the development of obesity-related insulin resistance. J Clin Invest 2003;112(12):1821–30. https://doi.org/10.1172/JCI200319451.

[121] Strissel KJ, Stancheva Z, Miyoshi H, Perfield JW, DeFuria J, Jick Z, Greenberg AS, Obin MS. Adipocyte death, adipose tissue remodeling, and obesity complications. Diabetes 2007;56(12):2910–8. https://doi.org/10.2337/db07-0767.

[122] Li X, Hastie AT, Peters MC, Hawkins GA, Phipatanakul W, Li H, Moore WC, Busse WW, Castro M, Erzurum SC, Gaston B, Israel E, Jarjour NN, Levy BD, Wenzel SE, Meyers DA, Fahy JV, Bleecker ER. Investigation of the relationship between IL-6 and type 2 biomarkers in patients with severe asthma. J Allergy Clin Immunol 2020;145(1):430–3. https://doi.org/10.1016/j.jaci.2019.08.031.

[123] Peters MC, McGrath KW, Hawkins GA, Hastie AT, Levy BD, Israel E, Phillips BR, Mauger DT, Comhair SA, Erzurum SC, Johansson MW, Jarjour NN, Coverstone AM, Castro M, Holguin F, Wenzel SE, Woodruff PG, Bleecker ER, Fahy JV. Plasma interleukin-6 concentrations, metabolic dysfunction, and asthma severity: a cross-sectional analysis of two cohorts. Lancet Respir Med 2016;4(7):574–84. https://doi.org/10.1016/S2213-2600(16)30048-0.

[124] Guler N, Kirerleri E, Ones U, Tamay Z, Salmayenli N, Darendeliler F. Leptin: does it have any role in childhood asthma? J Allergy Clin Immunol 2004;114(2):254–9. https://doi.org/10.1016/j.jaci.2004.03.053.

[125] Gurkan F, Atamer Y, Ece A, Kocyigit Y, Tuzun H, Mete N. Serum leptin levels in asthmatic children treated with an inhaled corticosteroid. Ann Allergy Asthma Immunol 2004;93(3):277–80. https://doi.org/10.1016/S1081-1206(10)61501-3.

[126] Kattan M, Kumar R, Bloomberg GR, Mitchell HE, Calatroni A, Gergen PJ, Kercsmar CM, Visness CM, Matsui EC, Steinbach SF, Szefler SJ, Sorkness CA, Morgan WJ, Teach SJ, Gan VN. Asthma control, adiposity, and adipokines among inner-city adolescents. J Allergy Clin Immunol 2010;125(3):584–92. https://doi.org/10.1016/j.jaci.2010.01.053.

[127] Mai XM, Böttcher MF, Leijon I. Leptin and asthma in overweight children at 12 years of age. Pediatr Allergy Immunol 2004;15(6):523–30. https://doi.org/10.1111/j.1399-3038.2004.00195.x.

[128] Nagel G, Koenig W, Rapp K, Wabitsch M, Zoellner I, Weiland SK. Associations of adipokines with asthma, rhinoconjunctivitis, and eczema in German schoolchildren. Pediatr Allergy Immunol 2009;20(1):81–8. https://doi.org/10.1111/j.1399-3038.2008.00740.x.

[129] Sood A, Cui X, Quails C, Beckett WS, Gross MD, Steffes MW, Smith LJ, Jacobs DR. Association between asthma and serum adiponectin concentration in women. Thorax 2008;63(10):877–82. https://doi.org/10.1136/thx.2007.090803.

[130] Sood A, Qualls C, Schuyler M, Thyagarajan B, Steffes MW, Smith LJ, Jacobs DR. Low serum adiponectin predicts future risk for asthma in women. Am J Respir Crit Care Med 2012;186(1):41–7. https://doi.org/10.1164/rccm.201110-1767OC.

[131] Ajuwon KM, Spurlock ME. Adiponectin inhibits LPS-induced NF-κB activation and IL-6 production and increases PPARγ2 expression in adipocytes. Am J Physiol Regul Integr Comp Physiol 2005;288(5):R1220−5. https://doi.org/10.1152/ajpregu.00397.2004.

[132] Masaki T, Chiba S, Tatsukawa H, Yasuda T, Noguchi H, Seike M, Yoshimatsu H. Adiponectin protects LPS-induced liver injury through modulation of TNF-α in KK-Ay obese mice. Hepatology 2004;40(1):177−84. https://doi.org/10.1002/hep.20282.

[133] Wulster-Radcliffe MC, Ajuwon KM, Wang J, Christian JA, Spurlock ME. Adiponectin differentially regulates cytokines in porcine macrophages. Biochem Biophys Res Commun 2004;316(3):924−9. https://doi.org/10.1016/j.bbrc.2004.02.130.

[134] Zhu L, Chen X, Chong L, Kong L, Wen S, Zhang H, et al. Adiponectin alleviates exacerbation of airway inflammation and oxidative stress in obesity-related asthma mice partly through AMPK signaling pathway. Int Immunopharm 2019;67:396−407. https://doi.org/10.1016/j.intimp.2018.12.030.

[135] Arita Y, Kihara S, Ouchi N, Takahashi M, Maeda K, Miyagawa JI, Hotta K, Shimomura I, Nakamura T, Miyaoka K, Kuriyama H, Nishida M, Yamashita S, Okubo K, Matsubara K, Muraguchi M, Ohmoto Y, Funahashi T, Matsuzawa Y. Paradoxical decrease of an adipose-specific protein, adiponectin, in obesity. Biochem Biophys Res Commun 1999;257(1):79−83. https://doi.org/10.1006/bbrc.1999.0255.

[136] Steffes MW, Gross MD, Schreiner PJ, Yu X, Hilner JE, Gingerich R, Jacobs DR. Serum adiponectin in young adults - interactions with central adiposity, circulating levels of glucose, and insulin resistance: the CARDIA study. Ann Epidemiol 2004;14(7):492−8. https://doi.org/10.1016/j.annepidem.2003.10.006.

[137] Suzukawa M, Koketsu R, Baba S, Igarashi S, Nagase H, Yamaguchi M, Matsutani N, Kawamura M, Shoji S, Hebisawa A, Ohta K. Leptin enhances ICAM-1 expression, induces migration and cytokine synthesis, and prolongs survival of human airway epithelial cells. Am J Physiol Lung Cell Mol Physiol 2015;309(8):L801−11. https://doi.org/10.1152/ajplung.00365.2014.

[138] Grotta MB, Squebola-Cola DM, Toro AADC, Ribeiro MAGO, Mazon SB, Ribeiro JD, Antunes E. Obesity increases eosinophil activity in asthmatic children and adolescents. BMC Pulm Med 2013;13(1). https://doi.org/10.1186/1471-2466-13-39.

[139] Zheng H, Zhang X, Castillo EF, Luo Y, Liu M, Yang XO. Leptin enhances TH2 and ILC2 responses in allergic airway disease. J Biol Chem 2016;291(42):22043−52. https://doi.org/10.1074/jbc.M116.743187.

[140] Muc M, Todo-Bom A, Mota-Pinto A, Vale-Pereira S, Loureiro C. Leptin and resistin in overweight patients with and without asthma. Allergol Immunopathol 2014;42(5):415−21. https://doi.org/10.1016/j.aller.2013.03.004.

[141] Sutherland ER, Goleva E, Strand M, Beuther DA, Leung DYM. Body mass and glucocorticoid response in asthma. Am J Respir Crit Care Med 2008;178(7):682−7. https://doi.org/10.1164/rccm.200801-076OC.

[142] Cardet JC, Ash S, Kusa T, Camargo CA, Israel E. Insulin resistance modifies the association between obesity and current asthma in adults. Eur Respir J 2016;48(2):403−10. https://doi.org/10.1183/13993003.00246-2016.

[143] Singh S, Bodas M, Bhatraju NK, Pattnaik B, Gheware A, Parameswaran PK, Thompson M, Freeman M, Mabalirajan U, Gosens R, Ghosh B, Pabelick C, Linneberg A, Prakash YS, Agrawal A. Hyperinsulinemia adversely affects lung structure and function. Am J Physiol Lung Cell Mol Physiol 2016;310(9):L837−45. https://doi.org/10.1152/ajplung.00091.2015.

[144] Leiria LOS, Arantes-Costa FM, Calixto MC, Alexandre EC, Moura RF, Folli F, Prado CM, Prado MA, Prado VF, Velloso LA, Donato J, Antunes E, Martins MA, Saad MJA. Increased airway reactivity and hyperinsulinemia in obese mice are linked by ERK signaling in brain stem cholinergic neurons. Cell Rep 2015;11(6):934−43. https://doi.org/10.1016/j.celrep.2015.04.012.

Chapter 19

Obesity and the brain: structural and functional imaging studies, and opportunities for large-scale imaging genetics

Ilona A. Dekkers[1], Janey Jiang[2], Hildo J. Lamb[1] and Philip Jansen[3,4,5]

[1]Department of Radiology, Cardio Vascular Imaging Group (CVIG), Leiden University Medical Center, Leiden, the Netherlands; [2]Department of Radiology, Haga Ziekenhuis, Den Haag, the Netherlands; [3]Department of Human Genetics, Amsterdam University Medical Centers, the Netherlands; [4]Department of Complex Trait Genetics, VU University Amsterdam, Amsterdam, the Netherlands; [5]Netherlands Institute for Neuroscience (NIN), an Institute of the Royal Academy of Arts and Sciences, Amsterdam, the Netherlands

Introduction

The burden of diseases associated with obesity has substantially increased over the past decades, making obesity and associated metabolic disorders one of the most challenging health problems to date [1]. The global obesity pandemic not only has led to a greater incidence of cardiovascular disease, hypertension, and type 2 diabetes [2], but has been associated with a concomitant rise in negative brain health outcomes, such as accelerated cognitive decline [3] and dementia [4]. A shared common component of these different diseases is the metabolic syndrome, which has been associated with low-grade systemic inflammation via complex intermediate pathways affecting various organs, including the liver, pancreas, adipose tissues, and also brain [5] (Fig. 19.1). Inflammatory responses in the central nervous system (CNS) with subtle glial cell activation in obesity, also referred to as neuroinflammation without peripheral immune cells, have been described in different brain structures, such as the hypothalamus [6]. Preclinical animal studies relating high-fat and high-sugar diet to neuroinflammatory changes in the brain have supported these observations [7]. Moreover, postmortem studies showing higher concentrations of Alzheimer's disease—associated hippocampal markers (e.g., amyloid beta and tau) in elderly obese patients compared with nonobese patients [8] also indicate a possible link between obesity and the brain. It has been hypothesized that brain structure is influenced negatively via systemic inflammation; however, alternatively, it is also possible that lower volume of brain regions or decreased microstructural integrity of tracts involved in the neuronal regulation of the food reward circuitry might also be associated with obesity. Functional imaging studies have been performed to investigate the responses in dopaminergic pathways that show interesting similarities between drug addiction and obesity, and of which the overlapping dysfunctional brain circuits may explain related behavioral deficits in obese individuals. With regard to the possible bidirectional relationship between obesity and the brain, there is an increasing interest to perform imaging genetic studies including via the use of Mendelian randomization (MR) to evaluate the potential causal direction of the found associations between obesity and brain structure on imaging.

Structural brain imaging and obesity

Over the past decades, an increasing number of studies have been performed that use imaging to evaluate the possible associated changes in the brain related to obesity. Possible detrimental influences of obesity on brain structure have mostly been assessed as part of small cohort studies and later in larger population-based imaging studies. In these studies, participants are often followed over time after initial extensive phenotyping using collection of baseline characteristics, physical examination, laboratory measurements, imaging, and genetic analysis.

Visceral and Ectopic Fat. https://doi.org/10.1016/B978-0-12-822186-0.00023-7

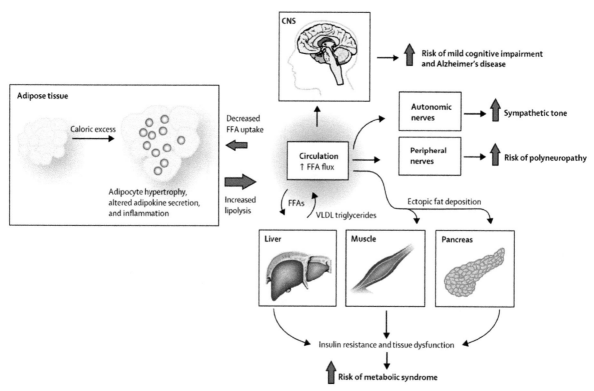

FIGURE 19.1 Possible pathophysiology of obesity and its adverse influences on the brain. The increased food intake leads to hypertrophy of adipocytes, which in particular in visceral fat leads to metabolic inflammation and adipose tissue dysfunction. The increase of free fatty acids (FFAs) has lipotoxic influences on peripheral tissues. Subsequent metabolic dysfunction is promoted by increased liver triglyceride production leading to dyslipidemia, skeletal muscle fat deposition leading to insulin resistance, and pancreatic fat deposition contributing to β-cell dysfunction. It is hypothesized that via the lipotoxic effects of dyslipidemia also, the brain is affected, and might contribute to mild cognitive impairment and possibly also the risk of Alzheimer's disease. *O'Brien PD, Hinder LM, Callaghan BC, Feldman EL. Neurological consequences of obesity. Lancet Neurol. 2017 Jun;16(6):465–477.*

For the assessment of volumetric differences, mostly three-dimensional magnetic resonance imaging (MRI) scans of the brain have been performed to derive quantitative brain metrics that allow for the assessment of global and regional brain volumes. MRI is particularly suited for the evaluation of brain structure because of its noninvasiveness and its clear delineation of white and gray matter using anatomical sequences (e.g., T1-weighted imaging). Moreover, in addition to more standard anatomical MRI sequences, techniques such as diffusion tensor imaging (DTI) enable more comprehensive assessment of in particular white matter structure. DTI is mainly used in research settings for the assessment of global and tract-specific white matter integrity by primarily fractional anisotropy (FA; directional coherence of water molecule diffusion) and mean diffusivity (MD; magnitude of water molecule diffusion) [9]. In this chapter, the focus is on studies that used structural imaging using T1-weighted sequences and DTI-based techniques.

Body Mass Index

Several studies have demonstrated that being overweight is a risk factor for dementia, in particular for Alzheimer's disease [10–12]. A longitudinal study in an urban sample of 392 Swedish nondemented elderly woman with 18 years of follow-up showed that being overweight at high age is a risk factor for dementia, particularly for Alzheimer's disease [11]. A subsequent study in 290 women with computed tomography scans of the brain of the same cohort found that high body mass index (BMI) was associated with temporal lobe atrophy [13], which is considered as an hallmark imaging finding for Alzheimer's disease [14,15]. Subsequent imaging studies in obese individuals have linked BMI to lower global brain volumes [16,17]. In addition, BMI has been associated with bilaterally decreased thickness of the parahippocampal and entorhinal cortices, and with increased thickness of parietal and occipital lobes, indicating a potential role of temporoparietal perceptual structures in obesity [18].

Moreover, also structural brain differences related to lower gray matter density have been described in obese subjects concerning brain regions (e.g., postcentral gyrus, frontal operculum, putamen, and middle frontal gyrus) that may play a role in the regulation of eating behavior (e.g., food reward circuitry) [19].

Fat distribution

In addition to imaging studies that focused on BMI as a measure of obesity, other studies have investigated the relationship with brain imaging findings and abdominal obesity. BMI differentiates poorly between body fat, muscle mass, and water, whereas there is a wide range of body fat distribution in both lean and obese adults. Abdominal or central obesity, reflected as waist circumference (WC) or waist-to-hip ratio (WHR), is a better marker of cardiometabolic risk and mortality than overall obesity as measured with BMI. Several studies focusing on obesity and structural changes in brain imaging have been performed that used waist circumference as a measure of abdominal obesity instead of BMI. An early brain imaging study in 112 older Latino individuals showed a negative association between higher levels of WHR and hippocampal volume, and a positive association between WHR and white matter hyperintensities [20]. Hippocampal atrophy and white matter hyperintensities are, in addition to temporal lobe atrophy, important brain imaging markers of dementia, of which the presence of white matter lesions has been particularly related to vascular dementia. Subsequent later studies have also shown an inverse association between waist circumference and gray matter volume [21,22]. In addition, a larger population-based study showed inverse association of abdominal fat with brain volume [23]. These findings were detectable not only in elderly subjects but also in middle-aged adults. Although WHR and WC are commonly used in obesity studies, these measures discriminate suboptimal between abdominal subcutaneous (aSAT) and visceral adipose tissue (VAT). This distinction is important since both compartments convey different cardiovascular risk factors that cluster together in the metabolic syndrome [24−26]. More recently, a large population-based imaging study investigated the association between total body fat (TBF) percentage and various volumetric measures of the brain and white matter microstructure [27]. This study was performed using cross-sectional anthropometric data and imaging data of 12.087 participants of the UK Biobank. This study found that in men, TBF was negatively associated with various subcortical gray matter volumes, including the globus pallidus and caudate nucleus, which have been associated with the reward circuitry of food-related stimuli [28]. In woman, TBF was solely negatively associated with globus pallidus volume. Fig. 19.2 shows an example of the illustrative brain imaging findings of two participants of the UK Biobank that were included in the study [29] and were of comparable age but strongly differing BMI and distinct brain volumes. A possible explanation of the described associations between obesity and lower gray matter volume [30] could be the suspected potential adverse effects of low-grade systemic inflammation, which has been considered to preferentially affect gray matter volume in contrast to white matter volume [31]. Findings from the Framingham Heart study support this notion, as several inflammatory bio-markers that are linked to obesity have also been associated with smaller brain volume [32]. Preclinical studies have linked high-fat diet to neuroinflammatory changes and neurodegeneration [33], which has supported the role of insulin resistance as a possible pathway of cognitive impairment in type 2 diabetes and Alzheimer's disease [34].

Diffusion tensor imaging

With regard to white matter microstructure, the cross-sectional analysis of the imaging data of the UK Biobank found that greater TBF percentages were linked to higher levels of white matter microstructure assessed by fractional anisotropy, and negative associations were found between body fat and mean diffusivity [29] (Fig. 19.3). These findings mean that a higher body fat percentage as a measure of general obesity is associated with a higher coherence but with a lower magnitude of water diffusion on diffusion tensor imaging. Interestingly, these observations were opposite to previously described findings in aging populations [35] and were not different with previously observed findings that showed negative associations between high BMI and fractional anisotropy [36,37]. Possible explanations are the differences in scan acquisition and postprocessing, such as a voxel-based approach and higher scan resolution. However, it should be noted that the earlier studies compared individuals with normal weight as compared with overweight and/or obese individuals. The clinical interpretation of the described associations between obesity and white matter integrity remains difficult as DTI findings as such cannot be directly translated to white matter histology.

Visceral fat

To date, several studies have been performed that had a specific focus on visceral fat in relation to brain imaging findings, rather than more generic measures such as BMI or TBF or anthropometric indices such as WHR or WC. In line with the earlier imaging studies that used more generic measures of obesity, these studies have shown that reduced cortical thickness is also associated with visceral fat [38,39]. Results that have been published thus far for visceral fat and white matter hyperintensities remain unclear with regard to the directionality of the found associations [40−42]. Few studies have been performed that evaluated hepatic fat as a specific fat compartment in relation to brain imaging findings.

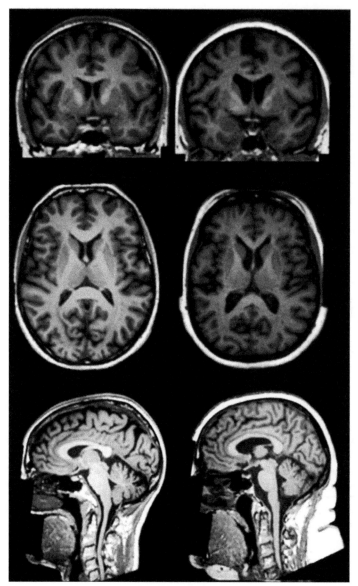

FIGURE 19.2   Example of T1-weighted brain MRI scans (coronal, axial, and sagittal plane) of two UK biobank participants (both female and 65 years old), one with a body fat percentage of 13% (left) and one with a body fat percentage of 49% (right) with the latter showing smaller volumes of subcortical gray matter structures in the individual with higher total body fat percentage [29].

Nonalcoholic fatty liver disease (NAFLD) is an archetypical example of ectopic fat accumulation in a visceral organ that causes organ-specific disease and affects risk of other related diseases such as type 2 diabetes and CVD [43]. A recent study showed an inverse relation for hepatic fat with cingulate gyrus and hippocampus gray matter volume [44]; however, no associations were found for hepatic steatosis on ultrasound and brain volumetric measurements [45]. More studies are needed to evaluate whether hepatic fat may indeed be a valuable marker of high-risk fat distribution in relation to "cerebrovascular metabolic disease."

Hypothalamic function

A particular focus in addition to global brain volumetric measures has been on the hypothalamus, which is a key brain area involved in energy homeostasis. Animal studies have demonstrated that a high-fat diet induces changes in the hypothalamic structure via an inflammatory response [46]. In humans, high BMI has been linked to the presence of hypothalamic gliosis in individuals with insulin resistance [47]. More recently, using two large samples of the general population, it was shown that a higher BMI was related to altered microstructure in the hypothalamus, independent from confounders such as

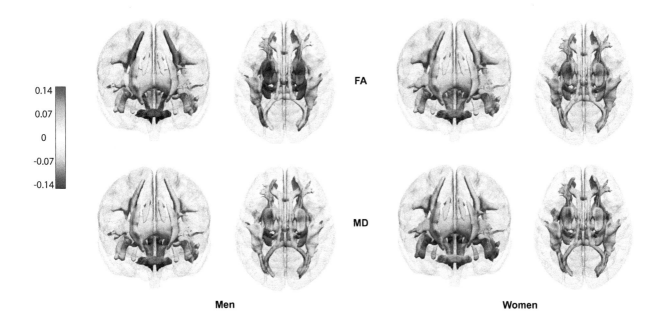

FIGURE 19.3   Overview of observed associations between total body fat, and tract fractional anisotropy (upper) and mean diffusivity (lower) on DTI for men and women. Colors represents standardized regression coefficients reflect the SD change in fractional anisotropy and mean diffusivity respectively per SD change in total body fat [29].

age, sex, and obesity-associated comorbidities [48]. In this study, hypothalamic volume and hypothalamic mean diffusivity derived by DTI were analyzed using state-of-the-art segmentation algorithms resulting in individual hypothalamic masks at the voxel level (Fig. 19.4) [48]. These findings show that the hypothalamus, as a main neuronal area involved in energy homeostasis, may undergo persisting microstructural changes in individuals with excessive weight and thereby affect brain eating behavior or energy regulation.

Although growing evidence indicates that obesity adversely affects the central nervous system and cognitive functioning, it should be noted that the majority of the published imaging studies involve observational studies with a cross-sectional design, which precludes causal inference. Additionally, most studies published have been focused on brain architecture rather than also taking into account associations with physical exercise, laboratory measurements, medication use, or cognitive functioning and could be possible sources of residual confounding. The availability of large population-based studies gives rise to detect subtle associations between obesity measures and brain structure and correction for relevant available covariates in these high-dimensional data sets.

Functional brain imaging studies and obesity

Aside from an influence of obesity on brain structure and functioning, a reverse direction of associations may also be plausible via neuronal influences on body weight regulation and eating behavior. Indeed, altered inhibitory control has been shown in obese individuals that shares clinical overlap and vulnerability with substance addiction [28]. Lower gray matter volumes of particularly the frontal and limbic brain areas in obesity may indicate that regulation of eating behavior could be influenced by altered inhibitory control via lower gray matter volume in these areas and associated affected signaling pathways of the corticolimbic tract [49]. The food reward circuitry has been studied in detail in various experimental studies that used positron emission tomography (PET) imaging combined with radioligands that specifically visualize the mesolimbic dopamine (DA) system [28]. By using radioligands that bind to dopamine 2 receptors (D2), the synaptic availability of DA neurotransmission can be studied, and in relation to responses to drugs and food in particular uptake in the striatum (e.g., caudate nucleus and lentiform nucleus) and prefrontal regions are of interest [50]. In morbidly obese individuals, D2 receptor availability was linked with brain glucose metabolism in the prefrontal regions, suggesting that a decrease in D2 receptors in obese individuals contributes to overeating, partly via deregulation of prefrontal regions that have been implicated to play a role in inhibitory control and emotional regulation (Fig. 19.5) [50,51]. This has been supported by functional imaging—demonstrated lower levels of striatal dopamine receptors in obese individuals (Fig. 19.6),

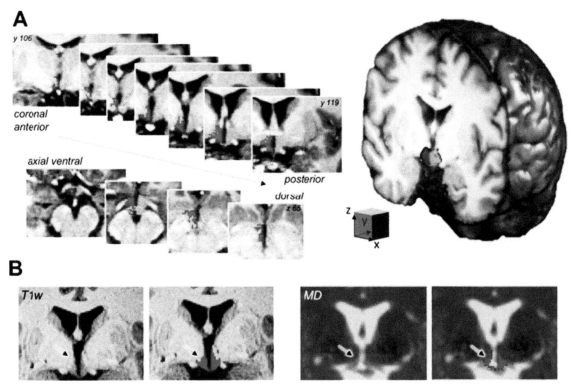

FIGURE 19.4 The hypothalamus analyzed using MRI in the coronal plane. (A) Semiautomated segmentation on anatomical images of the hypothalamus (right: red, left: orange). (B) Coregistration hypothalamus mask derived by T1-weighted (T1w) imaging to the mean diffusivity (MD) imaged based on diffusion-weighted imaging; arrows indicate sparing of hypothalamus voxels due to partial volume effects. *Reproduced under the terms of the Creative Commons CC BY license Thomas K, Beyer F, Lewe G, Zhang R, Schindler S, Schönknecht P, ... Witte AV (2019a). Higher body mass index is linked to altered hypothalamic microstructure. Sci Rep, 9(1). 1—11. https://doi.org/10.1038/s41598-019-53578-4*

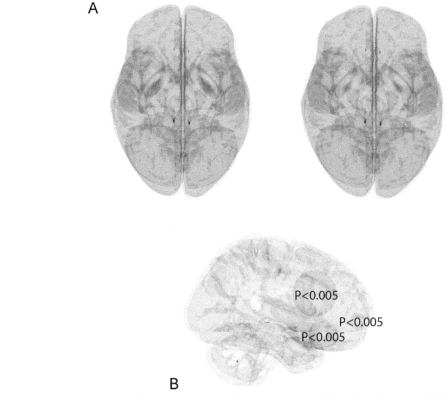

FIGURE 19.5 (A) Graphic summarising findings in positron emission tomography of dopamine 2 receptors (D2) measured with [11C]raclopride (a radioligand for D2) in controls (left) and morbidly obese individuals (right). (B) Graphic visualising the brain areas striatum, cingulate gyrus and orbitofrontal cortex where D2 receptors availability was associated with brain glucose metabolism assessed by [18F]fluorodeoxyglucose in obese individuals. *Adapted from Volkow N.D,, Wang G.J., Fowler J.S, Telang F. Overlapping neuronal circuits in addiction and obesity: evidence of systems pathology. Philos Trans R Soc Lond B Biol Sci. 2008 Oct 12;363(1507):3191—200.*

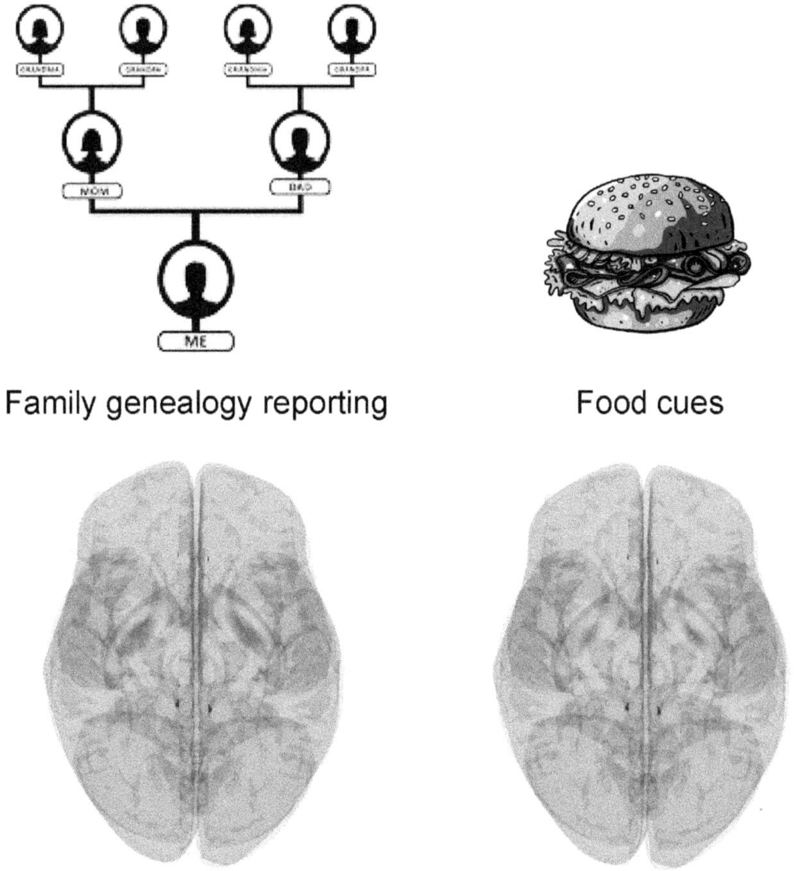

Family genealogy reporting   Food cues

FIGURE 19.6 Graphic summarising the averaged positron emission tomography images of dopamine 2 receptors (D2) measured with [^{11}C]raclopride in a group of controls tested while being interviewed on their family genealogy (neutral stimulus) or while being exposed to images of food (food cue stimulus), demonstrating differences in D2 receptor availability. To enhance the dopamine signal, participants were pretreated with oral methylphe-nidate to block dopamine transporters and so amplify the dopamine signal. *Adapted from Volkow N.D., Wang G.J, Fowler J.S, Telang F. Overlapping neuronal circuits in addiction and obesity: evidence of systems pathology. Philos Trans R Soc Lond B Biol Sci. 2008 Oct 12;363(1507):3191−200.*

which shows similarities to uptake patterns as described in addiction [50]. Similarly, differences in brain responses to food-related stimuli have been observed in obese individuals when compared with nonobese individuals [52]. Findings from functional brain imaging using PET suggest that obese individuals may have a dysfunctional dopaminergic pathway, which regulates neuronal systems that are associated with reward and motivation, as well as conditioning, impulse control, stress, and interoceptive awareness [28].

Ineffective insulin signaling, also referred to as insulin resistance, is a hallmark feature in type 2 diabetes and obesity and is increasingly studied in relation to neurodegenerative disorders such as Alzheimer's dementia. Increasing evidence indicates that the brain is an insulin sensitive organ, which has been highlighted by recent studies that have combined invasive insulin administration techniques with functional brain imaging such as magnetoencephalography (MEG) and functional MRI (fMRI) [53]. Examples of such invasive exogenous insulin administration techniques are hyperinsulinemic euglycemic clamp and intranasal insulin, while endogenous stimulation of insulin release is studied using tolerance tests (e.g., mixed meal, oral glucose, and intravenous glucose). Studies investigating the contribution of obesity-associated factors to brain insulin resistance by comparing neuronal activity in response to insulin using MEG and fMRI have revealed an attenuated response in overweight and obese individuals to both endogenous and exogenous insulin stimulation [53]. Long-term follow-up of individuals with brain insulin sensitivity determined by MEG who underwent a lifestyle intervention program showed that high brain insulin sensitivity at baseline was associated with a more pronounced reduction in total and visceral fat during the lifestyle intervention program (Fig. 19.7) [54]. In addition a cross-sectional cohort of 112 participants with precise fMRI of hypothalamic insulin sensitivity showed that strong insulin responsiveness of the hypothalamus is associated with less visceral fat, in contrast to subcutaneous fat (Fig. 19.8) [54]. These study findings demonstrate that high brain insulin sensitivity is linked to weight loss during lifestyle intervention and associated with a favorable body fat distribution, indicating the relevance to address brain insulin resistance in future therapeutic strategies.

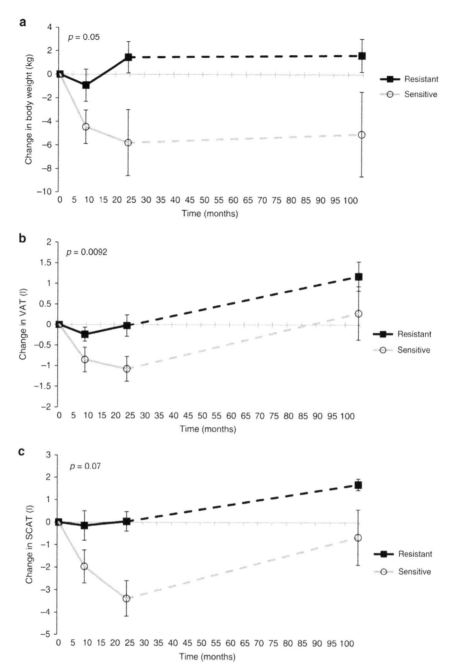

FIGURE 19.7 Changes in body composition over 9 years of lifestyle intervention for brain insulin resistant and sensitive individuals. (A) Body weight during follow-up (n = 15); (B) visceral adipose tissue (VAT) during follow-up (n = 12); (C) subcutaneous adipose tissue (SCAT) during follow-up (n = 12). Brain insulin sensitivity was assessed as change in the theta frequency band in response to insulin infusion, corrected for saline infusion by magnetoencephalography. *Reproduced under the terms of the Creative Commons CC BY license. Kullmann S, et al. Brain insulin sensitivity is linked to adiposity and body fat distribution. Nat Commun. 2020 Apr 15;11(1):1841.*

Genetic analyses of obesity and the brain

Genome-wide association studies

Analyses of genetic data have a strong potential to offer novel insights into the obesity–brain connection that cannot be obtained from traditional epidemiological studies alone. Genotypes can be integrated with molecular multiomics data such as functional annotation and gene expression to find mechanisms across different dimensions of system biology. Genome-wide association studies (GWASs) that link genetic variants to obesity identified the first susceptibility locus that

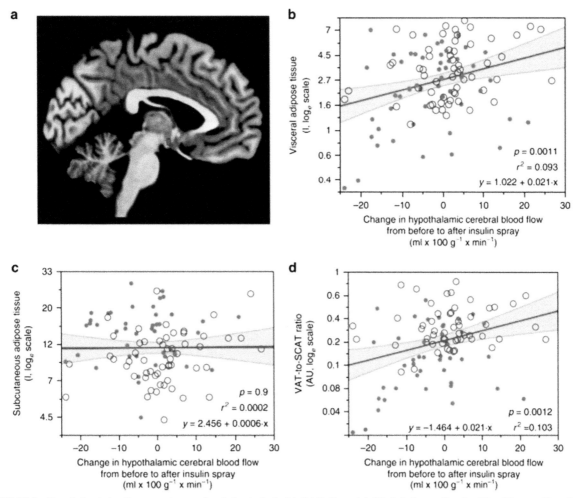

FIGURE 19.8 Hypothalamic insulin responsiveness in relation to body fat distribution; pink filled circles are females (N = 53), open blue circles are males (N = 59). (A) Change in cerebral blood flow in response to intranasal insulin administration was extracted for the hypothalamus. (B) Individuals with a strong insulin-induced suppression in hypothalamic blood flow had significantly less visceral adipose tissue. (C) Subcutaneous fat content was not associated with hypothalamic insulin sensitivity. (D) The ratio of visceral (VAT) to subcutaneous adipose tissue (SCAT) was lower in individuals with strong insulin-induced hypothalamic blood flow (d). Whole-brain fMRI experiments were conducted after an overnight fast and started under basal condition to quantify cerebral blood flow using arterial spin labeling. *Reproduced under the terms of the Creative Commons CC BY license. Kullmann S, et al. Nat Commun. 2020 Apr 15;11(1):1841. https://doi.org/10.1038/s41467-020-15686-y. PMID: 32296068; PMCID: PMC7160151.*

pinpointed the *FTO* locus [55], with many more risk genes following as sample size increased. Recent larger GWASs have been highly successful in identifying genetic variants that predispose to obesity [56] (ref), as collaborative efforts have now found over 700 genetic loci related to BMI [57]. In addition to these common genetic variants (i.e. with a population frequency >1%), exome-sequencing analysis that study rare genetic variants have found that mutations of strong effect in large sets of genes, such as MC4R and PCSK1. Interestingly, rare mutations in the GPR75 gene were shown to strongly protect against obesity, forming a potential new target for treatment development [58,59], and less so in other organs, showing that genetic predisposition for obesity mainly exerts its effects through mechanisms in the brain. Identified regions confirm known brain areas of importance such as the hypothalamus and pituitary, but also areas involved in cognition, including the hippocampus and frontal cortical areas [58,59]. On an even more fine-grained resolution of individual neurons, studies using single-cell RNA sequencing [60] have been able to find links of obesity genes with specific brain cell types of the hypothalamus, subthalamus, and midbrain, among other brain regions [61]. These studies complement large population-based imaging studies and generate hypotheses about new neurobiological pathways in obesity. Ultimately, these genetic studies of both common and rare variants in obesity may contribute to finding new targets that can be influenced by newly developed pharmacological treatment.

Polygenic risk scores

Building forth on recent large genetic studies of BMI, it has become possible to more accurately estimate an individuals' overall genetic predisposition to obesity based on large sets of known genetic variants. Polygenic risk scores (PRSs) are additive scores of large number of genetic risk variants found in GWASs and have shown to be a value tool for studying by estimating the overall genetic risk for obesity [62–64]. Combining genetic data and MRI data, studies have found that higher PRS (i.e. a higher genetic predisposition) of obesity are associated with lower surface area [65] and smaller prefrontal gray volumes of the cortex [66], showing that differences in genetic predisposition to obesity are reflected in differences in specific brain structures. As GWASs of obesity continue to increase, more accurate PRSs of obesity become available to study associations between obesity genetic factors and brain imaging phenotypes.

Mendelian randomization

Although associations between obesity and the brain have been extensively investigated in observational studies, these often cannot distinguish whether obesity causally affects the brain, or whether obesity results from aberrant brain structure and function. Genetic analyses can infer causality between different outcomes based on the genetic signal from GWASs. To this end, MR uses genetic variants identified from GWASs as instrumental variables, which are built on the assumption that genetic variants (predisposing for a risk factor) are randomly dispersed over the population [67]. MR studies have found that obesity predisposes to type 2 diabetes [68] and cardiovascular [69], but also less obvious causal associations with, e.g., multiple sclerosis [70]. MR analyses that explore causality between obesity and brain health are so far limited, but suggest that obesity is a causal factor for smaller global gray matter volume [23]. With available larger GWASs and more detailed analyses of specific brain regions, MR is a promising method to understand the brain–obesity association, and it is expected that exciting results will follow in the coming years (Fig. 19.9). Understanding these causal associations by use of genetic data is of great relevance for the effects of obesity prevention programs.

Future directions

Imaging studies discussed in this chapter have shown that obesity is associated with smaller cortical and subcortical gray matter volumes, and higher coherence but lower magnitude of white matter microstructure. These studies provide insights into the potential influences of obesity on the geometric organization of gray matter and white matter microstructure. Population-based imaging studies have led to a greater understanding of the relationship between obesity and the brain. The studies discussed were primarily based on the cross-sectional data of these large-scale epidemiological studies. As these population-based cohorts will be followed over time, also new insights will be become available that will prove an improved understanding of how brain architecture changes over time when exposed to obesity, and metabolic influences such as insulin resistance [34]. Moreover, studies that investigate brain structure in relation to metabolic responses (e.g., fasting and exercise, and eating and resting conditions) are needed [71]. Visceral fat volume in particular is of increasing interest, as this fat compartment particularly contributes to a low-grade systemic metabolic inflammation, and as such may lead to detrimental effects on brain structure and cognitive functioning [72]. The imaging studies discussed in

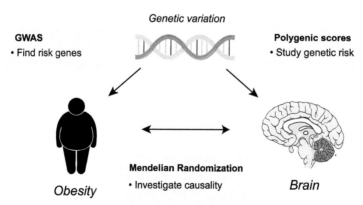

FIGURE 19.9 Overview of genetic methods used to investigate the brain–obesity axis. GWASs (genome-wide association studies) are able to find risk genes related to obesity, which can be linked to expression in the brain; polygenic risk scores are used to study links between genetic risk of obesity and the brain; Mendelian randomization can infer causality between obesity and the brain.

this chapter summarized findings that relate to volumetric and white matter indices. Functional brain imaging studies (e.g., nuclear metabolic studies and functional MRI studies) are in particular of interest for future studies as altered brain metabolism (e.g., brain insulin resistance) is possible underlying pathophysiologic pathway of the adverse effects of obesity on cognitive functioning. Finally, future studies are needed that evaluate whether stringent weight reduction and treatment of obesity-related metabolic disorders also benefit the potential neurologic consequences of obesity. In the field of obesity genetics, increasingly larger GWASs will further uncover the genes involved in obesity, and subsequently the brain areas and mechanisms that are influenced by these genes. This will lead to new hypotheses about the brain−obesity axis that can be further tested in experimental laboratory studies (e.g., neuronal cultures and animal models).

Conclusions

Observations from epidemiological studies have linked obesity with increased risk of dementia and provided a basis for subsequent imaging studies that investigated whether structural differences on brain imaging in obese individuals compared with individuals with a normal weight can be observed. With the increase of sample sizes of population-based imaging studies, there is a growing level of evidence indicating changes in brain structure in obesity such as brain atrophy and loss of white matter integrity. It can be concluded that multiple brain regions are involved in the obesity−brain axis rather than a single specific brain region. This reflects the complex etiology of obesity involving multiple factors such as, e.g., behavior, neuroendocrine, and metabolic and environmental influences. Although an increasing body of evidence indicates that obesity adversely affects the central nervous system and cognitive functioning, it should be noted that the majority of the published imaging studies involve observational studies with a cross-sectional design. However, increases in sample sizes of genetic studies and more sophisticated statistical methodologies such as MR can shed new light on causal links between obesity and the brain and uncover molecular pathways that explain a possible causal association.

References

[1] GBD 2015 Obesity Collaborators, Afshin A, Forouzanfar MH, Reitsma MB, Sur P, Estep K, Murray CJL. Health effects of overweight and obesity in 195 countries over 25 years. N Engl J Med 2017;377(1):13−27. https://doi.org/10.1056/NEJMoa1614362.

[2] The Emerging Risk Factors Collaboration, Wormser D, Kaptoge S, Di Angelantonio E, Wood AM, Pennells L, Danesh J. Separate and combined associations of body-mass index and abdominal adiposity with cardiovascular disease: collaborative analysis of 58 prospective studies. Lancet 2011;377(9771):1085−95. https://doi.org/10.1016/S0140-6736(11)60105-0.

[3] Gunstad J, Paul RH, Cohen RA, Tate DF, Spitznagel MB, Gordon E. Elevated body mass index is associated with executive dysfunction in otherwise healthy adults. Compr Psychiatr 2007;48(1):57−61. https://doi.org/10.1016/j.comppsych.2006.05.001.

[4] Whitmer RA, Gunderson EP, Barrett-Connor E, Quesenberry CP, Yaffe K. Obesity in middle age and future risk of dementia: a 27 year longitudinal population based study. BMJ 2005;330(7504):1360. https://doi.org/10.1136/bmj.38446.466238.E0.

[5] Lumeng CN, Saltiel AR. Inflammatory links between obesity and metabolic disease. J Clin Invest 2011;121(6):2111−7. https://doi.org/10.1172/JCI57132.

[6] Parimisetty A, Dorsemans A-C, Awada R, Ravanan P, Diotel N, Lefebvre d'Hellencourt C. Secret talk between adipose tissue and central nervous system via secreted factors−an emerging frontier in the neurodegenerative research. J Neuroinflamm 2016;13(1):67. https://doi.org/10.1186/s12974-016-0530-x.

[7] Guillemot-Legris O, Muccioli GG. Obesity-induced neuroinflammation: beyond the hypothalamus. Trends Neurosci 2017;40(4):237−53. https://doi.org/10.1016/j.tins.2017.02.005.

[8] Mrak RE. Alzheimer-type neuropathological changes in morbidly obese elderly individuals. Clin Neuropathol 2009;28(1):40−5. Retrieved from, http://www.ncbi.nlm.nih.gov/pubmed/19216219.

[9] Le Bihan D, Mangin JF, Poupon C, Clark CA, Pappata S, Molko N, Chabriat H. Diffusion tensor imaging: concepts and applications. J Magn Reson Imag 2001;13(4):534−46. https://doi.org/10.1002/jmri.1076.

[10] Beydoun MA, Beydoun HA, Wang Y. Obesity and central obesity as risk factors for incident dementia and its subtypes: a systematic review and meta-analysis. Obes Rev May 2008;9(3):204−18. https://doi.org/10.1111/j.1467-789X.2008.00473.x.

[11] Gustafson D, Rothenberg E, Blennow K, Steen B, Skoog I. An 18-year follow-up of overweight and risk of Alzheimer disease. Arch Intern Med 2003;163(13):1524−8. https://doi.org/10.1001/archinte.163.13.1524.

[12] Hassing LB, Dahl AK, Thorvaldsson V, Berg S, Gatz M, Pedersen NL, Johansson B. Overweight in midlife and risk of dementia: a 40-year follow-up study. Int J Obes 2009;33(8):893−8. https://doi.org/10.1038/ijo.2009.104.

[13] Gustafson D, Lissner L, Bengtsson C, Björkelund C, Skoog I. A 24-year follow-up of body mass index and cerebral atrophy. Neurology November 23, 2004;63(10):1876−81. https://doi.org/10.1212/01.WNL.0000141850.47773.5F.

[14] Jack CR, Dickson DW, Parisi JE, Xu YC, Cha RH, O'Brien PC, Petersen RC. Antemortem MRI findings correlate with hippocampal neuropathology in typical aging and dementia. Neurology 2002;58(5):750−7. https://doi.org/10.1212/WNL.58.5.750.

[15] Visser PJ, Verhey FRJ, Hofman PAM, Scheltens P, Jolles J. Medial temporal lobe atrophy predicts Alzheimer's disease in patients with minor cognitive impairment. J Neurol Neurosurg Psychiatry 2002;72(4):491−7. https://doi.org/10.1136/jnnp.72.4.491.

[16] Raji CA, Ho AJ, Parikshak NN, Becker JT, Lopez OL, Kuller LH, Thompson PM. Brain structure and obesity. Hum Brain Mapp 2009;31(3). https://doi.org/10.1002/hbm.20870. NA-NA.

[17] Ward MA, Carlsson CM, Trivedi MA, Sager MA, Johnson SC. The effect of body mass index on global brain volume in middle-aged adults: a cross sectional study. BMC Neurol 2005;5(1):23. https://doi.org/10.1186/1471-2377-5-23.

[18] Vainik U, Baker TE, Dadar M, Zeighami Y, Michaud A, Zhang Y, Dagher A. Neurobehavioral correlates of obesity are largely heritable. Proc Nat Acad Sci USA 2018;115(37):9312−7. https://doi.org/10.1073/PNAS.1718206115.

[19] Pannacciulli N, Del Parigi A, Chen K, Le DSNT, Reiman EM, Tataranni PA. Brain abnormalities in human obesity: a voxel-based morphometric study. Neuroimage 2006;31(4):1419−25. https://doi.org/10.1016/j.neuroimage.2006.01.047.

[20] Jagust W, Harvey D, Mungas D, Haan M. Central obesity and the aging brain. Arch Neurol 2005;62(10):1545−8. https://doi.org/10.1001/archneur.62.10.1545.

[21] Hayakawa YK, Sasaki H, Takao H, Yoshikawa T, Hayashi N, Mori H, Ohtomo K. The relationship of waist circumference and body mass index to grey matter volume in community dwelling adults with mild obesity. Obesity Sci Pract 2018;4(1):97−105. https://doi.org/10.1002/osp4.145.

[22] Janowitz D, Wittfeld K, Terock J, Freyberger HJ, Hegenscheid K, Völzke H, Grabe HJ. Association between waist circumference and gray matter volume in 2344 individuals from two adult community-based samples. Neuroimage 2015;122:149−57. https://doi.org/10.1016/j.neuroimage.2015.07.086.

[23] Debette S, Wolf C, Lambert JC, Crivello F, Soumaré A, Zhu YC, Elbaz A. Abdominal obesity and lower gray matter volume: a Mendelian randomization study. Neurobiol Aging 2014a;35(2):378−86. https://doi.org/10.1016/J.NEUROBIOLAGING.2013.07.022.

[24] Foster MC, Hwang SJ, Massaro JM, Hoffmann U, Deboer IH, Robins SJ, Fox CS. Association of subcutaneous and visceral adiposity with albuminuria: the framingham heart study. Obesity 2011;19(6):1284−9. https://doi.org/10.1038/oby.2010.308.

[25] Fox CS, Massaro JM, Hoffmann U, Pou KM, Maurovich-Horvat P, Liu CY, O'Donnell CJ. Abdominal visceral and subcutaneous adipose tissue compartments: association with metabolic risk factors in the framingham heart study. Circulation 2007;116(1):39−48. https://doi.org/10.1161/CIRCULATIONAHA.106.675355.

[26] Rosenquist KJ, Pedley A, Massaro JM, Therkelsen KE, Murabito JM, Hoffmann U, Fox CS. Visceral and subcutaneous fat quality and cardiometabolic risk. JACC (J Am Coll Cardiol): Cardiovas Imag 2013;6(7):762−71. https://doi.org/10.1016/j.jcmg.2012.11.021.

[27] Dekkers IA, de Mutsert R, de Vries APJ, Rosendaal FR, Cannegieter SC, Jukema JW, Lijfering WM. Determinants of impaired renal and vascular function are associated with elevated levels of procoagulant factors in the general population. J Thromb Haemostasis 2018;16(3):519−28. https://doi.org/10.1111/jth.13935.

[28] Volkow ND, Wise RA, Baler R. The dopamine motive system: implications for drug and food addiction. Nat Rev Neurosci 2017;18(12):741−52. https://doi.org/10.1038/nrn.2017.130.

[29] Dekkers IA, Jansen PR, Lamb HJ. Obesity, brain volume, and white matter microstructure at MRI: a cross-sectional UK biobank study. Radiology 2019;291(3):763−71. https://doi.org/10.1148/radiol.2019181012.

[30] Medic N, Ziauddeen H, Ersche KD, Farooqi IS, Bullmore ET, Nathan PJ, Fletcher PC. Increased body mass index is associated with specific regional alterations in brain structure. Int J Obes 2016;40(7):1177−82. https://doi.org/10.1038/ijo.2016.42.

[31] Vachharajani V, Granger DN. Adipose tissue: a motor for the inflammation associated with obesity. IUBMB Life 2009;61(4):424−30. https://doi.org/10.1002/iub.169.

[32] Jefferson AL, Massaro JM, Wolf PA, Seshadri S, Au R, Vasan RS, DeCarli C. Inflammatory biomarkers are associated with total brain volume: the Framingham Heart Study. Neurology 2007;68(13):1032−8. https://doi.org/10.1212/01.wnl.0000257815.20548.df.

[33] Granholm A-C, Bimonte-Nelson HA, Moore AB, Nelson ME, Freeman LR, Sambamurti K. Effects of a saturated fat and high cholesterol diet on memory and hippocampal morphology in the middle-aged rat. J Alzheim Dis 2008;14(2):133−45. https://doi.org/10.3233/JAD-2008-14202.

[34] Arnold SE, Arvanitakis Z, Macauley-Rambach SL, Koenig AM, Wang H-Y, Ahima RS, Nathan DM. Brain insulin resistance in type 2 diabetes and Alzheimer disease: concepts and conundrums. Nat Rev Neurol 2018;14(3):168−81. https://doi.org/10.1038/nrneurol.2017.185.

[35] Cox SR, Ritchie SJ, Tucker-Drob EM, Liewald DC, Hagenaars SP, Davies G, Deary IJ. Ageing and brain white matter structure in 3,513 UK Biobank participants. https://doi.org/10.1038/ncomms13629; 2016.

[36] Kullmann S, Schweizer F, Veit R, Fritsche A, Preissl H. Compromised white matter integrity in obesity. Obes Rev 2015;16(4):273−81. https://doi.org/10.1111/obr.12248.

[37] Xu J, Li Y, Lin H, Sinha R, Potenza MN. Body mass index correlates negatively with white matter integrity in the fornix and corpus callosum: a diffusion tensor imaging study. Hum Brain Mapp 2013;34(5):1044−52. https://doi.org/10.1002/hbm.21491.

[38] Cho J, Seo S, Kim WR, Kim C, Noh Y. Association between visceral fat and brain cortical thickness in the elderly: a neuroimaging study. Front Aging Neurosci 2021;13:358. https://doi.org/10.3389/fnagi.2021.694629.

[39] Veit R, Kullmann S, Heni M, Machann J, Häring HU, Fritsche A, Preissl H. Reduced cortical thickness associated with visceral fat and BMI. Neuroimage: Clin 2014;6:307−11. https://doi.org/10.1016/j.nicl.2014.09.013.

[40] Lampe L, Zhang R, Beyer F, Huhn S, Kharabian Masouleh S, Preusser S, Witte AV. Visceral obesity relates to deep white matter hyperintensities via inflammation. Ann Neurol 2019;85(2):194−203. https://doi.org/10.1002/ana.25396.

[41] Nam KW, Kwon H, Kwon HM, Park JH, Jeong HY, Kim SH, Hwang SS. Abdominal fatness and cerebral white matter hyperintensity. J Neurol Sci 2019;404:52−7. https://doi.org/10.1016/j.jns.2019.07.016.

[42] Portet F, Brickman AM, Stern Y, Scarmeas N, Muraskin J, Provenzano FA, Akbaraly TN. Metabolic syndrome and localization of white matter hyperintensities in the elderly population. Alzheimer's Dementia 2012;8(Suppl. 5). https://doi.org/10.1016/j.jalz.2011.11.007.

[43] Byrne CD. Ectopic fat, insulin resistance and non-alcoholic fatty liver disease. Proceedings of the Nutrition Society 2013;72:412−9. https://doi.org/10.1017/S0029665113001249.

[44] Beller E, Lorbeer R, Keeser D, Schoeppe F, Sellner S, Hetterich H, Stoecklein S. Hepatic fat is superior to BMI, visceral and pancreatic fat as a potential risk biomarker for neurodegenerative disease. Eur Radiol 2019;29(12):6662−70. https://doi.org/10.1007/s00330-019-06276-8.

[45] Yilmaz P. P3-339: Subclinical liver dysfunction IS associated with imaging markers of neurodegeneration, cerebral blood flow and cognitive decline: the Rotterdam study. Alzheimer's Dementia 2019;15:P1071−2. https://doi.org/10.1016/j.jalz.2019.06.3371.

[46] Thaler JP, Yi C-X, Schur EA, Guyenet SJ, Hwang BH, Dietrich MO, Schwartz MW. Obesity is associated with hypothalamic injury in rodents and humans. J Clin Invest 2012;122(1):153−62. https://doi.org/10.1172/JCI59660.

[47] Schur EA, Melhorn SJ, Oh S-K, Lacy JM, Berkseth KE, Guyenet SJ, Maravilla KR. Radiologic evidence that hypothalamic gliosis is associated with obesity and insulin resistance in humans. Obesity 2015;23(11):2142−8. https://doi.org/10.1002/oby.21248.

[48] Thomas K, Beyer F, Lewe G, Zhang R, Schindler S, Schönknecht P, Witte AV. Higher body mass index is linked to altered hypothalamic microstructure. Sci Rep 2019a;9(1):1−11. https://doi.org/10.1038/s41598-019-53578-4.

[49] Yokum S, Ng J, Stice E. Relation of regional gray and white matter volumes to current BMI and future increases in BMI: a prospective MRI study. Int J Obes 2012;36(5):656−64. https://doi.org/10.1038/ijo.2011.175.

[50] Volkow ND, Wang G-J, Fowler JS, Telang F. Overlapping neuronal circuits in addiction and obesity: evidence of systems pathology. Phil Trans Biol Sci 2008;363(1507):3191−200. https://doi.org/10.1098/rstb.2008.0107.

[51] Wang GJ, Volkow ND, Logan J, Pappas NR, Wong CT, Zhu W, Fowler JS. Brain dopamine and obesity. Lancet (London, England) 2001;357(9253):354−7. Retrieved from, http://www.ncbi.nlm.nih.gov/pubmed/11210998.

[52] Ziauddeen H, Farooqi IS, Fletcher PC. Obesity and the brain: how convincing is the addiction model? Nat Rev Neurosci 2012;13(4):279−86. https://doi.org/10.1038/nrn3212.

[53] Kullmann S, Heni M, Hallschmid M, Fritsche A, Preissl H, Häring H-U. Brain insulin resistance at the crossroads of metabolic and cognitive disorders in humans. Phys Rev 2016;96(4):1169−209. 2015.

[54] Kullmann S, Valenta V, Wagner R, Tschritter O, Machann J, Häring HU, Heni M. Brain insulin sensitivity is linked to adiposity and body fat distribution. Nat Commun 2020;11(1). https://doi.org/10.1038/S41467-020-15686-Y.

[55] Fawcett KA, Barroso I. The genetics of obesity: FTO leads the way. Trends Genet 2010;26(6):266. https://doi.org/10.1016/J.TIG.2010.02.006.

[56] Loos RJF, Yeo GSH. The genetics of obesity: from discovery to biology. Nat Rev Genet 2021;2021:1−14. https://doi.org/10.1038/s41576-021-00414-z.

[57] Yengo L, Sidorenko J, Kemper KE, Zheng Z, Wood AR, Weedon MN, Visscher PM. Meta-analysis of genome-wide association studies for height and body mass index in ∼700000 individuals of European ancestry. Hum Mol Genet 2018;27(20):3641. https://doi.org/10.1093/HMG/DDY271.

[58] Akbari P, Gilani A, Sosina O, Kosmicki JA, Khrimian L, Fang YY, Lotta LA. Sequencing of 640,000 exomes identifies GPR75 variants associated with protection from obesity. Science (New York, N.Y.) 2021;(6550):373. https://doi.org/10.1126/SCIENCE.ABF8683.

[59] Locke AE, Kahali B, Berndt SI, Justice AE, Pers TH, Day FR, Econs MJ. Genetic studies of body mass index yield new insights for obesity biology. Nature 2015;518(7538):197−206. https://doi.org/10.1038/nature14177. 2015 518:7538.

[60] Ofengeim D, Giagtzoglou N, Huh D, Zou C, Yuan J. Single-cell RNA sequencing: unraveling the brain one cell at a time. Trends Mol Med 2017;23(6):563−76. https://doi.org/10.1016/J.MOLMED.2017.04.006.

[61] Timshel PN, Thompson JJ, Pers TH. Genetic mapping of etiologic brain cell types for obesity. Elife 2020;9:1−45. https://doi.org/10.7554/ELIFE.55851.

[62] Khera AV, Chaffin M, Wade KH, Zahid S, Brancale J, Xia R, Kathiresan S. Polygenic prediction of weight and obesity trajectories from birth to adulthood. Cell 2019;177(3):587−596.e9. https://doi.org/10.1016/J.CELL.2019.03.028.

[63] Lewis CM, Vassos E. Polygenic risk scores: from research tools to clinical instruments. Genome Med 2020;12(1):1−11. https://doi.org/10.1186/S13073-020-00742-5/TABLES/2.

[64] Torkamani A, Topol E. Polygenic risk scores expand to obesity. Cell 2019;177(3):518−20. https://doi.org/10.1016/J.CELL.2019.03.051.

[65] Opel N, Thalamuthu A, Milaneschi Y, Grotegerd D, Flint C, Leenings R, Dannlowski U. Brain structural abnormalities in obesity: relation to age, genetic risk, and common psychiatric disorders : evidence through univariate and multivariate mega-analysis including 6420 participants from the ENIGMA MDD working group. Mol Psychiatr 2021;26(9). https://doi.org/10.1038/S41380-020-0774-9.

[66] Opel N, Redlich R, Kaehler C, Grotegerd D, Dohm K, Heindel W, Dannlowski U. Prefrontal gray matter volume mediates genetic risks for obesity. Mol Psychiatr 2017;22(5):703−10. https://doi.org/10.1038/MP.2017.51.

[67] Smith GD, Ebrahim S. Mendelian randomization: prospects, potentials, and limitations. Int J Epidemiol 2004;33(1):30−42. https://doi.org/10.1093/IJE/DYH132.

[68] Yuan S, Gill D, Giovannucci EL, Larsson SC. Obesity, type 2 diabetes, lifestyle factors, and risk of gallstone disease: a mendelian randomization investigation. Clin Gastroenterol Hepatol 2021. https://doi.org/10.1016/J.CGH.2020.12.034.

[69] Marini S, Merino J, Montgomery BE, Malik R, Sudlow CL, Dichgans M, Anderson CD. Mendelian randomization study of obesity and cerebrovascular disease. Ann Neurol 2020;87(4):516−24. https://doi.org/10.1002/ANA.25686.

[70] Mokry LE, Ross S, Timpson NJ, Sawcer S, Davey Smith G, Richards JB. Obesity and multiple sclerosis: a mendelian randomization study. PLoS Med 2016;13(6):e1002053. https://doi.org/10.1371/JOURNAL.PMED.1002053.

[71] Mattson MP, Moehl K, Ghena N, Schmaedick M, Cheng A. Intermittent metabolic switching, neuroplasticity and brain health. Nat Rev Neurosci 2018;19(2):63−80. https://doi.org/10.1038/nrn.2017.156.

[72] Klöting N, Blüher M. Adipocyte dysfunction, inflammation and metabolic syndrome. Rev Endocr Metab Disord 2014;15(4):277−87. https://doi.org/10.1007/s11154-014-9301-0.

Part V

Interventions

Chapter 20

The impact of very-low-calorie diets on ectopic fat deposition

Jennifer J. Rayner and Ines Abdesselam

Oxford Centre for Clinical Magnetic Resonance Research, Division of Cardiovascular Medicine, Radcliffe Department of Medicine, University of Oxford, Oxford, United Kingdom

Introduction

Very-low-calorie diets (VLCDs) are defined as providing 800 kcals per day or fewer [1], in contrast to "low-calorie diets," which include energy intake up to 1200 kcals, or "calorie-controlled diets," which merely aim to restrict calories below the total daily energy expenditure of the individual, hence inducing a calorie deficit and therefore gradual reduction in body fat. To achieve such a low-calorie intake, they are by default low-carbohydrate and low-fat, but maintain a high proportion of good-quality protein to maintain lean body mass while facilitating body fat reduction. The VLCD is often used in conjunction with ketogenic (very-low-carbohydrate) diets, or intermittent fasting, but this is not a mandatory component. They require vitamin and mineral supplementation, and the most commonly used approach is through a proprietary preparation of liquid supplements, consumed for each meal for the duration of the diet. The diet is equally valid using high-protein low-calorie dietary sources, but for convenience, the former approach is often preferred (Fig. 20.1).

The use of VLCDs was, until recently, considered to have peaked in the 1970s and 1980s, when their use fell out of favor following reports of sudden cardiac death [2,3]. While undeniably incredibly effective in terms of fat reduction, safety concerns persisted. However, with the increasing role of bariatric surgery, it began to become apparent that certain aspects of the surgical process led to huge metabolic improvements, even before the onset of significant subcutaneous fat reduction. Recent developments looking at the reversal of type II diabetes have led to a resurgence of interest in the use of modern, well-balanced VLCDs in the management of both ectopic fat deposition and its metabolic sequelae. In this chapter, we will endeavor to summarize this rapidly moving topic and communicate some of the excitement which is arising from the field.

While there is increasing evidence that the modern VLCD is safe [4], currently, they are only recommended for medical use for selected individuals under supervision [1]. However, there is no doubt that they are widely and increasingly used independently in the community, with no reports of adverse events. The historical deaths, which occurred related to the diets in the 1970s [3], were reported following use of low-quality protein supplementation, without sufficient attention to micronutrients, and following huge and rapid degrees of weight loss.

While VLCDs are certainly effective in terms of short-term weight loss [4–7], there has been additional controversy regarding the maintenance of results, with most [4], but not all [6–8], studies reporting significant weight regain following return to normal dietary patterns. Therefore, in terms of long-term overall body weight management, there does not seem to be pressing evidence of the superiority of this strategy.

However, when it comes to ectopic fat deposition, there is a significant body of evidence accumulating that VLCDs are an effective treatment not only for the excess adipose tissue itself but also for its metabolic consequences.

Visceral adipose tissue

A number of studies have reported effective reduction in visceral adipose tissue with VLCDs. These predominantly involve assessment of abdominal visceral fat with CT(9), MRI [9–15], or DEXA [8,15] before and after introduction

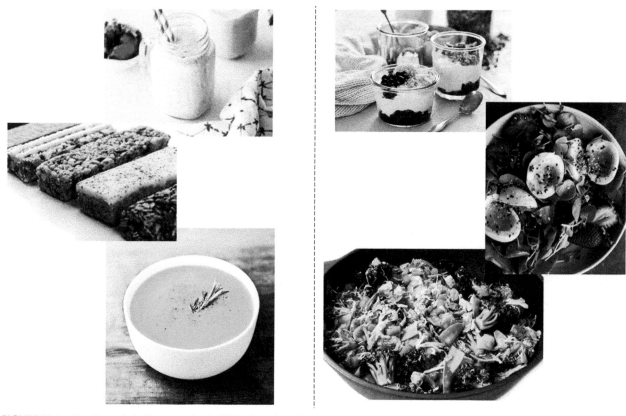

FIGURE 20.1 Very-low-calorie diets comprise 6–800 kcal per day, either of nutritionally balanced meal replacement products (left hand panel) or of low-calorie-density, high-protein foods (right hand panel).

of a VLCD (Fig. 20.2). Gomez-Arbelaez et al. [16] assessed reduction in visceral fat mass in response to a ketogenic VLCD over 4 months, using dual-energy X-ray absorptiometry, bioelectrical impedance, and air displacement plethysmography and noted strong correlation between the three alternative techniques. All these studies showed significantly greater reduction in visceral fat compared with whole-body fat mass over a short period of time, in keeping with the "overflow" hypothesis of fat storage [17].

One particularly elegant study was performed by Viljanen et al. [18], studying the impact of 6 weeks' VLCD intervention on otherwise-healthy obese individuals (Fig. 20.3). They not only investigated abdominal visceral and subcutaneous fat volume but also used PET imaging to study relative blood flow and glucose uptake. Interestingly, while VLCD was associated with greater proportion of visceral fat reduction consistent with previous studies, the results highlighted differential regulation of blood flow and glucose uptake between subcutaneous and visceral fat. Proportional perfusion and insulin-stimulated glucose uptake in the visceral fat depot was much greater, in keeping with its highly metabolic state. Resting blood supply to adipose tissue accounted for around 18% of cardiac output in an 100-kg obese individual. Weight loss leads to significant reduction in perfusion of both adipose depots, although there is no change in insulin-mediated glucose uptake in this healthy cohort.

A number of studies have also looked at thoracic visceral fat deposition in the form of pericardial or epicardial fat. These have demonstrated similar results to that seen in abdominal depots, with significant reduction in pericardial or epicardial fat induced by VLCD either measured on echo [19] or MRI [11,13] (Fig. 20.4). Snel et al. [11] reported an interesting finding in a cohort of obese individuals with type II diabetes mellitus, with VLCD leading to 17% reduction in pericardial fat volume over the first 16 weeks. They then followed up the cohort over 14 months of a regular diet, and while there was a near complete regain of total body weight, the reduction in pericardial fat was maintained, suggesting that some of the metabolic benefit of a VLCD may be maintained in the medium term.

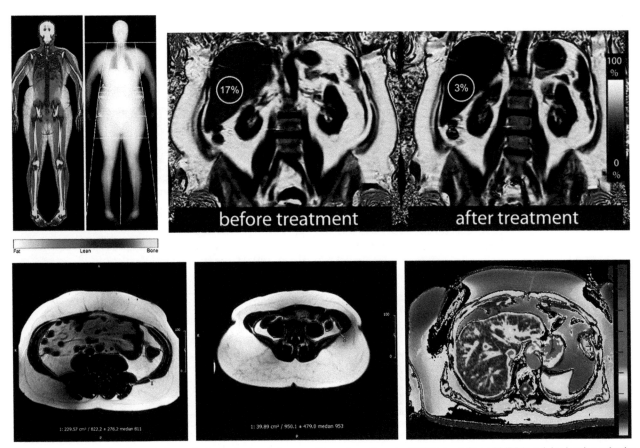

FIGURE 20.2 Visceral and ectopic fat can be imaged using dual-energy X-ray absorptiometry (DEXA; top left), and MRI (top right showing reduction in liver fat before and after VLCD; bottom left showing high visceral:subcutaneous fat ratio; bottom center showing low visceral:subcutaneous fat ratio; bottom right assessing liver inflammation as a result of steatohepatitis). *Top left figure reproduced with permission from Minetto et al., DXA-Derived Adiposity and Lean Indices for Management of Cardiometabolic and Musculoskeletal Frailty: Data Interpretation Tricks and Reporting Tips, Fron. Rehabilit. Sci. October 20, 2021 https://doi.org/10.3389/fresc.2021.712977; Top right figure reproduced with permission from Vogt LJ, Steveling A, Meffert PJ, Kromrey ML, Kessler R, Hosten N, et al. Magnetic Resonance Imaging of Changes in Abdominal Compartments in Obese Diabetics during a Low-Calorie Weight-Loss Program, PLoS One. 2016;11(4):e0153595.*

Hepatic ectopic fat

One of the first studies to comprehensively investigate the effect of a borderline VLCD (890 kcal per day) on metabolic health was carried out by Larson-Meyer et al. [9] in 2006. They used magnetic resonance spectroscopy techniques to demonstrate that caloric restriction led to significant reduction not only in total body fat (by $32 \pm 3\%$), but particularly in intrahepatic lipid (by $40 \pm 10\%$), even in overweight glucose-sensitive individuals. These findings have been borne out by a number of other studies in overweight and obese individuals, with VLCDs leading to rapid and pronounced reduction in hepatic fat deposition [10,13,20–23] (Figs. 20.2 and 20.4).

One of the main complications of hepatic ectopic lipid deposition is the progression from steatosis to steatohepatitis to cirrhosis, which is described by the umbrella term nonalcoholic fatty liver disease (NAFLD). This is a huge clinical concern for the future, given the burgeoning rates of obesity in the Western world. One key question is whether caloric restriction can not only reduce liver fat deposition but also reverse some of the end-organ damage associated with this. While a number of studies have demonstrated that body fat reduction is associated with improvement in established NAFLD [24,25], Scragg et al. demonstrated that a VLCD was not only feasible and safe in NAFLD but also associated with improvement in liver health as measured by liver function blood tests and liver stiffness [26].

Liver fat reduction resulting from VLCD has also been observed in individuals living with type II diabetes [11,12,14,27], alongside the parallel improvements in insulin sensitivity.

The metabolic consequences of this reduction in fat deposition were examined in an FDG-PET study in 2009 [22]. This found that a 6-week VLCD led to reduction in hepatic free fatty acid uptake as well as decreased fat content, with a

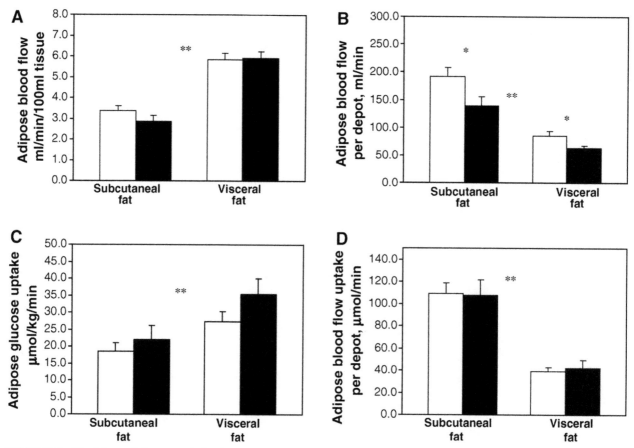

FIGURE 20.3 Blood flow and glucose uptake in adipose tissue. White bar is before and black bar is after the weight loss. *$P < .05$ compared between base line; **$P < .05$ compared between abdominal subcutaneous and visceral adipose tissue both at base line and after weight loss. *Reproduced with permission from Viljanen AP, Lautamaki R, Jarvisalo M, Parkkola R, Huupponen R, Lehtimaki T, et al. Effects of weight loss on visceral and abdominal subcutaneous adipose tissue blood-flow and insulin-mediated glucose uptake in healthy obese subjects. Ann Med. 2009;41(2):152−160.*

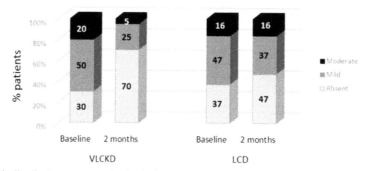

FIGURE 20.4 Very-low-calorie diets lead to a greater reduction in liver steatosis than a low-calorie diet. *Reproduced with permission from Cunha GM, Guzman G, Correa De Mello LL, Trein B, Spina L, Bussade I, et al. Efficacy of a 2-month very low-calorie ketogenic diet (VLCKD) compared to a standard low-calorie diet in reducing visceral and liver fat accumulation in patients with obesity. Front Endocrinol. 2020;11:607.*

significant fall in both hepatic endogenous glucose production and insulin resistance. It is this metabolic consequence of VLCDs that has driven some of the most exciting leaps in their therapeutic potential, as well as challenging our understanding about the pathophysiology of diabetes.

Very-low-calorie diet in the treatment of type II diabetes

The potential for caloric restriction to improve the control of blood sugar in type II diabetes is not a new finding [28]. However, the implications for widespread use of VLCDs to treat and even reverse diabetes have gained traction recently. One of the first signals that this may be a useful approach was highlighted by observations following bariatric surgery. It was known that gastric banding could lead to remission of relatively new-onset diabetes alongside weight loss in a significant proportion of individuals [29,30]. Detailed metabolic study in the immediate perioperative phase [31] raised the intriguing finding that diabetes "disappeared" with normalization of both insulin sensitivity and insulin secretion, in a matter of days following surgery, obviously preceding significant levels of whole-body fat loss.

The original hypothesis behind this was that the physical bypassing of sections of the gut, as well as acceleration of digestive transit into the distal intestinal tract, altered gastrointestinal hormone release, leading to improved insulin sensitivity and secretion. However, while bariatric surgery is associated with significant changes in gastrointestinal hormones, this was not found to be associated with the changes in insulin sensitivity [32].

At the same time, it was also found that the caloric restriction in the weeks immediately prior to bariatric surgery, initially to reduce the fat content and therefore volume of the liver to render laparoscopic surgery more technically straightforward [33], led to a marked reduction in hepatic fat [23]. This occurred in parallel with the improvements in insulin sensitivity, unsurprisingly given the effect of hepatic steatosis on the ability of insulin to suppress hepatic glucose production [34]. While this went some way to explain the improvement in insulin sensitivity, it could not account for the increase in insulin secretion.

Lim et al.'s study published in 2011 took a step further toward explaining this [35]. They used magnetic resonance spectroscopy, not only in the liver, but also in the pancreas, to document ectopic lipid deposition in type II diabetics before and during a VLCD. They found not only that early reduction of hepatic fat was associated with rapidly improved insulin sensitivity (Fig. 20.5), but also that a similar fall in pancreatic fat was linked to improved beta cell function over a slightly longer timeframe. This supported a "twin-cycle hypothesis" for the etiology of type II diabetes being linked to ectopic lipid deposition in both liver and pancreas.

These findings were further borne out by a series of studies by the same group, showing first that once normoglycemia had been induced through VLCD, that it could then be maintained through the transition to normal diet and weight maintenance [36], and thereafter in the randomized DiRECT trial [37]. This demonstrated that VLCD was a viable treatment option for diabetes and could be offered safely and effectively in the community, in contrast to the expensive, controlled environments required by some previous studies. Supporting results have now been published in subsequent studies [38,39], providing reassurance that a similar approach may be equally effective in different populations within different healthcare frameworks.

Fascinatingly, these studies provide further evidence for the existence of a personal threshold for lipid storage in the metabolic "sink," which is subcutaneous adipose tissue, beyond which excess lipid is deposited in visceral and ectopic depots with potential harmful consequences [40]. Weight loss in diabetes seems to be beneficial in different body sizes, with both nonobese individuals and those who lose weight but remain obese, improving their insulin sensitivity.

Finally, and excitingly for those of us working with the obese patient, the studies demonstrated that significant weight loss is achievable and potentially durable, in particular if it is being used to treat a disease process rather than as an arbitrary goal in itself.

Calorie restriction and cardiac lipid deposition

The impact of caloric restriction on intramyocardial lipid deposition has been more uncertain. It has been established that ectopic deposition of triglycerides within myocytes is associated with cardiac dysfunction [41,42] through a variety of mechanisms [43], including altered intracellular signaling and accumulation of toxic by-products of triglyceride

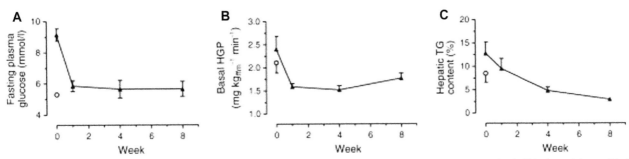

FIGURE 20.5 Very-low-calorie diets rapidly reduce plasma glucose, hepatic triglycerides, and hepatic glucose production in diabetic participants (black circles, compared with mean for matched nondiabetic controls (white circles)). *Reproduced with permission from Lim EL, Hollingsworth KG, Aribisala BS, Chen MJ, Mathers JC, Taylor R. Reversal of type 2 diabetes: normalisation of beta cell function in association with decreased pancreas and liver triacylglycerol. Diabetologia. 2011;54(10):2506—2514.*

metabolism. Therefore, it seems entirely logical that reducing intramyocardial fat deposition through calorie restriction would be beneficial [44], in a similar fashion to that seen in the liver.

However, one of the first changes induced by sudden calorie restriction is an increase in circulating free fatty acids (FFAs), through activation of lipoprotein lipase [10]. The heart is acutely sensitive to fluctuations in circulating substrate and will take up triglycerides in proportion to plasma concentrations [45]. A situation where myocardial lipid content is greater than the capacity for fatty acid oxidation has the potential to induce dysfunction, through diversion of triglyceride down nonoxidative pathways and accumulation of lipotoxic intermediate metabolites such as ceramide and diacyl glycerol. This not only further impairs FFA oxidation but also worsens intracellular insulin sensitivity, alters calcium handling [46], and favors accumulation of reactive oxygen species (ROS) [47], all of which impair cardiac function [41].

To investigate this further, van der Meer et al. [48] studied the impact of a brief VLCD in healthy volunteers on myocardial metabolism and function and found that over a period of 3 days, myocardial triglyceride content increased, with a parallel deterioration in diastolic function. A similar early deterioration was found in patients with type II diabetes [49]. However, if the diet was continued up to 16 weeks, a reduction in myocardial triglycerides was seen with an associated improvement in diastolic function [50]. This biphasic response, with early increase in MTGC and deterioration in function, followed by sustained fall in lipid content with functional improvement has now been seen in other studies including obese individuals without diabetes [10] (Fig. 20.6), and diabetics with cardiovascular complications [12,51]. Reassuringly, the improvement in myocardial function seems to be sustained even with the reintroduction of a normal diet, and a degree of reaccumulation of both overall body fat and MTGC [52], suggesting that the metabolic impact may be longstanding.

The mechanisms underlying these observed changes were elegantly demonstrated using FDG-PET imaging by Viljanen et al. [53], with weight loss induced through a 6-week VLCD leading to reduction in myocardial FFA uptake and triglyceride content, as well as reduction in mass and cardiac work. While whole-body insulin resistance fell, no change in myocardial glucose uptake was seen, supporting the preferential use of FFAs as fuel at rest, with the option of switching to glycolysis when required.

Obesity and diabetes are among the most significant risk factors for developing heart failure [54,55], and there is significant overlap in the metabolic abnormalities observed in the two conditions. While there is some evidence that modest calorie restriction is helpful in managing heart failure with preserved ejection fraction [56], the use of VLCDs or indeed weight management at all remains an active area of investigation.

Skeletal muscle lipid metabolism and very-low-calorie diets

Skeletal muscle is an additional focus for ectopic lipid deposition and one with significant metabolic importance given its role as a regulator of peripheral insulin sensitivity. Increased levels of intramyocellular lipid content (IMCL) can be associated with insulin resistance [57,58], although the picture is complicated by the observation that increased IMCLs are also observed in athletes [59], implicating a role for additional pathways in determining peripheral insulin sensitivity.

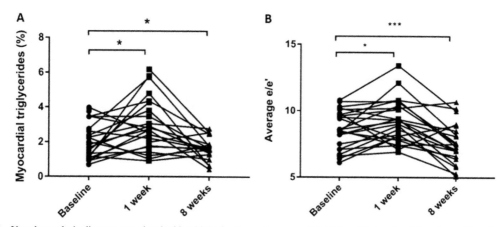

FIGURE 20.6 Very-low-calorie diets are associated with a biphasic change in myocardial triglyceride level and function, with early accumulation of myocardial triglyceride, and associated deterioration in diastolic myocardial function, but an overall improvement in both by 8 weeks. *Reproduced with permission from Rayner JJ, Abdesselam I, Peterzan MA, Akoumianakis I, Akawi N, Antoniades C, et al. Very low calorie diets are associated with transient ventricular impairment before reversal of diastolic dysfunction in obesity. Int J Obes. 2019;43(12):2536−2544.*

The short-term impact of a VLCD on skeletal muscle IMCLs in both obese and type II diabetics was demonstrated by Lara-Castro et al. [60], demonstrating significant reduction in both groups with associated increase in glucose disposal. Interestingly and in line with findings in other depots, the metabolic improvements were early, marked, and out of keeping with the degree of overall body fat change. While utilizing a low-calorie intervention (1000 kcal) rather than a VLCD, Nylen et al. [61] investigated the impact of calorie restriction on fatty acid metabolism pathways in skeletal muscle and found that genes promoting fatty acid uptake and utilization were enhanced.

In contrast, with a longer timeframe of weight maintenance following an early period of calorie restriction [9,14], there was no impact on IMCL concentration, highlighting perhaps that either the changes are time dependent or it is not only IMCL volume but also the pattern of lipid subspecies [61] as well as muscle oxidative capacity, which is important in determining insulin resistance.

Impact of very-low-calorie diet on bone marrow fat

Increased volume of adipose tissue within bone marrow has been associated with impairment of bone density and metabolism [62]. As part of a study looking at the effects of VLCD on disparate depots of adipose tissue deposition, Vogt et al. [14] found that in line with reduction in abdominal visceral fat volume, vertebral bone marrow fat content also fell.

Conclusion

In this chapter, we present evidence for the efficacy of VLCD intervention, not only on the volume of ectopic fat deposited in a variety of different depots, but also on the metabolic and functional consequences of this. Their use has extended our understanding of the pathophysiology underlying a number of different diseases (Fig. 20.7), as well as providing an exciting, cost-effective, and applicable treatment for metabolic disease in multiple organ systems.

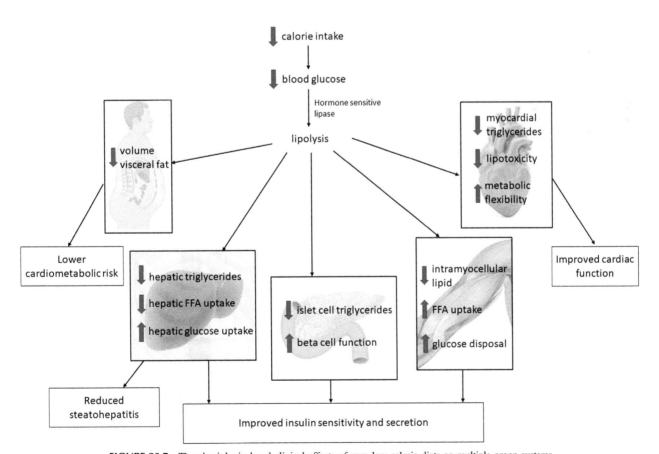

FIGURE 20.7   The physiological and clinical effects of very-low-calorie diets on multiple organ systems.

References

[1] Excellence NIfHaC. Obesity: identification, assessment and management (Clinical Guideline CG189) Available at: https://www.nice.org.uk/guidance/cg1892014.

[2] Isner JM, Sours HE, Paris AL, Ferrans VJ, Roberts WC. Sudden, unexpected death in avid dieters using the liquid-protein-modified-fast diet. Observations in 17 patients and the role of the prolonged QT interval. Circulation 1979;60(6):1401−12.

[3] Sours HE, Frattali VP, Brand CD, Feldman RA, Forbes AL, Swanson RC, et al. Sudden death associated with very low calorie weight reduction regimens. Am J Clin Nutr 1981;34(4):453−61.

[4] Tsai AG, Wadden TA. The evolution of very-low-calorie diets: an update and meta-analysis. Obesity 2006;14(8):1283−93.

[5] Mustajoki P, Pekkarinen T. Very low energy diets in the treatment of obesity. Obes Rev 2001;2(1):61−72.

[6] Larsen TM, Dalskov SM, van Baak M, Jebb SA, Papadaki A, Pfeiffer AF, et al. Diets with high or low protein content and glycemic index for weight-loss maintenance. N Engl J Med 2010;363(22):2102−13.

[7] Astbury NM, Piernas C, Hartmann-Boyce J, Lapworth S, Aveyard P, Jebb SA. A systematic review and meta-analysis of the effectiveness of meal replacements for weight loss. Obes Rev 2019;20(4):569−87.

[8] Moreno B, Crujeiras AB, Bellido D, Sajoux I, Casanueva FF. Obesity treatment by very low-calorie-ketogenic diet at two years: reduction in visceral fat and on the burden of disease. Endocrine 2016;54(3):681−90.

[9] Larson-Meyer DE, Heilbronn LK, Redman LM, Newcomer BR, Frisard MI, Anton S, et al. Effect of calorie restriction with or without exercise on insulin sensitivity, beta-cell function, fat cell size, and ectopic lipid in overweight subjects. Diabetes Care 2006;29(6):1337−44.

[10] Rayner JJ, Abdesselam I, Peterzan MA, Akoumianakis I, Akawi N, Antoniades C, et al. Very low calorie diets are associated with transient ventricular impairment before reversal of diastolic dysfunction in obesity. Int J Obes 2019;43(12):2536−44.

[11] Snel M, Jonker JT, Hammer S, Kerpershoek G, Lamb HJ, Meinders AE, et al. Long-term beneficial effect of a 16-week very low calorie diet on pericardial fat in obese type 2 diabetes mellitus patients. Obesity 2012;20(8):1572−6.

[12] van Eyk HJ, van Schinkel LD, Kantae V, Dronkers CEA, Westenberg JJM, de Roos A, et al. Caloric restriction lowers endocannabinoid tonus and improves cardiac function in type 2 diabetes. Nutr Diabetes 2018;8(1):6.

[13] Cunha GM, Correa de Mello LL, Hasenstab KA, Spina L, Bussade I, Prata Mesiano JM, et al. MRI estimated changes in visceral adipose tissue and liver fat fraction in patients with obesity during a very low-calorie-ketogenic diet compared to a standard low-calorie diet. Clin Radiol 2020;75(7):526−32.

[14] Vogt LJ, Steveling A, Meffert PJ, Kromrey ML, Kessler R, Hosten N, et al. Magnetic resonance imaging of changes in abdominal compartments in obese diabetics during a low-calorie weight-loss program. PLoS One 2016;11(4):e0153595.

[15] Goss AM, Gower B, Soleymani T, Stewart M, Pendergrass M, Lockhart M, et al. Effects of weight loss during a very low carbohydrate diet on specific adipose tissue depots and insulin sensitivity in older adults with obesity: a randomized clinical trial. Nutr Metab 2020;17:64.

[16] Gomez-Arbelaez D, Bellido D, Castro AI, Ordonez-Mayan L, Carreira J, Galban C, et al. Body composition changes after very-low-calorie ketogenic diet in obesity evaluated by 3 standardized methods. J Clin Endocrinol Metab 2017;102(2):488−98.

[17] Laurens C, Moro C. Intramyocellular fat storage in metabolic diseases. Horm Mol Biol Clin Investig 2016;26(1):43−52.

[18] Viljanen AP, Lautamaki R, Jarvisalo M, Parkkola R, Huupponen R, Lehtimaki T, et al. Effects of weight loss on visceral and abdominal subcutaneous adipose tissue blood-flow and insulin-mediated glucose uptake in healthy obese subjects. Ann Med 2009;41(2):152−60.

[19] Iacobellis G, Barbarini G, Letizia C, Barbaro G. Epicardial fat thickness and nonalcoholic fatty liver disease in obese subjects. Obesity 2014;22(2):332−6.

[20] Cunha GM, Guzman G, Correa De Mello LL, Trein B, Spina L, Bussade I, et al. Efficacy of a 2-month very-low-calorie ketogenic diet (VLCKD) compared to a standard low-calorie diet in reducing visceral and liver fat accumulation in patients with obesity. Front Endocrinol 2020;11:607.

[21] Viljanen AP, Iozzo P, Borra R, Kankaanpaa M, Karmi A, Lautamaki R, et al. Effect of weight loss on liver free fatty acid uptake and hepatic insulin resistance. J Clin Endocrinol Metab 2009;94(1):50−5.

[22] Hens W, Taeyman J, Cornelis J, Gielen J, Van Gaal L, Vissers D. The effect of lifestyle interventions on excess ectopic fat deposition measured by noninvasive techniques in overweight and obese adults: a systematic review and meta-analysis. J Phys Act Health 2016;13(6):671−94.

[23] Hollingsworth KG, Abubacker MZ, Joubert I, Allison ME, Lomas DJ. Low-carbohydrate diet induced reduction of hepatic lipid content observed with a rapid non-invasive MRI technique. Br J Radiol 2006;79(945):712−5.

[24] Thoma C, Day CP, Trenell MI. Lifestyle interventions for the treatment of non-alcoholic fatty liver disease in adults: a systematic review. J Hepatol 2012;56(1):255−66.

[25] Promrat K, Kleiner DE, Niemeier HM, Jackvony E, Kearns M, Wands JR, et al. Randomized controlled trial testing the effects of weight loss on nonalcoholic steatohepatitis. Hepatology 2010;51(1):121−9.

[26] Scragg J, Avery L, Cassidy S, Taylor G, Haigh L, Boyle M, et al. Feasibility of a very low calorie diet to achieve a sustainable 10% weight loss in patients with nonalcoholic fatty liver disease. Clin Transl Gastroenterol 2020;11(9):e00231.

[27] Petersen KF, Dufour S, Befroy D, Lehrke M, Hendler RE, Shulman GI. Reversal of nonalcoholic hepatic steatosis, hepatic insulin resistance, and hyperglycemia by moderate weight reduction in patients with type 2 diabetes. Diabetes 2005;54(3):603−8.

[28] Savage PJ, Bennion LJ, Flock EV, Nagulesparan M, Mott D, Roth J, et al. Diet-induced improvement of abnormalities in insulin and glucagon secretion and in insulin receptor binding in diabetes mellitus. J Clin Endocrinol Metab 1979;48(6):999−1007.

[29] Dixon JB, O'Brien PE, Playfair J, Chapman L, Schachter LM, Skinner S, et al. Adjustable gastric banding and conventional therapy for type 2 diabetes: a randomized controlled trial. JAMA 2008;299(3):316−23.

[30] Sjostrom CD, Lissner L, Wedel H, Sjostrom L. Reduction in incidence of diabetes, hypertension and lipid disturbances after intentional weight loss induced by bariatric surgery: the SOS intervention study. Obes Res 1999;7(5):477−84.

[31] Guidone C, Manco M, Valera-Mora E, Iaconelli A, Gniuli D, Mari A, et al. Mechanisms of recovery from type 2 diabetes after malabsorptive bariatric surgery. Diabetes 2006;55(7):2025−31.

[32] Salinari S, Bertuzzi A, Asnaghi S, Guidone C, Manco M, Mingrone G. First-phase insulin secretion restoration and differential response to glucose load depending on the route of administration in type 2 diabetic subjects after bariatric surgery. Diabetes Care 2009;32(3):375−80.

[33] Colles SL, Dixon JB, Marks P, Strauss BJ, O'Brien PE. Preoperative weight loss with a very-low-energy diet: quantitation of changes in liver and abdominal fat by serial imaging. Am J Clin Nutr 2006;84(2):304−11.

[34] Seppala-Lindroos A, Vehkavaara S, Hakkinen AM, Goto T, Westerbacka J, Sovijarvi A, et al. Fat accumulation in the liver is associated with defects in insulin suppression of glucose production and serum free fatty acids independent of obesity in normal men. J Clin Endocrinol Metab 2002;87(7):3023−8.

[35] Lim EL, Hollingsworth KG, Aribisala BS, Chen MJ, Mathers JC, Taylor R. Reversal of type 2 diabetes: normalisation of beta cell function in association with decreased pancreas and liver triacylglycerol. Diabetologia 2011;54(10):2506−14.

[36] Steven S, Hollingsworth KG, Al-Mrabeh A, Avery L, Aribisala B, Caslake M, et al. Very low-calorie diet and 6 months of weight stability in type 2 diabetes: pathophysiological changes in responders and nonresponders. Diabetes Care 2016;39(5):808−15.

[37] Lean ME, Leslie WS, Barnes AC, Brosnahan N, Thom G, McCombie L, et al. Primary care-led weight management for remission of type 2 diabetes (DiRECT): an open-label, cluster-randomised trial. Lancet 2018;391(10120):541−51.

[38] Umphonsathien M, Prutanopajai P, Aiam ORJ, Thararoop T, Karin A, Kanjanapha C, et al. Immediate and long-term effects of a very-low-calorie diet on diabetes remission and glycemic control in obese Thai patients with type 2 diabetes mellitus. Food Sci Nutr 2019;7(3):1113−22.

[39] Taheri S, Zaghloul H, Chagoury O, Elhadad S, Ahmed SH, El Khatib N, et al. Effect of intensive lifestyle intervention on bodyweight and glycaemia in early type 2 diabetes (DIADEM-I): an open-label, parallel-group, randomised controlled trial. Lancet Diabetes Endocrinol 2020;8(6):477−89.

[40] Cuthbertson DJ, Steele T, Wilding JP, Halford JC, Harrold JA, Hamer M, et al. What have human experimental overfeeding studies taught us about adipose tissue expansion and susceptibility to obesity and metabolic complications? Int J Obes 2017;41(6):853−65.

[41] Zhou YT, Grayburn P, Karim A, Shimabukuro M, Higa M, Baetens D, et al. Lipotoxic heart disease in obese rats: implications for human obesity. Proc Natl Acad Sci U S A 2000;97(4):1784−9.

[42] Ouwens DM, Boer C, Fodor M, de Galan P, Heine RJ, Maassen JA, et al. Cardiac dysfunction induced by high-fat diet is associated with altered myocardial insulin signalling in rats. Diabetologia 2005;48(6):1229−37.

[43] Sharma S, Adrogue JV, Golfman L, Uray I, Lemm J, Youker K, et al. Intramyocardial lipid accumulation in the failing human heart resembles the lipotoxic rat heart. Faseb J 2004;18(14):1692−700.

[44] Rider OJ, Francis JM, Ali MK, Petersen SE, Robinson M, Robson MD, et al. Beneficial cardiovascular effects of bariatric surgical and dietary weight loss in obesity. J Am Coll Cardiol 2009;54(8):718−26.

[45] Nelson RH, Prasad A, Lerman A, Miles JM. Myocardial uptake of circulating triglycerides in nondiabetic patients with heart disease. Diabetes 2007;56(2):527−30.

[46] Carvajal K, Balderas-Villalobos J, Bello-Sanchez MD, Phillips-Farfan B, Molina-Munoz T, Aldana-Quintero H, et al. Ca(2+) mishandling and cardiac dysfunction in obesity and insulin resistance: role of oxidative stress. Cell Calcium 2014;56(5):408−15.

[47] Vincent HK, Powers SK, Stewart DJ, Shanely RA, Demirel H, Naito H. Obesity is associated with increased myocardial oxidative stress. Int J Obes Relat Metab Disord 1999;23(1):67−74.

[48] van der Meer RW, Hammer S, Smit JW, Frolich M, Bax JJ, Diamant M, et al. Short-term caloric restriction induces accumulation of myocardial triglycerides and decreases left ventricular diastolic function in healthy subjects. Diabetes 2007;56(12):2849−53.

[49] Hammer S, van der Meer RW, Lamb HJ, de Boer HH, Bax JJ, de Roos A, et al. Short-term flexibility of myocardial triglycerides and diastolic function in patients with type 2 diabetes mellitus. Am J Physiol Endocrinol Metab 2008;295(3):E714−8.

[50] Hammer S, Snel M, Lamb HJ, Jazet IM, van der Meer RW, Pijl H, et al. Prolonged caloric restriction in obese patients with type 2 diabetes mellitus decreases myocardial triglyceride content and improves myocardial function. J Am Coll Cardiol 2008;52(12):1006−12.

[51] Jonker JT, Djaberi R, van Schinkel LD, Hammer S, Bus MT, Kerpershoek G, et al. Very-low-calorie diet increases myocardial triglyceride content and decreases diastolic left ventricular function in type 2 diabetes with cardiac complications. Diabetes Care 2014;37(1):e1−2.

[52] Jonker JT, Snel M, Hammer S, Jazet IM, van der Meer RW, Pijl H, et al. Sustained cardiac remodeling after a short-term very low calorie diet in type 2 diabetes mellitus patients. Int J Cardiovasc Imag 2014;30(1):121−7.

[53] Viljanen AP, Karmi A, Borra R, Parkka JP, Lepomaki V, Parkkola R, et al. Effect of caloric restriction on myocardial fatty acid uptake, left ventricular mass, and cardiac work in obese adults. Am J Cardiol 2009;103(12):1721−6.

[54] Kenchaiah S, Evans JC, Levy D, Wilson PW, Benjamin EJ, Larson MG, et al. Obesity and the risk of heart failure. N Engl J Med 2002;347(5):305−13.

[55] Ho JE, Enserro D, Brouwers FP, Kizer JR, Shah SJ, Psaty BM, et al. Predicting heart failure with preserved and reduced ejection fraction: the international collaboration on heart failure subtypes. Circ Heart Fail 2016;9(6).

[56] Kitzman DW, Brubaker P, Morgan T, Haykowsky M, Hundley G, Kraus WE, et al. Effect of caloric restriction or aerobic exercise training on peak oxygen consumption and quality of life in obese older patients with heart failure with preserved ejection fraction: a randomized clinical trial. JAMA 2016;315(1):36−46.

[57] Krssak M, Falk Petersen K, Dresner A, DiPietro L, Vogel SM, Rothman DL, et al. Intramyocellular lipid concentrations are correlated with insulin sensitivity in humans: a 1H NMR spectroscopy study. Diabetologia 1999;42(1):113−6.

[58] Phillips DI, Caddy S, Ilic V, Fielding BA, Frayn KN, Borthwick AC, et al. Intramuscular triglyceride and muscle insulin sensitivity: evidence for a relationship in nondiabetic subjects. Metabolism 1996;45(8):947—50.

[59] Klepochova R, Valkovic L, Hochwartner T, Triska C, Bachl N, Tschan H, et al. Differences in muscle metabolism between triathletes and normally active volunteers investigated using multinuclear magnetic resonance spectroscopy at 7T. Front Physiol 2018;9:300.

[60] Lara-Castro C, Newcomer BR, Rowell J, Wallace P, Shaughnessy SM, Munoz AJ, et al. Effects of short-term very low-calorie diet on intra-myocellular lipid and insulin sensitivity in nondiabetic and type 2 diabetic subjects. Metabolism 2008;57(1):1—8.

[61] Nylen C, Lundell LS, Massart J, Zierath JR, Naslund E. Short-term low-calorie diet remodels skeletal muscle lipid profile and metabolic gene expression in obese adults. Am J Physiol Endocrinol Metab 2019;316(2):E178—85.

[62] Patsch JM, Li X, Baum T, Yap SP, Karampinos DC, Schwartz AV, et al. Bone marrow fat composition as a novel imaging biomarker in post-menopausal women with prevalent fragility fractures. J Bone Miner Res 2013;28(8):1721—8.

Chapter 21

Intermittent fasting

Marjolein P. Schoonakker[1], Elske L. van den Burg[1], Petra G. van Peet[1], Hildo J. Lamb[2], Mattijs E. Numans[1] and Hanno Pijl[3]

[1]*Public Health and Primary Care, Leiden University Medical Center, Leiden, the Netherlands;* [2]*Department of Radiology, Cardio Vascular Imaging Group (CVIG), Leiden University Medical Center, Leiden, the Netherlands;* [3]*Internal Medicine, Leiden University Medical Center, Leiden, the Netherlands*

Abbreviations

ADF Alternate day fasting
CER Continuous energy restriction
FMD Fasting-mimicking diet
IER Intermittent energy restriction
PF Periodic fasting
SAT Subcutaneous adipose tissue
TRF Time-restricted feeding
VAT Visceral adipose tissue

Intermittent fasting methods

Intermittent fasting is rapidly gaining popularity as a contribution to a healthy lifestyle and a method to lose weight. The necessity for effective lifestyle interventions arises from the worldwide increasing problem of obesity and its related diseases. Since not all individuals seem to be able to adhere to continuous energy restriction (CER), it is interesting to look at other methods for lifestyle change. Ideally, healthcare providers should be able to offer patients a variety of effective lifestyle changes that have proven to be effective for prevention and treatment of these obesity-related diseases, to match an individual's needs and capabilities [1,2]. Intermittent fasting, in literature also known as intermittent energy restriction (IER), could be an interesting option [3].

IER is an overarching term for several dietary regimens [4]. It includes diets that apply water-only fasting for recurring periods, alternating with periods without dietary restrictions as well as diets alternating periods with reduced energy intake with periods without restrictions. Usually the low-calory periods allow a maximum of 25% of normal caloric intake. The periods of energy restriction are very diverse and differ from hours to several days. We will discuss most used IER regimens (Fig. 21.1).

Time-restricted feeding (TRF) refers to no energy intake, or a restricted amount of energy intake, for a period of 12−20 h a day. Early TRF refers to a period of reduced energy intake in the evening. When this period of reduced energy intake takes place in the morning, it is called late TRF. Alternate day fasting (ADF) is a regimen in which one day of eating ad libitum is alternated with a day of fasting or severe energy reduction. A minimum of two consecutive days of fasting or strongly reduced energy intake is referred to as periodic fasting (PF). Often used is the 5:2 diet, with two consecutive days of fasting and five days of no restrictions per week. A fasting-mimicking diet (FMD) comprises complex, fiber-rich carbohydrate and healthy fats, while it lacks refined carbohydrate and contains less than 10 energy% protein. Although an FMD typically offers some 25% of normal caloric intake, it induces a physiological response that mimics the response to water-only fasting because it provides just minute amounts of readily available glucose and amino acids. An FMD, however, does provide for essential nutrients such as vitamins and minerals [5,6]. The various IER methods are summarized in Fig. 21.1.

Visceral and Ectopic Fat. https://doi.org/10.1016/B978-0-12-822186-0.00025-0

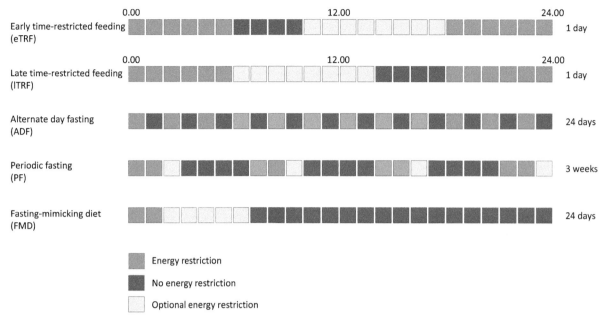

FIGURE 21.1 Intermittent energy restriction methods.

Physiology of intermittent energy restriction

Fasting activates several cellular and molecular mechanisms, leading to a "metabolic switch" in which the body switches from utilizing and storing glucose, to mobilizing fat [4,7]. Lipids in adipocytes are metabolized to free fatty acids and released in the blood, from where they are transported to hepatocytes and other tissues to serve as fuel [4] (Fig. 21.2). Moreover, hepatocytes convert free fatty acids into ketones, which become an important energy source alongside free fatty acids as an alternative to glucose. These processes usually start after 12—36 h of fasting, depending on several factors. First, hepatic glycogen stores must be depleted before significant amounts of ketones are produced. How long this takes depends on how extensive the initial glycogen content was at the beginning of the fast. Secondly, it depends on the level of energy expenditure during the fast. Besides being used as energy source, ketones are also potent signaling molecules activating several cellular pathways [7]. These activated pathways enhance intrinsic defense against oxidative and metabolic stress, facilitate the removal or repair of damaged molecules, promote DNA repair, stimulate mitochondrial biogenesis, and promote cell survival, while synthesis as well as growth and reproduction are minimized. Collectively, this improves resistance of cells and organs to stress. In a subsequent feeding period, tissue-specific processes of growth and plasticity are activated, and structural and functional tissue remodeling is initiated. The combination of fasting and refeeding periods facilitates systemic and cellular responses that carry over into the fed state and seem to improve physical and mental performance as well as resistance to disease [4,7—9].

Effect of intermittent energy restriction on health parameters in animal models

Several animal models have been used to study the effect of IER. In rodents, it has been shown that IER can have a beneficial effect on life span and several health parameters [6,10]. For example, the average life span of rats was increased by 30% when put on an ADF diet from the age of 10 weeks, compared with rats with an ad libitum diet [10]. Also in mice, extended longevity was seen when put on a bimonthly four-day FMD [6]. In lower species such as yeast, nematodes, and fruit flies, IER led to an increased life span as well [6,11]. The effects of IER on weight and fat, metabolic parameters, and other health parameters in animal models will be discussed in the following.

Effect of intermittent energy restriction on weight and fat in animal models

Overall, compared with controls fed ad libitum, mice on IER showed changes in body weight and/or fat distribution (Fig. 21.3). TRF prevented obesity and accumulation of lipids in the liver while retaining muscle mass in mice on a high-

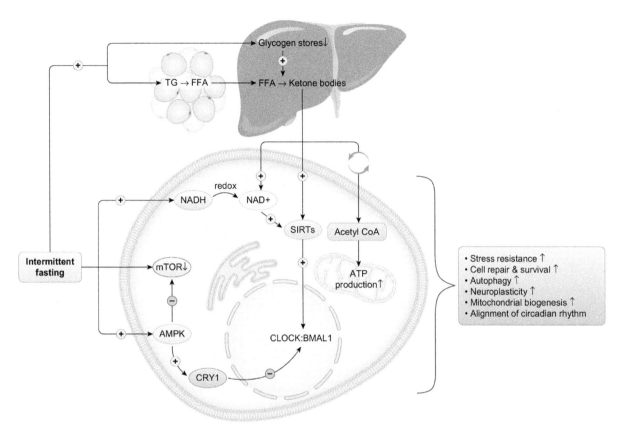

FIGURE 21.2 The effects of intermittent fasting. TG: triglycerides; FFA: free fatty acids; NAD: nicotinamide adenine dinucleotide; SIRT: sirtuins; mTOR: mammalian target of rapamycin; AMPK: adenosine monophosphate protein kinase; CRY1: Cryptochrome 1; CLOCK:BMAL1: circadian locomotor output cycles kaput: brain and muscle Arnt-like 1; acetyl CoA: acetyl coenzyme A; ATP: Adenosine triphosphate. Reprinted from Clinical Nutrition, 2021, Sep;40(9). Pages 5122-5132. Veldscholte K, Cramer ABG, Joosten KFM, Verbruggen SCAT. Intermittent fasting in paediatric critical illness: The properties and potential beneficial effects of an overnight fast in the PICU. *Reprinted from de Cabo R, Mattson MP. Effects of intermittent fasting on health, aging, and disease. New Engl J Med 2019;381(26):2541−2551.*

fat diet [4]. The same effects were observed in a study with mice on ADF combined with a high-fat diet [12]. Compared with the mice on ad libitum high-fat diet, weight gain was reduced, epididymal fat pads were smaller, and hepatic triglyceride content was lower. Concordant with these results, mice on a high-fat diet combined with IER showed decreased energy intake, body weight, fat mass, and fat cell size as well as reduced adipose tissue inflammation and fibrosis [13]. Mice on a high-fat diet combined with a 4-day FMD twice a month did not develop obesity. Compared with mice fed with the control diet, their body weight was 13.5% higher, whereas in mice fed with the obesogenic diet without FMD, body weight was 97.29% higher after 18 months [14]. The obesogenic diet without FMD also led to a significant accumulation of both visceral and subcutaneous fat compared with the control diet and obesogenic diet + FMD. The control and FMD group showed similar body fat content, and the FMD group had lower ratio of visceral adipose tissue (VAT) to subcutaneous adipose tissue (SAT) (percent VAT/SAT) compared with the obesogenic diet and control diet groups.

In another study with mice on an alternate-day modified fasting with 85% energy restriction, no significant change in bodyweight was observed [15]. Interestingly though, the proportion of subcutaneous fat increased, whereas the proportion of visceral fat decreased. This is in concordance with a study examining the plasticity of adipose tissue in response to fasting and refeeding in mice, where it was observed that during fasting, lipids were consumed in visceral adipose tissue, whereas during refeeding, lipids were predominantly recovered in subcutaneous tissues [16]. Mice on a 4-day FMD twice a month, with an ad libitum chow diet in between for 18 months, only demonstrated a trend for reduced total adipose tissue and a reduction in visceral fat deposits compared with a control group, with no change in subcutaneous adipose tissue volume [6]. Lean body mass remained the same in the intervention and control group. The effects were seen even though the total amount of calories consumed by the control mice on ad libitum diet and the mice on FMD was the same. FMD

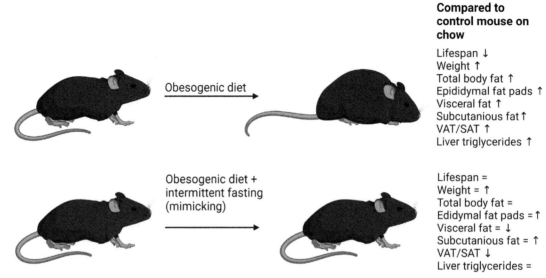

Compared to
control mouse on
chow

Lifespan ↓
Weight ↑
Total body fat ↑
Epididymal fat pads ↑
Visceral fat ↑
Subcutanious fat ↑
VAT/SAT ↑
Liver triglycerides ↑

Lifespan =
Weight = ↑
Total body fat =
Edidymal fat pads = ↑
Visceral fat = ↓
Subcutanious fat = ↑
VAT/SAT ↓
Liver triglycerides =

FIGURE 21.3 Effects of intermittent fasting regimes on body composition—related parameters in mice. *Created with BioRender.com.*

mice remained on the same weight for the first 4 months but did lose weight afterward. In mice on an ADF intervention, weight loss was also seen; however, no significant change in inguinal and epididymal adipose tissue mass was measured [17]. Though not tested, the authors proposed that the net weight loss was the result of skeletal muscle decrease. In this trial, adipocyte size was significantly reduced in both inguinal and epididymal adipose tissue, while total tissue mass had not changed, suggesting an increase in adipocyte number. Also, an increase in adipose tissue triglyceride metabolism was measured, with higher rates of lipolysis, increased plasma FFA concentrations, augmented gluconeogenesis, and de novo lipogenesis.

In conclusion, several IER regimes can prevent obesity, lipid accumulation in the liver, and fat accumulation in fat pads in mice on a high-fat diet. Furthermore, mice on IER exhibit an altered adipose tissue distribution, physiology, and structure, even in absence of weight loss (Fig. 21.3).

Effect of intermittent energy restriction on metabolic parameters in animal models

Besides the effects of IER on weight and fat distribution, effects of IER on plasma glucose and insulin levels, resting blood pressure and heart rate in mice and rats are also reported.

In a study with mice on ADF, reduced serum glucose and insulin levels were measured although overall food intake and body weight were similar, suggesting an effect of IER apart from caloric intake [18]. TRF can reverse high-fat food—induced obesity with impaired glucose tolerance, elevated plasma glucose, and insulin levels in mice [4]. Also, a 4-day FMD twice a month in nonobese mice reduced glucose and insulin levels [6]. However, these levels returned to normal within 7 days of refeeding. Compared with rats on an ad libitum diet, rats on ADF showed improved glucose metabolism [19]. Blood pressure and resting heart rate both progressively decreased during the first month and maintained the same level during the following 6 months. Furthermore when exposed to stressors, rats on ADF showed a smaller increase in blood pressure, heart rate, ACTH, corticosterone, and epinephrine levels compared with control rats on an ad libitum diet. Additionally, studies found favorable lipid profiles in rodents on ADF compared with the controls [4].

The results of the aforementioned studies indicate beneficial effects of IER on glucose tolerance, blood pressure, heart rate, and lipid profile in rodents (Fig. 21.4).

Effect of intermittent energy restriction on other health parameters in animal models

Other health parameters evaluated in animals on an IER diet include physical function, inflammation, cancer and skin lesion incidence, bone mineral density, mental health indicators, and gut microbiota composition.

Physical functions including running endurance, balance, and coordination are better in rats on ADF compared with ad libitum fed controls [7]. Mice on 4-day FMD cycles twice a month starting at middle age showed reduced tumor incidence,

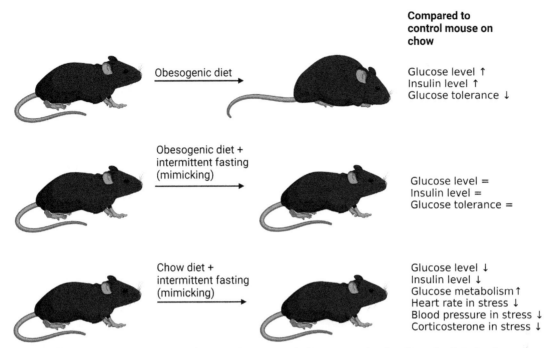

FIGURE 21.4   Effects of intermittent fasting regimes on metabolic parameters in mice. *Created with BioRender.com.*

delayed onset, and a major reduction in the number of skin lesions compared with controls [6]. The FMD group also had a reduced number of tissues with inflammation, less severe ulcerating dermatitis, and a higher femoral bone density.

In older mice on the same FMD, improved cognitive performance and hippocampal neurogenesis were found. Furthermore, brain neurons are protected against dysfunction and degeneration in different animal studies with ADF diets [4]. Animal models with epilepsy, Alzheimer disease, Parkinson disease, or stroke all show beneficial effects when put on ADF. Furthermore, ADF seems to improve cognitive performance, even when started later in life [4]. Cognitive function improvement was seen in multiple domains, including spatial memory, associative memory, and working memory [20].

IER also affects gut microbiome composition [21]. ADF shifts gut microbiome composition toward an abundance of Firmicutes, while most other phyla occur less, along with an elevation of the favorable fermentation products acetate and lactate. The authors suggested that it might be due to the change in microbiome that white adipose tissue browning was promoted, and metabolic homeostasis improved. In germ-free mice without gut microbiota, the beneficial effects of ADF on several indicators of metabolic function were less obvious. The metabolic effects of gut microbiota were also demonstrated in a study where germ-free mice received fecal transplants from obese and lean mice [22]. When receiving a fecal transplant from obese mice, their body and fat mass increased, and they developed the obesity-associated metabolic phenotype, whereas this effect was not seen when they received a fecal transplant from lean mice. These results suggest that alteration of the gut microbiome can influence the metabolic phenotype.

IER was also suggested to have positive immunomodulatory effects, at least partly mediated by the gut microbiome in multiple sclerosis mouse models [23].

Taken together, IER interventions result in positive effects on several health parameters including physical health, tumor incidence, cognitive function, skin lesions, bone mineral density, and immune disorders (Fig. 21.5). An alteration of the gut microbiome composition by IER possibly plays a role in the metabolic improvement. Fig. 21.6 gives an overview of some of the positive effects seen in literature upon using FMD, one of the IER methods.

Effect of intermittent energy restriction on health parameters in humans

In the past decades, more research has been performed exploring the effects of IER on body weight, fat mass as well as metabolic and other health parameters in humans. An overview of observed changes by use of IER in humans is illustrated in Fig. 21.7.

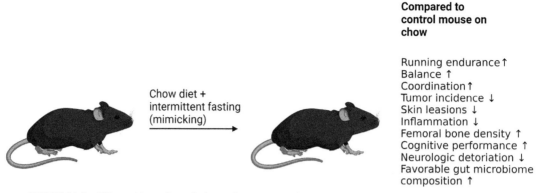

FIGURE 21.5 Effects of intermittent fasting regimes on several parameters in mice. *Created with BioRender.com.*

FIGURE 21.6 Graphical abstract. *Reprinted from Brandhorst S, Choi IY, Wei M, Cheng CW, Sedrakyan S, Navarrete G, et al. A periodic diet that mimics fasting promotes multi-system regeneration, enhanced cognitive performance, and healthspan. Cell Metab 2015;22(1):86–99 with permission from Elsevier.*

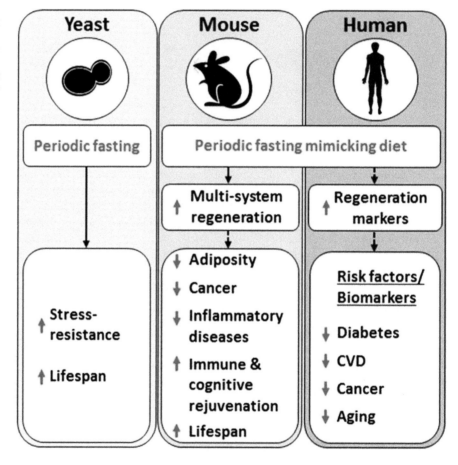

Effect of intermittent energy restriction on weight and fat in humans

In IER interventions in humans, fat mass loss is usually achieved along with weight loss. In a review including 40 studies implementing multiple forms of IER, 37 of the 40 studies demonstrated weight loss [24]. Three studies with lean participants showed no average weight loss.

Fat mass was reported in 23 trials, of which 20 reported a decrease. The other three trials tested lean persons or had only a decrease in one of the IER intervention arms. Fat-free mass was measured in 17 trials, and of these, nine reported a decrease and eight reported no change.

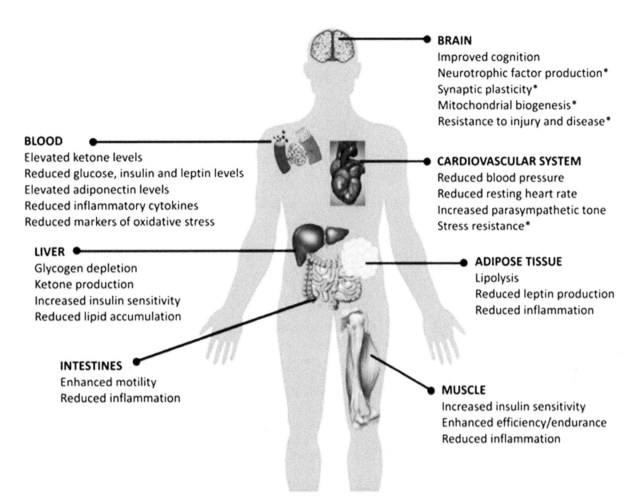

FIGURE 21.7   Examples of functional effects and major cellular and molecular responses of various organ systems to Intermittent Fasting (IF). In humans and rodents, IF results in decreased levels of circulating insulin and leptin, elevated ketone levels, and reduced levels of proinflammatory cytokines and markers of oxidative stress. Liver cells respond to fasting by generating ketones and by increasing insulin sensitivity and decreasing lipid accumulation. Markers of inflammation in the intestines are reduced by IF. The insulin sensitivity of muscle cells is enhanced, and inflammation is reduced in muscle cells in response to the metabolic switch triggered by fasting and exercise. Emerging findings further suggest that exercise training in the fasted state may enhance muscle growth and endurance. Robust beneficial effects of IF on the cardiovascular system have been documented and include reduced blood pressure, reduced resting heart rate, increased heart rate variability (improved cardiovascular stress adaptation), and resistance of cardiac muscle to damage in animal models of myocardial infarction. Studies of laboratory animals and human subjects have shown that IF can improve cognition (learning and memory); the underlying mechanisms may involve neurotrophic factors, stimulation of mitochondrial biogenesis and autophagy, and the formation of new synapses. IF also increases the resistance of neurons to stress and suppresses neuroinflammation. *Demonstrated in animal models but not yet evaluated in humans. *Reprinted from Mattson MP, Leeuwenburgh C, Mainous AG, et al. Flipping the metabolic switch: understanding and applying the health benefits of fasting. Obesity 2017;26(2):254—268.*

BMI and waist circumference were reported in 13 articles, 10 reported a decrease in BMI, and 12 reported a decrease in waist circumference. The three studies that measured hip circumference all showed that it was reduced by IER. This review shows that almost all IER interventions have a positive effect on both weight and fat, and only in lean persons, weight and fat remain similar.

Another review focused on the amount of weight and fat lost by different IER interventions. A body weight reduction of 3%—9% was achieved in 12—24 weeks in IER interventions with intermittent complete fasting 1—2 days per week [25]. Comparable effects were found in IER interventions with ADF with 25% of calories on fasting days with reductions in body weight reductions of 3%—7% in 3—12 weeks. Body fat was reduced by 3%—5.5% in these interventions, with most of the weight loss due to fat loss; however, a part of the weight loss was fat-free mass.

Part of the loss of total fat is the loss of visceral fat. A review summarizing the impact of seven IER interventions on visceral fat showed reductions of 4%—7% after 6—24 weeks treatment [26]. In these interventions, the visceral fat loss was mostly paralleled by the percentage of weight loss. It should be noted that visceral fat loss was not measured directly but estimated by measurements of waist circumference.

Proportionally in a study with three ADF interventions of eight weeks, an average weight loss of approximately 4 kg was due to 3 kg fat mass loss, 1 kg fat-free mass loss, and 0.075−0.135 kg visceral adipose tissue loss (measured by DXA) [27]. However, fat-free mass loss might be depending on the body composition of the subjects, because in obese women on IER, fat-free mass loss was approximately 10% of overall weight loss, whereas within nonobese subjects, it was as high as 30% [15,28,29].

Overall, almost all IER interventions result in weight loss, ranging from 3% to 9%, partly by loss of fat-free mass, but primarily by loss of fat. Concerning long-term effects, evidence is limited. One study with 6-month follow-up after the intervention reported no difference in weight regain between an IER and CER intervention [30]. More research is needed to draw conclusions. Studies of visceral fat measurements other than waist circumference are scarcely available at this moment, and to our knowledge, no data of IER on ectopic fat including hepatic, cardiac, and intramyocellular triglyceride stores is currently available.

More research with more defined mechanisms, for example, magnetic resonance imaging, will be necessary to gain more insight in the effect of IER on fat distribution.

Effect of intermittent energy restriction on metabolic parameters in humans

In addition to the positive effect of IER on fat mass, effects on different metabolic parameters have been observed.

Glucose homeostasis is one of them. In healthy individuals, IER regimes do not appear to affect fasting glucose levels [5,15,29,31]. However, patients with prediabetes on an ADF diet showed a 3%−6% reduction in fasting glucose [15,29,31]. A significant decrease in glucose of 11.8 ± 6.9 mg/dL was also observed in obese patients on an FMD (5). Studies with IER regimens ranging from 8 to 24 weeks also showed a decrease in fasting insulin levels of 11%−57% after 3−24 weeks [32]. The largest decrease in insulin levels was seen in the studies with the highest energy restriction. This effect on fasting insulin levels was independent of the prediabetes status of participants. Insulin resistance was also reduced by IER [32]. This effect was more pronounced in studies with greater weight loss. In type 2 diabetes patients on IER consisting of 75% energy restriction on five consecutive days every five weeks for 15 weeks, HbA1c was normalized in 47% of the patients [33]. IER consisting of energy restriction one day every week for 15 weeks led to a normalized HbA1c in 31% of the patients, compared with 8% in the control group. Although the differences between the groups were clinically relevant, they were not statistically significant. This beneficial effect on HbA1c was independent of the effects of IER on weight loss.

Variable results of the effect of IER are found on total and LDL cholesterol concentrations. Some trials report a reduction in total cholesterol of 6%−21% and LDL cholesterol from 7% to 32%, while others report no effect [32]. Significant reductions in total and LDL cholesterol were only found in studies in which participants had elevated cholesterol. Triglyceride concentrations decreased in the majority of IER studies, with reductions of 16%−42% [32]. This effect was dependent on the amount of weight loss.

Also, systolic and diastolic blood pressure decline in patients with borderline hypertension was dependent on weight loss [32]. Only IER interventions that achieved 6%−7% weight loss showed a decrease of 3%−8% in systolic blood pressure and 6%−10% in diastolic blood pressure after 6−24 weeks.

Taking all these results into account, IER interventions can have beneficial effects on glucose homeostasis, cholesterol, triglycerides, and blood pressure in patients with elevated baseline measures. Most effects seem to be weight loss related, except for effects on insulin levels and HbA1c levels, which have been shown to decline by IER independent of weight loss. More long-term trials should be conducted to draw conclusions regarding the sustainability of the effects. Results from a study in which long-term metabolic effects of an intermittent FMD for five consecutive days every month for 1 year in patients with type 2 diabetes will maybe shed new light on this subject [34].

Effect of intermittent energy restriction on other health parameters in humans

The effect of IER on many other health parameters has been examined, including inflammation-related diseases, cancer, and cognitive function. In one study with an ADF regimen in overweight patients with moderate asthma, pulmonary function and asthma symptoms improved [35]. This reduction in symptoms was associated with significant reduction in inflammatory and oxidative stress marker levels in the blood. In the autoimmune disease multiple sclerosis, only two small pilot studies have been conducted, which show improvement following IER on several scales concerning well-being and quality of life [36,37]. IER has not yet been studied in rheumatoid arthritis patients, but a review looking at short-term energy restriction interventions suggests a positive effect of fasting on subjective disease symptoms as well as rheumatoid arthritis activity [38].

Most clinical trials researching IER in cancer patients have so far focused on compliance and side effects, and only a few evaluated efficacy. Case studies suggest that IER can suppress tumor growth and extend survival [7]. Use of an FMD as an adjunct to neoadjuvant chemotherapy for breast cancer showed no difference in toxicity between the FMD and the control group, while the control group received additional dexamethasone [39]. A radiologically complete or partial response occurred significantly more often in the FMD group (OR 3.168). Also, a 90%−100% tumor cell loss was more likely to occur in patients on the FMD (OR 4.109). Cognitive function also can be positively influenced by use of IER, as several studies have demonstrated improvement in verbal memory, executive function, global cognition, and working memory in persons on IER [7].

Concerning psychological and psychiatric effects, an ADF regimen in patients with obesity had a small but statistically significant effect on binge eating and depression [40]. Purgative behavior and fear of fatness were unchanged, perceived body image was improved, and restrictive eating was increased.

Research of the effect of IER on the human gut microbiome is still in its infancy. An increase in the abundance of several protective microbial families including Bifidobacteriaceae, Lactobacillaceae, and Akkermansiaceae has been observed, suggesting fasting might be used to positively influence the gut microbiota [41].

In conclusion, relatively few studies have evaluated the impact of IER on inflammatory diseases, cancer, cognitive function, mental health, and gut microbiome composition. Although these studies yielded promising results, there is not enough evidence to date to draw definitive conclusions. Further exploration of the benefits of IER in the treatment of several diseases is warranted.

The effect of intermittent energy restriction versus continuous energy restriction on weight and fat in humans

IER is often compared with CER. Theoretically, IER could have advantages over CER concerning visceral fat loss, as IER produces more intense lipolytic stimuli compared with CER. Visceral adipocytes are more responsive to these stimuli compared with their subcutaneous counterparts; therefore, IER might induce proportionally more visceral fat loss [42,43].

A metaanalysis found a positive correlation between the ratio of visceral fat reduction and the degree of energy restriction, independent of weight loss. Since IER has periods with more energy restriction compared with CER, this might also favor IER [44].

There are some reviews and studies comparing the effect on weight and fat in IER and CER interventions. A review including 12 human trials concluded that the effect of IER appears to be comparable to CER with respect to weight loss, BMI, waist circumference, hip circumference, fat loss, and free fat loss [24]. Overall, most studies yielded no significant differences between the IER and CER interventions; some had better results with IER and others with CER. Another review also compared IER and CER interventions and categorized the trails in short duration (8−12 weeks), which included three IER interventions, and moderate duration (13−30 weeks) [42], which included two IER interventions. Weight loss was found to be less in IER compared with CER (4.5% vs. 8.8) in short-duration trials. In moderate-duration trials, however, weight loss was similar between IER and CER (10.0% vs. 8.8%). In two trials of 12 months, weight loss was not significantly different between the ADF and CER interventions. Relative to the control group, total weight loss of −6.0% was observed in the IER group and −5.3% in the CER group in one trial [45]. In the other trial, this was −6.8 kg in the IER groups versus −5.0 kg in the CER group [46]. Total fat reduction in short-duration studies was also less in IER compared with CER interventions (9.0% vs. 15.3%) [42]. In studies of moderate duration, IER reduced total fat mass more effectively than CER (18.0% vs. 14.8%). However, in long-term trials, no difference was found in total fat mass loss between both groups [45,46]. Visceral fat, estimated by waist circumference, was reduced comparably between short-term IER and CER (5.5% vs. 6.5%). In trials of moderate duration, IER showed a greater reduction in visceral fat compared with CER (9.0% vs. 6.2%) [42]. The effect on the ratio of waist circumference reduction to total fat mass reduction showed opposite results, with greater reduction of the ratio in IER than CER (0.67 vs. 0.42) diets in short-duration trials, and no effect in moderate-duration trials (0.45 for IER vs. 0.41 for CER). In the long-duration trials, also no significant difference in visceral fat loss was found between the two interventions [45,46].

Concluding, in short-duration trials, IER interventions seem less effective on weight and fat loss compared with CER interventions, in moderate-duration interventions, fat mass loss seems more effective in IER interventions, and in long-duration trials, no difference was found between groups in weight loss, fat loss, and visceral fat loss. No clear superiority of either IER or CER is apparent based on current data, but especially concerning visceral fat, too few studies have been conducted to draw hard conclusions.

Sustainability of intermittent energy restriction

Several factors are important for the sustainability of a lifestyle change such as IER. As persons are individually very different, one dietary regimen can be easy to follow for some but can be very hard to comply to for others. Adherence to CER often begins to decline at 6–8 weeks and progressively worsens thereafter [42]. Some patients found IER less demanding, as the diet was easier to understand and follow compared with CER [47]. Here, we will describe current knowledge for IER diets concerning dropout rates, adherence to the intervention, feeling hungry, effect on mood, and behavioral change over time.

Dropout can be an indicator of noncompliance. Fifteen IER interventions reported dropout rates ranging from 0% to 65%. Dropouts because of the inability to adhere to the diet were reported in 12 studies and ranged from 3% to 10% [24]. However, overall dropout was similar in IER and CER intervention studies [24,48]. The proportion of people dropping out due to inability to adhere to IER or CER was only mentioned in two studies. Both showed a greater dropout rate due to inability to adhere to CER compared with IER [3,49].

Although data concerning adherence are important for estimating sustainability of diets, to date these data are limited [50]. Self-reported adherence varied widely between studies, with percentages of 43%–97% after 3 months. In studies with one year of follow-up, self-reported adherence was 21%–44%. Dietary adherence did not significantly differ between IER and CER in a six-month ADF intervention [45].

Change in eating habits on the nonrestricted days when conducting an IER is interesting and important part of sustainability. Persons in a CER versus IER trial with a two to five IER regime consumed 23% less calories than the prescribed amount on nonrestricted days, which was comparable with the number of calories of the CER (3). This effect was also seen in an ADF intervention, where people ate less calories than instructed on the nonfasting days [45]. However, there was also a tendency of eating more than instructed on the fasting days.

Ability to adhere to IER might be better if people feel less hungry. Several studies report that subjects became habituated to the ADF regimen and felt very little hunger on the fast day, with no overeating on the feast day, even feeling an increase of fullness and satisfaction [29,31]. Not all studies report this effect. Out of ten trials describing appetite, four demonstrated an increase of appetite, and six demonstrated a decrease or no significant effect. However, in all studies, a significant weight loss was observed [24].

The effect of a diet on mood may also influence adherence. Unfortunately, only few trials report the impact on mood. Five trials showed that IER had a positive effect on mood, with bad temper being reported only in 3% of the participants; however, in a trial with lean participants, an overall worsening of mood was reported [24].

The combined results so far could indicate that for some persons CER is more suitable and for others IER is suitable, but overall, there is no evident superiority to either IER or CER regarding adherence to the diet.

IER interventions might be an option to try if former CER interventions were unsuccessful. Some participants felt less hungry and had a better mood on IER and experienced it less demanding than CER. Interindividual differences in response to a dietary treatment are likely due to a combination of behavioral, environmental, and psychosocial factors [50]. It will be interesting to investigate the effect of IER on behavioral context—and consequences—and to investigate which cognitive, environmental, or physiological factors influence adherence to IER. Conducting qualitative research with, for example, focus groups could therefore be useful. Furthermore, as not many trials incorporate treatment satisfaction or quality of life questionnaires, this could be an interesting and valuable addition to future research. Knowing more about the sustainability or IER can help doctors and patients in shared decision-making on dietary interventions.

Potential risks of intermittent energy restriction

While fasting, the human body has no or limited access to essential nutrients. After many weeks of continuous fasting (approximately 5–7 weeks in healthy adults), fasting converts into starvation, which causes vital organs and muscles to be consumed for energy [4,51]. Starvation has many effects on the body, including weight loss, diarrhea, delirium, and eventually death. Since IER only applies fasting periods for a limited period of time, these adverse events are prevented. In trials of shorter, more frequent fasts, including periodic fasting and ADF, severe events have not been reported [4]. More commonly, IER may cause mild adverse events such as dehydration, nausea, headaches, dizziness, syncope, weakness, feeling cold, feeling irritable, bad breath, low energy, and hunger pangs [9,40,51–53]. Usually, these side effects are mild and do not hinder participants in continuing the fasting period. In a review including nine IER trials, none of these trials reported any serious adverse events related to the dietary intervention [48]. Many side effects are linked to dehydration. It is important to hydrate well during any fasting regimen, because the fluids must be replaced that would normally be consumed in foods [53]. In general, when long-term intermittent fasting is undertaken, one must be aware of protein malnutrition and vitamin and mineral malnutrition [6,54]. If fasting is undertaken regularly, it might be necessary to use vitamin and/or mineral supplements [6,53].

There are specific populations that have to be extra careful while fasting [53]. Patients with diabetes should carefully consider if IER is the best suitable option for them and should not undertake this without the help of their physician. IER in combination with antidiabetic medication, especially sulfonylureas or insulin, can induce hypoglycemia. Treating physicians should adjust medication and, if necessary, plan additional glucose monitoring during the fasting periods, for example, flash glucose monitoring [55]. Other populations should refrain from fasting all together, such as pregnant and lactating women, young children, adults of advanced age, and frail older adults [9]. These groups have a higher risk of dehydration and not receiving the minimal amount of nutrients for growth and development.

Overall, for IER, only mild side effects have been reported, but there are some risks to consider.

Conclusion

Positive effects of IER on weight loss, fat mass loss, visceral fat loss, glucose tolerance, and many other parameters have been observed in both animal studies and clinical trials. Although several studies have indicated that benefits of IER are dissociated from the effects on weight loss [7], no overall superiority of IER over CER was demonstrated. For individuals who have tried a CER intervention unsuccessfully or who are unwilling to try a CER intervention, an IER intervention could be an option. Safety should always be considered. Several trials report positive effects of IER on multiple health parameters; however, further research is necessary to prove health improvement in the long term. Long-term studies and long-term follow-up are necessary to create a better understanding of various possible benefits and harms of using IER.

References

[1] Clifton P. Assessing the evidence for weight loss strategies in people with and without type 2 diabetes. World J Diabetes 2017;8(10):440−54.

[2] Franz MJ, Boucher JL, Evert AB. Evidence-based diabetes nutrition therapy recommendations are effective: the key is individualization. Diabetes Metab Syndr Obes 2014;7:65−72.

[3] Harvie M, Wright C, Pegington M, McMullan D, Mitchell E, Martin B, et al. The effect of intermittent energy and carbohydrate restriction v. daily energy restriction on weight loss and metabolic disease risk markers in overweight women. Br J Nutr 2013;110(8):1534−47.

[4] Anton SD, Moehl K, Donahoo WT, Marosi K, Lee SA, Mainous 3rd AG, et al. Flipping the metabolic switch: understanding and applying the health benefits of fasting. Obesity 2018;26(2):254−68.

[5] Wei M, Brandhorst S, Shelehchi M, Mirzaei H, Cheng CW, Budniak J, et al. Fasting-mimicking diet and markers/risk factors for aging, diabetes, cancer, and cardiovascular disease. Sci Transl Med 2017;9(377).

[6] Brandhorst S, Choi IY, Wei M, Cheng CW, Sedrakyan S, Navarrete G, et al. A periodic diet that mimics fasting promotes multi-system regeneration, enhanced cognitive performance, and healthspan. Cell Metab 2015;22(1):86−99.

[7] de Cabo R, Mattson MP. Effects of intermittent fasting on health, aging, and disease. N Engl J Med 2019;381(26):2541−51.

[8] Di Francesco A, Di Germanio C, Bernier M, de Cabo R. A time to fast. Science 2018;362(6416):770−5.

[9] Longo VD, Mattson MP. Fasting: molecular mechanisms and clinical applications. Cell Metab 2014;19(2):181−92.

[10] Goodrick CL, Ingram DK, Reynolds MA, Freeman JR, Cider NL. Differential effects of intermittent feeding and voluntary exercise on body weight and lifespan in adult rats. J Gerontol 1983;38(1):36−45.

[11] Hwangbo DS, Lee HY, Abozaid LS, Min KJ. Mechanisms of lifespan regulation by calorie restriction and intermittent fasting in model organisms. Nutrients 2020;12(4).

[12] Henderson CG, Turner DL, Swoap SJ. Health effects of alternate day fasting versus pair-fed caloric restriction in diet-induced obese C57Bl/6J male mice. Front Physiol 2021;12:641532.

[13] Liu B, Page AJ, Hatzinikolas G, Chen M, Wittert GA, Heilbronn LK. Intermittent fasting improves glucose tolerance and promotes adipose tissue remodeling in male mice fed a high-fat diet. Endocrinology 2019;160(1):169−80.

[14] Mishra A, Mirzaei H, Guidi N, Vinciguerra M, Mouton A, Linardic M, et al. Fasting-mimicking diet prevents high-fat diet effect on cardiometabolic risk and lifespan. Nat Metab 2021;3(10):1342−56.

[15] Varady KA, Hudak CS, Hellerstein MK. Modified alternate-day fasting and cardioprotection: relation to adipose tissue dynamics and dietary fat intake. Metabolism 2009;58(6):803−11.

[16] Tang HN, Tang CY, Man XF, Tan SW, Guo Y, Tang J, et al. Plasticity of adipose tissue in response to fasting and refeeding in male mice. Nutr Metab 2017;14:3.

[17] Varady KA, Roohk DJ, Loe YC, McEvoy-Hein BK, Hellerstein MK. Effects of modified alternate-day fasting regimens on adipocyte size, triglyceride metabolism, and plasma adiponectin levels in mice. J Lipid Res 2007;48(10):2212−9.

[18] Anson RM, Guo Z, de Cabo R, Iyun T, Rios M, Hagepanos A, et al. Intermittent fasting dissociates beneficial effects of dietary restriction on glucose metabolism and neuronal resistance to injury from calorie intake. Proc Natl Acad Sci U S A 2003;100(10):6216−20.

[19] Wan R, Camandola S, Mattson MP. Intermittent food deprivation improves cardiovascular and neuroendocrine responses to stress in rats. J Nutr 2003;133(6):1921–9.

[20] Wahl D, Coogan SC, Solon-Biet SM, de Cabo R, Haran JB, Raubenheimer D, et al. Cognitive and behavioral evaluation of nutritional interventions in rodent models of brain aging and dementia. Clin Interv Aging 2017;12:1419–28.

[21] Li G, Xie C, Lu S, Nichols RG, Tian Y, Li L, et al. Intermittent fasting promotes white adipose browning and decreases obesity by shaping the gut microbiota. Cell Metab 2017;26(4):672–685.e4.

[22] Ridaura VK, Faith JJ, Rey FE, Cheng J, Duncan AE, Kau AL, et al. Gut microbiota from twins discordant for obesity modulate metabolism in mice. Science 2013;341(6150):1241214.

[23] Cignarella F, Cantoni C, Ghezzi L, Salter A, Dorsett Y, Chen L, et al. Intermittent fasting confers protection in CNS autoimmunity by altering the gut microbiota. Cell Metab 2018;27(6):1222–1235.e6.

[24] Seimon RV, Roekenes JA, Zibellini J, Zhu B, Gibson AA, Hills AP, et al. Do intermittent diets provide physiological benefits over continuous diets for weight loss? A systematic review of clinical trials. Mol Cell Endocrinol 2015;418 Pt 2:153–72.

[25] Tinsley GM, La Bounty PM. Effects of intermittent fasting on body composition and clinical health markers in humans. Nutr Rev 2015;73(10):661–74.

[26] Barnosky AR, Hoddy KK, Unterman TG, Varady KA. Intermittent fasting vs daily calorie restriction for type 2 diabetes prevention: a review of human findings. Transl Res 2014;164(4):302–11.

[27] Hoddy KK, Kroeger CM, Trepanowski JF, Barnosky A, Bhutani S, Varady KA. Meal timing during alternate day fasting: impact on body weight and cardiovascular disease risk in obese adults. Obesity 2014;22(12):2524–31.

[28] Mattson MP, Longo VD, Harvie M. Impact of intermittent fasting on health and disease processes. Ageing Res Rev 2017;39:46–58.

[29] Varady KA, Bhutani S, Klempel MC, Kroeger CM, Trepanowski JF, Haus JM, et al. Alternate day fasting for weight loss in normal weight and overweight subjects: a randomized controlled trial. Nutr J 2013;12(1):146.

[30] Sundfør TM, Svendsen M, Tonstad S. Effect of intermittent versus continuous energy restriction on weight loss, maintenance and cardiometabolic risk: a randomized 1-year trial. Nutr Metab Cardiovasc Dis 2018;28(7):698–706.

[31] Klempel MC, Bhutani S, Fitzgibbon M, Freels S, Varady KA. Dietary and physical activity adaptations to alternate day modified fasting: implications for optimal weight loss. Nutr J 2010;9:35.

[32] St-Onge MP, Ard J, Baskin ML, Chiuve SE, Johnson HM, Kris-Etherton P, et al. Meal timing and frequency: implications for cardiovascular disease prevention: a scientific statement from the American heart association. Circulation 2017;135(9):e96–121.

[33] Williams KV, Mullen ML, Kelley DE, Wing RR. The effect of short periods of caloric restriction on weight loss and glycemic control in type 2 diabetes. Diabetes Care 1998;21(1):2–8.

[34] van den Burg EL, Schoonakker MP, van Peet PG, van den Akker-van Marle ME, Willems van Dijk K, Longo VD, et al. Fasting in diabetes treatment (FIT) trial: study protocol for a randomised, controlled, assessor-blinded intervention trial on the effects of intermittent use of a fasting-mimicking diet in patients with type 2 diabetes. BMC Endocr Disord 2020;20(1):94.

[35] Johnson JB, Summer W, Cutler RG, Martin B, Hyun DH, Dixit VD, et al. Alternate day calorie restriction improves clinical findings and reduces markers of oxidative stress and inflammation in overweight adults with moderate asthma. Free Radic Biol Med 2007;42(5):665–74.

[36] Choi IY, Piccio L, Childress P, Bollman B, Ghosh A, Brandhorst S, et al. A diet mimicking fasting promotes regeneration and reduces autoimmunity and multiple sclerosis symptoms. Cell Rep 2016;15(10):2136–46.

[37] Fitzgerald KC, Vizthum D, Henry-Barron B, Schweitzer A, Cassard SD, Kossoff E, et al. Effect of intermittent vs. daily calorie restriction on changes in weight and patient-reported outcomes in people with multiple sclerosis. Mult Scler Relat Disord 2018;23:33–9.

[38] Philippou E, Petersson SD, Rodomar C, Nikiphorou E. Rheumatoid arthritis and dietary interventions: systematic review of clinical trials. Nutr Rev 2021;79(4):410–28.

[39] de Groot S, Lugtenberg RT, Cohen D, Welters MJP, Ehsan I, Vreeswijk MPG, et al. Fasting mimicking diet as an adjunct to neoadjuvant chemotherapy for breast cancer in the multicentre randomized phase 2 DIRECT trial. Nat Commun 2020;11(1):3083.

[40] Hoddy KK, Kroeger CM, Trepanowski JF, Barnosky AR, Bhutani S, Varady KA. Safety of alternate day fasting and effect on disordered eating behaviors. Nutr J 2015;14:44.

[41] Llewellyn-Waters K, Abdullah MMH, editors. Intermittent fasting - a potential approach to modulate the gut microbiota in humans? A systematic review; 2021.

[42] Trepanowski J, Varady K. Intermittent versus daily calorie restriction in visceral fat loss. 2014. p. 181–8.

[43] Arner P. Differences in lipolysis between human subcutaneous and omental adipose tissues. Ann Med 1995;27(4):435–8.

[44] Chaston TB, Dixon JB. Factors associated with percent change in visceral versus subcutaneous abdominal fat during weight loss: findings from a systematic review. Int J Obes 2008;32(4):619–28.

[45] Trepanowski JF, Kroeger CM, Barnosky A, Klempel MC, Bhutani S, Hoddy KK, et al. Effect of alternate-day fasting on weight loss, weight maintenance, and cardioprotection among metabolically healthy obese adults: a randomized clinical trial. JAMA Intern Med 2017;177(7):930–8.

[46] Carter S, Clifton PM, Keogh JB. Effect of intermittent compared with continuous energy restricted diet on glycemic control in patients with type 2 diabetes: a randomized noninferiority trial. JAMA Netw Open 2018;1(3):e180756.

[47] Donnelly LS, Shaw RL, Pegington M, Armitage CJ, Evans DG, Howell A, et al. 'For me it's about not feeling like I'm on a diet': a thematic analysis of women's experiences of an intermittent energy restricted diet to reduce breast cancer risk. J Hum Nutr Diet 2018;31(6):773–80.

[48] Headland M, Clifton PM, Carter S, Keogh JB. Weight-loss outcomes: a systematic review and meta-analysis of intermittent energy restriction trials lasting a minimum of 6 months. Nutrients 2016;8(6).

[49] Harvie MN, Pegington M, Mattson MP, Frystyk J, Dillon B, Evans G, et al. The effects of intermittent or continuous energy restriction on weight loss and metabolic disease risk markers: a randomized trial in young overweight women. Int J Obes 2011;35(5):714−27.

[50] Rynders CA, Thomas EA, Zaman A, Pan Z, Catenacci VA, Melanson EL. Effectiveness of intermittent fasting and time-restricted feeding compared to continuous energy restriction for weight loss. Nutrients 2019;11(10).

[51] Horne BD, Muhlestein JB, Anderson JL. Health effects of intermittent fasting: hormesis or harm? A systematic review. Am J Clin Nutr 2015;102(2):464−70.

[52] Patterson RE, Sears DD. Metabolic effects of intermittent fasting. Annu Rev Nutr 2017;37:371−93.

[53] Grajower MM, Horne BD. Clinical management of intermittent fasting in patients with diabetes mellitus. Nutrients 2019;11(4).

[54] Mirzaei H, Suarez JA, Longo VD. Protein and amino acid restriction, aging and disease: from yeast to humans. Trends Endocrinol Metab 2014;25(11):558−66.

[55] Carter S, Clifton PM, Keogh JP. Flash glucose monitoring for the safe use of a 2-day intermittent energy restriction in patients with type 2 diabetes at risk of hypoglycaemia: an exploratory study. Diabetes Res Clin Pract 2019;151:138−45.

Chapter 22

Exercise

Joseph Henson, Emer M. Brady and Gaurav S. Gulsin

University of Leicester and the NIHR Leicester Biomedical Research Centre, Leicester, United Kingdom

Introduction

Regular physical activity is associated with a myriad of physiological benefits across the life course and is one of the cornerstone interventions for the prevention and management of over 20 chronic conditions and diseases [1]. Exercise training, irrespective of mode, provides an economically viable, nonpharmacological method for eliciting beneficial adaptations in markers of cardiometabolic risk. More specifically, several well-designed studies and meta-analyses that have examined the effects of aerobic activity (i.e., any activity that uses large muscle groups and is rhythmic in nature), resistance training (i.e., any activity that involves using your body weight or working against a force), or a combination of the two on ectopic and visceral adipose tissue. In this chapter, we detail current recommendations for physical activity to promote healthy living, explore mechanisms underlying the impact of exercise on visceral and ectopic adipose tissue with an emphasis on obesity and type 2 diabetes, and summarize the wealth of studies examining the effects of various modes of exercise.

Definition of key terms

In its most rudimentary form, physical activity is any substantial movement produced by skeletal muscles [2]. This includes a breadth of activities, spanning household chores and active transport. Conversely, exercise is considered a subcategory of physical activity that is typically planned, repetitive, and structured, with the purpose of improving or maintaining cardiorespiratory fitness [2], which is the ability of the circulatory and respiratory system to supply oxygen during sustained physical activity. Eliciting improvements in cardiorespiratory fitness has typically involved moderate- to vigorous-intensity aerobic exercise. More recently, there has been greater consideration of the full physical activity intensity spectrum. Although traditional guidelines promulgating at least 150 min of moderate-intensity physical activity and two resistance exercise sessions remain pivotal [1,3—5], there is also an increasing recognition that light-intensity exercise can have important effects on health (including visceral adipose tissue). At the other end of the spectrum, vigorous-intensity exercise can be undertaken using different approaches, including the use of near-maximal exercise through interval training. To aid interpretation and provide a frame of reference, examples of the commonly used terms, definitions, and examples used throughout this chapter are presented in Table 22.1 and Fig. 22.1.

Current recommendations

National (The UK Chief Medical Officers [CMO]), International (American College of Sports Medicine [ACSM] and World Health Organization [WHO]), and disease-specific (American Diabetes Association [ADA]) physical activity guidelines have been produced that apply to all age groups [1,3—5]. To discuss each component in detail is beyond the scope of this chapter. Therefore, a summary of the pertinent guidelines relating to this chapter can be found in Table 22.2.

Briefly, regular physical activity and structured exercise are recommended for all individuals, unless otherwise contraindicated. Across all guidance, 150 min/week of moderate-to-vigorous intensity is the recognized minimal amount of physical activity an adult (aged 16—65 years) should perform. Vigorous intensity can be substituted for moderate in those who are already physically active with a minimum of 75 min/week suggested. This should be supplemented with two-to-three resistance sessions/week [1,3—5]. The recently published WHO guidelines state that those with chronic disease

TABLE 22.1 Definitions and examples of commonly used terms.

		Sedentary behavior	Light intensity	Moderate intensity	Vigorous intensity	Resistance activities
Intensity	% VO$_2$ peak	–	37–40	46–63	64–90	–
	% HR max	–	57–63	64–76	77–95	–
	Borg RPE	6–8	9–11	12–13	14–17	9–15
	Metabolic equivalents (MET)	≤1.5	>1.5–2.9	3.0–5.9	≥6.0	2.0 - ≥6.0
	1-RM	–	30–49	50–69	≥70	40–60
	Practical definition	Any waking behavior characterized by a low energy expenditure ≤1.5 METs, while in a sitting, reclining or lying posture [6]	Activities that require standing up and moving around. Can also include activities of daily living	Can be defined by the "talk test": being able to talk but not sing indicates moderate intensity activity. Having difficulty talking without pausing is a sign of vigorous activity	An activity that requires a large amount of effort and causes rapid breathing and substantial increases in heart rate	Any activity that makes your muscles work harder than usual. Can involve using your body weight or working against a resistance

% VO$_2$ peak, peak oxygen consumption %; HR max, percentage of maximal heart rate; RPE, rating of perceived exertion [7]; MET, metabolic equivalent of task. One MET is defined as the energy used when at rest. Therefore, an activity with a MET value of 5 means exerting five times the energy than you would if you were sitting still. 1-RM, 1-repetition maximum is the heaviest weight that can be successfully lifted once through the complete range of motion.

Adapted from Garber CE, Blissmer B, Deschenes MR et al. American College of Sports Medicine position stand. Quantity and quality of exercise for developing and maintaining cardiorespiratory, musculo-skeletal, and neuromotor fitness in apparently healthy adults: guidance for prescribing exercise. Med Sci Sports Exerc 2011;43:1334–1359.

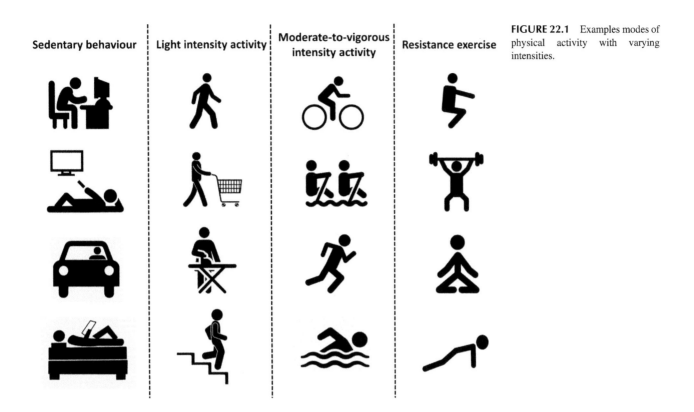

Sedentary behaviour	Light intensity activity	Moderate-to-vigorous intensity activity	Resistance exercise

FIGURE 22.1 Examples modes of physical activity with varying intensities.

(e.g., type 2 diabetes) may increase moderate-intensity aerobic activity to >300 min or >150 min of vigorous-intensity physical activity per week, for additional health benefits (including weight maintenance) [1].

Although individuals are encouraged to work toward the aforementioned recommendations, the absolute targets are somewhat arbitrary as physiological benefits can be achieved at levels below and above these thresholds (discussed later in this chapter). Importantly, the paradigm for the requirement for each bout of physical activity being 10 min or more to elicit benefit has shifted and is now more flexible, i.e., there is no requirement for bouts of activity or aiming to achieve the total minutes in a single dose. This subtle change in communication lends itself well to increasing the accessibility for a given person to achieve or work toward achieving the recommended guidelines.

It should also be emphasized that, although a higher intensity and duration of activity may elicit a greater range and magnitude of physiological adaptations, the dose–response relationship between physical activity and health outcomes is curvilinear, suggesting that the gains are especially significant for those currently doing the lowest levels of activity (fewer than 30 min per week), as the improvements in health per additional minute of physical activity will be proportionately greater [4].

Aerobic training interventions

Aerobic exercise is generally recognized as a safe and effective training modality that provides a powerful stimulus for inducing reductions in abdominal adipose tissue, in particular visceral adipose tissue [7–11]. For example, a 12-week exercise program designed to increase energy expenditure by 700 kcal/day in overweight men (while maintaining an isocaloric diet) reported an average weight loss of 7.5 kg and an average decrease in visceral adipose tissue of 6.9 cm^2/kg of weight loss [12]. Interestingly, this was similar to the diet-only group (700 kcal deficit) who also demonstrated a decrease of 5.9 cm^2/kg of weight loss. The relative reductions in visceral adipose tissue (expressed as % of total weight lost) across the trial arms are displayed in Fig. 22.2.

These findings are consistent with the STRRIDE (Studies Targeting Risk Reduction Intervention through Defined Exercise) study, where men in the high-amount exercise group experienced a visceral adipose tissue reduction of 5.6 cm^2/kg of weight loss [13]. This exercise training program ran for ∼8 months and targeted 23 kcal/kg/week at 75% peak VO$_2$, which is equivalent to jogging 20 miles/week. Similarly, Irwin et al. studied the effects of a 12-month exercise program,

TABLE 22.2 Current exercise recommendations.

	Physical activity (light/moderate/vigorous intensity)	Resistance activities
American College of Sports Medicine (ACSM) [5]		
Adults	150 min (2 h and 30 min) to 300 min (5 h) per week of moderate-intensity; or 75 min (1 h and 15 min) to 150 min (2 h and 30 min) a week of vigorous-intensity aerobic physical activity; or an equivalent combination of moderate- and vigorous-intensity aerobic activity. Where possible, aerobic activity should be spread throughout the week. Additional health benefits are gained >300 min (5 h) of moderate-intensity physical activity a week.	Muscle-strengthening activities of ≥moderate intensity that involve all major muscle groups on ≥2 days a week.
Chronic conditions (i.e., type 2 diabetes)	≥150 min a week (2 h and 30 min) to 300 min (5 h) a week of moderate-intensity; or 75 min (1 h and 15 min) to 150 min (2 h and 30 min) a week of vigorous-intensity aerobic physical activity; or an equivalent combination of moderate- and vigorous-intensity aerobic activity. Preferably, aerobic activity should be spread throughout the week. When adults with chronic conditions or disabilities are not able to meet the above key guidelines, they should engage in regular physical activity according to their abilities and should avoid inactivity.	Muscle-strengthening activities of ≥moderate intensity that involve all major muscle groups on ≥2 days a week.
American Diabetes Association (ADA) [3]		
Adults with type 2 diabetes	≥150 min of moderate- to vigorous-intensity activity weekly, spread over at least 3 days/week, with no more than two consecutive days without activity. Shorter durations (minimum 75 min/week) of vigorous intensity or interval training may be sufficient for younger and more physically fit individuals. Where possible, perform both aerobic and resistance exercise training. Increase total daily incidental (nonexercise) physical activity to gain additional health benefits. Even in brief (3−15 min) bouts. This should be encouraged as part of a whole-day approach. Participation in supervised training versus nonsupervised where feasible.	Two to three sessions/week of resistance exercise on nonconsecutive days.
UK Chief Medical Officers guidelines [4]		
Adults	Aim to be physically active every day ≥150 min (2 1/2 h) per week of moderate-intensity activity (such as brisk walking or cycling); or 75 min of vigorous-intensity activity (such as running); or even shorter durations of very vigorous-intensity activity (such as sprinting or stair climbing); or a combination of moderate-, vigorous-, and very-vigorous-intensity activity.	≥2 days/week muscle-strengthening activities at moderate or greater intensity involving all major muscle groups (upper and lower).
World Health Organization (WHO) [1]		
Adults	≥150−300 min of moderate-intensity aerobic physical activity per week; OR at least 75−150 min of vigorous-intensity aerobic physical activity; or an equivalent combination of moderate- and vigorous-intensity activity throughout the week. All adults and older adults should aim to do more than the recommended levels of moderate- to vigorous-intensity physical activity.	≥2 days/week muscle-strengthening activities at moderate or greater intensity involving all major muscle groups.

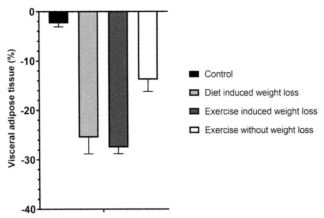

FIGURE 22.2   Relative reductions in visceral adipose tissue achieved with in a small (n = 52, mean BMI 31.3 ± 2.0 kg/m^2) randomized trial of 12-week interventions with diet-induced versus exercise-induced weight loss versus control. *Adapted from Ross R, Dagnone D, Jones PJ et al. Reduction in obesity and related comorbid conditions after diet-induced weight loss or exercise-induced weight loss in men. A randomized, controlled trial. Ann Intern Med 2000;133:92—103.*

consisting of at least 45 min of moderate-intensity exercise on 5 days/week for 12 months, in overweight postmenopausal women [8]. They reported a loss of 8.5 cm^2 of visceral adipose tissue and 1.3 kg of body weight, corresponding to a ratio of 6.5 cm^2/kg of weight change. In comparison, the women included in the high-amount exercise group in STRRIDE lost 6.9 cm^2 of visceral adipose tissue per kilogram of body weight [13].

Evidence from systematic review and metaanalytical studies have confirmed that aerobic exercise training is effective for reducing visceral adipose tissue in a dose—response manner [14,15], with an overall pooled effect size of −0.33 (95% CI: 0.52 to −0.14) [14]. When considering those participants with overweight and obesity, pooled estimates indicate that exercise training can decrease visceral adipose tissue by −0.50 (95% CI: 0.655 to −0.340) [15]. This finding may be particularly important from a clinical perspective, as these results are independent of meaningful weight loss, which is often difficult to achieve through exercise alone (see "Are exercise-induced changes in body weight necessary for reductions in visceral adipose tissue?").

This observation also extends to other measures of ectopic adipose tissue. For example, as little as 2 weeks of exercise training (either sprint interval or moderate to vigorous) has been shown to reduce pancreatic adipose tissue in healthy (from 4.4% to 3.6%) and dysglycemic individuals (from 8.7% to 6.7%) [16]. More broadly, a systematic review and meta-analysis (17 studies, n = 373) demonstrated that exercise training (moderate and high-intensity interval training [HIIT]) elicits an absolute reduction in intrahepatic triglycerides (IHTGs) of 3.3% (95% CI: −4.4, −2.2); with each week of training associated with ∼0.27% reduction [17]. Importantly, exercise reduces IHTG independent of significant weight change (−2.2% [95% CI: −2.9, −1.4]). That said, the benefits are substantially greater when weight loss occurs (−4.87% [95% CI: −6.6, −3.1]). Similarly, a systematic review and meta-analysis (33 studies, n = 1726) examined the effect of a lifestyle intervention (exercise conducted at 50%—80% VO$_2$ peak, hypocaloric diet or both) on ectopic adipose tissue storage (liver, heart, pancreas, and intramyocellular lipids [IMCL]) [18]. When considered together, there was a significant decrease in the liver, heart, and pancreas, with a trend toward a decrease in IMCL. When examined independently, exercise also decreased ectopic adipose tissue in the liver, with the effect being greater when combined with a low-calorie diet (Fig. 22.3) [14].

A recent systematic review and meta-analysis (10 studies, n = 521) also demonstrated that exercise (regardless of intervention duration) significantly reduces epicardial adipose tissue (Hedges' g = 0.82 [95% CI: 0.57—1.07]) in over-weight/obese adults [19]. When stratified by mode of exercise, however, the exercise benefits were only observed in aerobic interventions (6 studies, n = 287; 0.83 [95% CI: 0.52, 1.15]). This is largely due to insufficient data for studies examining the independent effect of resistance exercise training. These findings are broadly consistent with another systematic review and meta-analysis (24 studies, n = 1383), which examined the role of exercise and ectopic adipose tissue in those with type 2 diabetes [20]. Aerobic exercise (effect size = −0.23, 95% CI: 0.44, −0.03) (but not resistance training; effect size = −0.13; 95% CI: 0.37, 0.12) was effective for reducing visceral adipose tissue in overweight/obese adults with type 2 diabetes. There was a borderline-significant pooled effect size for intrahepatic adipose tissue storage reduction with exercise (effect size = −0.28; 95% CI: −0.57, 0.01). However, given the heterogeneity (duration, intensity, population) and methodological quality of the included studies, the results of these reviews should be interpreted with a degree of caution.

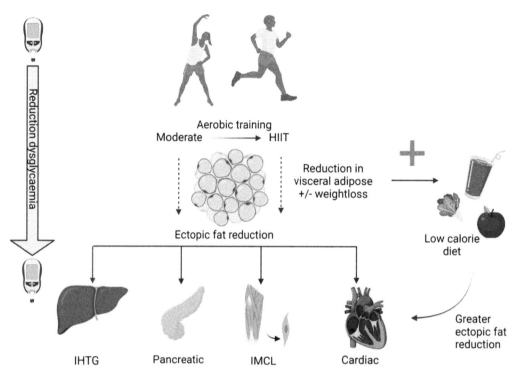

FIGURE 22.3 Beneficial effects of exercise training with and without dietary weight loss on glycemia and ectopic adipose tissue. A greater decrease in ectopic adipose tissue is evident when exercise is combined with dietary weight reduction. *HIIT*, high-intensity interval training; *IMCL*, intramyocellular lipids; *IHTGs*, intrahepatic triglycerides.

Resistance training interventions

In most cases, the influence of resistance exercise alone (see Fig. 22.1 for examples) upon total body weight is negligible. Therefore, calorie restriction and aerobic exercise are often promulgated. However, a recent meta-analysis including 34 studies and 2285 participants demonstrated that resistance training in the absence of calorie restriction may be effective for reducing visceral adipose tissue [21]. Although the effect size is small (−0.24; 95% CI: −0.34, −0.13), the results appear consistent across different intervention lengths, obesity classifications, and ages. Interestingly, the effects of resistance exercise plus calorie restriction were not significantly different from calorie restriction alone with regard to visceral adipose tissue outcomes. These findings are in contrast to a previous systematic review and meta-analysis, which suggested that resistance training was insufficient to reduce visceral adipose tissue [14]. However, the independent effect of resistance training was not assessed in this meta-analysis, as data were pooled from heterogenous studies, including those with and without dietary intervention(s).

Despite the statistically significant reductions in visceral adipose tissue, it is unclear if the magnitude of these changes is physiologically/clinically meaningful and in some cases whether they are independent of dietary modifications. To some extent, the clinical significance can be gauged by studying large prospective intervention studies examining the correlations between changes in visceral adipose tissue with exercise training and variables of cardiometabolic risk. In STRRIDE, the data suggest that a reduction of as little as 11 cm^2 in visceral adipose tissue is significantly related to changes in low-density lipoprotein (LDL) particle number, LDL size, and insulin sensitivity [22]. Therefore, the alterations in body composition (adipose tissue to muscle mass), coupled with the maintenance of muscle mass, still makes resistance training a viable method to reduced obesity-related risk factors—namely dyslipidemia, insulin resistance, and type 2 diabetes [11−13]. This is important, as Nieves et al. demonstrated that differences in visceral adipose tissue explain much of the atherogenic lipoprotein profile that is associated with obesity and insulin resistance [23]. Similarly, the authors of a Japanese prospective cohort study suggested that, irrespective of BMI, changes in visceral adipose tissue (estimated by bioelectrical impedance analysis) within 1 year correlated significantly with changes in the number of metabolic risk factors. In particular, men who reduced their visceral adipose tissue by 30 cm^2 decreased their metabolic risk by approximately 25% [24].

Aerobic and resistance training interventions

There has been limited data examining the combined effects of aerobic and resistance exercise on ectopic and visceral adipose tissue [14]. Despite a meta-analysis reporting that the synergistic effects result in a pooled effect versus control (effect size = −0.27; 95% CI: −0.46, −0.08), there was significant heterogeneity, and removing the one study with low precision and a large effect size attenuated the results. However, combining resistance training with aerobic exercise has been shown to be superior for body weight and adipose tissue loss and to result in greater lean body mass when compared with aerobic exercise training alone [25,26]. More broadly, resistance exercise with targeted weight loss through calorie restriction also provides a powerful anabolic stimulus that concomitantly improves muscle quality and muscle strength, increases muscle mass, and enhances physical fitness and function, with whole-body effects that remain unrivaled by any other lifestyle or pharmaceutical intervention [27,28]. This is also important as for every kilogram lost through intentional weight loss, around 25−30% is lean body mass (predominantly skeletal muscle) [29,30].

The role of intensity

Continuous moderate- to vigorous-intensity aerobic exercise (see Table 22.1 for definition) remains the most prevalent form of exercise training, due to its well-demonstrated efficacy and safety. However, low adherence to exercise training programs remains a major concern, in both research studies and the general population. Therefore, new and refined strategies are warranted to maximize effectiveness.

Maillard et al. suggested that HIIT (≥90% peak heart rate) is an effective method for reducing visceral adipose tissue, although interestingly they reported greater reductions in visceral adipose tissue were more likely at lower intensities (<90% peak heart rate) [31]. This is broadly consistent with a previous meta-analysis in overweight adults that suggested an intensity threshold of moderate (45−55% VO_2max) to vigorous ($\sim$70% VO_2max) exercise intensity to significantly decrease visceral adipose tissue [15]. This is similar to data from STRRIDE, which revealed that the middle-aged men and women in the inactive control group appeared to markedly increase visceral adipose tissue during the control period, whereas both of the low-amount exercise groups (14 kcal/kg body weight/week of exercise at either 50% peak VO_2, equivalent to walking 12 miles/week or 75% peak VO_2, equivalent to jogging 12 miles/week) prevented this increase, with no discernible effect of exercise intensity [13].

Conversely, the role of resistance training intensity is relatively scarce within the peer-reviewed scientific literature. Despite a network meta-analysis (32 studies, n = 1900) indicating that HIIT (standardized mean difference −0.39, 95% CI: −0.60 to −0.18) and aerobic exercise (−0.26, 95% CI: −0.38 to −0.13) of at least moderate intensity were beneficial for reducing visceral adipose tissue versus control, and no significant effects were found for resistance exercise [32]. That said, resistance training does appear to play an important role in preventing regain of visceral adipose tissue following weight loss. For example, following a 15% (12 kg) diet-induced weight loss, resistance training prevented regain of visceral adipose tissue, compared with those in the control group gaining 70% of their visceral adipose tissue lost [33].

How much is enough?

Given the interdependency of energy intake and expenditure, coupled with heterogeneity in study durations, training frequency, modality, and cohort characteristics, it is difficult to accurately predict the amount of additional exercise needed to result in ectopic or visceral adipose tissue reduction. However, Ross and Janssen reported that an increase in exercise is positively associated with a reduction in total adipose tissue in a dose−response manner in short-term interventions ($\nleqq$16 week), but not in long-term interventions ($\nleqq$26 week) [34]. It has also been suggested that at least 10 METs·h/w is required for significant visceral adipose tissue reduction [35], which equates to $\sim$150 min of brisk walking per week [36]. This is consistent with recommendations for adults with overweight or obesity, where a minimum of 60 min of at least moderate activity per day or 150 min of moderate-to-vigorous physical activity per week, respectively, in conjunction with energy restriction is promulgated [37].

Mechanisms underlying the effects of exercise on visceral and ectopic adipose tissue

Increasingly, it is recognized that visceral adipose tissue is a key mediator through which obesity and type 2 diabetes heighten cardiometabolic risk and drive cardiovascular disease. Although the mechanisms by which visceral adipose tissue mediates cardiovascular disease are not fully understood, local and system inflammation induced by visceral adipose tissue and increased insulin resistance are central to the pathophysiology [38]. Epicardial adipose tissue volume, for example, has been shown to correlate inversely with cardiac systolic strain rate in type 2 diabetes [39]. This mechanism is believed to be through the local secretion of proinflammatory cytokines and adipokines to the myocardium [40]. Insulin resistance, on the other hand, exerts multiple systemic effects that likely contribute to cardiovascular disease, including impaired vascular function, dysregulated cardiac energy substrate utilization, adverse cardiac remodeling, fibrosis, and inflammation [41]. It is likely that the modulation of visceral adipose tissue by exercise is a contributory mechanism driving the large-scale study observations that exercise improves cardiovascular health [42]. Indeed, multiple studies have demonstrated that exercise exerts anti-inflammatory effects. These include the release of interleukin-6 from contracting muscle fibers into the circulation (with subsequent increased levels of the interleukin-1 and interleukin-10 receptor antagonists), downregulation of Toll-like receptor expression on monocytes (causing inhibition of proinflammatory cytokine production, among other effects), and reduced macrophage infiltration into adipose tissue [43] (Fig. 22.4). Similarly, interventional studies have demonstrated a strong link between exercise training and both insulin-dependent and insulin-independent pathways causing improved glucose regulation, regardless of weight loss [44]. Given visceral adipose tissue is strongly linked to insulin resistance, it is likely that reductions in visceral adipose tissue promoted by exercise strongly contribute to improved insulin sensitivity.

Are exercise-induced changes in body weight necessary for reductions in visceral adipose tissue and how does this compare to other interventions?

Regular exercise plays an important role in maintaining a healthy weight across the life course—including the prevention of weight gain (even after weight loss). An increase in energy expenditure of 1500−2000 calories/week is associated with weight maintenance [45]. However, most, but not all, study data indicate that exercise alone plays a very small role in weight loss in those who are overweight [46,47].

Other treatment options for overweight or obese individuals include low-caloric diet, pharmacotherapy (or a combination of the two), and bariatric surgery. Previous studies have shown that bariatric surgery and low calorie diets lead to greater body weight loss and higher remission rates of type 2 diabetes in comparison with nonsurgical treatments of obesity (including exercise) [48,49]. However, such approaches do not necessarily lead to anticipated improvements in diastolic function, while also failing to address other important aspects of physical health, such as cardiorespiratory fitness [50]. When directly comparing methods, bariatric surgery and low-calorie diets may lead to greater reductions of visceral adipose tissue compared with exercise [49,51]. That said, a recent systematic review and metaanalysis including 34 studies (10 included in the metaanalysis) and 1502 participants demonstrated significant pooled effect sizes for the reduction in epicardial adipose tissue volume following weight loss (effect size = −0.89, 95% CI: 1.23 to −0.55, $P < .001$), pharmaceutical (effect size = −0.79, 95% CI: 1.37 to −0.21, $P < .01$), and exercise interventions (effect size = −1.11, 95% CI: 1.57 to −0.65, $P < .001$) [52]. Interestingly, the lowest heterogeneity was observed in the exercise interventions, suggesting it may be a modality with a particular specificity in targeting epicardial adipose tissue. These findings also corroborate with previous research illustrating the differential impacts of weight loss on adipose tissue of various locations after bariatric surgery, low-calorie diets, or exercise programs [51]. This is consistent with previous research, demonstrating that regular exercise has the advantage of ameliorating some of the negative health effects of obesity, even in the absence of weight loss. For example, a 13-week study in previously sedentary, lean men and in obese men with and without type 2 diabetes demonstrated that supervised aerobic exercise (five times per week for 60 min at a moderate intensity [∼60% peak oxygen uptake]) resulted in a marked reduction in visceral adipose tissue (∼17%), despite no weight loss [9]. This finding is consistent with previous observations in obese men [12] and women [53] and a multiethnic cohort across a wide range of adiposity classifications [54]. It is therefore important not to focus on the potential for weight loss as the sole outcome from increasing exercise levels, but rather to suggest that it may contribute to abdominal obesity reduction or weight maintenance efforts. This focus will reduce the likelihood of individuals using limitations of weight loss as a reason to discontinue their physical activity program.

The unique role of exercise in the prevention and management of chronic disease

The combination of weight loss (including visceral adipose tissue) and improved cardiometabolic health associated with surgery, pharmacological therapies, and novel dietary approaches is appealing, particularly given their independent and independent associations with a multitude of comorbidities. However, in terms of prevention and management of chronic disease, it is also important to understand the impact of these therapies on other markers of health, particularly physical function, frailty, and body composition. For example, type 2 diabetes not just is a disease of the cardiometabolic system but also represents a powerful physiological model of accelerated biological aging, increasing the risk of sarcopenia, impaired

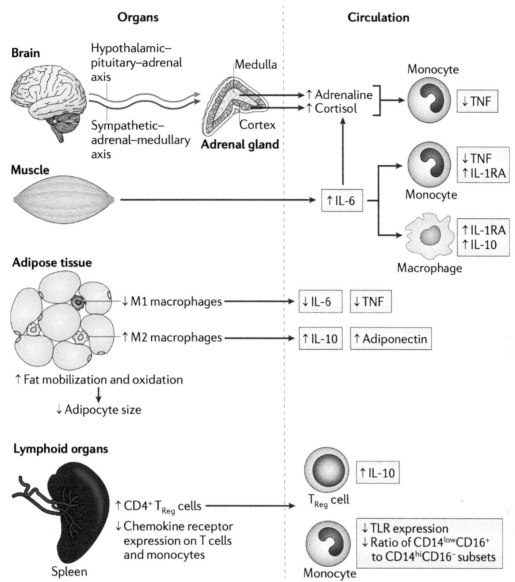

FIGURE 22.4 Potential mechanisms contributing to the antiinflammatory effects of exercise. Activation of the hypothalamic—pituitary—adrenal axis and the sympathetic nervous system (SNS) leads to the release of cortisol and adrenaline from the adrenal cortex and medulla, respectively. These hormones inhibit the release of tumor necrosis factor (TNF) by monocytes. Interleukin-6 (IL-6) produced by contracting skeletal muscle also down-regulates the production of TNF by monocytes and may stimulate further cortisol release. Acute elevations in IL-6 stimulate the release of IL-1 receptor antagonist (IL-1RA) from monocytes and macrophages, thus increasing the circulating concentrations of this antiinflammatory cytokine. Exercise training mobilizes regulatory T (TReg) cells (which are a major source of the anti-inflammatory cytokine IL-10) and decreases the ratio of inflammatory (CD14lowCD16+) monocytes to classical (CD14hiCD16−) monocytes. Following exercise, CD14hiCD16− monocytes express less Toll-like receptor 4 (TLR4) and thereby induce a reduced inflammatory response marked by lower levels of proinflammatory cytokines and reduced adipose tissue infiltration. Exercise also increases plasma concentrations of key inflammatory immune cell chemokines; repeated elevations of such chemokines may lead to a downregulation of their cellular receptors, resulting in reduced tissue infiltration. A reduction in adipose tissue mass and adipocyte size, along with reduced macrophage infiltration and a switch from an M1 to an M2 macrophage phenotype, may contribute to a reduction in the release of proin-flammatory cytokines (such as IL-6 and TNF) and an increase in the release of antiinflammatory cytokines (such as adiponectin and IL-10) from adipose tissue. *Reproduced with permission from Gleeson M, Bishop NC, Stensel DJ, Lindley MR, Mastana SS, Nimmo MA. The anti-inflammatory effects of exercise: mechanisms and implications for the prevention and treatment of disease. Nat Rev Immunol 2011;11:607—615.*

physical function, and impaired balance at a younger age [55—57]. Indeed, for every kilogram lost through a hypoenergetic diet, around 25%—30% is due to reductions in lean body mass (predominantly skeletal muscle) [29,30]. Combined aerobic and anaerobic exercise training provides a powerful anabolic stimulus that improves muscle quality and muscle strength, increases muscle mass, and enhances physical fitness and function, with whole-body effects that remain unrivalled by any other lifestyle or pharmaceutical intervention [27,28]. Weight loss without using exercise as an adjunct may limit the magnitude of longer-term benefits achieved with weight loss alone and leave those with type 2 diabetes at an increased risk of poor physical function, sarcopenia, and frailty in the future.

Conclusion

Despite the aerobic component of exercise interventions appearing central to exercised-induced ectopic and visceral adipose tissue modulation, evidence also suggests that resistance training attenuates visceral adipose tissue increases occurring over time, particularly following substantial weight loss. Although reducing ectopic and visceral adiposity in isolation is unlikely in most obese individuals, for whom multiple cardiometabolic risk factors are likely to be present, the evidence suggests that aerobic activity is likely to yield the greatest reduction in ectopic and visceral adipose tissue. That said, the combination of aerobic and resistance modalities with pharmacological therapies and novel dietary approaches may be beneficial in reducing and preventing the regain of visceral adipose tissue, while simultaneously improving overall health.

References

[1] Bull FC, Al-Ansari SS, Biddle S, et al. World Health Organization 2020 guidelines on physical activity and sedentary behaviour. Br J Sports Med 2020;54:1451−62.

[2] Caspersen CJ, Powell KE, Christenson GM. Physical activity, exercise, and physical fitness: definitions and distinctions for health-related research. Public Health Rep 1985;100:126−31.

[3] Colberg SR, Sigal RJ, Yardley JE, et al. Physical activity/exercise and diabetes: a position Statement of the American diabetes association. Diab Care 2016;39:2065−79.

[4] Care DHS. UK Chief medical Officers' physical activity guidelines. 2019.

[5] Medicine ACoS. Physical activity guidelines for Americans. 2nd ed. 2018.

[6] Garber CE, Blissmer B, Deschenes MR, et al. American College of Sports Medicine position stand. Quantity and quality of exercise for developing and maintaining cardiorespiratory, musculoskeletal, and neuromotor fitness in apparently healthy adults: guidance for prescribing exercise. Med Sci Sports Exerc 2011;43:1334−59.

[7] Giannopoulou I, Ploutz-Snyder LL, Carhart R, et al. Exercise is required for visceral fat loss in postmenopausal women with type 2 diabetes. J Clin Endocrinol Metab 2005;90:1511−8.

[8] Irwin ML, Yasui Y, Ulrich CM, et al. Effect of exercise on total and intra-abdominal body fat in postmenopausal women: a randomized controlled trial. JAMA 2003;289:323−30.

[9] Lee S, Kuk JL, Davidson LE, et al. Exercise without weight loss is an effective strategy for obesity reduction in obese individuals with and without Type 2 diabetes. J Appl Physiol 2005;99:1220−5.

[10] O'Leary VB, Marchetti CM, Krishnan RK, Stetzer BP, Gonzalez F, Kirwan JP. Exercise-induced reversal of insulin resistance in obese elderly is associated with reduced visceral fat. J Appl Physiol 2006;100:1584−9.

[11] Slentz CA, Houmard JA, Kraus WE. Exercise, abdominal obesity, skeletal muscle, and metabolic risk: evidence for a dose response. Obesity 2009;17(Suppl. 3):S27−33.

[12] Ross R, Dagnone D, Jones PJ, et al. Reduction in obesity and related comorbid conditions after diet-induced weight loss or exercise-induced weight loss in men. A randomized, controlled trial. Ann Intern Med 2000;133:92−103.

[13] Kraus WE, Torgan CE, Duscha BD, et al. Studies of a targeted risk reduction intervention through defined exercise (STRRIDE). Med Sci Sports Exerc 2001;33:1774−84.

[14] Ismail I, Keating SE, Baker MK, Johnson NA. A systematic review and meta-analysis of the effect of aerobic vs. resistance exercise training on visceral fat. Obes Rev 2012;13:68−91.

[15] Vissers D, Hens W, Taeymans J, Baeyens JP, Poortmans J, Van Gaal L. The effect of exercise on visceral adipose tissue in overweight adults: a systematic review and meta-analysis. PLoS One 2013;8:e56415.

[16] Heiskanen MA, Motiani KK, Mari A, et al. Exercise training decreases pancreatic fat content and improves beta cell function regardless of baseline glucose tolerance: a randomised controlled trial. Diabetologia 2018;61:1817−28.

[17] Sargeant JA, Gray LJ, Bodicoat DH, et al. The effect of exercise training on intrahepatic triglyceride and hepatic insulin sensitivity: a systematic review and meta-analysis. Obes Rev 2018;19:1446−59.

[18] Hens W, Taeyman J, Cornelis J, Gielen J, Van Gaal L, Vissers D. The effect of lifestyle interventions on excess ectopic fat deposition measured by noninvasive techniques in overweight and obese adults: a systematic review and meta-analysis. J Phys Act Health 2016;13:671−94.

[19] Saco-Ledo G, Valenzuela PL, Castillo-Garcia A, et al. Physical exercise and epicardial adipose tissue: a systematic review and meta-analysis of randomized controlled trials. Obes Rev 2021;22:e13103.

[20] Sabag A, Way KL, Keating SE, et al. Exercise and ectopic fat in type 2 diabetes: a systematic review and meta-analysis. Diabetes Metab 2017;43:195−210.

[21] Khalafi M, Malandish A, Rosenkranz SK, Ravasi AA. Effect of resistance training with and without caloric restriction on visceral fat: a systemic review and meta-analysis. Obes Rev 2021;22:e13275.

[22] Slentz CA, Aiken LB, Houmard JA, et al. Inactivity, exercise, and visceral fat. STRRIDE: a randomized, controlled study of exercise intensity and amount. J Appl Physiol 2005;99:1613−8.

[23] Nieves DJ, Cnop M, Retzlaff B, et al. The atherogenic lipoprotein profile associated with obesity and insulin resistance is largely attributable to intra-abdominal fat. Diabetes 2003;52:172−9.

[24] Okauchi Y, Nishizawa H, Funahashi T, et al. Reduction of visceral fat is associated with decrease in the number of metabolic risk factors in Japanese men. Diabetes Care 2007;30:2392−4.

[25] Cuff DJ, Meneilly GS, Martin A, Ignaszewski A, Tildesley HD, Frohlich JJ. Effective exercise modality to reduce insulin resistance in women with type 2 diabetes. Diabetes Care 2003;26:2977−82.

[26] Park SK, Park JH, Kwon YC, Kim HS, Yoon MS, Park HT. The effect of combined aerobic and resistance exercise training on abdominal fat in obese middle-aged women. J Physiol Anthropol Appl Human Sci 2003;22:129−35.

[27] Booth FW, Gordon SE, Carlson CJ, Hamilton MT. Waging war on modern chronic diseases: primary prevention through exercise biology. J Appl Physiol 2000;88:774−87.

[28] Booth FW, Thomason DB. Molecular and cellular adaptation of muscle in response to exercise: perspectives of various models. Physiol Rev 1991;71:541−85.

[29] Magkos F, Fraterrigo G, Yoshino J, et al. Effects of moderate and subsequent progressive weight loss on metabolic function and adipose tissue biology in humans with obesity. Cell Metab 2016;23:591−601.

[30] Heymsfield SB, Gonzalez MC, Shen W, Redman L, Thomas D. Weight loss composition is one-fourth fat-free mass: a critical review and critique of this widely cited rule. Obes Rev 2014;15:310−21.

[31] Maillard F, Pereira B, Boisseau N. Effect of high-intensity interval training on total, abdominal and visceral fat mass: a meta-analysis. Sports Med 2018;48:269−88.

[32] Chang YH, Yang HY, Shun SC. Effect of exercise intervention dosage on reducing visceral adipose tissue: a systematic review and network meta-analysis of randomized controlled trials. Int J Obes 2021;45:982−97.

[33] Hunter GR, Brock DW, Byrne NM, Chandler-Laney PC, Del Corral P, Gower BA. Exercise training prevents regain of visceral fat for 1 year following weight loss. Obesity 2010;18:690−5.

[34] Ross R, Janssen I. Physical activity, total and regional obesity: dose-response considerations. Med Sci Sports Exerc 2001;33:S521−7. discussion S528−9.

[35] Ohkawara K, Tanaka S, Miyachi M, Ishikawa-Takata K, Tabata I. A dose-response relation between aerobic exercise and visceral fat reduction: systematic review of clinical trials. Int J Obes 2007;31:1786−97.

[36] Ainsworth BE, Haskell WL, Herrmann SD, et al. Compendium of Physical Activities: a second update of codes and MET values. Med Sci Sports Exerc 2011 2011;43:1575−81.

[37] Disparities OHI. Physical activity: applying all Our health. Gov.uk; 2022.

[38] Levelt E, Gulsin G, Neubauer S, McCann GP. Mechanisms in endocrinology: diabetic cardiomyopathy: pathophysiology and potential metabolic interventions state of the art review. Eur J Endocrinol 2018;178:R127−39.

[39] Levelt E, Pavlides M, Banerjee R, et al. Ectopic and visceral fat deposition in lean and obese patients with type 2 diabetes. J Am Coll Cardiol 2016;68:53−63.

[40] Ayton SL, Gulsin GS, McCann GP, Moss AJ. Epicardial adipose tissue in obesity-related cardiac dysfunction. Heart 2022;108:339−44.

[41] Gulsin GS, Athithan L, McCann GP. Diabetic cardiomyopathy: prevalence, determinants and potential treatments. Ther Adv Endocrinol Metab 2019;10. 2042018819834869.

[42] Hamer M, O'Donovan G, Stamatakis E. Association between physical activity and sub-types of cardiovascular disease death causes in a general population cohort. Eur J Epidemiol 2019;34:483−7.

[43] Gleeson M, Bishop NC, Stensel DJ, Lindley MR, Mastana SS, Nimmo MA. The anti-inflammatory effects of exercise: mechanisms and implications for the prevention and treatment of disease. Nat Rev Immunol 2011;11:607−15.

[44] Hawley JA. Exercise as a therapeutic intervention for the prevention and treatment of insulin resistance. Diabetes Metab Res Rev 2004;20:383−93.

[45] Fogelholm M, Kukkonen-Harjula K. Does physical activity prevent weight gain–a systematic review. Obes Rev 2000;1:95−111.

[46] Franz MJ, VanWormer JJ, Crain AL, et al. Weight-loss outcomes: a systematic review and meta-analysis of weight-loss clinical trials with a minimum 1-year follow-up. J Am Diet Assoc 2007;107:1755−67.

[47] Johns DJ, Hartmann-Boyce J, Jebb SA, Aveyard P. Behavioural Weight Management Review G. Diet or exercise interventions vs combined behavioral weight management programs: a systematic review and meta-analysis of direct comparisons. J Acad Nutr Diet 2014;114:1557−68.

[48] Lean ME, Leslie WS, Barnes AC, et al. Primary care-led weight management for remission of type 2 diabetes (DiRECT): an open-label, cluster-randomised trial. Lancet 2017;391(10120):541−51.

[49] Cheng J, Gao J, Shuai X, Wang G, Tao K. The comprehensive summary of surgical versus non-surgical treatment for obesity: a systematic review and meta-analysis of randomized controlled trials. Oncotarget 2016;7:39216−30.

[50] Gulsin GS, Swarbrick DJ, Athithan L, et al. Effects of low-energy diet or exercise on cardiovascular function in working-age adults with type 2 diabetes: a prospective, randomized, open-label, blinded end point trial. Diabetes Care 2020;43(6):1300−10.

[51] Wu FZ, Huang YL, Wu CC, et al. Differential effects of bariatric surgery versus exercise on excessive visceral fat deposits. Medicine 2016;95:e2616.

[52] Launbo N, Zobel EH, von Scholten BJ, Faerch K, Jorgensen PG, Christensen RH. Targeting epicardial adipose tissue with exercise, diet, bariatric surgery or pharmaceutical interventions: a systematic review and meta-analysis. Obes Rev 2021;22:e13136.

[53] Ross R, Janssen I, Dawson J, et al. Exercise-induced reduction in obesity and insulin resistance in women: a randomized controlled trial. Obes Res 2004;12:789–98.

[54] Wilmore JH, Despres JP, Stanforth PR, et al. Alterations in body weight and composition consequent to 20 wk of endurance training: the heritage family study. Am J Clin Nutr 1999;70:346–52.

[55] Mickute M, Henson J, Rowlands AV, et al. Device-measured physical activity and its association with physical function in adults with type 2 diabetes mellitus. Diabet Med 2021;38:e14393.

[56] Abdelhafiz AH, Emmerton D, Sinclair AJ. Impact of frailty metabolic phenotypes on the management of older people with type 2 diabetes mellitus. Geriatr Gerontol Int 2021;21:614–22.

[57] Mesinovic J, Zengin A, De Courten B, Ebeling PR, Scott D. Sarcopenia and type 2 diabetes mellitus: a bidirectional relationship. Diabetes Metab Syndr Obes 2019;12:1057–72.

Chapter 23

Combined lifestyle interventions

Jena Shaw Tronieri[1], Karl Nadolsky[2] and Monica Agarwal[3]

[1]Department of Psychiatry, Perelman School of Medicine at the University of Pennsylvania, Philadelphia, PA, United States; [2]Department of Medicine, Michigan State University College of Human Medicine, Grand Rapids, MI, United States; [3]Department of Medicine, University of Alabama at Birmingham, Birmingham, AL, United States

Introduction

Obesity is a complex, progressive, and relapsing chronic disease that increases morbidity and mortality. A multimodal patient-centered approach to the prevention and treatment of obesity is required to combat the epidemic of obesity. The combined lifestyle interventions (ILI) of dietary changes, physical activity, and behavioral therapies are three main tenets of obesity management and are foundational for durable weight loss (Fig. 23.1). In addition, managing sleep and stress is important for weight management. Pharmacological therapy and bariatric surgery also require nutritional changes, physical activity, and psychological interventions for long-term success in managing excess weight.

Medical nutrition therapy

Introduction

Patients with obesity ought to be prescribed a dietary plan that creates an energy deficit (reduced calories) while following basic principles of healthy eating. Previous guidelines have recommended reducing usual intake by 500−750 kcal/d, estimating targets of 1200 to 1500 kcal/d for women or 1500 to 1800 kcal/d for men, or following one of the many dietary patterns with restrictions shown to create an energy deficit and weight loss [1,2]. Dietary patterns or strategies that have been shown to create an energy deficit leading to weight loss and health benefits include carbohydrate restriction (as little as 20 g/d), lower glycemic index/load, fat restriction, plant-based or vegetarian, high protein (often >25% of calories from protein), Mediterranean, and utilization of meal replacements. While caloric or energy quantity matters, quality remains very important for clinical health benefits and can support weight loss. Consuming whole foods rather than processed foods was shown to result in dramatically reduced ad libitum energy intake despite matched macronutrients in a tightly controlled inpatient trial [3].

Dietary patterns

Mediterranean diets are generally characterized by consumption of vegetables, fruits, legumes, whole grains, nuts/seeds, olive oil, and fish. This dietary pattern has been associated with cardiometabolic benefits including weight loss and improved cardiovascular outcomes [4−7]. The PREDIMED trial randomized subjects with obesity, type 2 diabetes mellitus (T2DM), and high cardiovascular risk to nuts or olive oil without energy restriction, resulting in more weight loss (including reductions in waist circumference) than reduced fat dietary recommendations, as well as reduced adverse cardiovascular events [8,9]. The incorporation of larger portions of low-energy-dense foods, such as fruits, vegetables, and legumes/pulses, provides essential fiber and phytonutrients while maintaining satiety and reducing energy intake [10−12].

The consumption of caloric or sugar-sweetened beverages does not increase satiety and increases calories consumed, and frequent consumption of these beverages may be a contributor to obesity and adiposity-based diseases [13]. Replacing sugar-sweetened beverages with zero-calorie drinks or water has shown to be beneficial despite observational concerns about non-nutritive sweeteners [14,15]. The optimal macronutrient distribution for weight loss has been frequently debated

FIGURE 23.1 Combined lifestyle interventions: the foundational changes of medical nutrition therapy, physical activity, and psychological interventions for obesity management.

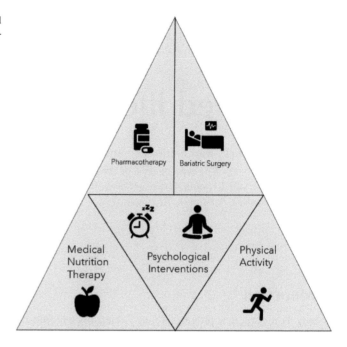

and remains controversial but ultimately comes down to adherence to a diet that produces an energy deficit [16,17]. It is most likely that one approach will not suit all patients. A meta-analysis of many popular diets including 48 unique trials revealed nearly identical weight loss results at 12 months for diets with different macronutrient profiles (7.25 kg with low carbohydrate and 7.27 kg for low-fat diets) [18], as did another meta-analysis of 14 macronutrient-based diets [19]. Finding potential targets in individuals' dietary habits for reducing energy intake, perhaps while increasing consumption of nutrient-dense whole foods, should be a focus of medical nutrition therapy.

Reducing dietary fat leads to an energy deficit and weight loss, as does reducing energy intake from carbohydrates, with some suggestion of a slight advantage of the lower-carbohydrate diets over low-fat diets in the short-term that is confounded by variable and poor adherence [20,21]. Randomized controlled studies have demonstrated greater weight loss at 6 months, albeit minimal difference by 1 year, with low-carbohydrate diets compared with low-fat diets [22]. A meta-analysis evaluating randomized controlled trials of low-fat and a variety of higher-fat dietary interventions for greater than 1 year showed no advantage, and weight loss was dependent upon the intensity of the interventions regardless of which arm [23]. A meta-analysis of tightly controlled feeding trials comparing low-carbohydrate/high-fat diets with high-carbohydrate/low-fat diets with higher protein consumption that held constant and isocaloric conditions (food provided to subjects) showed minimal differences but supported a slight statistically significant difference favoring the low-fat diets in terms of energy expenditure and weight [24]. Genetic variability has been hypothesized as a reason for the variable individual responses to differing dietary prescriptions, similar to baseline insulin dynamics supported by preliminary research. This observation illustrates the emergent science of nutrient—gene interactions relevant to obesity research. The DIETFITS trial randomized over 600 adults with obesity to "healthy low-fat" versus "healthy low-carbohydrate" diets in the context of evaluating whether three single-nucleotide polymorphism multilocus genotype responsiveness patterns or insulin secretion (30 min post glucose challenge) were associated with weight loss. There was no significantly different weight loss between macronutrient groups (−5.3 kg for low fat; 6 kg for low carbohydrate), and neither genotype pattern nor baseline insulin secretion was associated with the different diets' effects on weight loss [25].

Several studies have suggested that diets higher in protein (25%−30%) improve satiety and support lower caloric intake in free-living environments along with a slight "metabolic advantage," resulting in weight loss [26−29]. Dietary protein is beneficial for maintaining fat-free mass during weight loss and even during weight gain [30]. A large trial randomized over 800 adults with obesity to one of four diets of similar foods differing in ratios of fat, protein, and carbohydrate (20%, 15%, and 65%; 20%, 25%, and 55%; 40%, 15%, and 45%; and 40%, 25%, and 35%, respectively) plus counseling for 2 years. After an average of 7% of initial weight was lost across all four groups at 6 months, weight regain began after 1 year. By 2 years, the average weight lost was 4% in all macronutrient groups, with adherence having the strongest association with treatment response [31]. It was shown, however, that those who achieved the largest protein intake per urinary nitrogen excretion did indeed lose more weight [32]. A meta-analysis suggested that short-term benefits of higher protein interventions may linger for weight maintenance, again with better adherence as the critical factor [33]. Higher protein diets are generally thought to support the retention of muscle mass during weight loss interventions, although there are some subtle contradictory results [34]. High protein consumption may accelerate chronic kidney disease (CKD) and should be cautiously personalized in patients with baseline elevated creatinine and estimated glomerular filtration rate (eGFR) consistent with CKD. Modest protein restriction (0.8 g/kg) may slightly slow the progression of that disease and has been recommended historically [35]. Recent data have suggested otherwise, including a cohort of patients enrolled in a French high-protein weight loss plan that had no adverse changes in eGFR and a recent PRCT of 68 patients with obesity and normal renal function at baseline that failed to demonstrate any adverse effect on renal function of a very-low (4%)-carbohydrate diet with 35% protein [36,37]. Subanalysis of participants with prediabetes in a high-protein, low-energy meal replacement diet did not reveal an association with creatinine clearance, eGFR, albumin/Cr ratio, or serum creatinine [38]. High protein consumption in those without kidney disease, even very high levels in trained athletes, has not been shown to be detrimental [39]. Recent guidance has suggested maintaining a protein intake of 0.8 g protein/kg (weight)/day for those with diabetes mellitus and CKD not treated with dialysis [40].

Very-low-calorie diets (VLCDs; <800 kcal/d) often coined "protein-supplemented modified fasts" and low-calorie diets (LCDs; 800−1500 kcal/d) are linked with comparable rates of long-term weight loss, albeit more rapid initially with VLCDs [41]. In a large, multicenter study involving 1389 patients followed up for at least 1 year on a VLCD providing 600−800 calories per day, mean weight loss was −6.9 ± 2.6 kg at 1 month, −12.3 ± 5.3 kg at 3 months, and −13.1 ± 8.0 kg at 12 months primarily from fat loss per bioimpedance analysis [42]. VLCDs have been shown to rapidly improve or even reverse T2DM when followed by sustainable weight loss maintenance program [43]. VLCDs require protein sources of high nutritional value and supplementation of vitamins and micronutrients, including sodium, potassium, calcium, iron, and magnesium. VLCDs are safest when monitored by a physician as part of a comprehensive weight reduction program and are contraindicated in pregnancy/lactation, major psychiatric disease, severe systemic disease, and type 1 diabetes [44]. The European Association for the Study of Obesity recently published guidelines based upon a meta-analysis of "very-low-calorie ketogenic diets" (VLCKD) concluding that "VLCKD can be recommended as an effective dietary treatment for individuals with obesity after considering potential contraindications," keeping in mind personalization [45].

A popular strategy in obesity treatment is the use of commercial meal replacements (liquid shakes or bars) to improve adherence to a low- or very-low-calorie dietary plan. Meal replacements serve as both a nutritional and a behavioral strategy, as they provide calorie- and portion-controlled meals, generally fortified with vitamins and minerals, and they eliminate the need to make food choices. They are typically used to replace one or two meals daily. A meta-analysis of six controlled trials found that subjects on a diet plan that included liquid meal replacements lost 2.54 kg more at 3 months and 2.44 kg more at 1 year than did those on a reduced energy food-based plan [46]. Another meta-analysis reported similar benefits of formula meal replacements regardless of whether a VLCD or LCD goal was provided, and regardless of whether or not patients had T2DM [47]. A pragmatic randomized trial comparing a 810 kcal/d formula prescription for 3 months followed by 1 month of food reintroduction led to nearly 11% weight loss at 1 year compared with 3% in a standard nurse-led behavioral support program with modest energy restriction [48]. Recent trials have shown that initial intensive weight loss using a meal replacement strategy as part of a comprehensive program can markedly improve cardiometabolic markers with return to "normoglycemia" in prediabetes and remission of T2DM [49,50]. A 2021 meta-analysis of 22 studies involving 24 interventions and nearly 2000 patients suggested that meal replacement−based low-energy diets are superior to food-based low-energy diets, especially if ≥ 60% of total daily energy intake was from the meal replacements [51]. Similarly, a recent multicenter randomized trial with nearly 500 participants with obesity and cardiometabolic risk factors suggested that a liquid meal replacement plan combined with intensive lifestyle intervention (ILI) reduced weight and improved cardiovascular risk surrogates more than lifestyle alone [52].

While published meta-analyses of hypocaloric diets for weight management in people with type 2 diabetes do not support any macronutrient profile or dietary recommendation over others, very-low-energy diets and formula meal replacements appear the most effective approaches, generally providing less energy than self-administered food-based diets. Programs including a hypocaloric formula "total diet replacement" induction phase were most effective for type 2 diabetes remission [53]. Meal replacements have also been shown to be a potentially useful tool to assist with weight loss maintenance. This was illustrated in a trial of knee arthritis patients with obesity who completed a 68-week ILI averaging 10% weight loss who were then randomized to either intermittent use of meal replacements (5 weeks every 4 months) or daily use (one to two meals) for 3 years. In that study, there was slight but nonsignificant weight regain on average with no significant difference between groups [54].

TABLE 23.1 The dietary patterns/modifications for weight loss and additional benefits beyond weight loss.

Dietary pattern (prescriptive changes are *not* mutually exclusive for individuals)	Description (generalized descriptions as definitions vary in literature)	Benefits beyond weight loss
Replacing ultraprocessed or refined foods with "whole food" is a common denominator[a]	Reduced intake of energy-dense, nutrient- poor processed foods including sugar- sweetened beverages. Consume vegetables, fruit, legumes, whole grains, lean animal protein, nuts/seeds, dairy.	• Associated with reduced mortality
Carbohydrate restriction	Spectrum of carbohydrate (sugar and starch) ranging from very-low-carbohydrate ketogenic diets (20–50 gm carbohydrate daily or < 26% of calories) to inclusion of fruit.	• Acute and chronic glycemic improvement • Improved blood pressure • Improved triglycerides
Fat restriction	Restricts intake of naturally occurring animal or plant fats in addition to restricting added fats and oils. Encourages low-fat protein and veggies, legumes, fruit, and grains.	• Reduced LDL-c • Improved blood pressure • Reduced dysglycemic progression
Animal protein restriction (vegetarian)	Restricts intake of animal protein ranging from "flexitarian" (occasional animal consumption) to veganism (avoid all animal products).	• Reduced LDL-c • Improved glycemia • Improved blood pressure
Mediterranean	Encourages veggies, fruit, and whole grains with low-fat animal protein and emphasis on nuts/seeds and olive oil.	• Reduced cardiovascular events • Improved glycemia • Improved blood pressure
Paleolithic	Consumption of food theoretically available prior to agricultural revolution including veggies, fruit, animals, nuts, and eggs.	• Generally improved glycemia • Likely depends upon other aspects
Meal replacements	Replacement of usual meals with energy- controlled formulations, often in the form of protein drinks or bars.	• Improved glycemia • Diabetes prevention/remission • Improved blood pressure
Intermittent fasting (IF) time-restricted feeding	IF includes dramatic caloric restriction some days with usual intake other days (i.e., alternate day or 5:2 as examples). Time- restricted feeding limits time frame of eating.	• Mixed data on cardiometabolic health • Generally dependent on weight loss

[a]*Ultraprocessed diet definition [60].*

Periods of prolonged fasting, popularly coined "intermittent fasting" or "alternate day fasting" among others, have proven to be a viable method for energy restriction, leading to weight loss and metabolic benefits [55,56]. There are a variety of ways to incorporate bouts of energy restriction interspaced by habitual energy intake to create an energy deficit in weight loss, and the intermittent pattern is hypothesized to improve adherence. A small trial comparing continuous with intermittent energy restriction, controlled for macronutrients, resulted in similar weight loss and subjective appetite ratings with marginal differences in metabolic rate, exercise efficiency, and overall appetite-regulating hormone changes [57]. A 1-year trial comparing 2 days weekly of 400/600 kcal/d (women/men, respectively) showed similar weight loss of 8 versus 9 kg, respectively, similar cardiometabolic marker improvements, and minimal weight regain (1.1 vs. 0.4 kg, respectively) but higher hunger scores in the intermittent fasting group [58]. This strategy also appears to have similar weight and glycemic benefits for those with obesity complicated by T2DM [59]. Table 23.1 summarizes the various dietary patterns for weight management.

Summary

Overall, the available evidence from meta-analyses suggest that intermittent fasting paradigms produce equivalent weight loss when compared with continuous energy restriction plans without differences between groups in weight or body fat loss [61]. There is a concern regarding intermittent fasting and time-restricted feeding about skipping breakfast due to historical data correlating breakfast eating to better weight and health, but a metaanalysis of 13 randomized trials examining the

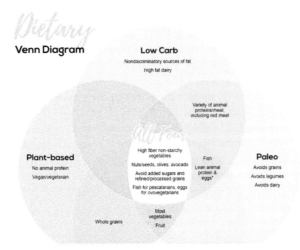

FIGURE 23.2   An energy deficit must be created to result in weight loss and improved health and can be accomplished through a variety of methods that should include replacing processed foods with whole foods and can integrate aspects of the plethora of macronutrient restrictive diets and dietary patterns, which notably share many aspects without being mutually exclusive.

effect of breakfast on weight change and/or on energy intake found minimal difference and actually slightly favored those assigned to skip breakfast for energy intake [62]. Nutrition therapy can be individualized but must ultimately create an energy deficit to result in weight loss and improved adiposity-based diseases. This can be accomplished through a variety of methods that include replacing processed foods with whole foods and can integrate aspects of the plethora of macronutrient restrictive diets and dietary patterns while also incorporating meal replacement strategies and meal timing strategies without being mutually exclusive (Fig. 23.2).

Physical activity

Introduction

Physical inactivity was characterized as a global pandemic and a major leading cause of death worldwide in 2012 [63]. Sedentary times of 9.5 h or more are associated with a higher risk for death [64]. In addition, physical inactivity is responsible for a significant economic burden of at least $67.5 billion per year [65]. Global estimates show that one in four (27.5%) adults and more than three-quarters (81%) of adolescents do not meet the recommendations for aerobic exercise as outlined by the 2010 Global Recommendations on Physical Activity for Health [66]. The COVID-19 pandemic has further contributed to physical inactivity and sedentary behavior [67].

In the Multi-Ethnic Study of Atherosclerosis (MESA) cohort of 6795 men and women free of cardiovascular disease at baseline, physical activity was inversely related to cardiometabolic risk associated with obesity and central obesity [68]. Furthermore, physical activity and cardiorespiratory fitness are associated with reduced risk for all-cause mortality independently of body mass index (BMI) [69]. In addition, pooled data from six studies have shown that meeting the minimum 2008 Physical Activity Guidelines for Americans of either 75 min of vigorous-intensity or 150 min of moderate-intensity activities (7.5 metabolic-equivalent [MET] hours per week) was associated with longevity benefit with 3–5 times the recommended leisure-time physical activity minimum and no excess risk at 10 or more times the recommended minimum [70]. Furthermore, physical activity is associated with reduced risk for premature mortality at any intensity with reduced sedentary time, evidenced by a nonlinear dose–response pattern in middle-aged and older adults [71]. In another study of 1.4 million participants, leisure-time physical activity was associated with a lower risk of 10 cancers after BMI adjustment [72].

Benefits of physical activity

Obesity incidence has increased dramatically over the past 50 years. Physical activity levels have been declining globally, potentially contributing to the obesity epidemic. Obesity is the driver for type 2 diabetes and cardiovascular disease, among other noncommunicable diseases. Physical activity is the cornerstone for preventing and treating obesity and obesity-related complications such as type 2 diabetes. It can improve mental health and foster wellness. The U.S. Diabetes

Prevention Program (DPP) multicenter trial utilized ILIs (dietary restriction and moderate-intensity physical activity for >150 min per week supported by behavioral therapy) to achieve 7% weight loss to prevent and delay type 2 diabetes [73]. The DPP showed that ILIs were more effective than metformin in preventing diabetes; the ILI group had a 58% reduction in incidence compared to placebo, while the metformin group had a 31% reduction [73]. Although weight loss was the dominant predictor of reduced diabetes incidence with a 16% reduction for every kilogram weight loss, among participants who did not meet the weight loss goal at year 1, those who achieved the physical activity goal had 44% lower diabetes incidence [74]. Furthermore, the DPP outcomes study with a follow-up of 15 years revealed that cumulative incidence of type 2 diabetes was still lower in the original ILI group [75]. There also was a 6% decrease in diabetes incidence per six MET-h/week in time-dependent physical activity over an average of 12 years (controlled for age, sex, baseline physical activity, and weight) [76]. Physical activity was inversely related to the incidence of diabetes among the DPP participants, underscoring the importance of physical activity in the prevention of diabetes. The Action for Health in Diabetes (Look AHEAD) trial showed that ILI participants had better hemoglobin A1c, greater improvements in fitness, and in all cardiovascular risk factors except for low-density lipoprotein cholesterol [77]. Although ILI did not reduce the occurrence of a composite CVD outcome, the participants had reduced the incidence of obesity-related complications and lowered healthcare costs over a decade [78]. Regular physical activity is associated with a lower prevalence of cardiovascular risk factors and has been proven to prevent and treat noncommunicable diseases such as heart disease, stroke, and diabetes. Although the weight loss from regular physical activity may be modest, maintaining regular physical activity alleviates insulin resistance, lowers cardiometabolic risk, promotes cardiorespiratory fitness, and reduces mortality [79]. The Whole Health Organization Global action plan 2018–30 aims to reduce physical inactivity by 15% by 2030 in adults and adolescents (WHO policy).

Recommendations for physical activity

The American College of Sports Medicine (ACSM) recommends a program of regular exercise that includes cardiorespiratory, resistance, flexibility, and neuromotor exercise training beyond activities of daily living to improve and maintain physical fitness and health [80]. The 2018 update of the Physical Activity Guidelines recommended that adults do at 150–300 min per week of moderate-intensity or 75–150 min a week of vigorous-intensity aerobic physical activity, or an equivalent combination of moderate- and vigorous-intensity aerobic activity for substantial health benefits [81] (Fig. 23.3). There could be additional benefits of engaging in moderate-intensity physical activity beyond the recommended time. The aerobic activity should be spread throughout the week. Furthermore, adults should also engage in moderate- or greater-intensity muscle-strengthening activities that involve all major muscle groups on two or more days a week, as these activities provide additional health benefits [81]. Older adults should do multicomponent physical activity that includes

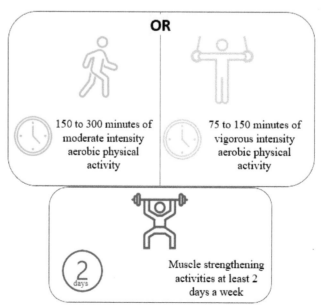

FIGURE 23.3 Recommendations for physical activity for adults for health living and weight management.

balance training and aerobic and muscle-strengthening activities. Although evidence was insufficient to quantify a sedentary behavior threshold, reducing sedentary behaviors is recommended across all age groups and abilities [66]. The American Association of Clinical Endocrinology (AACE) Obesity guidelines recommend that resistance training should be prescribed to patients with overweight and obesity undergoing weight loss therapy to aid in fat loss while preserving fat-free mass. The goal should be resistance training two to three times per week, consisting of single-set exercises that use the major muscle groups [82]. In addition, an increase in nonexercised and active leisure activities should be encouraged to reduce sedentary behaviors [82]. The American Diabetes Association (ADA) Standard of Medical Care in Diabetes recommends that those who achieve weight loss goals have a higher level of aerobic moderate-intensity physical activity 200–300 min/week for weight maintenance [83]. Collectively, all the guidelines affirm the importance of regular aerobic activity and resistance training to improve overall health. There is a positive relationship between the amount of physical activity and the prevention of weight regain, but there is limited evidence of the dose–response relationship between physical activity and the risk of weight gain in adults [84]. Exercise programs should be individualized, considering an individual's physical fitness, health status, exercise response, and stated goals [80]. A pre-exercise medical evaluation is not needed in individuals with type 2 diabetes planning to participate in the low- to moderate-intensity physical activity unless symptoms of cardiovascular disease or microvascular complications are present [85]. Medical clearance is recommended in sedentary individuals with type 2 diabetes before participating in moderate- to high-intensity physical activity [85]. Preexercise medical clearance remains controversial, and recommendations should be tailored to the individual [66,85]. Gradual progression in intensity, duration, and exercise frequency should be considered.

In a review of 46 randomized control trials involving approximately 16,000 participants worldwide, physical activity interventions delivered in primary care settings effectively increased participation in self-reported moderate to vigorous physical activity [86]. Most individuals visit their primary care professionals at least annually. This could be an opportunity to emphasize regular physical activity to prevent and treat noncommunicable diseases and improve overall health in the primary care setting. Multiple contacts are needed to increase participation in physical activity, so all healthcare professionals (primary care and specialists) should counsel for physical activity when applicable.

Adipose tissue and physical activity

Obesity is commonly assessed using body mass index, but BMI cannot distinguish between fat mass and fat-free mass. A pooled analysis of seven cohorts showed a J-shaped association between fat mass and mortality, with a 50% increased mortality risk in high versus low levels of fat mass [87]. In contrast, fat-free mass was associated with a 30% decrease in mortality risk in high versus low levels. Waist circumference is a better predictor of abdominal adiposity and cardiometabolic risk [88]. The abdominal fat distribution defines distinct obesity subphenotype. Visceral (VAT) and subcutaneous (SAT) adipose tissues contribute to obesity but may have different diabetogenic and atherogenic risk profiles [89]. VAT is associated with a more adverse cardiometabolic and atherogenic obesity phenotype than SAT, a more favorable phenotype. Excess VAT is a marker of dysfunctional SAT, associated with lipid deposition in organs such as the liver, heart, pancreas, and skeletal muscle, thereby forming ectopic fat depots [90]. Aerobic exercise compared with resistance training results in greater VAT reduction, and volume and intensity of the exercise type may also affect VAT [91]. Although dietary changes have a greater effect on weight loss, exercise tends to have superior effects in reducing VAT, and total body weight loss may not reflect the change in VAT and may be a poor maker when evaluating the benefits of ILIs [92]. Aerobic exercise without a hypocaloric diet can reduce VAT, even after 12 weeks [93]. In addition to reducing VAT and ectopic fat, exercise also induces molecular adaptations in white adipose tissue that improve insulin sensitivity [94]. Moderate and vigorous physical activities aid in reducing abdominal visceral fat and ectopic fat even in the absence of weight loss. It favors the maintenance of fat-free mass during the weight loss and weight maintenance phase and increases cardiorespiratory fitness [79,95].

Type and duration of physical activity

Evidence of several RCTs suggests that an increase in exercise is associated with a significant reduction in waist circumference, independent of the intensity of exercise, and a reduction in waist circumference can be observed with or without weight loss [88]. Therefore, routine measurement of waist circumference as an anthropometric measure can be a useful tool in determining the efficacy of exercise in reducing abdominal obesity. Ten weeks of high-intensity interval training (HIIT) and moderate-intensity exercise training can reduce body fat by ∼ 2 kg and waist circumference by ∼ 3 cm without body mass change [96]. Short-term moderate-intensity to high-intensity exercise training can induce modest improvement in body composition in people with overweight and obesity without accompanying body weight changes [96]. In a review of 149 studies, exercise led to a weight loss of -1.5 to -3.5 kg, fat loss from 1.3 to 2.6 kg, and visceral fat loss of $0.33-0.56$, and there was no difference in weight, fat, and visceral loss between aerobic and HIIT as long as energy expenditure was equal [97]. In another meta-analysis, high-intensity training resulted in greater improvement of cardiorespiratory fitness and a greater reduction of % body fat compared with traditional exercise, but the overall effect for BMI was not different in high-intensity and traditional exercise [98]. In a meta-analysis reviewing the effect of interval training versus moderate-intensity continuous training, patterns of the intensity of effort and duration during endurance exercise had minimal influence on longitudinal changes in fat mass and fat-free mass [99]. In another study of 3964 participants for different training types (aerobic, resistance, combined aerobic plus resistance, and HIIT), the maximal oxygen consumption increased in all types of training [100]. HIIT was most effective in increasing maximal oxygen consumption, and resistance training was most effective for increasing muscle strength.

National weight control registry data showed that physical activity is vital for long-term weight loss maintenance, and sustained moderate to vigorous physical activity of >10 min in duration may aid in weight management [101]. A study assessing moderate-to-vigorous physical activity (MVPA) by accelerometer confirmed the association between physical activity and all-cause mortality, with hazard ratios of 0.28 for 5-minute bouts and 0.35 for 10-min bouts highest versus lowest quartiles [102]. Sporadic and bouted MVPA, even in bouts of $5-10$ min, is associated with reduced mortality. Furthermore, physical activity of any bout duration is associated with improved health outcomes, including all-cause mortality [66,94].

Recommendations

The most common motivators among individuals for physical activity are weight management, physical fitness, and social support, and the most common barriers are lack of self-discipline/motivation, pain or physical discomfort, and lack of time [103]. Furthermore, participation in physical activity may be limited due to lack of access to facilities and attributable to social and environmental determinants and must be addressed to maximize participation [85]. Since exercise adherence is vital, personal preference should guide exercise prescription, and any bout duration of physical activity should be encouraged. Typical exercise prescription should include type, duration, intensity, and frequency of exercise. There is significant variability in the effects of physical activity due to environmental influences and individual factors, such as habitual physical activity, fitness, genetic and physiological factors, and social and psychological factors [80]. Therefore, expectations for weight loss with physical activity in the absence of caloric restriction should be realistic.

Four vital signs, (1) waist circumference, (2) cardiorespiratory fitness, (3) level of reported physical activity, and (4) overall diet quality, should be considered for cardiometabolic risk assessment in people with overweight/obesity [90]. Three of these can be modified by regular physical activity, and the fourth can be addressed with dietary changes. Therefore, a multimodality approach using a combination of dietary changes, regular physical activity, and behavioral changes should be considered in the management of obesity.

Sleep

Introduction

Sleep duration is affected by age and several other factors, including psychological, behavioral, environmental, and social aspects. Sleep duration has decreased worldwide, likely resulting in part from over-use of social media, lifestyle choices, and mobile technology. There is a significant relationship between hours of sleep and obesity among infants, children, and adolescents [104]. Sleep duration is an essential predictor of obesity, and the findings are consistent across different populations. Sleep debt in the early stages of life has a significant impact on physical and psychological wellbeing. A later bedtime is a strong predictor of short sleep duration, which can contribute to more time for food consumption and increased screen time. Furthermore, short sleep duration is associated with fatigue, mood changes, impaired judgment, and decreased impulse control. Individuals who restrict sleep over prolonged periods may compromise their health and wellbeing. The altered thermoregulation and fatigue associated with sleep deprivation can cause reduced energy expenditure and decreased physical activity [105]. Shift work causes circadian misalignment and is a risk factor for overweight and obesity [106]. The duration of the night shift, frequency, and intensity of night shift work seem to determine risk for weight gain. Shift workers are more likely to develop cardiometabolic disorders, including obesity, type 2 diabetes, and hypertension, due to disruption of biological and environmental rhythms, including sleep deprivation and change in dietary and lifestyle behaviors [107].

The possible mechanisms of the relationship between insufficient or poor sleep and obesity include changes in appetite control, increased hunger, and insulin and glucose metabolism [108]. There are also changes in cortisol, growth hormone, and thyroid hormone with reduced sleep duration. In one study, 2 days of sleep restriction were associated with reductions in the anorexigenic hormone leptin, elevations in the orexigenic factor ghrelin, increased hunger, and increased appetite for calorie-dense foods with high carbohydrate content [109]. In a meta-analysis, short sleep duration was associated with increased ghrelin levels, and sleep deprivation had significant effect of both leptin and ghrelin [113].

Obstructive sleep apnea

Obstructive sleep apnea (OSA) is a common adiposity-based chronic disease linked to obesity. OSA is characterized by repeated episodes of partial or complete loss of the respiratory airflow during sleep due to narrowing or closure of the upper airway. In one study, the overall prevalence of OSA ranged from 9% to 30% in the general adult population, 13%−33% in men, and 6%−10% among women [110]. The prevalence is higher in older ages, males, and those with higher BMI. There is a bidirectional link between obesity, T2DM, and OSA. Reduced secretion of melatonin, a neurohormone, which is a risk factor for diabetes, has been reported in OSA [111]. In addition, sleep apnea causes intermittent hypoxia and sleep fragmentation, which results in further weight gain and which causes worsening of OSA through direct weight-dependent (increased neck circumference, narrowed airway, increased mechanical load) and indirect weight-dependent mechanisms such as leptin resistance, hyperglycemia, and hyperinsulinemia [112]. Therefore, weight loss, healthy eating, and regular physical activity are essential for preventing and treating OSA and are standard treatments for OSA in addition to therapeutic interventions such as continuous positive airway pressure (CPAP). There are other rare sleep disorders such as obesity hypoventilation syndrome and narcolepsy, which are associated with obesity [113].

Recommendations

Like a healthy diet and physical activity, sleep is vital for physical, cognitive, and emotional health. Encouraging sufficient sleep time is essential in managing obesity. The National Sleep Foundation in the United States recommends that young adults between ages 18 and 25 years and adults between ages 26 and 64 years have 7−9 h of sleep and older adults >65 years have 7−8 h of sleep [114].

Behavioral interventions

Guidelines for treating obesity consistently recommend that the dietary and physical activity recommendations discussed above be offered alongside behavioral strategies designed to facilitate adherence to treatment goals [115−117]. These multicomponent behavioral weight loss programs, which often are referred to as *lifestyle interventions*, produce larger mean weight losses than interventions that provide diet and activity recommendations alone [118].

Treatment structure

The behavioral treatment component of an ILI is delivered through regular individual or group meetings with a trained interventionist. Cost considerations generally favor the use of group treatment, given the approximately equivalent weight losses produced by the two approaches [119]. Interventionists typically are health professionals, including dietitians or psychologists, but laypersons also have been successfully trained in treatment delivery [116]. The strongest evidence supports the efficacy of interventions delivered in-person or by telephone (with or without video conferencing) [116]. Digital interventions are often used to complement these traditional approaches and may eventually supplant them.

Although ILIs may be delivered flexibly, most of the programs that have been evaluated in clinical trials have followed a predefined protocol in which a new topic related to weight control is introduced in each session. Interventions can vary in intensity, but the largest weight losses are produced by high-intensity treatments that offer at least 14 sessions (meetings) in the first 6 months [116,120]. This initial treatment period may be followed by additional sessions, typically at a reduced frequency, to facilitate the maintenance of lost weight.

Behavior therapy principles

Behavioral principles derived from classical conditioning were first applied to the modification of eating and weight in the 1960s and were expanded in the 1980s to also incorporate cognitive techniques [121]. Key components of behavior

TABLE 23.2 Behavior therapy principles commonly included in lifestyle interventions for weight loss.

Principle	Definition	Example
Goal setting	Identifying specific, measurable goals that the patient believes are likely to be achievable.	"I will take a 30-min walk on Monday, Wednesday, and Friday in the evening after I get home from work. If it is raining I will do a yoga video."
Self-monitoring	Recording food intake, physical activity, body weight, and other targets for change. Self-monitoring allows patients to assess progress with meeting their identified goals. Records also may include information about factors that support goal achievement. Most patients now use smartphone apps or other digital devices to aid self-monitoring.	Food records typically list the food type, amount or portion size, timing of eating, and calorie content of the food. Patients may track other goals related to macronutrient intake, and most apps also display vitamin and mineral content. Patients are encouraged to keep a running total throughout the day to help them to meet their overall dietary targets.
Problem solving	Identifying environmental, social, cognitive, or emotional factors that may have contributed to suboptimal goal achievement. Patient (and provider) brainstorm potential solutions to address each contributing factor, select the intervention with the greatest likelihood of success, and evaluate its efficacy.	"I am less likely to go to the gym once I go home and begin to relax, so I will bring my gym clothes to the office so that I can go directly there after work."
Stimulus control	Limiting exposure to cues that are associated with behaviors that the patient wishes to change or adding cues associated with desired behaviors.	"I will limit the number of high-calorie snacks that I bring into my home and store the ones that I do purchase on a low shelf where they are out of eyesight."
Cognitive restructuring	Identifying and challenging negative or maladaptive thoughts that could interfere with behavior change.	"I will respond to thoughts that a 1 lb weight gain means that I will never be able to lose weight by reminding myself that small weight fluctuations are normal and that sticking to my healthy eating and activity routine has the greatest likelihood of helping me to reach my weight loss goals."

therapy for weight loss, including goal setting, self-monitoring, stimulus control, problem-solving, and cognitive restructuring, are described in the following. Detailed descriptions can be obtained by reviewing the treatment protocols for the Diabetes Prevention Program [122] or the Look AHEAD (Action for Health in Diabetes) study [123], as well as published manuals tailored for brief session delivery in primary care settings [124] (Table 23.2).

Goal setting

In behavioral weight loss treatments, patients are encouraged to select specific, measurable behaviors that they wish to adopt and to identify when, where, how, and with whom they will engage in each behavior [125]. In addition to specific targets for diet (e.g., caloric intake) and physical activity (e.g., exercise minutes per week), interventionists encourage patients to set goals that focus on changing their environment (e.g., removing high-calorie foods from the home) and building habits that facilitate adherence to diet and activity targets (e.g., bringing gym clothes to work). Progress with meeting the identified goals is reviewed with the interventionist (and group members, if applicable) at subsequent treatment sessions. These check-ins create an opportunity for the interventionist to provide positive reinforcement when goals are achieved [126]. If a goal has not been met, the interventionist or group can help the patient to address barriers.

Self-monitoring

Self-monitoring (i.e., recording) of food intake, physical activity, and body weight is the cornerstone of behavioral treatment because it provides critical information about goal progress. Records also can help individuals to identify behavioral patterns and additional targets for change. A high frequency of self-monitoring is associated with better short- and long-term weight loss [127,128]. Most ILIs provide specific goals for self-monitoring, and barriers to record-keeping are likely to be addressed directly in session. Although many programs have used paper journals, a number of smartphone applications ("apps") and devices (e.g., fitness trackers, "smart" scales) now exist to facilitate self-monitoring.

Problem-solving

Participants are taught to identify factors that may have contributed to suboptimal goal achievement, including both situational and cognitive or emotional antecedents. Linking these preceding events, and their consequences, to form a "behavior chain" can allow a patient to identify opportunities to "break the chain" on future occasions by intervening to alter the sequence of events [125]. For example, a patient might identify that not bringing healthy snacks to work, particularly when combined with high job stress, increases their likelihood of consuming high-calorie snack foods from an office vending machine. The patient is taught to brainstorm potential solutions to address each contributing factor and then to select the intervention with the greatest likelihood of success (early in the chain, if possible), implement it, and evaluate its efficacy. For example, the aforementioned patient might decide to pack healthy snacks, employ skills to cope with negative emotions (e.g., deep breathing, talk to a friend), or both to support their consumption of fewer high-calorie snack foods (Fig. 23.4).

Cognitive techniques

Many psychological treatments emphasize the role of cognition (thought) in determining a person's emotions and behavior. A number of lifestyle modification programs incorporate strategies derived from cognitive behavioral therapy that are designed to directly address thinking patterns that could interfere with behavior change. For example, a patient who responds to an overeating episode by either minimizing (e.g., "Eating a few more won't matter") or magnifying its impact (e.g., "I've already blown it; I might as well eat whatever I want") might be slow to resume efforts to meet their diet and activity goals. Cognitive restructuring techniques help patients to identify maladaptive or unrealistic thoughts, evaluate the validity of those thoughts, and respond in a manner that increases the likelihood that they will behave consistently with their goals. For example, a patient might respond to thoughts about a dietary lapse by reminding him/herself that a temporary setback does not undo previous progress and emphasizing the importance of getting back on track as soon as possible. Alternative psychological techniques, such as those derived from acceptance-based treatments or motivational interviewing, also have shown promise as adjuncts to standard behavioral strategies [130].

Efficacy of multicomponent behavioral interventions

After 6−12 months of treatment, intensive lifestyle interventions (with at least 14 sessions in the first 6 months) produce mean losses of 5%−10% of initial weight (5−10 kg) that are significantly larger than those produced by usual care [116,127]. Moderate-intensity programs that provide one to two sessions per month are associated with smaller mean losses of 2%−4% of initial weight. Sustained weight losses of as little as 3% can produce clinically meaningful health benefits, including improvements in triglycerides, blood glucose, hemoglobin A1c, and the risk of developing type 2

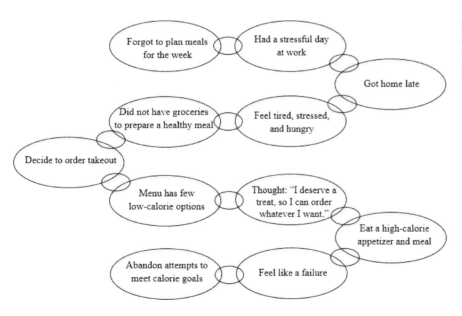

FIGURE 23.4 A behavior chain, in which situations, feelings, and thoughts that lead to or result from a given behavior (i.e., antecedents and consequences) are linked to help a patient to identify opportunities for intervention. Additional behavior chain examples can be found in Ref. [129].

diabetes [116]. Losses of more than 5% of initial weight are also associated with improvements in blood pressure, cholesterol, and lipids, as well as quality of life and depression. Across these health outcomes, larger weight losses are associated with greater improvements [131].

Weight regain continues to temper the long-term benefits of lifestyle modification. On average, one-third of lost weight is regained in the year following treatment [132]. However, weight losses remain superior to usual care at most long-term follow-up points [116]. Although improvements in some cardiometabolic risk factors are reversed or diminished by weight regain, other benefits may outlast the initial weight loss. For example, the intensive ILI in the Diabetes Prevention Program treatment trial produced an initial loss of 7.1 kg at 6—12 months. After a mean follow-up of 2.8 years, the 5.6 kg weight loss maintained by the lifestyle group was associated with a 58% lower incidence in the development of type 2 diabetes, compared with placebo [133]. At 10 years posttreatment, weight loss no longer differed between the groups (2 kg for ILI and 1 kg for placebo), but the ILI group maintained a 34% lower incidence of type 2 diabetes [134].

The provision of ongoing behavioral treatment sessions improves long-term weight loss outcomes [116,132]. In a review of 13 studies assessing the effect of ongoing treatment on weight loss maintenance [132], participants who received lifestyle sessions in the year after a short-term program maintained on average 96.3% of their initial weight loss (10.3 kg of an initial 10.7 kg mean loss). Comparison groups without extended contact maintained 66.5% (6.6 kg) of their initial loss. In longer-term extended treatment, attendance begins to decline, and some weight regain occurs. At 2 years, treated patients maintain 65.8% of their initial loss, compared with 38.3% for patients not receiving follow-up sessions [132]. Treated patients continue to maintain about 50% of their initial weight loss after 3—5 years of extended treatment [133,135].

The challenge of dissemination

The majority of the findings described before come from large, funded trials in which treatment was delivered in person by experienced providers working in academic medical centers. Providers in other settings often lack the time and training to deliver intensive ILIs. These treatments also can be time-consuming and costly for participants, and many individuals, particularly those in rural communities or economically disadvantaged urban areas, have limited access to care. Identifying methods to disseminate effective lifestyle modification to the millions of people who would benefit from it is thus a key priority.

Patient access can be improved by delivering ILIs in community, primary care, or workplace settings, and such programs are associated with lower program and participant costs. Of these, behavioral treatments delivered in community centers have produced outcomes that are most similar to those achieved in academic medical centers [136]. High-intensity lifestyle programs delivered in-person or by phone in primary care settings also produce clinically meaningful weight losses (4—7 kg) [137]. However, intensive programs can be difficult to integrate into medical practices due to their demand on provider time, as well as inadequate provider training and reimbursement. Less intensive counseling may be more feasible in primary care settings but produces smaller weight losses (1—2 kg). Worksite programs also typically produce modest mean losses (1—2 kg) [136].

Delivering ILIs by telephone, Internet, or mobile phone is another alternative for improving accessibility. Telephone appears to be equally effective to in-person delivery for both weight loss and maintenance, and it substantially reduces travel costs to the participant (but not clinic costs) [138]. Internet (e.g., Website, email), mobile phone (e.g., text message), and app-based treatments have the widest availability and lowest costs. These digital interventions typically produce smaller mean losses than in-person treatments but are superior to control groups in some studies [139]. Comprehensive digital platforms that offer a structured program of diet, physical activity, and behavioral strategies and provide interventionist feedback produce the strongest results (a mean 2.1 kg loss in meta-analysis) [139]. Comprehensive digital programs also provide a low-cost option for facilitating weight loss maintenance. Several studies have reported minimal to no differences in weight regain with online versus in-person maintenance treatment [136]. Unfortunately, the majority of commercially available monitoring and weight loss apps include only a small percentage of behavioral treatment strategies, and most do not provide tailored feedback [140]. Such programs are not likely to induce significant weight loss for most individuals, and user engagement declines rapidly without interventionist support [141].

As technology continues to advance, new opportunities will likely emerge to develop effective, fully automated digital weight loss interventions. The provision of enhanced features, such as integration with social media, virtual reality, online games, or tracking devices has shown the potential to increase user engagement and improves personalized feedback, which may enhance weight loss [142]. Also in development are just-in-time adaptive interventions that use machine learning to identify individual risk factors for behavioral lapses and provide intervention strategies at the times when an individual is most at risk [143]. Although the outcomes of digital interventions have been mixed thus far, they remain an important direction for future development due to their wide reach and low cost.

Behavioral intervention and antiobesity medication

Antiobesity medications such as orlistat, liraglutide, phentermine-topiramate, and naltrexone-bupropion produce placebo-subtracted weight losses of 3−8 kg [144]. The newly approved semaglutide produces a larger placebo-subtracted loss of 12.7 kg [145]. Antiobesity medications and behavioral interventions have potentially complementary mechanisms of action. Medications modify internal factors such as appetite (or nutrient absorption), while behavioral treatments help patients modify external factors including the food environment and lifestyle habits [127]. However, in most pharmaco-therapy trials, patients are provided with minimal- or low-intensity diet and activity counseling.

In a pivotal trial, Wadden and colleagues [127] demonstrated that prescribing sibutramine (withdrawn from the market in 2010), alongside intensive lifestyle intervention, produced larger mean weight losses than either treatment alone. Participants who received sibutramine alone lost 5.0 kg, and those receiving lifestyle modification alone lost 6.7 kg. A third group that received both treatments lost 12.1 kg, roughly equivalent to the sum of the weight losses in the other two groups. A study of ILI with liraglutide also suggested that combined treatment could produce weight losses equivalent to the additive benefit of the two treatment components [146]. A subsequent study again found that liraglutide improved weight loss when compared with intensive lifestyle treatment with placebo [142]. However, the placebo-subtracted benefit in the latter study (3.4% of initial weight) was somewhat smaller than the average benefit of liraglutide when combined with lower-intensity treatment (5.2 kg in metaanalysis [147]). A trial evaluating semaglutide with ILI achieved mean weight losses of 16.0% that were only slightly larger than those achieved by patients treated with less intensive counseling in a separate trial (14.9%) [145,148]. However, only a randomized trial comparing different treatment intensities can truly determine whether intensive ILI enhances the efficacy of this medication.

Pharmacotherapy could play an even more important role in obesity management by facilitating the maintenance of lost weight, potentially by counteracting unfavorable changes in appetite-related hormones and energy expenditure that occur with weight loss [144]. Several trials have shown that the provision of antiobesity medication after either behavioral or pharmacologic weight loss induction improves long-term outcomes [149,150]. This approach has been likened to the treatment of other chronic health conditions that require long-term pharmacologic intervention. Overall, these findings suggest that adding antiobesity medication to lifestyle modification has the potential to increase both initial and long-term weight reduction, which may result in larger improvements in health and greater satisfaction with weight loss than either intervention alone.

Behavioral intervention and bariatric surgery

Bariatric surgery is the most effective treatment option for individuals with class 3 obesity (BMI ≥40) or class 2 obesity (BMI ≥35) accompanied by obesity-related comorbidities. Although at 10 years patients continue to have a larger mean losses than those achieved by other interventions (about 16%−25% of initial weight, depending on surgical type), they have regained about a third of their maximum weight loss [151,152]. As with behavioral and pharmacologic interventions, weight loss is variable and a minority of patients will have a suboptimal response to surgical treatment.

Behavioral factors are thought to play a role in these postsurgical weight loss outcomes. Patients who have had bariatric surgery are advised to follow a number of postoperative dietary and physical activity recommendations to optimize treatment outcomes, and several studies have found that behavioral and psychosocial factors are associated with post-surgical weight loss [153]. However, the use of behavioral treatments to enhance the efficacy of bariatric surgery has produced mixed results. A recent systematic review of 44 studies found that cognitive behavioral interventions produced significant changes in postsurgical eating psychopathology (e.g., binge eating) and improved mood and quality of life [154]. However, over two-thirds of these interventions did not enhance weight loss. The programs that did improve weight tended to occur during the postoperative (vs. preoperative) period were initiated within 12 months of surgery and included a relatively high number of treatment visits, suggesting a potential role for intensive behavioral treatment during the immediate postoperative period.

Summary

Obesity is a complex, progressive, and relapsing chronic disease characterized by abnormal or excess adiposity that impairs health. A multimodal approach of medical nutrition therapy, physical activity, behavioral therapy, pharmacotherapy, and surgery is needed to manage obesity. In addition, periodic surveillance and counseling are necessary to prevent obesity at all stages of life, including childhood, adolescence, adulthood, and older age.

References

Nutrition

[1] Garvey WT, et al. American association of clinical endocrinologists and American college of endocrinology comprehensive clinical practice guidelines for medical care of patients with obesity. Endocr Pract 2016;22(Suppl. 3):1—203.

[2] American College of Cardiology/American Heart Association Task Force on Practice Guidelines, Obesity Expert Panel. Executive summary: guidelines (2013) for the management of overweight and obesity in adults: a report of the American college of cardiology/American heart association task force on practice guidelines and the obesity society published by the obesity society and American college of cardiology/American heart association task force on practice guidelines. Based on a systematic review from the the obesity expert panel, 2013. Obesity (Silver Spring) 2014 2013;22(Suppl. 2):S5—39.

[3] Hall KD, Ayuketah A, Brychta R, et al. Ultra-processed diets cause excess calorie intake and weight gain: an inpatient randomized controlled trial of ad libitum food intake. Cell Metabol October 6, 2020;32(4):690.

[4] Nordmann AJ, et al. Meta-analysis comparing Mediterranean to low-fat diets for modification of cardiovascular risk factors. Am J Med 2011;124(9):841—51.

[5] Schwingshackl L, et al. Adherence to a Mediterranean diet and risk of diabetes: a systematic review and meta-analysis. Publ Health Nutr 2015;18(7):1292—9.

[6] Esposito K, et al. Mediterranean diet and weight loss: meta-analysis of randomized controlled trials. Metab Syndr Relat Disord 2011;9(1):1—12.

[7] Liyanage T, et al. Effects of the Mediterranean diet on cardiovascular outcomes—systematic review and meta-analysis. PLoS One 2016;11(8):e0159252.

[8] Estruch R, et al. PREDIMED Study Investigators. Effect of a high-fat Mediterranean diet on bodyweight and waist circumference: a prespecified secondary outcomes analysis of the PREDIMED randomised controlled trial. Lancet Diabetes Endocrinol 2016;4(8):666—76.

[9] Estruch R, et al. PREDIMED Study Investigators. Primary prevention of cardiovascular disease with a Mediterranean diet supplemented with extra-virgin olive oil or nuts. N Engl J Med 2018;378(25):e34.

[10] Ello-Martin JA, et al. The influence of food portion size and energy density on energy intake: implications for weight management. Am J Clin Nutr 2005;82(1 Suppl. l):236S—41S.

[11] Viguiliouk E, et al. Can pulses play a role in improving cardiometabolic health? Evidence from systematic reviews and meta-analyses. Ann N Y Acad Sci 2017;1392(1):43—57.

[12] Li SS, et al. Dietary pulses, satiety and food intake: a systematic review and metaanalysis of acute feeding trials. Obesity 2014;22(8):1773—80.

[13] DellaValle DM, et al. Does the consumption of caloric and non-caloric beverages with a meal affect energy intake? Appetite 2005;44:187—93.

[14] Rogers PJ, et al. Does low-energy sweetener consumption affect energy intake and body weight? A systematic review, including meta-analyses, of the evidence from human and animal studies. Int J Obes 2016;40(3):381—94. https://doi.org/10.1038/ijo.2015.177.

[15] Nadolsky KZ. COUNTERPOINT: artificial sweeteners for obesity-better than sugary alternatives; potentially a solution. Endocr Pract October 2021;27(10):1056—61.

[16] Dansinger ML, et al. Comparison of the Atkins, Ornish, Weight Watchers, and Zone diets for weight loss and heart disease risk reduction: a randomized trial. JAMA 2005;293(1):43—53.

[17] Alhassan S, et al. Dietary adherence and weight loss success among overweight women:results from the A TO Z weight loss study. Int J Obes 2008;32(6):985—91.

[18] Johnston BC, et al. Comparison of weight loss among named diet programs in overweight and obese adults: a meta-analysis. JAMA 2014;312(9):923—33.

[19] Ge L, Sadeghirad B, Ball GDC, da Costa BR, et al. Comparison of dietary macronutrient patterns of 14 popular named dietary programmes for weight and cardiovascular risk factor reduction in adults: systematic review and network meta-analysis of randomised trials. BMJ April 1, 2020;369:m696.

[20] Hooper L, et al. Effects of total fat intake on body weight. Cochrane Database Syst Rev 2015;8:CD011834.

[21] Bueno NB, et al. Very-low-carbohydrate ketogenic diet v. low-fat diet for long-term weight loss: a metaanalysis of randomised controlled trials. Br J Nutr 2013;110(7):1178—87.

[22] Nordmann AJ, et al. Effects of low-carbohydrate vs low-fat diets on weight loss and cardiovascular risk factors: a meta-analysis of randomized controlled trials. Arch Intern Med 2006;166(3):285—93.

[23] Tobias DK, et al. Effect of low-fat diet interventions versus other diet intervention on long-term weight change in adults: a systematic review and meta-analysis. Lancet Diabetes Endocrinol 2015;3(12):968—79.

[24] Hall KD, et al. Obesity energetics: body weight regulation and the effects of diet composition. Gastroenterology 2017;152(7):1718—1727.e3.

[25] Gardner CD, et al. Effect of low-fat vs low-carbohydrate diet on 12-month weight loss in overweight adults and the association with genotype pattern or insulin secretion: the DIETFITS Randomized Clinical Trial. JAMA 2018;319(7):667—79.

[26] Belza A, et al. Contribution of gastroenteropancreatic appetite hormones to protein induced satiety. Am J Clin Nutr 2013;97:980–9. 0004386957.INDD 377 8/26/2019 9:15:47 PM.

[27] Mikkelsen PB, et al. The effect of fat-reduced diets on 24-h energy expenditure: comparisons between animal protein, vegetable protein, and carbohydrate. Am J Clin Nutr 2000;72:1135–41.

[28] Wycherley TP, et al. Effects of energy-restricted high-protein, low-fat compared with standard-protein, low-fat diets: a meta-analysis of randomized controlled trials. Am J Clin Nutr 2012;96:1281–98.

[29] Oliveira CLP, Boulé NG, Sharma AM, et al. A high-protein total diet replacement increases energy expenditure and leads to negative fat balance in healthy, normal-weight adults. Am J Clin Nutr February 2, 2021;113(2):476–87.

[30] Krieger JW, et al. Effects of variation in protein and carbohydrate intake on body mass and composition during energy restriction: a meta-regression. Am J Clin Nutr 2006;83:260–74.

[31] Sacks FM, et al. Comparison of weight-loss diets with different compositions of fat, protein, and carbohydrates. N Engl J Med 2009;360(9):859–73.

[32] Bray GA, et al. Markers of dietary protein intake are associated with successful weight loss in the POUNDS Lost trial. Clin Obes 2017;7(3):166–75.

[33] Clifton PM, et al. Long term weight maintenance after advice to consume low carbohydrate, higher protein diets—a systematic review and meta analysis. Nutr Metabol Cardiovasc Dis 2014;24(3):224–35.

[34] Kim JE, O'Connor LE, Sands LP, Slebodnik MB, Campbell WW. Effects of dietary protein intake on body composition changes after weight loss in older adults: a systematic review and meta-analysis. Nutr Rev 2016;74:210–24.

[35] Kidney Disease: Improving Global Outcomes (KDIGO) CKD Work Group. KDIGO clinical practice guideline for the evaluation and management of chronic kidney disease. Kidney Int Suppl 2013;3:1–150.

[36] Truche AS, Bailly S, Fabre O, Legrand R, Zaoui P. A specific high-protein weight loss program does not impair renal function in patients who are overweight/obese. Nutrients January 17, 2022;14(2):384.

[37] Brinkworth GD, et al. Renal function following long-term weight loss in individuals with abdominal obesity on a very-low carbohydrate diet vs high carbohydrate diet. J Am Diet Assoc 2010;110:633–8.

[38] Møller G, et al. Higher protein intake is not associated with decreased kidney function in pre-diabetic older adults following a one-year intervention—a preview sub-study. Nutrients 2018;10(1). pii: E54.

[39] Jäger R, et al. International society of Sports nutrition position stand: protein and exercise. J Int Soc Sports Nutr 2017;14:20.

[40] de Boer IH, Caramori ML, Chan JCN, et al. Executive summary of the 2020 KDIGO Diabetes Management in CKD Guideline: evidence-based advances in monitoring and treatment. Kidney Int October 2020;98(4):839–48.

[41] Tsai AG, et al. The evolution of very-low-calorie diets: an update and meta-analysis. Obesity 2006;14(8):1283–93.

[42] Zahouani A, et al. Short- and long-term evolution of body composition in 1,389 obese outpatients following a very low calorie diet (Pro'gram18 VLCD). Acta Diabetol 2003;40(Suppl. 1):S149–50.

[43] Steven S, et al. Very low-calorie diet and 6 months of weight stability in type 2 diabetes: pathophysiological changes in responders and non-responders. Diabetes Care 2016;39(5):808–15.

[44] Gonzalez-Campoy JM. Bariatric endocrinology and very-low-calorie meal plans. Endocr Pract 2017;23(6):741–4.

[45] Muscogiuri G, El Ghoch M, Colao A, et al. Obesity management task force (OMTF) of the European Association for the Study of Obesity (EASO). European guidelines for obesity management in adults with a very low-calorie ketogenic diet: a systematic review and meta-analysis. Obes Facts 2021;14(2):222–45.

[46] Heymsfield SB, et al. Weight management using a meal replacement strategy meta- and pooling analysis from six studies. Int J Obes Relat Metab Disord 2003;27:537–49.

[47] Leslie WS, et al. Weight losses with low-energy formula diets in obese patients with and without type 2 diabetes: systematic review and meta-analysis. Int J Obes 2017;41(6):997.

[48] Astbury NM, et al. Doctor Referral of Overweight People to Low Energy total diet replacement Treatment (DROPLET): pragmatic randomised controlled trial. BMJ 2018;362:k3760.

[49] Christensen P, et al. Men and women respond differently to rapid weight loss: metabolic outcomes of a multi-centre intervention study after a low-energy diet in 2500 overweight, individuals with pre diabetes (PREVIEW). Diabetes Obes Metabol 2018;20(12):2840–51. https://doi.org/10.1111/dom.13466.

[50] Lean ME, et al. Primary care-led weight management for remission of type 2 diabetes (DiRECT): an open-label, cluster-randomised trial. Lancet 2018;391(10120):541–51.

[51] Min J, Kim SY, Shin IS, Park YB, Lim YW. The effect of meal replacement on weight loss according to calorie-restriction type and proportion of energy intake: a systematic review and meta-analysis of randomized controlled trials. J Acad Nutr Diet August 2021;121(8):1551–1564.e3.

[52] Halle M, Röhling M, Banzer W, et al. ACOORH study group. Meal replacement by formula diet reduces weight more than a lifestyle intervention alone in patients with overweight or obesity and accompanied cardiovascular risk factors-the ACOORH trial. Eur J Clin Nutr April 2021;75(4):661–9.

[53] Churuangsuk C, Hall J, Reynolds A, et al. Diets for weight management in adults with type 2 diabetes: an umbrella review of published meta-analyses and systematic review of trials of diets for diabetes remission. Diabetologia January 2022;65(1):14–36.

[54] Christensen P, et al. Long-term weight-loss maintenance in obese patients with knee osteoarthritis: a randomized trial. Am J Clin Nutr 2017;106(3):755–63.

[55] Horne BD, et al. Health effects of intermittent fasting: Hormesis or harm? A systematic review. Am J Clin Nutr 2015;102(2):464—70.

[56] Harris L, et al. Intermittent fasting interventions for treatment of overweight and obesity in adults: a systematic review and meta-analysis. JBI Database System Rev Implement Rep 2018;16(2):507—47.

[57] Coutinho SR, et al. Compensatory mechanisms activated with intermittent energy restriction: a randomized control trial. Clin Nutr 2018;37(3):815—23.

[58] Sundfør TM, et al. Effect of intermittent versus continuous energy restriction on weight loss, maintenance and cardiometabolic risk: a randomized 1-year trial. Nutr Metabol Cardiovasc Dis 2018;28(7):698—706.

[59] Carter S, et al. Effect of intermittent compared with continuous energy restricted diet on glycemic control in patients with type 2 diabetes: a randomized noninferiority trial. JAMA Netw Open 2018;1(3):e180756.

[60] Gibney MJ. Ultra-processed foods: definitions and policy issues. Curr Develop Nutr 2019;3(2):nzy077.

[61] Rynders CA, Thomas EA, Zaman A, Pan Z, Catenacci VA, Melanson EL. Effectiveness of intermittent fasting and time-restricted feeding compared to continuous energy restriction for weight loss. Nutrients October 14, 2019;11(10):2442.

[62] Sievert K, Hussain SM, Page MJ, Wang Y, Hughes HJ, Malek M, et al. Effect of breakfast on weight and energy intake: systematic review and meta-analysis of randomised controlled trials. BMJ January 30, 2019;364:l42.

Physical activity

[63] Kohl 3rd HW, Craig CL, Lambert EV, Inoue S, Alkandari JR, Leetongin G, et al. The pandemic of physical inactivity: global action for public health. Lancet 2012;380(9838):294—305.

[64] Ekelund U, Tarp J, Steene-Johannessen J, Hansen BH, Jefferis B, Fagerland MW, et al. Dose-response associations between accelerometry measured physical activity and sedentary time and all cause mortality: systematic review and harmonised meta-analysis. BMJ 2019:366.

[65] Ding D, Lawson KD, Kolbe-Alexander TL, Finkelstein EA, Katzmarzyk PT, Van Mechelen W, et al. The economic burden of physical inactivity: a global analysis of major non-communicable diseases. Lancet 2016;388(10051):1311—24.

[66] Bull FC, Al-Ansari SS, Biddle S, Borodulin K, Buman MP, Cardon G, et al. World Health Organization 2020 guidelines on physical activity and sedentary behaviour. Br J Sports Med 2020;54(24):1451—62.

[67] Hall G, Laddu DR, Phillips SA, Lavie CJ, Arena R. A tale of two pandemics: how will COVID-19 and global trends in physical inactivity and sedentary behavior affect one another? Prog Cardiovasc Dis 2021;64:108.

[68] McAuley PA, Chen H, Lee DC, Artero EG, Bluemke DA, Burke GL. Physical activity, measures of obesity, and cardiometabolic risk: the Multi-Ethnic Study of Atherosclerosis (MESA). J Phys Activ Health 2014;11(4):831.

[69] Pedersen BK. Body mass index-independent effect of fitness and physical activity for all-cause mortality. Scand J Med Sci Sports 2007;17(3):196—204.

[70] Arem H, Moore SC, Patel A, Hartge P, De Gonzalez AB, Visvanathan K, et al. Leisure time physical activity and mortality: a detailed pooled analysis of the dose-response relationship. JAMA Intern Med 2015;175(6):959—67.

[71] Ekelund U, Tarp J, Steene-Johannessen J, Hansen BH, Jefferis B, Fagerland MW, et al. Dose-response associations between accelerometry measured physical activity and sedentary time and all cause mortality: systematic review and harmonised meta-analysis. Bmj 2019:366.

[72] Moore SC, Lee IM, Weiderpass E, Campbell PT, Sampson JN, Kitahara CM, et al. Association of leisure-time physical activity with risk of 26 types of cancer in 1.44 million adults. JAMA Intern Med 2016;176(6):816—25.

[73] Knowler WC, Barrett-Connor E, Fowler SE, Hamman RF, Lachin JM, Walker EA, et al. Reduction in the incidence of type 2 diabetes with lifestyle intervention or metformin. 2002.

[74] Hamman RF, Wing RR, Edelstein SL, Lachin JM, Bray GA, Delahanty L, et al. Effect of weight loss with lifestyle intervention on risk of diabetes. Diabetes Care 2006;29(9):2102—7.

[75] Diabetes Prevention Program Research Group. Long-term effects of lifestyle intervention or metformin on diabetes development and microvascular complications over 15-year follow-up: the Diabetes Prevention Program Outcomes Study. Lancet Diabetes Endocrinol 2015;3(11):866—75.

[76] Kriska AM, Rockette-Wagner B, Edelstein SL, Bray GA, Delahanty LM, Hoskin MA, et al. The impact of physical activity on the prevention of type 2 diabetes: evidence and lessons learned from the diabetes prevention program, a long-standing clinical trial incorporating subjective and objective activity measures. Diabetes Care 2021;44(1):43—9.

[77] Look AHEAD Research Group. Cardiovascular effects of intensive lifestyle intervention in type 2 diabetes. N Engl J Med 2013;369(2):145—54.

[78] Pi-Sunyer X. The look AHEAD trial: a review and discussion of its outcomes. Curr Nutr Rep 2014;3(4):387—91.

[79] Gaesser GA, Angadi SS. Obesity treatment: weight loss versus increasing fitness and physical activity for reducing health risks. iScience 2021;24(10):102995.

[80] Garber CE, Blissmer B, Deschenes MR, Franklin BA, Lamonte MJ, Lee IM, et al. Quantity and quality of exercise for developing and maintaining cardiorespiratory, musculoskeletal, and neuromotor fitness in apparently healthy adults: guidance for prescribing exercise. 2011.

[81] Piercy KL, Troiano RP, Ballard RM, Carlson SA, Fulton JE, Galuska DA, et al. The physical activity guidelines for Americans. JAMA 2018;320(19):2020—8.

[82] Garvey, W. T., Mechanick, J. I., Brett, E. M., Garber, A. J.,American association of clinical endocrinologists and American college of endocrinology comprehensive clinical practice guidelines formedical care of patients with obesity. Endocr Pract, 22, 1-203

[83] American Diabetes Association Professional Practice Committee, American Diabetes Association Professional Practice Committee. 8. Obesity and weight management for the prevention and treatment of type 2 diabetes: standards of medical care in diabetes—2022. Diabetes Care 2022;45(Supplement_1):S113—24.

[84] Jakicic JM, Powell KE, Campbell WW, Dipietro L, Pate RR, Pescatello LS, et al. Physical activity and the prevention of weight gain in adults: a systematic review. Med Sci Sports Exerc 2019;51(6):1262.

[85] Kanaley JA, Colberg SR, Corcoran MH, Malin SK, Rodriguez NR, Crespo CJ, et al. Exercise/physical activity in individuals with type 2 diabetes: a consensus statement from the American College of Sports medicine. Med Sci Sports Exerc 2022.

[86] Kettle VE, Madigan CD, Coombe A, Graham H, Thomas JJ, Chalkley AE, et al. Effectiveness of physical activity interventions delivered or prompted by health professionals in primary care settings: systematic review and meta-analysis of randomised controlled trials. BMJ 2022:376.

[87] Sedlmeier AM, Baumeister SE, Weber A, Fischer B, Thorand B, Ittermann T, et al. Relation of body fat mass and fat-free mass to total mortality: results from 7 prospective cohort studies. Am J Clin Nutr 2021;113(3):639—46.

[88] Ross R, Neeland IJ, Yamashita S, Shai I, Seidell J, Magni P, et al. Waist circumference as a vital sign in clinical practice: a consensus statement from the IAS and ICCR working group on visceral obesity. Nat Rev Endocrinol 2020;16(3):177—89.

[89] Neeland IJ, Ayers CR, Rohatgi AK, Turer AT, Berry JD, Das SR, et al. Associations of visceral and abdominal subcutaneous adipose tissue with markers of cardiac and metabolic risk in obese adults. Obesity 2013;21(9):E439—47.

[90] Chartrand DJ, Murphy-Després A, Alméras N, Lemieux I, Larose E, Després JP. Overweight, obesity, and CVD risk: a focus on visceral/ectopic fat. Curr Atherosclerosis Rep 2022:1—11.

[91] Rao S, Pandey A, Garg S, Park B, Mayo H, Després JP, et al. Effect of exercise and pharmacological interventions on visceral adiposity: a systematic review and meta-analysis of long-term randomized controlled trials. In: Mayo clinic proceedings, vol. 94. Elsevier; February 2019. p. 211—24. No. 2.

[92] Verheggen RJHM, Maessen MFH, Green DJ, Hermus ARMM, Hopman MTE, Thijssen DHT. A systematic review and meta-analysis on the effects of exercise training versus hypocaloric diet: distinct effects on body weight and visceral adipose tissue. Obes Rev 2016;17(8):664—90.

[93] Vissers D, Hens W, Taeymans J, Baeyens JP, Poortmans J, Van Gaal L. The effect of exercise on visceral adipose tissue in overweight adults: a systematic review and meta-analysis. PLoS One 2013;8(2):e56415.

[94] Gaesser GA, Angadi SS. Obesity treatment: weight loss versus increasing fitness and physical activity for reducing health risks. iScience 2021;24(10):102995.

[95] Boulé NG, Prud'homme D. Canadian adult obesity clinical practice guidelines: physical activity in obesity management. Available from: https://obesitycanada.ca/guidelines/physicalactivity. [Accessed 10 January 2022].

[96] Wewege M, Van Den Berg R, Ward RE, Keech A. The effects of high-intensity interval training vs. moderate-intensity continuous training on body composition in overweight and obese adults: a systematic review and meta-analysis. Obes Rev 2017;18(6):635—46.

[97] Bellicha A, van Baak MA, Battista F, Beaulieu K, Blundell JE, Busetto L, et al. Effect of exercise training on weight loss, body composition changes, and weight maintenance in adults with overweight or obesity: an overview of 12 systematic reviews and 149 studies. Obes Rev 2021;22:e13256.

[98] Türk Y, Theel W, Kasteleyn MJ, Franssen FME, Hiemstra PS, Rudolphus A, et al. High intensity training in obesity: a meta-analysis. Obesity Sci & Pract 2017;3(3):258—71.

[99] Steele J, Plotkin D, Van Every D, Rosa A, Zambrano H, Mendelovits B, et al. Slow and steady, or hard and fast? A systematic review and meta-analysis of studies comparing body composition changes between interval training and moderate intensity continuous training. Sports 2021;9(11):155.

[100] Van Baak MA, Pramono A, Battista F, Beaulieu K, Blundell JE, Busetto L, et al. Effect of different types of regular exercise on physical fitness in adults with overweight or obesity: systematic review and meta-analyses. Obes Rev 2021;22:e13239.

[101] Catenacci VA, Ogden LG, Stuht J, Phelan S, Wing RR, Hill JO, Wyatt HR. Physical activity patterns in the national weight control registry. Obesity 2008;16(1):153—61.

[102] Saint-Maurice PF, Troiano RP, Matthews CE, Kraus WE. Moderate-to-vigorous physical activity and all-cause mortality: do bouts matter? J Am Heart Assoc 2018;7(6):e007678.

[103] Baillot A, Chenail S, Barros Polita N, Simoneau M, Libourel M, Nazon E, et al. Physical activity motives, barriers, and preferences in people with obesity: a systematic review. PLoS One 2021;16(6):e0253114.

Sleep

[104] Miller MA, Kruisbrink M, Wallace J, Ji C, Cappuccio FP. Sleep duration and incidence of obesity in infants, children, and adolescents: a systematic review and meta-analysis of prospective studies. Sleep 2018;41(4):zsy018.

[105] Patel SR, Hu FB. Short sleep duration and weight gain: a systematic review. Obesity 2008;16(3):643—53.

[106] Sun M, Feng W, Wang F, Li P, Li Z, Li M, et al. Meta-analysis on shift work and risks of specific obesity types. Obes Rev 2018;19(1):28—40.

[107] Hemmer A, Mareschal J, Dibner C, Pralong JA, Dorribo V, Perrig S, et al. The effects of shift work on cardio-metabolic diseases and eating patterns. Nutrients 2021;13(11):4178.

[108] Spiegel K, Tasali E, Leproult R, Van Cauter E. Effects of poor and short sleep on glucose metabolism and obesity risk. Nat Rev Endocrinol 2009;5(5):253—61.

[109] Spiegal K, Tasali E, Penev P, Van Cauter E. Sleep curtailment in healthy young men is associated with decreased leptin levels, elevated ghrelin levels and increased hunger and appetite. Ann Intern Med 2004;141(11):846—50.

[110] Senaratna CV, Perret JL, Lodge CJ, Lowe AJ, Campbell BE, Matheson MC, et al. Prevalence of obstructive sleep apnea in the general population: a systematic review. Sleep Med Rev 2017;34:70—81.

[111] Reutrakul S, Siwasaranond N, Nimitphong H, Saetung S, Chirakalwasan N, Chailurkit LO, et al. Associations between nocturnal urinary 6-sul-fatoxymelatonin, obstructive sleep apnea severity and glycemic control in type 2 diabetes. Chronobiol Int 2017;34(3):382–92.

[112] Pugliese G, Barrea L, Laudisio D, Salzano C, Aprano S, Colao A, et al. Sleep apnea, obesity, and disturbed glucose homeostasis: epidemiologic evidence, biologic insights, and therapeutic strategies. Curr Obes Rep 2020;9(1):30–8.

[113] Lin J, Jiang Y, Wang G, Meng M, Zhu Q, Mei H, et al. Associations of short sleep duration with appetite-regulating hormones and adipokines: a systematic review and meta-analysis. Obes Rev 2020;21(11):e13051.

[114] Hirshkowitz M, Whiton K, Albert SM, Alessi C, Bruni O, DonCarlos L, et al. National Sleep Foundation's updated sleep duration recommendations. Sleep Health 2015;1(4):233–43.

Behavioral therapy

[115] Curry S, Krist A, Owens D, Barry M, Caughey A, Davidson K, et al. Behavioral weight loss interventions to prevent obesity-related morbidity and mortality in adults: US Preventive Services Task Force recommendation statement. JAMA 2018;320(11):1163–71.

[116] Jensen MD, Ryan DH, Apovian CM, Ard JD, Comuzzie AG, Donato KA, et al. 2013 AHA/ACC/TOS guideline for the management of overweight and obesity in adults: a report of the American college of cardiology/American heart association task force on practice guidelines and the obesity society. J Am Coll Cardiol 2014;63(25 Pt B):2985.

[117] Durrer Schutz D, Busetto L, Dicker D, Farpour-Lambert N, Pryke R, Toplak H, et al. European practical and patient-centred guidelines for adult obesity management in primary care. Obes Facts 2019;12(1):40–66.

[118] Shaw K, O'Rourke P, Del Mar C, Kenardy J. Psychological interventions for overweight or obesity. Cochrane Database Syst Rev 2005;(2):CD003818.

[119] Renjilian DA, Perri MG, Nezu AM, McKelvey WF, Shermer RL, Anton SD. Individual versus group therapy for obesity: effects of matching participants to their treatment preferences. J Consult Clin Psychol 2001;69(4):717–21.

[120] Perri MG, Limacher MC, Castel-Roberts K, Daniels MJ, Durning PE, Janicke DM, et al. Comparative effectiveness of three doses of weight-loss counseling: two-year findings from the rural LITE trial. Obesity 2014;22(11):2293–300.

[121] Wadden TA, Foster GD. Behavioral treatment of obesity. Med Clin 2000;84(2):441–61.

[122] The Diabetes Prevention Program Research Group. The diabetes prevention program (DPP): description of lifestyle intervention. Diabet Care 2002;25(12):2165–71.

[123] Wadden TA, West DS, Delahanty L, Jakicic J, Rejeski J, Williamson D, et al. The Look AHEAD Study: a description of the lifestyle intervention and the evidence supporting it. Obesity 2006;14(5):737–52.

[124] Wadden TA, Tsai AG, Tronieri JS. A protocol to deliver intensive behavioral therapy (IBT) for obesity in primary care settings: the MODEL-IBT program. Obesity 2019;27(10):1562–6.

[125] Wadden TA, Crerand CE, Brock J. Behavioral treatment of obesity. Psychiatr Clin 2005;28(1):151–70.

[126] Wadden TA, Tronieri JS, Butryn ML. Lifestyle modification approaches for the treatment of obesity in adults. Am Psychol 2020;75(2):235–51.

[127] Wadden TA, Berkowitz RI, Womble LG, Sarwer DB, Phelan S, Cato RK, et al. Randomized trial of lifestyle modification and pharmacotherapy for obesity. N Engl J Med 2005;353(20):2111–20.

[128] Tronieri JS, Wadden TA, Walsh O, Berkowitz RI, Alamuddin N, Chao AM. Measures of adherence as predictors of early and total weight loss with intensive behavioral therapy for obesity combined with liraglutide 3.0 mg. Behav Res Ther 2020;131:103639.

[129] Brownell KD. LEARN program for weight management. 10th ed. Dallas, TX: American Health Publishing Company; 2004.

[130] Butryn ML, Schumacher LM, Forman EM. Alternative behavioral weight loss approaches: acceptance and commitment therapy and motivational interviewing. In: Wadden TA, Bray GA, editors. Handbook of obesity treatment. 2nd ed. New York, NY: The Guilford Press; 2018. p. 508–21.

[131] Wing RR, Lang W, Wadden TA, Safford M, Knowler WC, Bertoni AG, et al. Benefits of modest weight loss in improving cardiovascular risk factors in overweight and obese individuals with type 2 diabetes. Diabetes Care 2011;34(7):1481–6.

[132] Perri MG, Corsica JA. Improving the maintenance of weight lost in the behavioral treatment of obesity. In: Wadden TA, Stunkard AJ, editors. Handbook of obesity treatment. 1st ed. New York, NY: Guilford Press; 2002. p. 465–79.

[133] Knowler WC, Barrett-Connor E, Fowler SE, Hamman RF, Lachin JM, Walker EA, et al. Reduction in the incidence of type 2 diabetes with lifestyle intervention or metformin. N Engl J Med 2002;346(6):393–403.

[134] Diabetes Prevention Program Research Group. 10-year follow-up of diabetes incidence and weight loss in the Diabetes Prevention Program Outcomes Study. Lancet 2009;374(9702):1677–86.

[135] Wadden TA, Neiberg RH, Wing RR, Clark JM, Delahanty LM, et al. Four-year weight losses in the Look AHEAD study: factors associated with long-term success. Obesity 2011;19(10):1987–98.

[136] Butryn ML, Webb V, Wadden TA. Behavioral treatment of obesity. Psychiatr Clin 2011;34(4):841–59.

[137] Tronieri JS, Wadden TA, Chao AM, Tsai AG. Primary care interventions for obesity: review of the evidence. Cur Obes Rep 2019;8(2):128–36.

[138] Donnelly JE, Goetz J, Gibson C, Sullivan DK, Lee R, Smith BK, et al. Equivalent weight loss for weight management programs delivered by phone and clinic. Obesity 2013;21(10):1951–9.

[139] Sherrington A, Newham JJ, Bell R, Adamson A, McColl E, et al. Systematic review and meta-analysis of internet-delivered interventions providing personalized feedback for weight loss in overweight and obese adults. Obes Rev 2016;17(6):541–51.

[140] Pagoto S, Schneider K, Jojic M, DeBiasse M, Mann D. Evidence-based strategies in weight-loss mobile apps. Am J Prev Med November 2013, 2013;45(5):576–82.

[141] Laing B, Mangione C, Tseng C, Leng M, Vaisberg E, Mahida M, et al. Effectiveness of a smartphone application for weight loss compared with usual care in overweight primary care patients: a randomized, controlled trial. Ann Intern Med 2014;161(10):S5−12.

[142] Wadden TA, Tronieri JS, Sugimoto D, Lund MT, Auerbach P, Jensen C, et al. Liraglutide 3.0 mg and intensive behavioral therapy (IBT) for obesity in primary care: the SCALE IBT randomized controlled trial. Obesity 2020;28(3):529−36.

[143] Forman EM, Schumacher LM, Crosby R, Manasse SM, Goldstein SP, Butryn ML, et al. Ecological momentary assessment of dietary lapses across behavioral weight loss treatment: characteristics, predictors, and relationships with weight change. Ann Behav Med 2017;51(5):741−53.

[144] Apovian CM, Aronne LJ, Bessesen DH, McDonnell ME, Murad MH, Pagotto U, et al. Pharmacological management of obesity: an Endocrine Society clinical practice guideline. J Clin Endocrinol Metab 2015;100(2):342−62.

[145] Wilding JP, Batterham RL, Calanna S, Davies M, Van Gaal LF, Lingvay I, et al. Once-weekly semaglutide in adults with overweight or obesity. N Engl J Med 2021;384(11):989−1002.

[146] Wadden TA, Walsh OA, Berkowitz RI, Chao AM, Alamuddin N, Gruber KA, et al. Intensive behavioral therapy for obesity combined with liraglutide 3.0 mg: a randomized controlled trial. Obesity 2019;27(1):75−86.

[147] Khera R, Murad MH, Chandar AK, Dulai PS, Wang Z, Prokop LJ, et al. Association of pharmacological treatments for obesity with weight loss and adverse events: a systematic review and meta-analysis. JAMA 2016;315(22):2424−34.

[148] Wadden TA, Bailey TS, Billings LK, Davies M, Frias JP, Koroleva A, et al. Effect of subcutaneous semaglutide vs placebo as an adjunct to intensive behavioral therapy on body weight in adults with overweight or obesity: the STEP 3 randomized clinical trial. JAMA 2021;325(14):1403−13.

[149] Smith SR, Weissman NJ, Anderson CM, Sanchez M, Chuang E, Stubbe S, et al. Multicenter, placebo-controlled trial of lorcaserin for weight management. N Engl J Med 2010;363(3):245−56.

[150] Wadden T, Hollander P, Klein S, Niswender K, Woo V, Hale P, et al. Weight maintenance and additional weight loss with liraglutide after low-calorie-diet-induced weight loss: the SCALE Maintenance randomized study. Int J Obes 2013;37(11):1443−51.

[151] Pories WJ, MacDonald Jr KG, Morgan EJ, Sinha MK, Dohm GL, Swanson MS, et al. Surgical treatment of obesity and its effect on diabetes: 10-y follow-up. Am J Clin Nutr 1992;55(2):582S−5S.

[152] Sjöström L, Lindroos A, Peltonen M, Torgerson J, Bouchard C, Carlsson B, et al. Lifestyle, diabetes, and cardiovascular risk factors 10 years after bariatric surgery. N Engl J Med 2004;351(26):2683−93.

[153] Sheets CS, Peat CM, Berg KC, White EK, Bocchieri-Ricciardi L, Chen EY, et al. Post-operative psychosocial predictors of outcome in bariatric surgery. Obes Surg 2015;25(2):330−4.

[154] David LA, Sijercic I, Cassin SE. Preoperative and post-operative psychosocial interventions for bariatric surgery patients: a systematic review. Obes Rev 2020;21(4):e12926.

Chapter 24

Medical therapy

Janina Senn and Stefan Fischli

Luzerner Kantonsspital, Division of Endocrinology, Diabetes and Clinical Nutrition, Luzern, Switzerland

Introduction

This chapter about medical therapy will focus mainly on EU-approved medicaments for the treatment of type 2 diabetes mellitus and obesity. In essence, it summarizes actual data on existing and the newest therapeutic agents with proven cardiovascular benefits, including metformin, orlistat, GLP-1 receptor agonists (GLP-1-RA), and sodium glucose cotransporter-2 inhibitors (SGLT-2 inhibitors), which currently represent important pillars of modern diabetes and obesity treatment as well as have multiple effects on cardiovascular parameters and on ectopic and visceral fat.

Thiazolidinediones (so-called "insulin sensitizers") were used very often a few years ago and also have proven benefits on different adipose tissues. The unfavorable side effect profile, including weight gain, reduction in bone density, and the still open questions regarding cardiovascular safety, has led to a very restricted use of these medicaments. Therefore, from a clinical point of view, the authors decided not to include thiazolidinediones in this chapter.

Whereas orlistat is used only for weight reduction, metformin, GLP-1-RA, and SGLT-2 inhibitors are antidiabetic medicaments for the treatment of type 2 diabetes mellitus, a condition characterized by a state of insulin resistance, visceral adiposity, and ectopic fat deposition in different organs (Fig. 24.1). These substances affect glucose metabolism in different ways, either directly by increasing insulin secretion, reducing glucagon secretion and stimulating renal glucose excretion, or indirectly by reducing insulin resistance in target tissues leading to reduced hepatic glucose production, enhancing peripheral glucose uptake and suppressing lipolysis. Glucose and fat metabolism (i.e., visceral and ectopic fat) are closely linked together. Reduction in fat mass, especially visceral and ectopic fat, always will result in improvements of insulin secretion and insulin sensitivity, explaining the different effects of these medicaments on glucoregulation and lipid metabolism (Fig. 24.2).

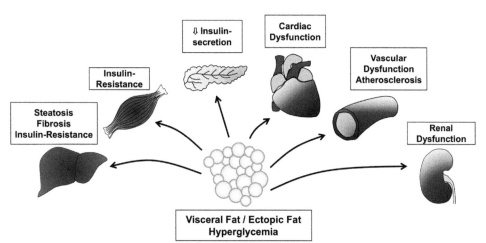

FIGURE 24.1 Clinical consequences of obesity/type 2 diabetes mellitus.

Visceral and Ectopic Fat. https://doi.org/10.1016/B978-0-12-822186-0.00014-6

FIGURE 24.2 Medicaments—direct effects on glucose regulation; indirect effects on visceral/ectopic fat. GLP-1-RA, GLP-1 receptor agonist; SGLT-2 inhibitors, sodium glucose cotransporter-2 inhibitors.

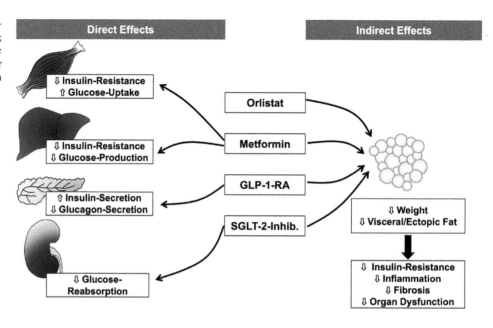

Metformin

Mechanism of action/side effects

Due to its glucose lowering properties, metformin is still to this day considered the initial and background treatment of choice (in combination with other antidiabetics) in patients with type 2 diabetes mellitus.

Metformin is a derivate of galegine, an isoprenyl derivative of guanidine, originally derived from the plant *Galega officinalis*. In 1950, metformin was synthesized in the form of a biguanide (containing two N-linked molecules of guanidine) with a much lower rate of hepato- and renotoxicity than its precursors [1,2].

vvAlthough metformin has some weight-reducing effects and prevents diabetes mellitus [3], it is approved for neither weight reduction nor the prevention of type 2 diabetes mellitus. Even though it has been in clinical use for more than 60 years, the mechanisms of how metformin acts on metabolism are complex and have not been fully explored and understood.

One of the main sites of action is the liver where uptake of metformin into the hepatocytes is promoted by the organic cation transporter-1 (OCT1). After accumulation within the mitochondria, the compound inhibits complex I of the respiratory chain and glycerophosphate dehydrogenase (mGPD), thereby promoting activation of AMP-activated protein kinase (AMPK) and inhibition of adenylate cyclase, leading to multiple downstream inhibitory effects on gluconeogenesis and glucagon action [1,2]. Metformin-induced AMPK-activation inhibits lipid synthesis in muscle and the liver, reducing intracellular/intravascular lipid content and improving insulin sensitivity [4]. Metformin also has an effect on weight, food intake, and appetite [5] (Fig. 24.3).

Some data show beneficial cardiovascular outcomes in patients treated with metformin [6–8]. However, evidence is weak, and a direct comparison with the results of the newer cardiovascular outcome trials (i.e., GLP-1-RA and SGLT-2 inhibitors) is difficult due to different study designs and sample sizes.

Generally, metformin is considered a safe medication with no risk of hypoglycemia. Approximately, 30%–50% of patients on metformin report mild and dose-related gastrointestinal (GI) side effects, including abdominal pain, nausea, diarrhea, and vomiting [9]. GI side effects can be minimized by stepwise up-titration and use of extended-release dosing forms. A very rare but frightening complication with an estimated incidence of about 4.3 events/100,000 person years [10] is lactic acidosis, which is caused by enhanced hepatic lactate production as a consequence of complex I inhibition. Lactic acidosis is preventable in most of the cases through different measures such as not giving a prescription in case of advanced renal insufficiency and stopping the medication in states with volume depletion. Chronic treatment with metformin can lead to vitamin B12 deficiency, which warrants regular control of B12 stores [11].

Clinical efficacy

Average HbA1c lowering with metformin is about −1.0% [12], but it should be noted that the individual potential for HbA1c reduction in daily clinical practice is sometimes much higher. Metformin causes only a slight reduction

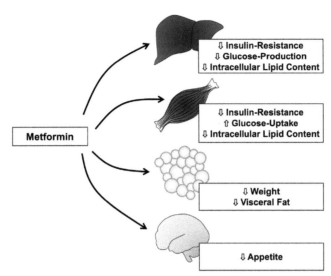

FIGURE 24.3 Metformin—mechanisms of action.

(1–2 kg) or stabilization in weight [13] in patients with diabetes but also has proven weight-reducing effects in persons without diabetes [14].

The Diabetes Prevention Program Research Group conducted one of the largest studies on metformin treatment and long-term safety, tolerability, and weight loss. Over 2 years, patients with metformin lost 2.1 kg ± 5.7% of their weight compared with the placebo group with 0.02 kg ± 5.5% ($P < .001$). Metformin was also better at reducing waist circumference versus placebo (metformin group 2.1 cm ± 7.1 cm vs. placebo group 0.79 cm ± 6.5 cm ($P < .001$)). Weight loss remained stable and significantly higher in the metformin group with 2.0% versus the placebo group with 0.2% in the 10-year follow-up study [15].

There is some evidence of a positive effect on hepatic steatosis/nonalcoholic fatty liver disease (NFLD), but there is a paucity of data and conflicting results for monotherapy as well as a lack of placebo-controlled studies [16]. However, there may be the potential for new combination treatment regimens of metformin together with SGLT-2 inhibitors and GLP-1-RA (see the following).

Orlistat

Mechanism of actions/side effects

Orlistat reduces fat intake, leading to weight reduction, which consequently improves glucose metabolism. It is approved for weight reduction, but not for the prevention of type 2 diabetes mellitus.

Orlistat (tetrahydrolipstatin) is a chemically synthetic derivative of lipstatin, a naturally occurring product from *Streptomyces toxytricini*. It inhibits irreversible and specific gastric and pancreatic lipases through the formation of a covalent bond with the active serine site of the lipases within the GI lumen. As a consequence, ingested fat in the form of triglycerides cannot be hydrolyzed into free fatty acids and glycerol and, therefore, is absorbed by the intestinal endothelium. The unhydrolyzed triglycerides are excreted with the feces, which causes a reduction in caloric intake without creating an increased appetite [17–19] (Fig. 24.4).

In general, orlistat is well tolerated. The main side effects are primarily of a GI nature and explained by the mechanism of action. The higher amount of triglycerides in the feces results in oily stools (27.1%), oily spotting (13.7%), fecal urgency (9.0%), fecal incontinence (6.1%), hyperdefecation (5.3%), and flatus with discharge (4.1%) [20].

It is suggested that these GI side effects usually occur early in the treatment and decrease with long-term use. This was shown in the XENDOS study where 91% of patients in the orlistat group had at least one GI event in the first year (vs. placebo 65%), but the event rate was reduced in the fourth year of treatment to 36% (vs. placebo 23%) [21]. Patients are therefore advised to avoid a high-fat diet to reduce occurrence of GI side effects.

Orlistat-induced fat malabsorption also bears the risk of a deficiency in fat-soluble vitamins (vitamins A, D, E, K) with long-term use of orlistat. Therefore, levels of these vitamins should be checked on a regular basis and replaced in case of deficiency [20].

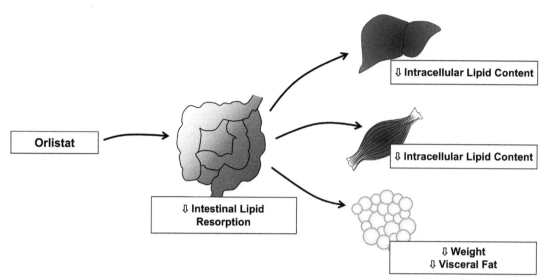

FIGURE 24.4 Orlistat—mechanisms of action.

Clinical efficacy

The long-term effect and safety of orlistat were evaluated in the XENDOS study [22]. The study investigated if orlistat in combination with lifestyle changes has a significant influence on body weight and on the progression of type 2 diabetes over 4 years in obese patients (BMI $\geq$30 kg/m^2) without diabetes, but with either normal glucose tolerance or impaired glucose tolerance. The mean weight loss after 1 year and 4 years was significantly higher in the orlistat group compared with the placebo group (10.6 vs. 6.2 kg and 5.8 vs. 3.0 kg, respectively). Compared with placebo, orlistat significantly reduced the progression to type 2 diabetes (cumulative incidence rates after 4 years: 9.0% vs. 6.2%). Further improvements in the orlistat group were seen in waist circumference, insulin sensitivity, blood pressure, and lipids.

A few studies investigated the effect of orlistat on body fat distribution and ectopic fat. In the XENDOS study [22], orlistat led to a significant reduction in visceral fat. Applying the visceral fat:subcutaneous ratio [23], the effect on different fat depots with a treatment of 60 mg orlistat daily compared with placebo was investigated. At the end of the study, a reduction in visceral adipose tissue (VAT), loss of total fat mass as well as a reduction in intramuscular adipose tissue and liver fat was significantly higher in the orlistat group.

The benefit of orlistat in NAFLD was shown in the study of Filippatos et al. [24], where therapy with orlistat led to a reduction in the level of aminotransferases and a reduction in steatosis of the liver (determined by ultrasound).

Glucagon-like peptide 1 receptor agonists

Mechanisms of action/side effects

Glucagon-like peptide 1 receptor agonists (GLP-1-RAs) lower blood glucose through different mechanisms. They represent the antidiabetic class with the most pronounced weight reduction and also have profound effects on visceral and ectopic fat. GLP-1-RAs are approved for the therapy of type 2 diabetes mellitus, and some are approved for the treatment of obesity (liraglutide).

GLP-1-RAs are analogs of the gut-derived incretin hormone glucagon-like peptide 1, which is secreted after ingestion of food. Endogenous GLP-1 stimulates glucose-dependent insulin secretion, suppresses glucagon, and delays gastric emptying. Via direct action on the hypothalamus, it promotes satiety and reduces energy intake. GLP-1 exerts a variety of other actions on the immune, cardiovascular, and cerebral system as well as on hepatic, muscular, and adipose tissue [25] (Fig. 24.5). GLP-1-RAs can be grouped according to their structure (exendin-4- or human GLP-1-backbone), half-life (several hours to several days) and molecular weight. GLP-1-RAs with a shorter half-life have an impact on gastric emptying, thereby reducing primary postprandial glucose levels, whereas GLP-1-RAs with a longer half-life (days) mainly lead to a reduction in fasting plasma glucose levels.

Due to their peptide hormone structure, GLP-1-RAs have to be applied by subcutaneous injection. However, recently, an oral preparation of a GLP-1-RA has been approved (semaglutide). In cardiovascular outcome trials, several GLP-1-RAs have shown to reduce cardiovascular endpoints [26—28].

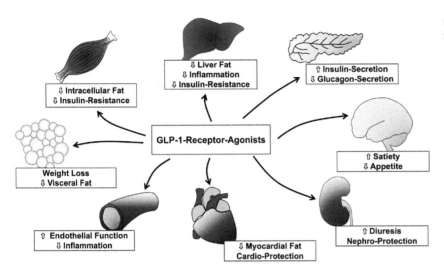

FIGURE 24.5 GLP-1 receptor agonists—mechanisms of action.

GLP-1-RAs lack hypoglycemia risk unless they are combined with sulfonylureas or insulin. Frequent side effects include GI symptoms (nausea, vomiting, or diarrhea). The symptoms appear in up to 60% of patients but are mainly transient and can be reduced by a stepwise up-titration of the dose. Treatment with GLP-1-RA is associated with an increased frequency of gallbladder- and bile-duct-stone formation [29] and retinopathy in patients treated with semaglutide [27]. GLP-1-RA can be combined with other oral antidiabetic medicaments or insulin.

Clinical efficacy

When compared in head-to-head studies, GLP-1-RAs demonstrate a wide range of efficacy in the reduction of HbA1c and weight. This is mainly due to the different characteristics of the substances (cf. above). It seems that GLP-1-RAs with a longer half-life are more potent in lowering HbA1c and weight. The reduction in HbA1c and weight ranges were from −0.78% to −1.8% and −0.64 to −5.8 kg, respectively [30].

Liraglutide has been approved for the treatment of obesity. Compared with placebo treatment with liraglutide, 3.0 mg/day led to a dose-related weight loss of 6.0−8.8 kg [31] and reduced the risk of progression to type 2 diabetes mellitus [32]. The weight loss with semaglutide is even more pronounced. In a phase III study, a 68-week therapy with 2.4 mg semaglutide once weekly resulted in a weight loss of −15.3 kg [33].

Most of the studies carried out with GLP-1-RA in patients with type 2 diabetes mellitus show a reduction in fat mass [34,35], and most of the results are consistent with a significant reduction in visceral fat mass [36−38], a reduction in insulin resistance, and an improvement in type 2 diabetes mellitus. Several investigations also show a reduction in epicardial fat [39,40], representing one of the possible causative factors for the cardioprotective properties of these agents.

The GLP-1-RA liraglutide reduces intrahepatic fat stores in overweight patients with type 2 diabetes mellitus and NAFLD [41,42]. Several randomized and controlled trials with liraglutide and semaglutide have shown a positive impact on liver enzymes, hepatic steatosis [43,44], and resolution or improvement of histological markers of NAFLD [45,46].

Sodium glucose cotransporter-2 inhibitors

Mechanisms of action/side effects

SGLT-2 inhibitors are newer antidiabetic medications, which block renal glucose reabsorption in the proximal tubule, leading to glucosuria, mild diuresis, and natriuresis. Apart from their direct glucose-lowering effects, newer studies demonstrate cardio- [47−49] and renoprotective [50,51] properties, even in patients without diabetes [52,53]. They are approved for the treatment of type 2 diabetes mellitus and in patients with heart failure with reduced ejection fraction (HFrEF).

Today, SGLT-2 inhibitors are a mainstay in the treatment of diabetic patients. The safety profile is favorable, the substances lack intrinsic risk of hypoglycemia, and they promote weight loss. Common side effects include urogenital

FIGURE 24.6   SGLT-2 inhibitors—mechanisms of action.

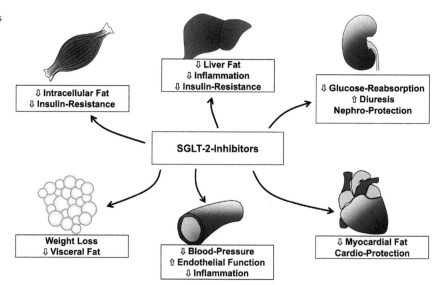

infections (i.e., mycoses and urinary tract infections) due to glucosuria. In rare cases, complicated urinary tract infections (i.e., pyelonephritis or urosepsis) can occur. Euglycemic diabetic ketoacidosis and a probable association with a higher risk for lower extremity amputation represent very rare but potential fatal adverse events [54,55].

SGLT-2 inhibitors promote weight loss and affect adipose tissue metabolism in different ways. Glucosuria leads to calorie loss, lowers glucose and insulin concentrations, and raises glucagon levels. The reduced insulin:glucagon ratio stimulates lipolysis and hepatic ketone production [56]. The diuretic effect of SGLT-2 inhibitors is only modest. Therefore, loss of fat components is the main factor contributing to weight reduction. In a clinical study comparing the effects of the SGLT-2 inhibitor dapagliflozin versus placebo on fat tissue metabolism, dapagliflozin reduced total body weight mainly by reducing the amount of visceral and subcutaneous adipose tissue [57].

In addition, SGLT-2 inhibitors induce energy expenditure by the browning of white adipose tissue and thermogenesis in brown adipose tissue, and they reduce accumulation of ectopic fat and adipose tissue inflammation [58]. The later effects probably provide a partial explanation for the cardiovascular protective characteristics of SGLT-2 inhibitors (Fig. 24.6).

Clinical efficacy

Reduction in weight is modest and ranges from −1.74 kg compared with placebo (monotherapy) to −1.8 kg compared with other antidiabetic medicaments [59]. Waist circumference is reduced by about −1.20 cm [60]. The effect of SGLT-2 inhibitors on weight reduction is lower than could be anticipated by the glucosuria-induced negative calorie balance. Adaptive mechanisms in appetite regulation and energy uptake counteract and limit the effect of these substances on weight loss [61]. Therefore, the combination of SGLT-2 inhibitors with other substances can exert synergistic effects on weight. For example, dual therapy with SGLT-2 inhibitors and GLP-1-RA demonstrates greater weight loss than the corresponding monotherapy [62−64].

There is growing evidence that SGLT-2 inhibitors reduce intrahepatic lipid content. Several studies in patients with type 2 diabetes mellitus treated with different SGLT-2 inhibitors have demonstrated, apart from a reduction in the visceral fat mass, a lower liver fat content, improvement of liver enzymes, and better glycemic control [65−69]. The effects in patients with NAFLD are comparable with treatment with thiazolidines (TZD), with the difference being that compared with the weight-gaining properties of TZD, SGLT-2 inhibitors promote weight loss [70].

The data regarding the impact of SGLT-2 inhibitor treatment on epi- and myocardial fat in patients with type 2 diabetes mellitus are somewhat conflicting. Some studies [39,71,72] show a significant reduction in cardial fat, whereas others [73,74] do not. Possible explanations for this dichotomy are differences in study designs and treatment durations, diverging characteristics of patients (i.e., duration of diabetes, presence of micro- and or macrovascular complications, and HbA1c values at inclusion) and different methods of evaluating epi- and myocardial fat.

Conclusions

Obesity and type 2 diabetes mellitus are two conditions associated with profound perturbations in glucose and lipid metabolism. Excessive visceral fat and ectopic fat deposition in virtually every organ (i.e., pancreas, liver, kidney, heart, brain, and blood vessels) leads—in concert with chronic elevated blood glucose levels and other cardiovascular risk factors—to a variety of severe clinical consequences (i.e., aggravation of insulin resistance, cardiovascular dysfunction, renal insufficiency, and hepatic steatosis/fibrosis). The effects of the so-called "lipo- and glucotoxicity" are manifold, accounting for the high morbidity and mortality rates in this patient population. Therapy today is always multimodal, combining different compounds to treat cardiovascular risk factors (i.e., high blood pressure and dyslipidemia), lowering blood glucose and reducing visceral and ectopic fat. A growing body of evidence demonstrates that this treatment approach effectively reduces long-term complications and end-organ damage as well as ultimately decreases morbidity and mortality in these persons.

References

[1] Foretz M, et al. Understanding the glucoregulatory mechanisms of metformin in type 2 diabetes mellitus. Nat Rev Endocrinol 2019;15(10):569—89. https://doi.org/10.1038/s41574-019-0242-2.

[2] Rena G, et al. The mechanisms of action of metformin. Diabetologia 2017;60(9):1577—85. https://doi.org/10.1007/s00125-017-4342-z.

[3] The Diabetes Prevention Program. Design and methods for a clinical trial in the prevention of type 2 diabetes. Diabetes Care 1999;22:623—34.

[4] Pernicova I, Korbonits M. Metformin—mode of action and clinical implications for diabetes and cancer. Nat Rev Endocrinol 2014;10:143—56.

[5] Yerevanian A, et al. Metformin: mechanisms in human obesity and weight loss. Curr Obes Rep 2019;8(2):156—64. https://doi.org/10.1007/s13679-019-00335-3.

[6] UKPDS study group. Effect of intensive blood-glucose control with metformin on complications in overweight patients with type 2 diabetes (UKPDS 34). UK Prospective Diabetes Study (UKPDS) Group. Lancet 1998;352:854—65.

[7] Maruthur NM, Tseng E, Hutfless S, Wilson LM, Suarez-Cuervo C, Berger Z, Chu Y, Iyoha E, Segal JB, Bolen S. Diabetes medications as monotherapy or metformin-based combination therapy for type 2 diabetes: a systematic review and meta-analysis. Ann Intern Med 2016;164:740—51.

[8] Han Y, Xie H, Liu Y, Gao P, Yang X, Shen Z. Effect of metformin on all-cause and cardiovascular mortality in patients with coronary artery diseases: a systematic review and an updated meta-analysis. Cardiovasc Diabetol 2019;18:96.

[9] Sanchez-Rangel E, et al. Metformin: clinical use in type 2 diabetes. Diabetologia 2017;60(9):1586—93. https://doi.org/10.1007/s00125-017-4336-x.

[10] Salpeter SR, Greyber E, Pasternak GA, Salpeter EE. Risk of fatal and nonfatal lactic acidosis with metformin use in type 2 diabetes mellitus. Cochrane Database Syst Rev 2010:CD002967.

[11] Kim J, Ahn CW, Fang S, Lee HS, Park JS. Association between metformin dose and vitamin B12 deficiency in patients with type 2 diabetes. Medicine 2019;98:e17918.

[12] Hirst JA, Farmer AJ, Ali R, Roberts NW, Stevens RJ. Quantifying the effect of metformin treatment and dose on glycemic control. Diabetes Care 2012;35:446—54.

[13] Golay A. Metformin and body weight. Int J Obes 2005 2008;32:61—72.

[14] Seifarth C, Schehler B, Schneider HJ. Effectiveness of metformin on weight loss in non-diabetic individuals with obesity. Exp Clin Endocrinol Diabetes Off J Ger Soc Endocrinol Ger Diabetes Assoc 2013;121:27—31.

[15] 10-year follow-up of diabetes incidence and weight loss in the diabetes prevention program outcomes study. Lancet 2009;374:1677—86.

[16] Pinyopornpanish K, Leerapun A, Pinyopornpanish K, Chattipakorn N. Effects of metformin on hepatic steatosis in adults with nonalcoholic fatty liver disease and diabetes: insights from the cellular to patient levels. Gut Liver 2021. https://doi.org/10.5009/gnl20367.

[17] Tak YJ, Lee SY. Long-term efficacy and safety of anti-obesity treatment: where do we stand? Metabolism 2020. https://doi.org/10.1007/s13679-020-00422-w.

[18] Heck AM, Pharm D, et al. Orlistat, a new lipase inhibitor for the management of obesity. Pharmacotherapy 2000;20(3):270—9. https://doi.org/10.1592/phco.20.4.270.34882.

[19] Henness S, et al. Orlistat: a review of its use in the management of obesity. Drugs 2006;66(12):1625—56. https://doi.org/10.2165/00003495-200666120-00012.

[20] Pilitsi E, et al. Pharmacotherapy of obesity: available medications and drugs under investigation. Metab Clin Exp 2018;92:170—92. https://doi.org/10.1016/j.metabol.2018.10.010.

[21] Torgerson JS, et al. XENical in the prevention of diabetes in obese subjects (XENDOS) study: a randomized study of orlistat as an adjunct to lifestyle changes for the prevention of type 2 diabetes in obese patients. Diabetes Care 2004;27(1):155—61. https://doi.org/10.2337/diacare.27.1.155.

[22] Tiikkainen M, et al. Effects of equal weight loss with orlistat and placebo on body fat and serum fatty acid composition and insulin resistance in obese women. Am J Clin Nutr 2004;79(1):22—30. https://doi.org/10.1093/ajcn/79.1.22.

[23] Smith SR, et al. Orlistat 60 mg reduces visceral adipose tissue: a 24-week randomized, placebo-controlled, multicenter trial. Obesity 2011;19(9):1769—803. https://doi.org/10.1038/oby.2011.143.

[24] Filippatos TD, et al. Orlistat-associated adverse effects and drug interactions: a critical review. Drug Saf 2008;31(1):53–65. https://doi.org/10.2165/00002018-200831010-00005.

[25] Drucker DJ. The cardiovascular biology of glucagon-like peptide-1. Cell Metab 2016;24:15–30.

[26] Marso SP, Daniels GH, Brown-Frandsen K, et al. Liraglutide and cardiovascular outcomes in type 2 diabetes. N Engl J Med 2016;375:311–22.

[27] Marso SP, Bain SC, Consoli A, et al. Semaglutide and cardiovascular outcomes in patients with type 2 diabetes. N Engl J Med 2016;375:1834–44.

[28] Gerstein HC, Colhoun HM, Dagenais GR, et al. Dulaglutide and cardiovascular outcomes in type 2 diabetes (REWIND): a double-blind, randomised placebo-controlled trial. Lancet 2019;394:121–30.

[29] Faillie J-L, Yu OH, Yin H, Hillaire-Buys D, Barkun A, Azoulay L. Association of bile duct and gallbladder diseases with the use of incretin-based drugs in patients with type 2 diabetes mellitus. JAMA Intern Med 2016;176:1474–81.

[30] Trujillo JM, Nuffer W, Ellis SL. GLP-1 receptor agonists: a review of head-to-head clinical studies. Ther Adv Endocrinol Metab 2015;6:19–28.

[31] Pi-Sunyer X, Astrup A, Fujioka K, et al. A randomized, controlled trial of 3.0 mg of liraglutide in weight management. N Engl J Med 2015;373:11–22.

[32] le Roux CW, Astrup A, Fujioka K, et al. 3 years of liraglutide versus placebo for type 2 diabetes risk reduction and weight management in individuals with prediabetes: a randomised, double-blind trial. Lancet 2017;389:1399–409.

[33] Wilding JPH, Batterham RL, Calanna S, et al. Once-weekly semaglutide in adults with overweight or obesity. N Engl J Med 2021;384:989.

[34] Jendle J, Nauck MA, Matthews DR, Frid A, Hermansen K, Düring M, Zdravkovic M, Strauss BJ, Garber AJ, LEAD-2 and LEAD-3 Study Groups. Weight loss with liraglutide, a once-daily human glucagon-like peptide-1 analogue for type 2 diabetes treatment as monotherapy or added to metformin, is primarily as a result of a reduction in fat tissue. Diabetes Obes Metab 2009;11:1163–72.

[35] Morano S, Romagnoli E, Filardi T, Nieddu L, Mandosi E, Fallarino M, Turinese I, Dagostino MP, Lenzi A, Carnevale V. Short-term effects of glucagon-like peptide 1 (GLP-1) receptor agonists on fat distribution in patients with type 2 diabetes mellitus: an ultrasonography study. Acta Diabetol 2015;52:727–32.

[36] Ishii S, Nagai Y, Sada Y, Fukuda H, Nakamura Y, Matsuba R, Nakagawa T, Kato H, Tanaka Y. Liraglutide reduces visceral and intrahepatic fat without significant loss of muscle mass in obese patients with type 2 diabetes: a prospective case series. J Clin Med Res 2019;11:219–24.

[37] Suzuki D, Toyoda M, Kimura M, et al. Effects of liraglutide, a human glucagon-like peptide-1 analogue, on body weight, body fat area and body fat-related markers in patients with type 2 diabetes mellitus. Intern Med 2013;52:1029–34.

[38] van Eyk HJ, Paiman EHM, Bizino MB, de Heer P, Geelhoed-Duijvestijn PH, Kharagjitsingh AV, Smit JWA, Lamb HJ, Rensen PCN, Jazet IM. A double-blind, placebo-controlled, randomised trial to assess the effect of liraglutide on ectopic fat accumulation in South Asian type 2 diabetes patients. Cardiovasc Diabetol 2019;18:87.

[39] Iacobellis G, Mohseni M, Bianco SD, Banga PK. Liraglutide causes large and rapid epicardial fat reduction. Obesity 2017;25:311–6.

[40] Iacobellis G, Villasante Fricke AC. Effects of semaglutide versus dulaglutide on epicardial fat thickness in subjects with type 2 diabetes and obesity. J Endocr Soc 2020;4:bvz042.

[41] Petit J-M, Cercueil J-P, Loffroy R, Denimal D, Bouillet B, Fourmont C, Chevallier O, Duvillard L, Vergès B. Effect of liraglutide therapy on liver fat content in patients with inadequately controlled type 2 diabetes: the Lira-NAFLD study. J Clin Endocrinol Metab 2017;102:407–15.

[42] Yan J, Yao B, Kuang H, et al. Liraglutide, sitagliptin, and insulin glargine added to metformin: the effect on body weight and intrahepatic lipid in patients with type 2 diabetes mellitus and nonalcoholic fatty liver disease. Hepatology 2019;69:2414–26.

[43] Astrup A, Rössner S, Van Gaal L, Rissanen A, Niskanen L, Al Hakim M, Madsen J, Rasmussen MF, Lean MEJ, NN8022-1807 Study Group. Effects of liraglutide in the treatment of obesity: a randomised, double-blind, placebo-controlled study. Lancet 2009;374:1606–16.

[44] Armstrong MJ, Houlihan DD, Rowe IA, Clausen WHO, Elbrønd B, Gough SCL, Tomlinson JW, Newsome PN. Safety and efficacy of liraglutide in patients with type 2 diabetes and elevated liver enzymes: individual patient data meta-analysis of the LEAD program. Aliment Pharmacol Ther 2013;37:234–42.

[45] Armstrong MJ, Gaunt P, Aithal GP, et al. Liraglutide safety and efficacy in patients with non-alcoholic steatohepatitis (LEAN): a multicentre, double-blind, randomised, placebo-controlled phase 2 study. Lancet 2016;387:679–90.

[46] Newsome PN, Buchholtz K, Cusi K, Linder M, Okanoue T, Ratziu V, Sanyal AJ, Sejling A-S, Harrison SA, NN9931-4296 Investigators. A placebo-controlled trial of subcutaneous semaglutide in nonalcoholic steatohepatitis. N Engl J Med 2021;384:1113–24.

[47] Zinman B, Wanner C, Lachin JM, et al. Empagliflozin, cardiovascular outcomes, and mortality in type 2 diabetes. N Engl J Med 2015;373:2117–28.

[48] Neal B, Perkovic V, Mahaffey KW, et al. Canagliflozin and cardiovascular and renal events in type 2 diabetes. N Engl J Med 2017. https://doi.org/10.1056/NEJMoa1611925.

[49] Wiviott SD, Raz I, Bonaca MP, et al. Dapagliflozin and cardiovascular outcomes in type 2 diabetes. N Engl J Med 2019;380:347–57.

[50] Perkovic V, Jardine MJ, Neal B, et al. Canagliflozin and renal outcomes in type 2 diabetes and nephropathy. N Engl J Med 2019;380:2295–306.

[51] Heerspink HJL, Stefánsson BV, Correa-Rotter R, et al. Dapagliflozin in patients with chronic kidney disease. N Engl J Med 2020;383:1436–46.

[52] McMurray JJV, Solomon SD, Inzucchi SE, et al. Dapagliflozin in patients with heart failure and reduced ejection fraction. N Engl J Med 2019;381:1995–2008.

[53] Packer M, Anker SD, Butler J, et al. Cardiovascular and renal outcomes with empagliflozin in heart failure. N Engl J Med 2020;383:1413–24.

[54] Taylor SI, Blau JE, Rother KI. SGLT2 inhibitors may predispose to ketoacidosis. J Clin Endocrinol Metab 2015;100:2849–52.

[55] Ueda P, Svanström H, Melbye M, Eliasson B, Svensson A-M, Franzén S, Gudbjörnsdottir S, Hveem K, Jonasson C, Pasternak B. Sodium glucose cotransporter 2 inhibitors and risk of serious adverse events: nationwide register based cohort study. BMJ 2018;363:k4365.

[56] Pereira MJ, Eriksson JW. Emerging role of SGLT-2 inhibitors for the treatment of obesity. Drugs 2019;79:219–30.

[57] Bolinder J, Ljunggren Ö, Kullberg J, Johansson L, Wilding J, Langkilde AM, Sugg J, Parikh S. Effects of dapagliflozin on body weight, total fat mass, and regional adipose tissue distribution in patients with type 2 diabetes mellitus with inadequate glycemic control on metformin. J Clin Endocrinol Metab 2012;97:1020−31.

[58] Xu L, Ota T. Emerging roles of SGLT2 inhibitors in obesity and insulin resistance: focus on fat browning and macrophage polarization. Adipocyte 2018;7:121−8.

[59] Vasilakou D, Karagiannis T, Athanasiadou E, Mainou M, Liakos A, Bekiari E, Sarigianni M, Matthews DR, Tsapas A. Sodium-glucose cotransporter 2 inhibitors for type 2 diabetes: a systematic review and meta-analysis. Ann Intern Med 2013;159:262−74.

[60] Musso G, Gambino R, Cassader M, Pagano G. A novel approach to control hyperglycemia in type 2 diabetes: sodium glucose co-transport (SGLT) inhibitors: systematic review and meta-analysis of randomized trials. Ann Med 2012;44:375−93.

[61] Ferrannini G, Hach T, Crowe S, Sanghvi A, Hall KD, Ferrannini E. Energy balance after sodium-glucose cotransporter 2 inhibition. Diabetes Care 2015;38:1730−5.

[62] Frías JP, Hardy E, Ahmed A, Öhman P, Jabbour S, Wang H, Guja C. Effects of exenatide once weekly plus dapagliflozin, exenatide once weekly alone, or dapagliflozin alone added to metformin monotherapy in subgroups of patients with type 2 diabetes in the DURATION-8 randomized controlled trial. Diabetes Obes Metab 2018;20:1520−5.

[63] Ludvik B, Frías JP, Tinahones FJ, Wainstein J, Jiang H, Robertson KE, García-Pérez L-E, Woodward DB, Milicevic Z. Dulaglutide as add-on therapy to SGLT2 inhibitors in patients with inadequately controlled type 2 diabetes (AWARD-10): a 24-week, randomised, double-blind, placebo-controlled trial. Lancet Diabetes Endocrinol 2018;6:370−81.

[64] Zinman B, Bhosekar V, Busch R, Holst I, Ludvik B, Thielke D, Thrasher J, Woo V, Philis-Tsimikas A. Semaglutide once weekly as add-on to SGLT-2 inhibitor therapy in type 2 diabetes (SUSTAIN 9): a randomised, placebo-controlled trial. Lancet Diabetes Endocrinol 2019;7:356−67.

[65] Kuchay MS, Krishan S, Mishra SK, et al. Effect of empagliflozin on liver fat in patients with type 2 diabetes and nonalcoholic fatty liver disease: a randomized controlled trial (E-LIFT trial). Diabetes Care 2018;41:1801−8.

[66] Koshizaka M, Ishikawa K, Ishibashi R, et al. Comparing the effects of ipragliflozin versus metformin on visceral fat reduction and metabolic dysfunction in Japanese patients with type 2 diabetes treated with sitagliptin: a prospective, multicentre, open-label, blinded-endpoint, randomized controlled study (PRIME-V study). Diabetes Obes Metab 2019;21:1990−5.

[67] Ohta A, Kato H, Ishii S, Sasaki Y, Nakamura Y, Nakagawa T, Nagai Y, Tanaka Y. Ipragliflozin, a sodium glucose co-transporter 2 inhibitor, reduces intrahepatic lipid content and abdominal visceral fat volume in patients with type 2 diabetes. Expert Opin Pharmacother 2017;18:1433−8.

[68] Johansson L, Hockings PD, Johnsson E, Dronamraju N, Maaske J, Garcia-Sanchez R, Wilding JPH. Dapagliflozin plus saxagliptin add-on to metformin reduces liver fat and adipose tissue volume in patients with type 2 diabetes. Diabetes Obes Metab 2020;22:1094−101.

[69] Phrueksotsai S, Pinyopornpanish K, Euathrongchit J, Leerapun A, Phrommintikul A, Buranapin S, Chattipakorn N, Thongsawat S. The effects of dapagliflozin on hepatic and visceral fat in type 2 diabetes patients with non-alcoholic fatty liver disease. J Gastroenterol Hepatol 2021. https://doi.org/10.1111/jgh.15580.

[70] Ito D, Shimizu S, Inoue K, Saito D, Yanagisawa M, Inukai K, Akiyama Y, Morimoto Y, Noda M, Shimada A. Comparison of ipragliflozin and pioglitazone effects on nonalcoholic fatty liver disease in patients with type 2 diabetes: a randomized, 24-week, open-label, active-controlled trial. Diabetes Care 2017;40:1364−72.

[71] Bouchi R, Terashima M, Sasahara Y, et al. Luseogliflozin reduces epicardial fat accumulation in patients with type 2 diabetes: a pilot study. Cardiovasc Diabetol 2017;16:32.

[72] Fukuda T, Bouchi R, Terashima M, et al. Ipragliflozin reduces epicardial fat accumulation in non-obese type 2 diabetic patients with visceral obesity: a pilot study. Diabetes Ther Res Treat Educ Diabetes Relat Disord 2017;8:851−61.

[73] Hiruma S, Shigiyama F, Hisatake S, Mizumura S, Shiraga N, Hori M, Ikeda T, Hirose T, Kumashiro N. A prospective randomized study comparing effects of empagliflozin to sitagliptin on cardiac fat accumulation, cardiac function, and cardiac metabolism in patients with early-stage type 2 diabetes: the ASSET study. Cardiovasc Diabetol 2021;20:32.

[74] Gaborit B, Ancel P, Abdullah AE, et al. Effect of empagliflozin on ectopic fat stores and myocardial energetics in type 2 diabetes: the EMPACEF study. Cardiovasc Diabetol 2021;20:57.

Chapter 25

Gastric volume reduction interventions and effects on visceral fat and metabolic biomarkers

Sean M. O'Neill[1] and Stacy A. Brethauer[2]

[1]*Department of Surgery, Division of Minimally Invasive Surgery, University of Michigan, Ann Arbor, MI, United States;* [2]*Department of Surgery, Division of GI and General Surgery, The Ohio State University Wexner Medical Center, Columbus, OH, United States*

Introduction

Bariatric surgery has been shown to be highly effective and safe for weight loss and resolution of obesity-related comorbidities. However, many eligible patients do not receive bariatric surgery for any of a variety of reasons. As a result, there has been sustained interest in developing less invasive, endoluminal interventions to achieve the same goals of weight reduction and comorbidity resolution.

Endobariatrics is a growing field, with several new procedures and devices introduced in the past 10 years. Several of the most well-described techniques include endoscopic sleeve gastroplasty (ESG), primary obesity surgery endoluminal procedure (the POSE and POSE-2 procedures), and intragastric balloons (IGBs) (Table 25.1 and Fig. 25.1). As with laparoscopic bariatric surgery, the primary outcome of interest with endobariatric interventions is sustained weight loss over time. However, the long-term positive health impact of these interventions is due more to the resolution of obesity-related comorbidities, particularly type 2 diabetes mellitus, hypertension, obstructive sleep apnea, osteoarthritis, polycystic ovarian syndrome, hyperlipidemia, and many others, than due solely to weight loss per se. As a result, studies of endobariatric procedures have assessed a wide range of clinical outcomes and biochemical markers (Table 25.2). As with any procedure, these interventions are not without adverse effects, both mild and severe (Table 25.3).

TABLE 25.1 Endobariatric interventions.

	Intervention types	Specific interventions
ESG	Endoscogic sleeve gastroplasty	Restore device
		OverStitch
POSE	Primary obesity surgery endoluminal	POSE-1
		POSE-2
IGB	Intragastric balloon	Orbera
		Obalon
		Elipse
		ReShape Duo
		Spatz

Visceral and Ectopic Fat. **https://doi.org/10.1016/B978-0-12-822186-0.00005-5**

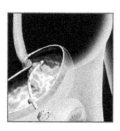
Aspire Assist

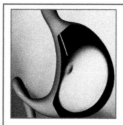
Ellipse Balloon

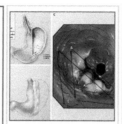
Endoscopic Sleeve Gastoplasy Apollo Device

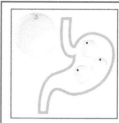
Obalon Balloon

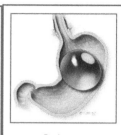
Orbera

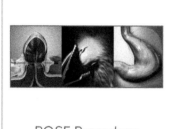
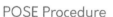
POSE Procedure

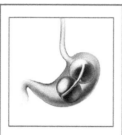
Reshape

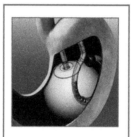
Spatz Balloon

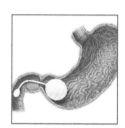
Transpyloric Shuttle

FIGURE 25.1 Currently available endoluminal procedures and devices for weight loss. Endoscopic sleeve gastroplasty (ESG), POSE, and intragastric balloons (IGBs) are highlighted in orange, green, and red, respectively. *With permission from Elsevier, Mechanick JI, Apovian C, Brethauer S, et al. Clinical practice guidelines for the perioperative nutrition, metabolic, and nonsurgical support of patients undergoing bariatric procedures—2019 update: cosponsored by American Association of Clinical Endocrinologists/American College of Endocrinology, The Obesity Society, American Society for Metabolic & Bariatric Surgery, Obesity Medicine Association, and American Society of Anesthesiologists. Surg Obes Relat Dis. February 2020;16(2):175–247.*

Therefore, in this chapter, we will review the three most well-described types of endoluminal interventions (ESG, POSE, and IGB) that work through the mechanism of gastric volume reduction, which means reducing the intraluminal space to induce earlier satiety and consequent weight loss (Fig. 25.4). For each of these interventions, we will briefly describe the procedure, then review the existing evidence for each. We first look to randomized controlled trials for evidence, followed by meta-analyses of observational trials, and finally observational case series. The structures and outcomes of these studies are heterogeneous, so direct comparisons on a wide range of outcomes is not possible. The most commonly reported outcome is percent total body weight loss (%TBWL), so that will serve as the primary comparative metric between these different approaches. Additional metabolic biomarkers are published with much less regularity, making comparisons challenging, but we will highlight certain markers of interest for each intervention. Finally, reporting of serious adverse events is relatively consistent, allowing for direct comparisons across intervention types. The end result of this survey is an evidence map (Table 25.4) which can serve as both a guide to the current evidence as well as a roadmap for future areas of investigation in this relatively new and evolving field.

Endoscopic sleeve gastroplasty

The concept of endoscopic suturing to achieve gastric volume reduction is not new. Since the first reports of sleeve gastrectomy were published in 2003 [1], investigators have sought to achieve similar results with less invasive endoscopic techniques, which have continued to evolve over the past two decades.

The first attempts to plicate the stomach using a suction-based suturing device (Restore device, Bard, Franklin Lakes, NJ) were shown to be technically feasible [2] and were able to achieve short-term weight loss (average BMI reduction of 4.0 kg/m2; %TBWL not reported), but these benefits were not durable. The sutures used in this device were partial-thickness, which resulted in 13 of 18 patients losing the plications at 1-year follow-up [3]. Despite these early technical obstacles, however, the stage was set for newer devices that could provide more durable results.

TABLE 25.2 Measures for possible effects of endobariatric interventions.

Measures of visceral and ectopic fat	Abbreviation
Total body weight loss (%)	%TBWL
Excess weight loss (%)	%EWL
Weight (kg)	
Body Mass index (kg/m2)	BMI
Waist circumference (cm)	WC
Waist-to-hip ratio	WHR
Metabolic biomarkers	**Abbreviation**
Systolic and diastolic blood pressure (mean)	SBP/DBP
Satiety threshold	
Leptin	
Ghrelin	
Glucagon-like peptide	GLP-1
Peptide YY	PYY
Adiponectin	
Blood glucose	BG
C-reactive protein	CRP
Resting metabolic rate	RMR
Resting metabolic rate adjusted for mass	RMR/Mass
Resting metabolic rate adjusted for fat-free mass	RMR/FFM
Homeostatic model assessment for insulin resistance	HOMA-IR
Liver function tests	LFTs
Liver volume	
Hepatic steatosis/Fibrosis	
Nonalcoholic fatty liver disease activity score	NAS

The current evolution of this approach is called ESG (Fig. 25.2). This procedure utilizes an endoscopic suturing device (OverStitch, Apollo Endosurgery, Austin, TX) to plicate the greater curve and reduce intragastric volume by up to 70%. This is performed under general anesthesia as a same-day procedure [4]. Early case series reported promising weight loss results, with TBWL results ranging between 14.9% and 18.7% [4–8]. From a technical standpoint, several variations of ESG exist, depending on the suture pattern and length of greater curvature included in the plication [7–11].

Meta-analyses

Two major systematic reviews with meta-analyses have been published on ESG (Table 25.4). Singh et al. [12] pooled eight studies (all observational, no controlled or randomized controlled trials) with a total of 1859 patients. TBWL was 14.9% [95% CI: 13.8–15.9] at 6 months, 16.4% [15.2–17.6] at 12 months, and 20.0% [16.9–23.1] at 24 months. Severe adverse events (SAEs) occurred in 2.3% [95% CI: 1.3–4.0] of cases, and included upper gastrointestinal bleeding (0.8%), perigastric fluid collection (0.7%), severe abdominal pain (0.7%), perforation (0.5%), and postprocedure fever (0.5%). Three patients from one study (0.16%) required reversal of ESG due to persistent symptoms. Hedjoudje et al. [13] pooled 8 studies (three retrospective cohort, five prospective cohort, no controlled or randomized controlled trials) with a total of 1772 patients. TBWL was 15.1% [95% CI, 14.3–16.0] at 6 months, 16.5% [15.2–17.8] at 12 months, and 17.2% [14.6–19.7] at 18–24 months. SAEs occurred in 2.2% [95% CI, 1.6–3.1] of cases, and included pain/nausea requiring hospitalization (1.1%), upper gastrointestinal bleeding (0.6%), and perigastric leak or fluid collection (0.5%).

TABLE 25.3 Adverse effects of endobariatric interventions.

Mild adverse effects

Heartburn

Bloating

Nausea/vomiting

Abdominal pain

Constipation

Balloon loss (due to emesis or deflation)

Diarrhea

Severe adverse effects

Fever

Severe pain

Esophagitis

Intraluminal bleeding

Extraluminal bleeding

Gastric microperforation/perigastric fluid collection

Gastric perforation/peritonitis

Pleural effusion

Liver abscess

Readmission

Need for repeat procedure

Need for reversal of procedure

Small bowel obstruction

Death

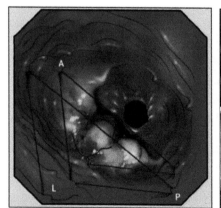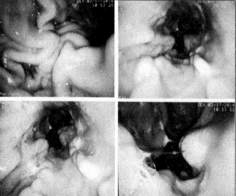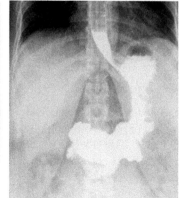

FIGURE 25.2 Illustration of suture pattern, endoscopic and radiographic views of endoscopic sleeve gastroplasty (ESG). *With permission of Revista Española de Enfermedades Digestivas. From López-Nava Breviere G, Bautista-Castaño I, Fernández-Corbelle JP, Trell M. Endoscopic sleeve gastroplasty (the Apollo method): a new approach to obesity management. Rev Esp Enferm Dig. 2016 April;108(4):201-6. doi: 10.17235/reed.2016.3988/ 2015. PMID: 26900986.*

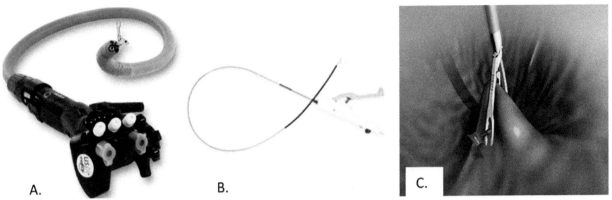

FIGURE 25.3 Instrumentation and creation of a single plication for the POSE procedure. *With permission from Elsevier, López-Nava G, Bautista-Castaño I, Jimenez A, de Grado T, Fernandez-Corbelle JP. The Primary Obesity Surgery Endolumenal (POSE) procedure: 1-year patient weight loss and safety outcomes. Surg Obes Relat Dis. July–August 2015;11(4):861–865.*

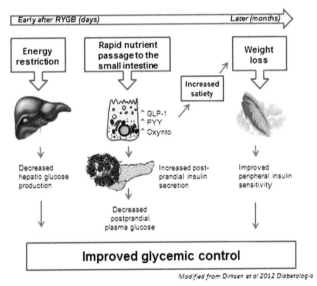

FIGURE 25.4 Mechanisms for weight loss and diabetes amelioration after bariatric surgery. *With permission from Elsevier, Holst JJ, Madsbad S, Bojsen-Møller KN, Svane MS, Jørgensen NB, Dirksen C, Martinussen C. Mechanisms in bariatric surgery: Gut hormones, diabetes resolution, and weight loss. Surg Obes Relat Dis. May 2018;14(5):708–714. doi: 10.1016/j.soard.2018.03.003. Epub 2018 Mar 8. PMID: 29776493; PMCID: PMC5974695.*

Case series

Follow-up results up to 5 years have recently been published by Sharaiha et al. [14], who reported on 216 patients in a single-center prospective cohort undergoing ESG between 2013 and 2019. Five-year follow-up was available for 38 patients with mean TBWL of 15.9% [95% CI: 11.7–20.5], with 90% of patients maintaining 5% TBWL and 61% of patients maintaining 10% TBWL. Patient compliance with follow-up, endoscopist experience, TBWL at 1 month, and younger age were associated with greater TBWL outcomes. Adjunct pharmacotherapy was added in 27% of patients at a median of 5 months (IQR: 3–9 months) post-procedure after showing weight regain. Repeat ESG was performed in 6% of patients for weight regain or stabilization at a median of 24 months (range: 12–51 months); in these patients, their mean TBWL at the time of repeat ESG was 21.5% [SD: 11%] with a mean weight regain of 2.3% TBWL. The most common mild adverse events were heartburn for up to 3 weeks (25% of patients), nausea/vomiting requiring antiemetics or intravenous hydration (19%), epigastric pain persisting after 24 h (31%), and constipation requiring over-the-counter laxatives (29%). Moderate adverse events occurred in three (1.3%) patients, including pain requiring endoscopic reversal of the ESG (n = 1) and perigastric leak managed with antibiotics or percutaneous drainage (n = 2). There were no severe or fatal adverse events reported in this series.

TABLE 25.4 Evidence map of endobariatric interventions.

| Outcome | Intervention | Evidence type | | Notable observational case series |
		Randomized controlled trials (RCTs)	Meta-analyses	
%TBWL	Overstitch	None	20.0% at 24 months (n = 1859 pts, 8 studies) [12]	15.9% at 60 months (n = 213 pts) [14]
	POSE-1	5.0% versus 1.4% (P = .23) at 12 months (n = 332) [23]	17.2% at 18–24 months (n = 1772 pts, 8 studies) [13]	
		13.0% versus 5.3% (P < .01) at 12 months (n = 39) [26]	12.7% at 12–15 months (n = 613 pts, 7 studies) [24]	
	POSE-2	None	None	17.8% at 12 months (n = 46 pts) [22]
	Orbera	None	13.2% at 6 months (n = 5549 pts, 44 studies) [27]	
	Obalon	7.1% versus 5.1% (P = .008) at 6 months (n = 387 pts) [28]	None	
	Elipse	None	10.9% at 12 months (n = 2013 pts, 6 studies) [29]	
			12.0% at 4 months (n = 2152 pts, 7 studies) [30]	
SAEs	Overstitch	None	**2.3% (gastric perforation, bleeding, microperforation, fever) [12]**	
	POSE-1	9.5% versus 8.1% (P = .84) (bleeding, liver abscess) [23]	2.2% (severe pain/nausea, bleeding, microperforation) [13]	
	POSE-2	None	2.8% (bleeding, abscess, severe pain) [24]	8.6% (perforation, bleeding) [22]
	Orbera	None	None	
	Obalon	0.3% (bleeding ulcer) [28]	Esophagitis (2%–9%), balloon migration (0.5%–2.3%), Ulcer [27]	
	Elipse	None	0.2% (gastric perforation, small bowel obstruction) [29]	

Mild adverse events	Overstitch	None	**Pain (31%), constipation (29%), heartburn (25%), nausea/vomiting (19%) [14]**
	POSE-1	78% versus 55% (P < .001) (pain, nausea, vomiting) [23]	Pain (44%), Sore throat (26%), nausea (20%), vomiting (17%) [24]
	POSE-2	None	None
	Orbera	None	Early removal, reflux [27]
	Obalon	91% (pain 73%, nausea 56%, vomiting 17%, bleeding 5%) [28]	None
	Elipse	None	Early removal due to emesis or spontaneous deflation (< 0.1%) [29]
			Abdominal pain (38%), vomiting (30%), diarrhea (15%) [30]
			Not reported [22]

The largest single series in the literature comes from Alqahtani et al. [15] and included 1000 patients with 18 months of follow-up. Mean (SD) TBWL was 14.8% (8.5%). Significant weight loss of 5% TBWL was maintained at 1 year in 90% of patients completing follow-up. Adverse events included fever (0.5%), perigastric fluid collections with associated pleural effusions (0.4%), blood loss requiring IV hydration or transfusion (0.4%), and severe abdominal pain requiring readmission with conservative management (0.5%) or reversal of ESG (0.3%). The mechanisms for weight loss with ESG are not fully understood. Interestingly, multiple observations from repeat ESG procedures note that in many cases, the stitches are no longer intact, even if gastric volume remains reduced and weight loss is maintained [15,16]. Several case reports of nonfatal severe complications exist, including gastric perforation requiring emergent surgical intervention [17,18] and gallbladder perforation [19].

Metabolic effects

In regard to the effect of ESG (and all endobariatric procedures) on metabolic biomarkers, various mechanisms have been proposed, and this remains an active area of scientific inquiry. For example, bariatric surgery is very well established, but our understanding of its variable biomarker effects and mechanisms for weight loss and resolution of comorbidities remains incomplete (Fig. 25.5). Therefore, in endobariatrics, it remains to be seen to what extent these mechanisms may be similar or different to those for traditional bariatric surgery.

One human study has reported findings related to the metabolic and physiologic effects of ESG. Lopez-Nava et al. [20] compared ESG to laparoscopic sleeve gastrectomy (LSG) at baseline and 6 months in a nonrandomized cohort of 24 patients. LSG achieved greater TBWL than ESG (24.4% vs. 13.3%, $P < .001$), and the biochemical profiles of each procedure differed. Both ESG and LSG produced a significant decline in leptin levels at 6 months. Ghrelin, which is

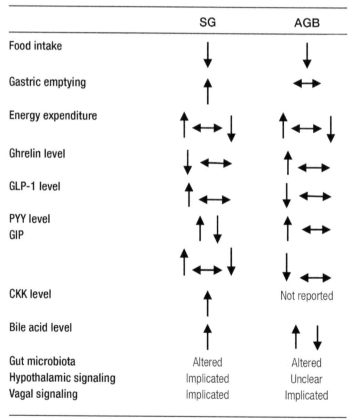

FIGURE 25.5 Effects on metabolic biomarkers after sleeve gastrectomy (SG) and adjustable gastric banding (AGB) surgery. *With permission from Wiley, Wang Y, Guo X, Lu X, Mattar S, Kassab G. Mechanisms of weight loss after sleeve gastrectomy and adjustable gastric banding: far more than just restriction. Obesity. November 2019;27(11):1776–1783. doi: 10.1002/oby.22623. Epub 2019 Sep 23. PMID: 31545007.*

Data obtained from both human and animal studies. More than one arrow means data are conflicting.
AGB, adjustable gastric banding; CKK, cholecystokinin; GIP, glucose-dependent insulinotropic peptide; GLP-1, glucagon-like peptide 1; PYY, peptide YY; SG, sleeve gastrectomy; ↑, increased; ↔ no change; ↓, decreased.

produced in the gastric fundus and rises in response to fasting and falls postprandially was examined in this study as it serves as a driver of hunger and is a potential mechanism adding to successful long-term weight loss. Despite leaving the gastric fundus intact, ESG prevented a compensatory increase in fasting ghrelin level after weight loss; a possible mechanism could be due to satiation-induced early meal termination and delay in gastric emptying. With LSG, ghrelin levels were significantly reduced, which is a well-established effect attributed to removal of the fundus. In contrast to ESG, which slows gastric emptying, LSG increases gastric emptying due to high intragastric pressure and faster propagation of antral propulsion waves. This delivers nutrients to the small bowel sooner and induces release of Glucagon-like peptide (GLP-1) and peptide YY (PYY). Lopez-Nava et al. [20] found increases in GLP-1 and PYY after LSG, but not after ESG. In ESG, therefore, a blunted incretin response was observed compared to LSG. Independent of the incretin response, the first phase insulin response and overall insulin sensitivity were also blunted in ESG compared to LSG. Adiponectin is a hormone produced primarily in adipose tissue (adipokine) that is involved in glucose regulation and fatty acid breakdown. Adiponectin decreases in obesity and increases during caloric restriction and, in this study, levels increased after LSG but not significantly following ESG. The significance of these findings is yet to be fully explained.

Primary obesity surgery endoluminal (POSE) procedure

The POSE procedure utilizes an endoscopic platform (USGI Medical, San Clemente, CA) to produce full-thickness plications of the gastric wall (Fig. 25.3). The original POSE procedure (POSE-1) created plications of the fundus and body [21]; this has been refined to both narrow the gastric diameter and shorten the vertical length of the stomach (referred to as the POSE-2 procedure) [22]. Motivation for the change in technique came from the results of the ESSENTIAL randomized controlled trial [23] which compared POSE-1 to sham endoscopy, and resulted in mean (SD) TBWL of 4.95% (7.04%) for intervention patients, which was not statistically significant when compared to TBWL of 1.38% (5.58%) for controls. The POSE-1 intervention arm did show a significant improvement in fasting blood glucose at 1 year compared to the control arm, but there were no differences seen in blood pressure, hemoglobin A1c, cholesterol, or triglycerides. With POSE-2, Lopez-Nava et al. reported mean (SD) TBWL of 17.8% (9.5%) at 12 months in an observational study of 46 patients [22].

Meta-analysis

Amid this evolution in the technique, one systematic review with meta-analysis has been published (Table 25.4). Singh et al. [24] conducted a meta-analysis assessing the original POSE (POSE-1). They included seven studies (two RCTs, five observational) with a total of 613 patients. Pooled mean TBWL at 12—15 months was 12.7% (95% CI: 8.1—17.2). The incidence of SAEs was 2.8%, including GI bleeding, extra-gastric bleeding, hepatic abscess, and severe pain, nausea, and vomiting. This was felt to fulfill the American Society for Gastrointestinal Endoscopy (ASGE) joint task force thresholds for safety and efficacy. Pooled analysis of POSE-2 outcomes has yet to be performed, as relatively few studies utilizing the revised technique have been published to date.

Metabolic effects

Espinos et al. [25] evaluated several physiologic, hormonal, and metabolic markers at 2, 6, and 15 months following POSE-1 in 18 patients with Class 1 or 2 obesity. Mean (SD) TBWL at 15 months was 19.1% (6.6%). Mean caloric intake capacity (as measured by standardized protein drink intake to the point of maximal satiation) was reduced from 901 kcal/meal at baseline to 473 kcal/meal at 2 months ($P < .001$), and trended upward but remained significantly reduced at 574 kcal/meal at 6 months ($P < .001$). Gastric emptying as assessed by scintigraphy at 2 month follow-up was delayed during the first postprandial hour; however, this reverted to normal at the 6-month mark. Leptin and fasting glucose levels were significantly reduced at the 2- and 6-month marks. Fasting ghrelin was significantly increased at both follow-up intervals, likely related to weight loss. Postprandial peptide-YY, a satiety-producing hormone released by the distal bowel that acts on the hypothalamus, increased at 2 and 6 months following POSE, and patients with postprandial PYY increase at 2 months were more likely to experience significant weight loss at 15 months. The MILEPOST randomized controlled trial [26] demonstrated significant reductions in satiety thresholds at 12 months in a 3:1 randomized set of 44 patients following POSE (n = 34) or diet/exercise only (n = 10). Mean TBWL at 12 months was 13.0% for POSE versus 5.3% for controls ($P = .01$). Satiety thresholds on POSE patients were reduced from 1176 kcal at baseline to 473 kcal at 2 months and 568 kcal at 12 months ($P < .001$). Thresholds in control patients were also significantly reduced from 861 kcal at baseline to 520 kcal at 12 months ($P < .05$). Between POSE and control groups, however, satiety thresholds did not differ significantly at any time point.

Intragastric balloon therapy

In contrast to the endoscopic plication approaches taken by ESG and POSE, intragastric balloon (IGB) interventions have a much longer and varied history, dating back to the 1980s in various forms. The current era of balloon therapy in the United States includes two FDA-approved IGBs still on the market (Orbera, Obalon) and one newer IGB in preapproval phase (Elipse) (Fig. 25.1). The ReShape Duo dual-balloon IGB is FDA-approved but is no longer marketed after its acquisition by Apollo Endosurgery, the maker of Orbera.

IGB types

Orbera is a single balloon that is placed under conscious sedation and filled with 400−700 mL of saline through a thin catheter under endoscopic vision. It is designed to be left in place for 6 months. Removal is performed endoscopically, with puncture aspiration of the fluid, and retrieval with a large grasper.

Obalon comprises up to three nitrogen gas-filled balloons (up to 250 mL volume each) that are placed in awake patients under fluoroscopic vision. The patient swallows a large capsule attached to a catheter, and X-ray confirms intragastric position. The balloon is then inflated to a pressure of 9−13 kPa, and the catheter is withdrawn. One to two additional balloons can be placed in the same manner in the following weeks. All 3 balloons are to be removed endoscopically at 6 months; they are first punctured for desufflation and then retrieved with a grasper.

The Elipse system is a bioabsorbable balloon consisting of a capsule connected to a thin catheter that is swallowed by awake patients in the outpatient setting. An X-ray confirms intragastric position, and the balloon is then filled with 550 mL of fluid. After approximately 4 months, the balloon dissolves and is passed through the gastrointestinal tract.

Meta-analyses and controlled trials

There have been multiple trials assessing the different intragastric balloon systems. The Orbera system has been studied in one meta-analysis and one randomized controlled trial. One RCT assessing the Obalon system has been published. Two meta-analyses have been published specifically examining the Elipse system. We will briefly review the evidence for each platform (Table 25.4).

Orbera

In the largest meta-analysis of the Orbera system, Kumar et al. [27] examined 44 studies with a pooled total of 5549 patients. Mean TBWL at 6 months was 13.2% [95% CI: 12.3−14.0]. The Orbera can accommodate a balloon filling volume (BFV) between 400 and 700 mL, and the studies in this analysis featured BFVs ranging between 500 and 700 mL. No significant effect of BFV was found in regard to weight loss outcomes; however, BFV greater than 600 mL was associated with significantly less esophagitis (2.4% vs. 9.4%, $P < .001$) and less device migration (0.5% vs. 2.3%, $P = .004$) compared to BFV less than 600 mL. The mechanism underlying the esophagitis effect is not clear, but may relate to a heavier balloon sitting differently in the stomach which results in less gastroesophageal reflux. The authors of this study concluded that a BFV of at least 600 mL is advisable for optimal outcomes with Orbera IGBs.

Obalon

The SMART trial [28] was a multicenter randomized sham-controlled trial of the Obalon system in 387 patients. Mean (SD) %TBWL at therapy completion was 7.1% (5.0%) in the intervention arm and 3.6% (5.1%) in the control arm, a statistically significant finding ($P = .0085$). Nonserious adverse events occurred in 91% of intervention patients, most commonly abdominal pain (73%), nausea (56%), vomiting (17%), and dyspepsia (17%).

Elipse

Vantanasiri et al. [29] and Ramai et al. [30] published meta-analyses of the Elipse system. Vantanasiri et al. pooled six studies with 2013 patients, finding a mean 6-month %TBWL of 12.8% (95% CI: 11.6%−13.9%) and 12-month %TBWL of 10.9% (95% CI: 5.0%−13.9%). The serious adverse event rate was 0.2%. One patient required surgical intervention for gastric perforation, and three developed small bowel obstruction requiring laparoscopic or endoscopic intervention. Three patients expelled their balloons early due to emesis, and nine patients experienced early spontaneous deflation. Ramai et al. pooled seven studies with a total of 2152 patients. Mean %TBWL at 4 months was 12% (95% CI: 10.1%−14.3%). Adverse events in both studies were rare and included. Nonserious adverse events included abdominal pain (38%), vomiting (30%), and diarrhea (15%).

Metabolic and visceral fat effects of intragastric balloons

There are a wide variety of IGB studies examining a wide variety of measures of metabolism, biomarkers, and body composition, making comparative analysis exploratory at this point. However, one particularly active area of interest with balloon interventions is in treating nonalcoholic fatty liver disease (NAFLD) and nonalcoholic steatohepatitis (NASH). These patients, particularly those with cirrhosis and bleeding diatheses, may be poor candidates for laparoscopic surgery, so an endoluminal intervention with minimal blood loss is a potentially beneficial and relatively low-risk option. Several other studies have assessed a variety of biochemical and physiologic characteristics. It should be noted that the metabolic effects of IGB are related to the degree of weight loss achieved and, to date, there are no other mechanisms (gut hormones, incretins) that are altered directly as a result of balloon placement.

NAFLD and NASH

Chandan et al. [31] pooled nine studies using the Orbera system, with a total of 442 intragastric balloon placements. Six-month outcomes demonstrated improvement in liver steatosis in 79% (95%CI: 66%−88%) of patients in three studies, and improvement in NAFLD Activity Score (NAS) in 84% (95% CI: 61%−94%) of patients in two studies. Radiographic reduction in liver volume was seen in 94% (95% CI: 81%−98%) of patients in three studies. The Homeostatic Model Assessment for Insulin Resistance (HOMA-IR) score, which measures insulin resistance, was improved in 65% (95% CI: 54%−74%) of patients in three studies. Liver enzymes, including AST, ALT, and GGT, tended to decrease post-intervention, but pooled results were not statistically significant. Bazerbachi et al. [32] studied 21 patients with nonalcoholic steatohepatitis undergoing Orbera placement at a single center. Pre- and post-intervention liver biopsies were obtained, in addition to measurement of NAS (Range: 0−5), weight, transaminases, lipid levels, fasting glucose, hemoglobin A1c, and hepatic steatosis and early fibrosis measured with magnetic resonance elastography (MRE). All patients had histologic liver fibrosis at baseline, but none had cirrhosis. NAS improved from a median of 4 (range: 2−5) to 1 (range: 0−4) after the intervention. Histologic fibrosis improved in 15% of patients, was unchanged in 60%, and worsened in 25%. There was no significant difference in waist-to-hip ratio. The authors report that when applying FDA criteria for resolution of NASH (lack of fatty liver disease or simple steatosis without steatohepatitis, NAS score of 0−1 for inflammation, NAS score of 0 for ballooning, and no progression of hepatic fibrosis), 50% of the study patients were able to achieve these goals post-intervention.

Metabolism and body composition

Gazdzinska et al. [33] assessed 21 patients with mean (SD) BMI 49.5 (7.3) at a single-center undergoing placement of the Orbera balloon, and assessed changes at 6 months in body composition, resting metabolic rate (RMR), and RMR adjusted for mass and fat-free mass (RMR/FFM). With IGB therapy, they noted statistically significant mean decreases in BMI of 9.4%, in body mass of 9.5%, in fat content of 13.8% and in fat-free mass of 5.4%. Mean RMR also decreased from 2500 kcal/day to 2140 kcal/day. RMR/mass and RMR/FFM did not change significantly.

Guedes et al. [34] studied 42 patients at a single center undergoing Orbera or Spatz (a fluid-filled, adjustable IGB not available in the United States) therapy for 6 months. Significant reductions were seen in levels of leptin, high-sensitivity CRP, glucose, insulin, HOMA-IR, and triglycerides. Waist-to-hip ratio decreased 3.7% ($P = .0001$).

Reimao et al. [35] examined 40 patients undergoing Orbera placement, and found significant reductions in mean (SD) body fat mass (36 (5) kg at baseline versus 25 (8) kg at 6 months, $P < .001$), fat area (161 (22) versus 124 (27) cm2, $P < .001$), and weight (90 (12) versus 76 (15) kg, $P < .001$), with no significant change in lean body mass (49 (13) versus 47 (15) kg, $P = .31$) or fat-free body mass (53 (12) versus 52 (11) kg, $P = .48$).

Conclusion

Interventional treatment of obesity and metabolic disorders continues to evolve, and the full range of possible therapies has begun to include an increasing number of endoscopic and nonsurgical treatments that work by reducing the effective volume of the gastric reservoir. The primary outcome of interest remains TBWL, although resolution of comorbidities and metabolic biomarkers are an important and active area of research.

To briefly summarize the three major approaches, TBWL with ESG is 15%−20% after 2−5 years, with a severe adverse event rate of 2.3%. TBWL with POSE has a wider range (5%−17%) as the technique has evolved, with a severe adverse event rate of 2.8%. The Obalon balloon demonstrated 7% TBWL in a randomized controlled trial, while meta-analyses of observational data for the Orbera and Elipse yielded 13.2% and 10.9% TBWL, respectively. Most intragastric balloon patients (90%) experience mild adverse events, most commonly abdominal pain, nausea, vomiting and bloating. SAEs with IGB devices appear to be less common than with ESG or POSE as there is a lower risk of gastric perforation, although balloon migration and bowel obstruction have been described.

The relative effects of ESG, POSE and IGBs on metabolic parameters, fat content, and body composition have yet to be fully elucidated in the literature. Ultimately, the goal of these interventions is not just to reduce body adiposity, but to resolve comorbidities. Several studies have assessed a variety of metabolic markers. Both ESG and POSE delay gastric emptying, at least temporarily, as opposed to LSG, which increases gastric emptying and therefore provides early stimulation of the hindgut and L-cell mass that produce GLP-1 and PYY. ESG, POSE, and LSG all decrease leptin levels and fasting glucose, likely as a response to weight loss. LSG is well-known to decrease ghrelin levels due to fundectomy; in limited studies, ESG appeared to prevent an increase in ghrelin, while POSE resulted in ghrelin increase. Additionally, GLP-1, PYY, and adiponectin were all increased after LSG but not after ESG. PYY increased after POSE.

The role of IGBs in halting the progression or reversing nonalcoholic fatty liver disease and NASH remains an area of close interest, as single studies suggest that up to 50% of well-selected patients are able to achieve resolution of early-stage NASH; however, further study of this effect in randomized controlled trials is needed. Studies of body composition and metabolic rate changes after IGB placement have shown results that are to be expected given the degree of weight loss achieved with IGBs.

First-line treatment for obesity and obesity-related comorbidities remains adhering to a disciplined diet and regular physical activity. Although these can be highly effective in the short term, particularly with intensive, face-to-face programs, weight regain after these programs is nearly universal, as it is difficult to maintain such behaviors after the body's homeostatic set point has become accustomed to the obese state. Medications for obesity can only be prescribed for finite periods of time, although they too can be highly effective in the short run. Bariatric surgery is highly effective and durable, although in the United States, fewer than 1% of qualifying individuals actually go on to receive bariatric surgery. This is for a wide variety of reasons, including insurance restrictions, reluctance of providers to refer patients for these interventions, and reluctance on the part of patients to pursue an elective operation. Given this landscape, endoluminal gastric volume reduction interventions offer an intriguing new therapeutic modality for those patients who have tried and failed behavioral and medical therapies and who are not a candidate for bariatric surgery. In particular, patients with severe comorbidities placing them at heightened perioperative risk are the ideal candidates for these interventions. The field of endobariatrics continues to evolve, and as the evidence continues to grow, our understanding of which intervention is the right one for each patient will continue to evolve as well.

References

[1] Regan JP, Inabnet WB, Gagner M, Pomp A. Early experience with two-stage laparoscopic Roux-en-Y gastric bypass as an alternative in the super-super obese patient. Obes Surg December 2003;13(6):861–4.

[2] Brethauer SA, Chand B, Schauer PR, Thompson CC. Transoral gastric volume reduction for weight management: technique and feasibility in 18 patients. Surg Obes Relat Dis November–December 2010;6(6):689–94.

[3] Brethauer SA, Chand B, Schauer PR, Thompson CC. Transoral gastric volume reduction as intervention for weight management: 12-month follow-up of TRIM trial. Surg Obes Relat Dis May–June 2012;8(3):296–303.

[4] Sartoretto A, Sui Z, Hill C, Dunlap M, et al. Endoscopic sleeve gastroplasty (ESG) is a reproducible and effective endoscopic bariatric therapy suitable for widespread clinical adoption: a large, international multicenter study. Obes Surg 2018;28(7):1812–21.

[5] Sharaiha RZ, Kumta NA, Saumoy M, Desai AP, et al. Endoscopic sleeve gastroplasty significantly reduces body mass index and metabolic complications in obese patients. Clin Gastroenterol Hepatol 2017;15(4):504–10.

[6] Lopez-Nava G, Sharaiha RZ, Vargas EJ, Bazerbachi F, et al. Endoscopic sleeve gastroplasty for obesity: a multicenter study of 248 patients with 24 months follow-up. Obes Surg 2017;27(10):2649–55.

[7] Kumar N, Abu Dayyeh BK, Lopez-Nava Breviere G, Galvao Neto MP, et al. Endoscopic sutured gastroplasty: procedure evolution from first-in-man cases through current technique. Surg Endosc 2018;32(4):2159–64.

[8] Graus Morales J, Crespo Pérez L, Marques A, Marín Arribas B, et al. Modified endoscopic gastroplasty for the treatment of obesity. Surg Endosc 2018;32(9):3936–42.

[9] de Moura DTH, de Moura EGH, Thompson CC. Endoscopic sleeve gastroplasty: from whence we came and where we are going. World J Gastrointest Endosc May 16, 2019;11(5):322–8.

[10] Marrache MK, Al-Sabban A, Itani MI, Sartoretto A, Kumbhari V. Endoscopic sleeve gastroplasty by use of a novel suturing pattern, which allays concerns for revisional bariatric surgery. VideoGIE February 7, 2020;5(4):133–4.

[11] Jain D, Bhandari BS, Arora A, Singhal S. Endoscopic sleeve gastroplasty - a new tool to manage obesity. Clin Endosc 2017;50:552–61.

[12] Singh S, Hourneaux de Moura DT, Khan A, Bilal M, Ryan MB, Thompson CC. Safety and efficacy of endoscopic sleeve gastroplasty worldwide for treatment of obesity: a systematic review and meta-analysis. Surg Obes Relat Dis February 2020;16(2):340–51.

[13] Hedjoudje A, Abu Dayyeh BK, Cheskin LJ, Adam A, Neto MG, Badurdeen D, Morales JG, Sartoretto A, Nava GL, Vargas E, Sui Z, Fayad L, Farha J, Khashab MA, Kalloo AN, Alqahtani AR, Thompson CC, Kumbhari V. Efficacy and safety of endoscopic sleeve gastroplasty: a systematic review and meta-analysis. Clin Gastroenterol Hepatol May 2020;18(5):1043–53. e4.

[14] Sharaiha RZ, Hajifathalian K, Kumar R, Saunders K, Mehta A, Ang B, Skaf D, Shah S, Herr A, Igel L, Dawod Q, Dawod E, Sampath K, Carr-Locke D, Brown R, Cohen D, Dannenberg AJ, Mahadev S, Shukla A, Aronne LJ. Five-year outcomes of endoscopic sleeve gastroplasty for the treatment of obesity. Clin Gastroenterol Hepatol October 2020;;1:S1542–3565. https://doi.org/10.1016/j.cgh.2020.09.055 (20)31385–9.

[15] Alqahtani A, Al-Darwish A, Mahmoud AE, Alqahtani YA, Elahmedi M. Short-term outcomes of endoscopic sleeve gastroplasty in 1000 consecutive patients. Gastrointest Endosc June 2019;89(6):1132–8.

[16] Runge TM, Yang J, Fayad L, Itani MI, Dunlap M, Koller K, Mullin GE, Simsek C, Badurdeen D, Kalloo AN, Khashab MA, Kumhbari V. Anatomical configuration of the stomach post-endoscopic sleeve gastroplasty (ESG)-What are the sutures doing? Obes Surg May 2020;30(5):2056–60.

[17] Whitfield EP, Leeds SG, Kerlee KR, Ward MA. Endoscopic sleeve gastroplasty requiring emergent partial gastrectomy. SAVE Proc. June 22, 2020;33(4):635–6.

[18] Surve A, Cottam D, Medlin W, Richards C, Belnap L. A video case report of gastric perforation following endoscopic sleeve gastroplasty and its surgical treatment. Obes Surg October 2019;29(10):3410–1.

[19] de Siqueira Neto J, de Moura DTH, Ribeiro IB, Barrichello SA, Harthorn KE, Thompson CC. Gallbladder perforation due to endoscopic sleeve gastroplasty: a case report and review of literature. World J Gastrointest Endosc March 16, 2020;12(3):111–8.

[20] Lopez-Nava G, Negi A, Bautista-Castaño I, Rubio MA, Asokkumar R. Gut and metabolic hormones changes after endoscopic sleeve gastroplasty (ESG) vs. Laparoscopic sleeve gastrectomy (LSG). Obes Surg July 2020;30(7):2642–51.

[21] Espinós JC, Turró R, Mata A, Cruz M, da Costa M, Villa V, Buchwald JN, Turró J. Early experience with the incisionless operating Platform™ (IOP) for the treatment of obesity : the primary obesity surgery endolumenal (POSE) procedure. Obes Surg September 2013;23(9):1375–83.

[22] Lopez Nava G, Asokkumar R, Laster J, Negi A, Normand E, Fook-Chong S, Bautista-Castaño I. Primary obesity surgery endoluminal (POSE-2) procedure for treatment of obesity in clinical practice. Endoscopy November 2021;53(11):1169–73. https://doi.org/10.1055/a-1324-8498. Epub November 27, 2020. PMID: 33246352].

[23] Sullivan S, Swain JM, Woodman G, Antonetti M, De La Cruz-Muñoz N, Jonnalagadda SS, Ujiki M, Ikramuddin S, Ponce J, Ryou M, Reynoso J, Chhabra R, Sorenson GB, Clarkston WK, Edmundowicz SA, Eagon JC, Mullady DK, Leslie D, Lavin TE, Thompson CC. Randomized sham-controlled trial evaluating efficacy and safety of endoscopic gastric plication for primary obesity: the ESSENTIAL trial. Obesity February 2017;25(2):294–301.

[24] Singh S, Bazarbashi AN, Khan A, Chowdhry M, Bilal M, de Moura DTH, Jirapinyo P, Thakkar S, Thompson CC. Primary obesity surgery endoluminal (POSE) for the treatment of obesity: a systematic review and meta-analysis. Surg Endosc February 1, 2021. https://doi.org/10.1007/s00464-020-08267-z. Epub ahead of print. PMID: 33523277].

[25] Espinós JC, Turró R, Moragas G, Bronstone A, Buchwald JN, Mearin F, Mata A, Uchima H, Turró J, Delgado-Aros S. Gastrointestinal physiological changes and their relationship to weight loss following the POSE procedure. Obes Surg May 2016;26(5):1081–9.

[26] Miller K, Turró R, Greve JW, Bakker CM, Buchwald JN, Espinós JC. MILEPOST multicenter randomized controlled trial: 12-month weight loss and satiety outcomes after pose [SM] vs. Medical therapy. Obes Surg February 2017;27(2):310–22.

[27] Kumar N, Bazerbachi F, Rustagi T, McCarty TR, Thompson CC, Galvao Neto MP, Zundel N, Wilson EB, Gostout CJ, Abu Dayyeh BK. The influence of the Orbera intragastric balloon filling volumes on weight loss, tolerability, and adverse events: a systematic review and meta-analysis. Obes Surg September 2017;27(9):2272–8.

[28] Sullivan S, Swain J, Woodman G, Edmundowicz S, Hassanein T, Shayani V, Fang JC, Noar M, Eid G, English WJ, Tariq N, Larsen M, Jonnalagadda SS, Riff DS, Ponce J, Early D, Volckmann E, Ibele AR, Spann MD, Krishnan K, Bucobo JC, Pryor A. Randomized sham-controlled trial of the 6-month swallowable gas-filled intragastric balloon system for weight loss. Surg Obes Relat Dis December 2018;14(12):1876–89.

[29] Vantanasiri K, Matar R, Beran A, Jaruvongvanich V. The efficacy and safety of a procedureless gastric balloon for weight loss: a systematic review and meta-analysis. Obes Surg September 2020;30(9):3341–6.

[30] Ramai D, Singh J, Mohan BP, Madedor O, Brooks OW, Barakat M, et al. Influence of the Elipse intragastric balloon on obesity and metabolic profile: a systematic review and meta-analysis. J Clin Gastroenterol 2021;55(10):836–41. https://doi.org/10.1097/MCG.0000000000001484.

[31] Chandan S, Mohan BP, Khan SR, Facciorusso A, Ramai D, Kassab LL, Bhogal N, Asokkumar R, Lopez-Nava G, McDonough S, Adler DG. Efficacy and safety of intragastric balloon (IGB) in non-alcoholic fatty liver disease (NAFLD): a comprehensive review and meta-analysis. Obes Surg January 6, 2021. https://doi.org/10.1007/s11695-020-05084-0 [Epub ahead of print].

[32] Bazerbachi F, Vargas EJ, Rizk M, Maselli DB, Mounajjed T, Venkatesh SK, Watt KD, Port JD, Basu R, Acosta A, Hanouneh I, Gara N, Shah M, Mundi M, Clark M, Grothe K, Storm AC, Levy MJ, Abu Dayyeh BK. Intragastric balloon placement induces significant metabolic and histologic improvement in patients with nonalcoholic steatohepatitis. Clin Gastroenterol Hepatol January 2021;19(1):146–54. https://doi.org/10.1016/j.cgh.2020.04.068. e4.

[33] Gaździńska AP, Mojkowska A, Zieliński P, Gazdzinski SP. Changes in resting metabolic rate and body composition due to intragastric balloon therapy. Surg Obes Relat Dis January 2020;16(1):34–9.

[34] Guedes MR, Fittipaldi-Fernandez RJ, Diestel CF, Klein MRST. Impact of intragastric balloon treatment on adipokines, cytokines, and metabolic profile in obese individuals. Obes Surg August 2019;29(8):2600–8.

[35] Reimão SM, da Silva MER, Nunes GC, Mestieri LHM, Dos Santos RF, de Moura EGH. Improvement of body composition and quality of life following intragastric balloon. Obes Surg June 2018;28(6):1806–8.

[36] Holst JJ, Madsbad S, Bojsen-Møller KN, Svane MS, Jørgensen NB, Dirksen C, Martinussen C. Mechanisms in bariatric surgery: Gut hormones, diabetes resolution, and weight loss. Surg Obes Relat Dis May 2018;14(5):708−14. https://doi.org/10.1016/j.soard.2018.03.003. Epub 2018 Mar 8. PMID: 29776493; PMCID: PMC5974695.

[37] Wang Y, Guo X, Lu X, Mattar S, Kassab G. Mechanisms of weight loss after sleeve gastrectomy and adjustable gastric banding: far more than just restriction. Obesity November 2019;27(11):1776−83. https://doi.org/10.1002/oby.22623. Epub 2019 Sep 23. PMID: 31545007.

Chapter 26

Roux-en-Y gastric bypass: influence on adipose tissue and metabolic homeostasis

Christopher P. Menzel, Charles R. Flynn and Wayne J. English

Vanderbilt University Medical Center, Department of Surgery, Nashville, TN, United States

Introduction

Obesity is a complex disease that is increasing at an ominously high rate worldwide. The Centers for Disease Control (CDC) in the United States reported a prevalence of obesity of 42.4% in 2018 [1]. The World Health Organization (WHO) reported in 2016 that nearly 40% of the worldwide population are overweight and 13% are obese. This number has tripled over the past four decades. In all regions, aside from sub-Saharan Africa and certain regions of Asia, overweight individuals outnumber underweight individuals decisively [2].

Obesity exerts deleterious effects on overall health, longevity, and quality of human life, and with the increasing numbers of overweight and obese individuals, health professionals worldwide have been confronted with increasing burden of managing obesity-related comorbidities including heart disease, type 2 diabetes mellitus, stroke, and certain types of cancer. Without doubt, we are amid an epidemic that silently began nearly half a century ago.

Patients undergoing bariatric surgery can achieve durable sustained weight loss that can lead to significant reduction or resolution of obesity-related comorbidities. Because of the profound improvements on obesity-related metabolic conditions, these surgical procedures are frequently referred to as metabolic and bariatric procedures. Obese individuals have increased lipolytic activity in visceral fat contributing to increased cardiovascular and metabolic risk. This chapter will explore mechanisms by which the gold standard of metabolic and bariatric operations, Roux-en-Y gastric bypass (RYGB), can reverse the deleterious effects of adiposopathy and provide metabolic benefits.

RYGB procedure description

RYGB is considered a restrictive and malabsorptive surgery of the stomach, duodenum, and jejunum within the small intestine (Fig. 26.1). It involves creating a small gastric pouch measuring approximately 15–30 mL causing a restriction in oral intake.

Malabsorption is also seen due to reconfiguring the small intestine resulting in nutrient diversion to the small intestine, thus bypassing the duodenum and proximal jejunum. The jejunum, approximately 50 cm distal to the ligament of Treitz, is divided, and the proximal end is reconnected 100–150 cm distally to reestablish bile and pancreatic enzyme flow into the distal small intestine. The gastrojejunostomy is then created by attaching the initially divided distal end of the jejunum to the gastric pouch. The small intestine from the ligament of Treitz to the jejunojejunostomy is referred to as the biliopancreatic limb, or nonalimentary limb. The segment of intestine between the gastric pouch and jejunojejunostomy is known as the Roux limb, or alimentary limb (Fig. 26.2). The remaining small intestine from the jejunojejunostomy to the ileocecal valve is referred to as the common channel.

Mechanisms of RYGB

The mechanisms by which the RYGB causes weight loss is threefold: calorie restriction, malabsorption, and hormonal influences [3]. The calorie restriction is due to creating an approximately 25 mm anastomosis in which the gastric pouch

Visceral and Ectopic Fat. https://doi.org/10.1016/B978-0-12-822186-0.00001-8

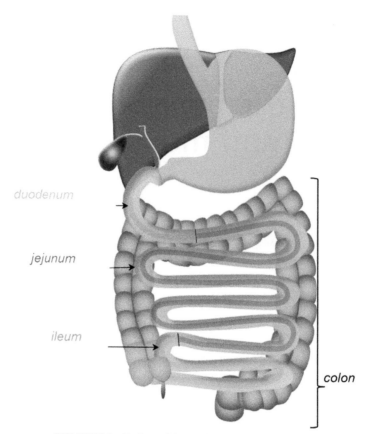

FIGURE 26.1 Regions of the small intestine before surgery.

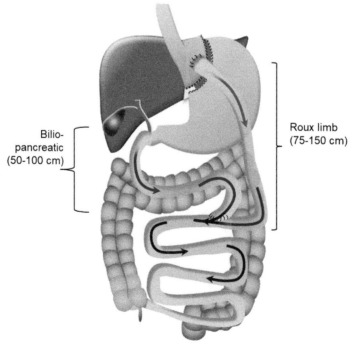

FIGURE 26.2 The RYGB surgery involves the creation of a gastric pouch, a biliopancreatic limb, a jejunojejunostomy, and a gastrojejunostomy that reroute the flow of food (alimentary flow; blue arrow) and reroute more distally the flow of gallbladder bile and pancreatic secretions nonalimentary flow; red arrow) such that food and bile meet more distally (purple) down the cephalocaudal axis.

holds approximately one ounce of fluid before reaching the anastomosis resulting in restrictive outflow that prohibits consumption of larger than about 1—2 ounces after surgery.

Restriction results in limited gastric pouch distensibility, which has been implicated in a neural pathway involved with the baroreceptor, or stretch, reflex that signals to decrease the physiologic receptive relaxation seen in native, uncut gastric tissue. It has been reported that a greater degree of gastric pouch distention and increased gastrojejunostomy anastomosis size are factors that are associated with weight regain [3].

The second mechanism is malabsorption. There is typically between 150 and 200 cm of small intestine bypassed in the RYGB, and the common channel is the only segment of the small intestine that possesses the ability for absorption due to the changes in anatomy. This results in decreased ability to absorb fats, carbohydrates, proteins, vitamins, and micronutrients, which ultimately leads to increased utilization of stored calories from glycogen, predominantly in the liver and muscle, and adipose tissue. The diversion of gastric secretions and bile immediately into the midjejunal segment results in complex neurohormonal, bile acid, and microbiome alterations that affect hunger, satiety, insulin sensitivity, and glucose homeostasis (Fig. 26.3).

Finally, and most importantly, is the gastrointestinal hormonal alteration seen affecting the gut—brain axis, which is now believed to be the predominant mechanism for weight loss and cardiometabolic improvements after RYGB. Two hypotheses have been proposed to explain the effects of RYGB on T2DM, the foregut and hindgut theory (Fig. 26.4). The foregut theory proposes that exclusion of the proximal segment of the small intestine reduces or suppresses the secretion of antiincretin hormones, leading to improvement of glucose homeostasis. The hindgut theory proposes that T2DM control results from the more rapid delivery of nutrients to the distal small intestine, thereby enhancing the release of incretin hormones such as glucagon-like peptide-1 (GLP-1) [4].

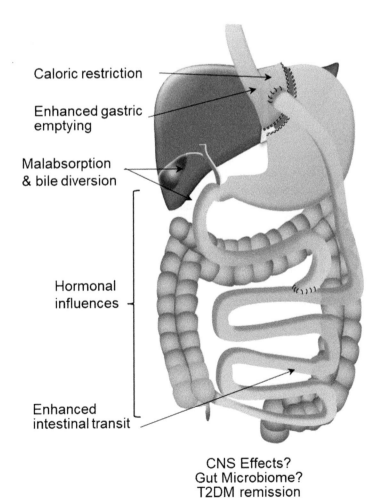

Caloric restriction

Enhanced gastric emptying

Malabsorption & bile diversion

Hormonal influences

Enhanced intestinal transit

CNS Effects?
Gut Microbiome?
T2DM remission

FIGURE 26.3 RYGB remodels several aspects of gut anatomy that serve to both impart and reinforce a reduction of food intake (caloric restriction and enhanced gastric emptying), modify how food is digested (distal bile diversion), alter gastrokine and enterokine secretion (hormonal influences), and enhance the transit of food.

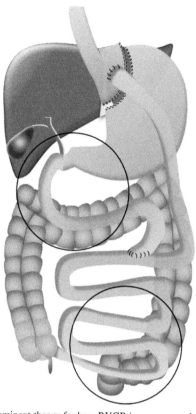

Foregut theory :
Exclusion of alimentary
flow reduces or
suppressed secretion
of anti-incretins

Hindgut theory:
A more rapid delivery of undigested
nutrients to the distal small
intestine and colon
enhances incretin
secretion

FIGURE 26.4 In one prominent theory for how RYGB improves metabolic control and instills weight loss, the foregut theory describes decreased or suppressed secretion of antiincretins that negatively affect insulin secretion. In the hindgut theory, the amplified delivery of bile and food to the small bowel enhances incretin secretion.

Multiple studies have outlined that, through multiple mechanisms, intestinal hormone such as glucagon-like peptide 1 (GLP-1), peptide YY (PYY), and gastric inhibitory peptide (GIP) drastically change in concentration immediately after RYGB and exert their respective effects on insulin resistance, neurohormonal feedback, and adipose tissue utilization, among other mechanisms [5]. Dozens of peptides, hormones, and transcription factors have been shown to be specifically affected, and many more are thought to play a major role in adipocyte function including various adipokines, bile acids, and inflammatory-modulating cytokines [6].

Endocrine and neural signaling alterations occur by creating a small gastric pouch. The gastric fundus and body are separated from the gastric pouch, which divide vagal nerve fibers that begin to decussate from the anterior and posterior vagal nerve trunks at the hiatus. The resulting disruption in neuroendocrine communication have been reported to impact appetite and satiety.

These complex mechanisms together lead to not only significant weight loss but also resolution or significant improvement of obesity-related comorbidities.

RYGB—effect on weight loss and obesity-related comorbidities

RYGB is considered the gold standard of metabolic operations, even though sleeve gastrectomy (SG) is more commonly performed in the United States and worldwide (Fig. 26.5). Patients undergoing RYGB have been shown to experience higher percent weight loss, superior comorbidity resolution, and comparably low short- and long-term complications when compared with patients undergoing SG. RYGB has been shown to be associated with better sustained type 2 diabetes remission compared with SG [7]. On average, between 70% and 80%, excess body weight loss (EBWL) is observed at 12−18 months postoperatively with RYGB. Patients undergoing RYGB also experience less weight regain in the short-term compared with medical therapy or other metabolic and bariatric surgery procedures, such as adjustable gastric band (AGB), proving success and durability of the procedure [8]. Maintenance of long-term weight loss has been shown to be determined by many patient factors, including younger age and fewer obesity-related comorbid conditions [9].

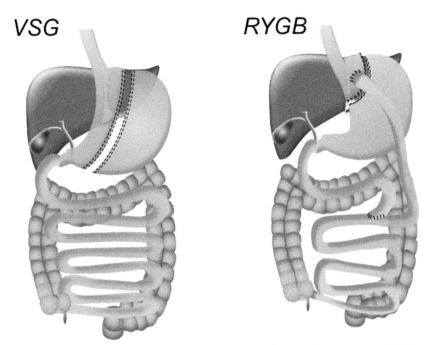

FIGURE 26.5   Schematics of sleeve gastrectomy (SG) and Roux-en-Y gastric bypass (RYGB).

Pathogenesis of obesity through adipose tissue

Obesity is characterized by an increase in adipose tissue (Fig. 26.6). In addition to its role in energy storage, adipose tissue is an active endocrine and immune organ. Fat accumulation in the obese state occurs by both an increase in the number of fat cells (hyperplasia) and an increase in size of native fat cells (hypertrophy). In obesity, this process is dysregulated, and hypertrophy becomes pathophysiologic, which causes adipocytes to be unable to perform basic cellular functions properly. This dysfunction causes structural cell damage, which subsequently triggers a local stress reaction causing a systemic release of inflammatory molecules triggering adverse endocrine and neurohumoral responses. This impaired adipogenesis observed in obesity prompted the term "adiposopathy," or sick fat, as defined by many endocrinologists to represent the imbalance of these biochemical factors and disruption of the metabolic balance seen in obesity [10]. Furthermore, adiposopathy leads to the development of insulin resistance, amplified adipogenesis resulting in increased visceral and peripheral fat stores, and the eventual development of the metabolic syndrome [11].

Molecular markers in obesity have changed quantities after RYGB

Impaired adipogenesis in obese individuals disallows physiologic release of antiinflammatory modulators and thus results in a proinflammatory state. There are multiple proteins responsible for adipocyte molecular function, and concentrations of these are observed to be altered in obesity. Many of them, however, significantly change after RYGB.

Adiponectin, a polypeptide released from normal adipocytes, plays an important antiinflammatory role in the body. It has been found to be downregulated and exists in lower concentrations in obese individuals. Patients undergoing RYGB have been shown to increase adiponectin levels with weight loss [10].

Other such polypeptides include C-reactive protein and tumor necrosis factor-alpha. Concentrations of these factors are known to decrease after RYGB and have been associated with a significant reduction in cardiometabolic risks [6].

Acylation-stimulating protein (ASP), a potent adipose storage factor, is found to be upregulated in obesity and causes increased differentiation of adipocytes and increased storage within adipocytes. After bariatric surgery, adipocyte-derived ASP is significantly downregulated [12].

Molecular concentrations of ghrelin and leptin, two of the primary regulators of hunger and satiety, similarly increase and decrease, respectively, after RYGB. Overall, these metabolic changes are partly responsible for the improvement of insulin resistance after RYGB and correlates with increased adiponectin levels [12,13].

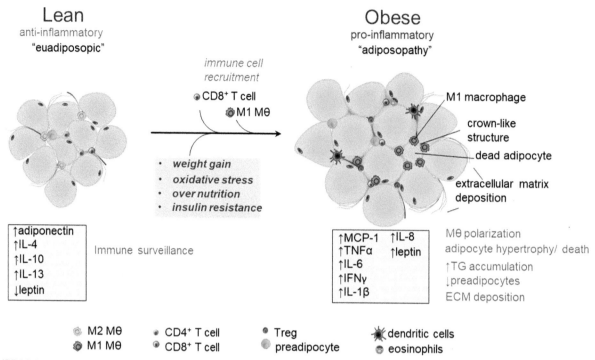

FIGURE 26.6 Adipose tissue expansion is accompanied by numerous cellular, structural, and hormonal changes. In lean individuals, adipose tissue is in an antiinflammatory or "euadiposopic" state characterized by increased levels of adiponectin, interleukin 4 (IL-4), IL-10, IL-13, and decreased leptin. In settings of weight gain, precipitated by overnutrition and/or hormonal imbalance, oxidative stress, insulin resistance, and inflammation ensue, the latter characterized by a loss of M2 macrophages (M2 Mθ), and an infiltration of CD8$^+$ T cells and M1 macrophages (M1 Mθ). The resulting obese adipose tissue assumes a proinflammatory or "adiposopathic" phenotype characterized by increased secretion of inflammatory cytokines such as monocyte chemoattractant protein 1 (MCP-1), tumor necrosis factor alpha (TNFα), IL-6, interferon gamma (IFNγ), IL-1β, IL-8, and leptin and decreased adiponectin. Hallmarks of proinflammatory processes are crown-like structures that are foci of dying adipocytes surrounded by macrophages, neutrophils, and eosinophils derived from monocytes in blood. There additionally is a decrease in preadipocyte frequency and an increase in extracellular matrix deposition.

Changes in adipose tissue

Bariatric surgery causes adipose tissue loss through a variety of mechanisms (Fig. 26.7). Reduction of adipose tissue mass reduces the effects of several hormones including leptin, adiponectin, resistin, visfatin, and retinol-binding protein-4 on appetite, glucose and lipid metabolism, and energy balance. The reduction of adipocyte size and a reduction in visceral adiposity is thought to be a key reason how bariatric surgery reverses the deleterious effects of adiposopathy [11]. On a

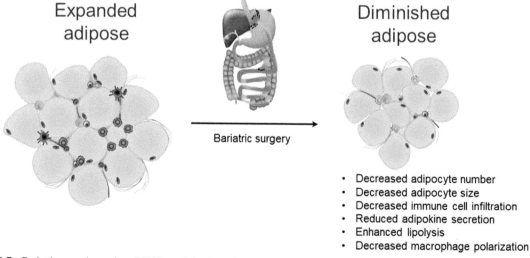

FIGURE 26.7 Bariatric surgeries such as RYGB result in visceral, subcutaneous, and ectopic adipose tissue remodeling that diminishes the inflammatory phenotype. Enhanced lipolysis resulting from decreased caloric intake reduces adipocyte number, decreases adipocyte size and immune cell content, and reduces inflammatory adipokine secretion.

cellular level, the decreased size of adipocytes and decreased volume of fat within adipocytes themselves decrease the stress condition, inflammatory response, and the unchecked, unhealthy metabolic activity of the sick adipose cells [14].

Another important beneficial effect seen after bariatric surgery is a significant reduction in hepatic fat volume. This can be explained by the utilization of fat stores from adipose tissue and therefore less free circulating fatty acids being delivered to the liver [15]. Saturated free fatty acids themselves have been implicated in causing lipotoxicity to the liver, pancreas, and muscle, all of which contribute to the observed insulin resistance in obesity. For instance, lipotoxicity to the liver would cause impaired glucose utilization and therefore increased output of glucose from the liver into the circulation, causing insulin resistance. Similarly, impaired beta cell function in the pancreas and accumulation of lipids within myocytes can both contribute to insulin resistance as well [16]. Metabolic and bariatric surgery has been shown to significantly decrease levels of FFAs and improve hepatic steatosis [17]. These changes improve insulin resistance and reverse the consequence of metabolic syndrome.

Bile acids and metabolic and bariatric surgery

Bile acids are another important factor component of metabolic regulation in obesity. As described by the hindgut theory mentioned earlier, there is a shortened route for bile acids to reach the ileum, which is the primary area for bile reabsorption, after RYGB. Thus, reabsorption back into the enterohepatic circulation increases ore bile acid reabsorption, which leads to upregulated synthesis and effects on energy expenditure, glucose utilization, and management, among other mechanisms. Notably, the same changes in bile acid concentrations are not seen in studies on the vertical sleeve gastrectomy. This makes sense based on the anatomical differences seen with each operation and the resultant mechanisms of weight loss and metabolic improvement [18].

Bile acids have long been a subject of interest as a hypothetical treatment modality in obesity. Mice models have demonstrated weight loss and various measures of metabolic improvement equal between an RYGB and distal ileum biliary diversion (through creating a gallbladder—ileal anastomosis). Interestingly, the same studies did not show similar results if the bile was diverted to the jejunum or duodenum (controls). Despite similar results in weight loss and metabolic improvement, the mechanisms between a bile diversion and RYGB are significantly different. In biliary diversion, nutrition passes through the GI tract in the usual order, with the only difference being bile being emptied in the distal ileum. After RYGB, bile still enters the GI tract in the duodenum through the biliary system, while ingested contents bypass the foregut and enter more distally. Bile acids meet the alimentary contents at the jejunojejunostomy, which is located at midjejunum. Another interesting discrepancy between the ileal bile diversion and RYGB mouse models was that in the bile diversion group, circulating conjugated bile acid levels were tenfold higher than controls, whereas the RYGB mice had near normal levels of bile acids [19]. This emphasizes the mechanistic difference between these strategies in obesity treatment and warrants further review in humans to determine if this is clinically relevant.

The mechanisms by which bile acids cause weight loss and metabolic gains are through their ability to function as signaling molecules to increase energy metabolism, insulin release and glycemic control and regulate its own synthesis (Fig. 26.8). Additionally, it has been observed, in animal models with enzyme deficiencies related to bile acid synthesis and gene transcription (farnesoid X receptor FXR), that glucose tolerance and weight loss from bariatric surgery are reversed, further emphasizing the important role that bile acids may have in obesity treatment and weight loss [20].

Visceral fat

There is little debate that visceral obesity leads to increased risk for type 2 diabetes mellitus, hypertension, dyslipidemia, and sleep apnea [21]. Prevailing theories suggest that one of the key mechanisms in developing all these metabolic derangements is elevated free fatty acids (FFAs). Studies show there is a failure to suppress FFA metabolism in response to meal ingestion in patients with obesity. This is partially attributable to insulin resistance in the liver, muscle, and adipose tissues. Still, if FFA concentrations are compared between lean and obese subjects, those with increased visceral obesity had excess FFA and inflammatory mediator delivery to the liver, directly causing impairment of FFA metabolism [15].

Greater lipolytic activity in the liver is seen in patients with obesity and is associated with increased cardiometabolic disease. One hypothesis proposed to explain this is the "Portal Theory" in which increased FFA elaborated from visceral fat increases uptake, via the portal vein, directly into the liver, which significantly alters glucose and lipid metabolism (Fig. 26.9). One study looking at visceral adipose tissue samples taken during RYGB demonstrated higher lipolytic activity in patients with metabolic syndrome compared with patients without metabolic syndrome [22].

Visceral fat has been demonstrated to be the most hormonally active and pathogenic fat in the body. Increased deposition of visceral fat is correlated with increased incidence in hepatic-mediated metabolic disease, such as

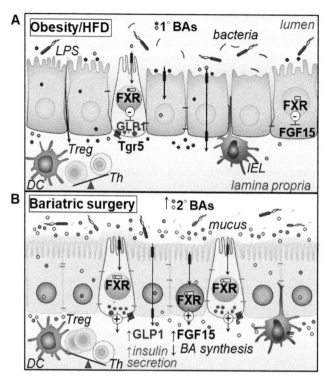

FIGURE 26.8 (A) The intestinal epithelium in obesity and with high-fat feeding exhibits functional impairments that decrease fidelity of cell—cell junctions and increase epithelial permeability to inflammatory commensal bacteria and bacterial metabolites such as lipopolysaccharide (LPS). Obesity is accompanied by an increase in primary (1 degree) bile acid (BA) synthesis and an immune cell balance in the lamina propria that favors diminished T regulatory (Treg) and enhanced T helper (Th) cell abundances as well as functional changes to intraepithelial lymphocytes (IELs). In obesity the nuclear BA receptor farnesoid X receptor (FXR) in absorptive enterocytes (pink) is activated, and expression of the atypical fibroblast growth factor, FGF15/19 (FGF15 in mice and FGF19 in humans), is increased. However, circulating levels of FGF15/19 that enter systemic circulation and normally act on the liver to inhibit hepatic BA synthesis are decreased by mechanisms not understood. In enteroendocrine L cells (green), activated FXR suppresses the transcription of the incretin glucagon-like polypeptide 1 (GLP-1). BAs also act on another BA receptor, Takeda G protein—coupled receptor 5 (Tgr5) to regulate GLP-1 secretion through cAMP-mediated G protein—coupled signaling. (B) After bariatric surgery, an increase in gut microbial diversity, secondary BA formation, and restoration of intestinal epithelium integrity are accompanied by mucus deposition, a strengthening of cell—cell junctions, and a switch in the Treg cell/Th cell balance. There is also an increase in the number of enteroendocrine cells and released FXR-mediated inhibition of GLP-1 and FGF15/19 release concomitant with enhanced insulin secretion and decreased hepatic BA synthesis.

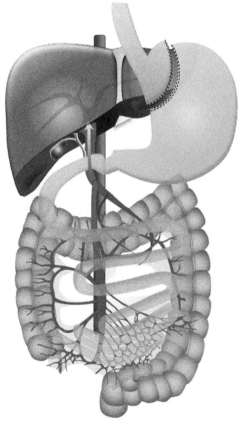

FIGURE 26.9 The Portal Theory in which increased FFA elaborated from visceral fat increases uptake, via the portal vein, directly into the liver which significantly alters glucose and lipid metabolism.

steatohepatitis, T2DM, and dyslipidemia. RYGB has been shown to reduce visceral, ectopic, and subcutaneous fat; however, it is the reduction of visceral fat that is most associated with improvement in metabolic conditions after weight loss [23]. RYGB causes higher visceral adipose tissue loss compared with nonsurgical treatment and may explain one of the primary reasons why reversal of metabolic comorbidities is seen in a significantly high percentages of patients undergoing RYGB.

The visceral adiposity index (VAI), which is a model that uses parameters including waist circumference, high density cholesterol, and triglyceride levels to assess fat function, was applied in one study to obese patients undergoing RYGB. This study concluded significant weight change, enhanced glycemic control, and more favorable lipid profiles after surgery. VAI decreased from baseline level of 4.41 to 1.74 3 months after surgery and continued to decrease significantly over time. A higher VAI was shown to be associated higher rate of T2DM remission [24].

The omentum, which has long been known to have immunologic significance, harbors a significant amount of visceral fat in the obese state. Since visceral fat is known to have such pathologic consequences on the body, it has been hypothesized that omentectomy during RYGB may accelerate the metabolic change that occurs after surgery. As fat cell number and volume decrease, hormones produced by fat change in composition and the chronic inflammatory condition characterized by obesity is reversed. Though early studies were conflicting, multiple randomized, double-blind controlled trials comparing the effects on weight loss, insulin sensitivity, and other metabolic improvements have refuted the benefit of omentectomy at the time of RYGB [25−28].

RYGB has been shown to be the superior weight loss modality to eliminate visceral fat when compared with obese subjects employing exercise as weight loss therapy alone. Obese patients undergoing RYGB lose statistically significantly more visceral fat at 3 months [29]. Studies comparing RYGB to other nonsurgical interventions have drawn similar conclusions at 2 years [30].

Ectopic fat

Adipose tissue plays an important physiologic role to most organs systems in the body. Hence, its location surrounding most organs in the body is appropriate. Ectopic fat is defined as excess adipose tissue in locations not typically associated with adipose tissue storage. Ectopic fat has been found to exert both systemic and local effects on tissues.

Systemic effects include impaired FFA metabolism, promotion of insulin resistance on B-islets and target tissues alike, and a proinflammatory, dysregulated metabolic syndrome. Conversely, ectopic fat deposits around the heart, renal sinuses, and blood vessels have been shown to predominantly exert local effects. Ectopic pericardial fat can be further broken down into epicardial fat, which is adipose tissue between the surface of the myocardium and the visceral layer of the pericardium, and paracardial fat, which is the adipose tissue situation on the outer surface of the partial pericardium. Dysregulated adipose hypertrophy increases the release of macrophages and upregulation of inflammatory adipokines into the viscera and its borders. These cells infiltrate the myocardium and vessel walls and inflict inflammatory damage. The Framingham Heart study demonstrated that epicardial fat content was associated with coronary artery calcium. Epicardial fat has also been shown to release bioactive molecules and inflammatory mediators including free fatty acids, which interact with cardiac vascular cells. Increased epicardial adipose tissue deposition has also been associated with heart disease, and this increased volume suggests that epicardial fat contributes to atherosclerosis. These results were supported by showing an association between epicardial fat and incident coronary heart disease, in addition to decreased cardiac function. Thus, the results of specifically epicardial fat on the development of arteriosclerosis and heart disease by local cytotoxic means present yet another problem and association with obesity [31].

RYGB has been shown to decrease cardiovascular mortality by 50% in patients with severe obesity [32]. Studies show a significantly larger decrease in paracardial fat after RYGB when compared with dietary managed weight loss. Interestingly, though RYGB showed decreases in both paracardial and epicardial fat, there was a much greater difference in paracardial fat loss compared with the nonsurgical group than what was seen with epicardial fat loss [33]. Given what we know about the association between epicardial fat and cardiovascular pathology, it is curious that RYGB does not lead to a larger decrease in epicardial fat given the cardioprotective qualities exhibited by RYGB. The reason why epicardial fat content changes less than visceral and paracardial fat after RYGB is unknown. One theory proposes epicardial fat may be resistant to weight loss given its different embryologic origin from paracardial and visceral fat [29]. Another suggests epicardial fat may be cardioprotective to balance against inflammatory effects of free fatty acids and cytokines released from infiltrative macrophages in paracardial fat. Despite showing only a modest decrease in epicardial fat content, weight loss after RYGB is still associated with superior epicardial fat loss when compared with other nonsurgical weight loss methods [33]. Additional studies are needed to better understand the physiologic function, mechanisms, and pathogenicity of epicardial fat.

Subcutaneous fat

Subcutaneous fat mass is substantially higher in patients with obesity as well. Though it is not as deleterious as visceral fat is toward end-organ function, subcutaneous adipose tissue is hormonally active and causes pathophysiologic changes in fat. In attempting to quantify subcutaneous fat's role in cardiometabolic disease, multiple studies have shown lower concentrations of bioactive inflammatory markers in subcutaneous fat when compared with visceral fat. Consequently, subcutaneous fat is not thought to be as detrimental to patients with obesity [34].

Multiple studies looked at the effects of subcutaneous fat reduction by performing panniculectomy during, or after, RYGB to determine if the removal of substantial volume of subcutaneous fat was associated with cardiometabolic benefit. Though cosmetic and quality of life outcomes were shown to improve in patients with concurrent or subsequent panniculectomy, there is no data illustrating metabolic benefit specifically attributable to panniculectomy [35]. This supports the theory that visceral fat is a more hormonally active and relevant in the development of metabolic syndrome and the subsequent resolution with decreased visceral fat seen after RYGB.

Additional studies have demonstrated increased adiponectin levels after subcutaneous fat removal alone. In patients undergoing procedures that involve subcutaneous fat removal, such as abdominoplasty and mammoplasty, there are statistically significant increases in adiponectin, improvement in HDL cholesterol, and decreased fasting glucose noted in the short term. However, subcutaneous fat removal procedures have not been shown to improve obesity-related comorbidities, but these studies did not look at differences in parameters based on body mass index [36]. Regardless, these results demonstrate that subcutaneous fat remains hormonally active and works in tandem with visceral and ectopic fat as part of obesity's pathogenesis.

One study looking at visceral, subcutaneous, epicardial, and liver fat measurements after RYGB demonstrated an association with long-term remission and incidence of diabetes, dyslipidemia, and hypertension. Fat depots in patients up to 14 years after RYGB were obtained by noncontrast computed tomography and compared with patients who did not undergo surgery. Significantly lower visceral, subcutaneous, and epicardial fat was demonstrated (42%, 20%, 30% lower, respectively), and liver-to-spleen density ratio was 9% higher at follow-up in the bariatric surgery group compared with the nonsurgery group. Lower visceral fat at follow-up exam was significantly associated with increased remission and decreased incidence of diabetes, hypertension, and dyslipidemia. The liver-to-spleen ratio was associated with the remission and incidence of hypertriglyceridemia, but not with other fat depots. Epicardial fat was related to incidence of elevated low-density lipoprotein cholesterol and low high-density lipoprotein cholesterol [37]. Notably, subcutaneous fat was not associated with the presence of obesity-related comorbid disease. It has also been demonstrated that there is no difference in lipolytic activity in subcutaneous fat when comparing patients with, and without, metabolic syndrome undergoing RYGB. These results demonstrate that subcutaneous fat may not be associated with increased risk for cardiometabolic disease [22].

Overview of metabolic benefits after RYGB

Insulin resistance plays a significant role in the development of T2DM and metabolic syndrome from prolonged impaired adipogenesis and resultant insulin resistance. Approximately 90% of patients with T2DM are obese and overweight. T2DM resolution after RYGB has consistently been reported to occur in approximately 70%−80% of cases, and in some studies up to 90% [38]. Bariatric surgery has been identified to achieve comorbidity resolution across many other conditions related to the metabolic syndrome, including hypertension (up to 92% resolution), dyslipidemia (65% resolution), nonalcoholic steatohepatitis-related steatosis (90% resolution), and obstructive sleep apnea (74%−98% resolution). Quality of life improvement of 95% and 5-year mortality risk reduction of 89% have been observed in patients undergoing metabolic and bariatric surgery. Other metabolic benefits include improvement or resolution in depression, asthma, pulmonary function, gastroesophageal reflux disease, gout, and degenerative joint disease (Table 26.1) [39].

A weight loss nadir is typically achieved approximately 12−24 months after RYGB, and weight regain of approximately 5%−7% of total weight can be seen thereafter [40]. One could predict a resurgence of cardiometabolic disease after weight regain, but interestingly, patients who regain weight after RYGB have been shown to remain metabolically healthy. There is no significant association between weight regain after RYGB and the recurrence of cardiometabolic disease, suggesting a protective mechanism related to the altered anatomy created during RYGB and resultant morphological and functional changes seen in adipose tissue after RYGB.

TABLE 26.1 Comorbidity resolution following metabolic and bariatric surgery.

Comorbidity	Percent resolution
Migraine headache	57%
Depression	55%
Benign intracranial hypertension	96%
Obstructive sleep apnea	74%—98%
Hypercholesterolemia	63%
Asthma	82% improvement
Hypertension	52%—92%
Nonalcoholic fatty liver disease	90% improvement; 37% resolution of inflammation
Metabolic syndrome	80%
Gastroesophageal reflux disease	72%—98%
Type 2 diabetes mellitus	83%
Polycystic ovarian syndrome	79%—hirsutism; 100%—menstrual dysfunction
Urinary stress incontinence	44%—88%
Degenerative joint disease	44%—88%
Venous stasis disease	95%

Class 1 obesity and metabolic and bariatric surgery

The immense weight loss and comorbidity resolution benefit of RYGB on patients with obesity has been emphasized thus far. However, the data discussed earlier in this chapter are limited to patients undergoing RYGB with class 2, and 3, obesity (BMI >35 kg/m^2, BMI >40 kg/m^2, respectively) (Table 26.2). Class 2 obesity requires a comorbid condition, while class 3 obesity does not require a comorbid condition to qualify for metabolic and bariatric surgery.

Patients with class 1 obesity (BMI 30—35 kg/m^2) have been shown to fail nonsurgical therapy, which further illustrates that the obesity problem is not being addressed adequately [41].

Additionally, superior treatment to improve or resolve T2DM after RYGB is being denied in patients with BMI <35 kg/m^2. The American Society for Metabolic and Bariatric Surgeons (ASMBS) published a position paper, referencing multiple randomized controlled trials and reviews from data collected from 2013 to 2018, outlining the superiority of bariatric surgery (specifically RYGB and SG) to nonsurgical therapy in the treatment of class 1 obesity for weight loss, T2DM remission, and resolution of other comorbidities. Furthermore, RYGB is proven to be cost-effective in the long term [41]. Hopefully, it will only be a matter of time before all classes of obesity can be offered metabolic and bariatric surgery treatment options.

TABLE 26.2 Obesity classes.

Weight class	Body mass index (BMI)	Ideal weight (exemplary 5 ft 7 in individual)
Healthy weight	18.0—24.9 kg/m^2	121—153 lb (54.9—69.4 kg)
Overweight	25.0—29.9 kg/m^2	159—185 lb (72.1—83.9 kg)
Class I obesity	30.0—34.9 kg/m^2	191—223 lb (86.6—101.2 kg)
Class II obesity	35.0—39.9 kg/m^2	224—249 lb (101.6—112.9 kg)
Class III obesity	≥40.0 kg/m^2	255—344 lb (115.7—156 kg)

Conclusion

Several studies have now shown that RYGB produces greater weight loss and sustained improvements in glycemic control and cardiometabolic risk compared with intensive lifestyle and medical intervention management. RYGB is superior to most other surgical interventions for weight loss with the exception of duodenal switch, which has been shown to impart greater cardiometabolic risk reduction, but has greater postoperative complication rates and increased risk of malnutrition/malabsorption [42]. Alternatives to bariatric surgery including endoscopic procedures that reduce gastric volume (gastric plication, gastric balloon), duodenal mucosal resurfacing, and novel pharmacotherapies (e.g., semaglutide) vary in the degree of weight loss, glucoregulation, and cardiovascular risk reduction and are emerging, but are not the mainstay therapy.

RYGB produces overwhelming beneficial weight loss outcomes and comorbidity resolution for patients with obesity, especially for those patients with increased visceral fat and metabolic syndrome. Cardiometabolic improvements seen after RYGB are due to numerous factors, including calorie restriction, malabsorption due to nutritional rerouting, changes in adipose tissue size and lipolytic activity, and gastrointestinal hormone alterations.

References

[1] Control CD. Adult obesity facts. 2021. https://www.cdc.gov/obesity/data/adult.html. [Accessed 19 May 2021].

[2] Organization WH. Obesity and overweight fact sheet. 2021. https://www.who.int/news-room/fact-sheets/detail/obesity-and-overweight. [Accessed 19 May 2021].

[3] Maleckas A, Gudaitytė R, Petereit R, Venclauskas L, Veličkienė D. Weight regain after gastric bypass: etiology and treatment options. Gland Surg 2016;5(6):617−24.

[4] Mingrone G, Castagneto-Gissey L. Mechanisms of early improvement/resolution of type 2 diabetes after bariatric surgery. Diabetes Metab 2009;35(6 Pt 2):518−23.

[5] Pournaras DJ, le Roux CW. Obesity, gut hormones, and bariatric surgery. World J Surg 2009;33(10):1983−8.

[6] Frikke-Schmidt H, O'Rourke RW, Lumeng CN, Sandoval DA, Seeley RJ. Does bariatric surgery improve adipose tissue function? Obes Rev 2016;17(9):795−809.

[7] Schauer PR, Bhatt DL, Kirwan JP, et al. Bariatric surgery versus intensive medical therapy for diabetes - 5-year outcomes. N Engl J Med 2017;376(7):641−51.

[8] Maciejewski ML, Arterburn DE, Van Scoyoc L, et al. Bariatric surgery and long-term durability of weight loss. JAMA Surg 2016;151(11):1046−55.

[9] Shantavasinkul PC, Omotosho P, Corsino L, Portenier D, Torquati A. Predictors of weight regain in patients who underwent Roux-en-Y gastric bypass surgery. Surg Obes Relat Dis 2016;12(9):1640−5.

[10] Linscheid P, Christ-Crain M, Stoeckli R, et al. Increase in high molecular weight adiponectin by bariatric surgery-induced weight loss. Diabetes Obes Metabol 2008;10(12):1266−70.

[11] Bays HE, Laferrère B, Dixon J, et al. Adiposopathy and bariatric surgery: is 'sick fat' a surgical disease? Int J Clin Pract 2009;63(9):1285−300.

[12] Faraj M, Havel PJ, Phélis S, Blank D, Sniderman AD, Cianflone K. Plasma acylation-stimulating protein, adiponectin, leptin, and ghrelin before and after weight loss induced by gastric bypass surgery in morbidly obese subjects. J Clin Endocrinol Metab 2003;88(4):1594−602.

[13] Vendrell J, Broch M, Vilarrasa N, et al. Resistin, adiponectin, ghrelin, leptin, and proinflammatory cytokines: relationships in obesity. Obes Res 2004;12(6):962−71.

[14] Löfgren P, Andersson I, Adolfsson B, et al. Long-term prospective and controlled studies demonstrate adipose tissue hypercellularity and relative leptin deficiency in the postobese state. J Clin Endocrinol Metab 2005;90(11):6207−13.

[15] Verna EC, Berk PD. Role of fatty acids in the pathogenesis of obesity and fatty liver: impact of bariatric surgery. Semin Liver Dis 2008;28(4):407−26.

[16] Blüher M. Adipose tissue dysfunction in obesity. Exp Clin Endocrinol Diabetes 2009;117(6):241−50.

[17] Klein S, Mittendorfer B, Eagon JC, et al. Gastric bypass surgery improves metabolic and hepatic abnormalities associated with nonalcoholic fatty liver disease. Gastroenterology 2006;130(6):1564−72.

[18] Wang W, Cheng Z, Wang Y, Dai Y, Zhang X, Hu S. Role of bile acids in bariatric surgery. Front Physiol 2019;10:374.

[19] Flynn CR, Albaugh VL, Abumrad NN. Metabolic effects of bile acids: potential role in bariatric surgery. Cell Mol Gastroenterol Hepatol 2019;8(2):235−46.

[20] Watanabe M, Horai Y, Houten SM, et al. Lowering bile acid pool size with a synthetic farnesoid X receptor (FXR) agonist induces obesity and diabetes through reduced energy expenditure. J Biol Chem 2011;286(30):26913−20.

[21] Jensen MD. Role of body fat distribution and the metabolic complications of obesity. J Clin Endocrinol Metab 2008;93(11 Suppl. 1):S57−63.

[22] Andersson DP, Löfgren P, Thorell A, Arner P, Hoffstedt J. Visceral fat cell lipolysis and cardiovascular risk factors in obesity. Horm Metab Res 2011;43(11):809−15.

[23] Pontiroli AE, Frigè F, Paganelli M, Folli F. In morbid obesity, metabolic abnormalities and adhesion molecules correlate with visceral fat, not with subcutaneous fat: effect of weight loss through surgery. Obes Surg 2009;19(6):745−50.

[24] Ke Z, Li F, Gao Y, et al. The use of visceral adiposity index to predict diabetes remission in low BMI Chinese patients after bariatric surgery. Obes Surg 2021;31(2):805–12.

[25] Andersson DP, Eriksson-Hogling D, Bäckdahl J, et al. Omentectomy in addition to bariatric surgery-a 5-year follow-up. Obes Surg 2017;27(4):1115–8.

[26] Andersson DP, Thorell A, Löfgren P, et al. Omentectomy in addition to gastric bypass surgery and influence on insulin sensitivity: a randomized double blind controlled trial. Clin Nutr 2014;33(6):991–6.

[27] Dillard TH, Purnell JQ, Smith MD, et al. Omentectomy added to Roux-en-Y gastric bypass surgery: a randomized, controlled trial. Surg Obes Relat Dis 2013;9(2):269–75.

[28] Lee Y, Pedziwiatr M, Major P, Brar K, Doumouras AG, Hong D. The effect of omentectomy added to bariatric surgery on metabolic outcomes: a systematic review and meta-analysis of randomized controlled trials. Surg Obes Relat Dis 2018;14(11):1766–82.

[29] Wu FZ, Huang YL, Wu CC, et al. Differential effects of bariatric surgery versus exercise on excessive visceral fat deposits. Medicine 2016;95(5):e2616.

[30] Gloy VL, Briel M, Bhatt DL, et al. Bariatric surgery versus non-surgical treatment for obesity: a systematic review and meta-analysis of randomised controlled trials. BMJ 2013;347:f5934.

[31] Rosito GA, Massaro JM, Hoffmann U, et al. Pericardial fat, visceral abdominal fat, cardiovascular disease risk factors, and vascular calcification in a community-based sample: the Framingham Heart Study. Circulation 2008;117(5):605–13.

[32] Aminian A, Zajichek A, Arterburn DE, et al. Association of metabolic surgery with major adverse cardiovascular outcomes in patients with type 2 diabetes and obesity. JAMA 2019.

[33] van Schinkel LD, Sleddering MA, Lips MA, et al. Effects of bariatric surgery on pericardial ectopic fat depositions and cardiovascular function. Clin Endocrinol 2014;81(5):689–95.

[34] Torriani M, Oliveira AL, Azevedo DC, Bredella MA, Yu EW. Effects of Roux-en-Y gastric bypass surgery on visceral and subcutaneous fat density by computed tomography. Obes Surg 2015;25(2):381–5.

[35] Colabianchi V, de Bernardinis G, Giovannini M, Langella M. Panniculectomy combined with bariatric surgery by laparotomy: an analysis of 325 cases. Surg Res Pract 2015;2015:193670.

[36] Vinci V, Valaperta S, Klinger M, et al. Metabolic implications of surgical fat removal: increase of adiponectin plasma levels after reduction mammaplasty and abdominoplasty. Ann Plast Surg 2016;76(6):700–4.

[37] Hunt SC, Davidson LE, Adams TD, et al. Associations of visceral, subcutaneous, epicardial, and liver fat with metabolic disorders up to 14 Years after weight loss surgery. Metab Syndr Relat Disord 2021;19(2):83–92.

[38] Nandagopal R, Brown RJ, Rother KI. Resolution of type 2 diabetes following bariatric surgery: implications for adults and adolescents. Diabetes Technol Therapeut 2010;12(8):671–7.

[39] Fouse T, Brethauer S. Resolution of comorbidities and impact on longevity following bariatric and metabolic surgery. Surg Clin 2016;96(4):717–32.

[40] Sjöström L. Review of the key results from the Swedish Obese Subjects (SOS) trial - a prospective controlled intervention study of bariatric surgery. J Intern Med 2013;273(3):219–34.

[41] Aminian A, Chang J, Brethauer SA, Kim JJ, Committee ASfMaBSCI. ASMBS updated position statement on bariatric surgery in class I obesity (BMI 30-35 kg/m. Surg Obes Relat Dis 2018;14(8):1071–87.

[42] Skogar M, Holmback U, Hedberg J, Riserus U, Sundbom M. Preserved fat-free mass after gastric bypass and duodenal switch. Obes Surg 2017;27(7):1735–40.

Chapter 27

Fecal transplant

M.M. Ruissen[1], J.J. Keller[2] and Maarten E. Tushuizen[3]
[1]*Department of Internal Medicine, Leiden University Medical Center, Leiden, the Netherlands;* [2]*Department of Gastroenterology, Haaglanden Medical Center, The Hague, the Netherlands;* [3]*Department of Gastroenterology & Hepatology, Leiden University Medical Center, Leiden, the Netherlands*

The gut microbiome

The term gut microbiota is defined as the whole population of bacteria, viruses, parasites, and fungi colonizing the intestinal tract [1]. The composition of the gut microbiome impacts food absorption, the enterohepatic circulation of bile acids, intestinal permeability, systemic inflammation, immunity, and the role of microbial-related metabolites. In addition, it is linked to the so-called the gut—liver axis and gut—brain axis [2]. A disturbed microbiome seems to play a role in the pathogenesis of a wide range of diseases.

The gut microbiome harbors distinct microbial features, microbial variety, and composition per mammalian species [3]. Furthermore, the composition of the gut microbiome differs greatly across individuals [1], There are about 10^{14} bacterial cells within the human body, of which most are located within the gastrointestinal tract [4]. There are about 15,000—36,000 different bacterial species colonizing the human population, and each individual harbors about 500—1500 different species. The microbiome mainly consists of bacteria from the phyla Bacteriodes and Firmicutes, with in lesser extent bacteria from other phyla such as Proteobacteria, Actinobacteria, Verrucomicrobia, and Fusobacteria [5]. After a dynamic composition of the developing microbiome during infancy, from adulthood on the gut microbiome has shown to be remarkably stable over time in composition and function during adulthood [6,7]. The complex composition of bacterial species plays an important role in the fermentation of indigestible food components into absorbable metabolites, the synthesis of essential vitamins [8], the removal of toxic compounds, the outcompetition of pathogens, the strengthening of the intestinal barrier, and the stimulation and regulation of the immune system within the host [9—11].

Differences in microbiome constitution across individuals can be related to microbiome-intrinsic and microbiome-extrinsic factors [12]. Microbiome-intrinsic factors are mainly the result of the state of the host, such as lifetime. Microbiome-extrinsic factors are referring to various environmental factors that influence the host by interacting with or impacting the gut microbiome [12]. Host-related factors further enhance the variation of the gut microbiome. They are classified as host-extrinsic factors (e.g., diet [13,14], lifestyle [15,16], BMI(17) and medication [17]), host-intrinsic factors (e.g., genetics [18,19]), and environmental factors (e.g., vertical transmission of microbiome strains from mother to neonate [12]). These factors overlap and interact with each other. Altogether, microbiome- and host-related factors only account for 10%—15% of the microbiome variation between individuals [12]. The remaining variation is accounted for by factors associated with the functionality of the gut microbiome, which does not translate directly to the taxonomic microbiome composition. The functional variability and sensitivity to perturbation has shown to be significantly larger compared with the metagenomic variability [20]. Also the transit time of the feces [21] and the stool consistency [22] have shown to be associated to the composition of the gut microbiome and gut microbiome functionality. However, how functionality and metagenomics are linked together still remains largely unknown.

Multiple studies have shown that instability and dysbiosis of the gut microbiome and microbiota alterations are associated to a variety of medical disorders, including, for example, inflammatory bowel disease [23], obesity [24,25], irritable bowel syndrome, and type 2 diabetes [26]. In particular, an overall reduction in microbiome diversity was found in patients with ulcerative colitis [27], Crohn's disease [27,28], rheumatoid arthritis [29], type 2 diabetes [30], and obesity [31]. In patients with obesity, this reduction in microbial diversity was found to be correlated with the severity of obesity [32]. While the exact pathophysiological link between the composition of the gut microbiome and the wide variety of expected

Visceral and Ectopic Fat. https://doi.org/10.1016/B978-0-12-822186-0.00010-9

associated diseases remains unknown, it was found that in patients with obesity, low microbial gene richness appears to be associated on a functional level with a proinflammatory status [33], an increase in lipopolysaccharide (LPS) production that is related to insulin resistance and adverse lipidomic profile [34]. Additionally, specific microbiota can produce pro- or antiinflammatory metabolites, potentially protecting or damaging tissues, organs, or entire organ systems. Recently, studies have shown that *Klebsiella pneumoniae* is able to produce high levels of ethanol, resulting in clinical presentations similar to those associated with alcohol (ab)use, without any alcohol being consumed [35]. On the other hand, short-chain fatty acids (SCFAs) are known for their ability to protect the body and relieve oxidative stress, but SCFAs were found to be dramatically reduced in patients with obesity and type 2 diabetes [30,31]. Increasing the butyrate production, an SCFA formed as a metabolite by microbial fermentation, has been implicated to alleviate obesity and related comorbidities [36] and protect against the development of type 1 diabetes mellitus [37] and cancer [38].Given the associations with a great variety of diseases, it is expected that modulation of the gut microbiome becomes a versatile therapeutic target in the future [12].

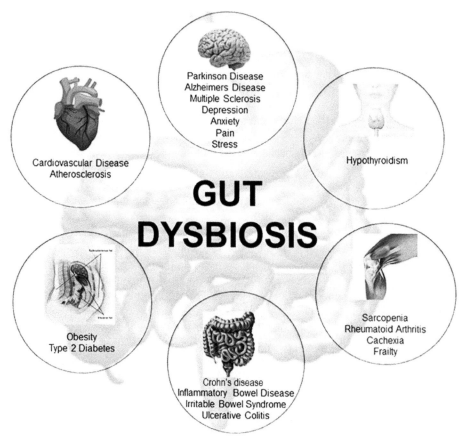

GUT DYSBIOSIS AND DISEASE. *ADJUSTED FIGURE FROM: HTTPS://DOI.ORG/10.3389/FNUT.2020.00017.*

Gut microbiome modulation

There are different strategies to modulate the gut microbiome (Fig. 27.1). First, the composition of the gut microbiome is modulated by diet [39]. Alterations in diet or weight loss through diet are therefore also associated with alterations of the gut microbiome [13,40]. Dietary modification of the gut microbiome may also be supported by prebiotics, which are "nondigestible food ingredients that promote the growth of beneficial microorganisms in the intestines." Another way to modulate the gut microbiome is the use of probiotics [41]. Probiotics are "live microorganisms that, when administered in adequate amounts, confer a health benefit on the host." Importantly, the effects of probiotics are strain dependent and disease specific, which means that for each disorder a specific probiotic strain or mixture needs to be identified. Unfortunately, convincing evidence for broad use of probiotics is lacking currently. However, the results of several studies are promising. For example, two randomized RCTs have showed that a cocktail of probiotics can significantly reduce the

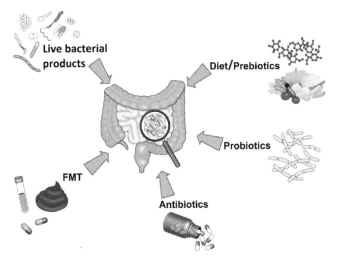

FIGURE 27.1 Potential treatment strategies for gut microbiota modulation. *Adjusted figure from https://doi.org/10.1016/j.semcancer.2020.06.006*

amount of liver fat, improve liver enzymes, and reduce plasma liver enzymes after 12 weeks [42], although major variability was found between the participants.

Furthermore multiple drugs have shown to modulate the gut microbiome. Antibiotics are well known for their dramatic reduction in microbial diversity and specific shifts in microbial species [43,44], but may also be used to modulate the gut microbiome in a beneficial way, for example, in patients with hepatic encephalopathy that are treated with rifaximin. Also nonantibiotic drugs have shown to impact the composition of the gut microbiome [45]. For example, metformin, a glucose-lowering drug, showed to induce strong microbiome shifts in patients with type 2 diabetes mellitus (T2DM), with depletion of butyrate-producing taxa [46]. In addition, the use of proton pump inhibitors was found to be associated to a decrease in microbial diversity and changes in 20% of the taxa of the gut microbiome [47], and NSAIDs and atypical antipsychotics both showed to result in enrichness of certain specific bacterial species [48,49].

Other medical interventions that modulate or affect the gut microbiome are bowel cleansing [50], with often a recovery of the microbial composition after 14 days, and abdominal surgery. For example, Roux-and-Y gastric bypass surgery [51] caused an increase in Firmicutes and a decrease in Proteobacteria compared with BMI-matched obese patients.

A promising method to alter the gut microbiome composition, aiming to restore a healthy homeostasis, is fecal microbiome transplantation (FMT) from healthy donors to patients, providing a widely available, noninvasive, nonchemical, and cost-effective therapeutic strategy for a large variety of medical conditions. In the future, FMT will eventually be replaced by the introduction of new, standardized, sophisticated live bacterial products.

Fecal microbiome transplantation

Fecal material is a highly biologically active, complex mixture of microbia and living organisms. It forms an independent organ within the individual and is therefore transmittable from individual to individual. Fecal microbiome transplantation is the introduction of a fecal suspension of a healthy donor into the gastrointestinal tract of a recipient. It is a way to modulate the composition and function of the gut microbiome. Several studies have shown FMT to be followed by an increased alpha diversity in the recipients microbiome and a shift toward the microbial composition of the donor [52]. FMT can be performed via gastroscopy or nasoduodenal tube [53], colonoscopy [54], or oral capsules [55].

After FMT is performed, the bacterial strains of the donor and recipient coexist within the gut, with conspecific strains surviving longer than new species [56]. A study on FMT as a treatment for recurrent *Clostridium difficile* infections showed a dramatic increase of the patient's microbiota diversity after FMT (Fig. 27.2) [53]. The success of the FMT treatment relies mostly on the richness of the gut microbiome of the donor [57]. Recent research has shown the survival of the donor microbiome to be up to 3 months after FMT [58]; however, data of further long-term survival are still lacking [56].

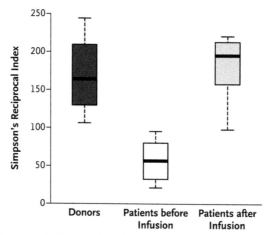

FIGURE 27.2 Microbiota diversity in patients before and after infusion of donor feces, as compared with diversity in healthy donors [53].

Fecal transplantations—murine models

Murine models provide unique opportunities for controlled experiments with genetically modified mouse models with low maintenance costs, high reproductive rates, and a short life cycle [58,59]. While more than 85% of the genomic sequences and regulatory networks among transcription factors between mouse and human are conserved, the overall gene expression and regulation has shown to be considerably different [60]. Additionally, the anatomy and physiology of the gastrointestinal tract of the mouse shows a lot of similarities, but also has some prominent differences reflecting their diverging diets, feeding patterns, body sizes, and metabolic requirements [58,59]. With the total average ratio of the gut surface area to body surface being comparable between mice and humans, the length and surface area differ greatly over the different parts of the small and large intestine. Mice have a nonglandular forestomach lined with keratinizing squamous mucosa and biofilm of *Lactobacillus* spp., which is used for food storage [58]. The cecum in mice is relatively large, because it plays an important in the fermentation of plant materials and the production of vitamin B and K, which mice reabsorb through coprophagy [59]. Also the intestinal architecture differs, with the intestines of mice showing no haustra, longitudinal folds within the distal colon and a different architecture of the villi, potentially in an effort to compensate for the lack of surface enlarging folds [61,62]. These differences in colonic microcompartmentalization and structuring might contribute to the creation of diverse ecological microniches hosting differing microbial communities [59]. The differences in genetic expression and regulation as well as the differences in anatomy and physiology of the gastrointestinal tract between mice and humans hamper the extrapolation of study findings to humans; however, to date, murine models remain the first step in research practice [12,58].

The role of the gut microbiome in metabolism and modulation of the gut microbiome by FMT was firstly studied in murine cohousing experiments focused on the development of nonalcoholic fatty liver disease (NAFLD) [63]. In these experiments, FMT was performed from metabolically altered mice into germ-free mice. This resulted in some histologic features characteristic for NAFLD. FMT from conventional mice on high-fat diet (HFD) showing metabolic alterations characteristic for NAFLD together with steatosis hepatis, into germ-free mice, showed to result in a threefold increase in hepatic triglyceride content and increased expression of genes associated to hepatic lipogenesis in recipients. When performing FMT from obese weight-matched mice without steatosis to germ-free mice, the recipients maintained a healthy liver. This shows that there are specific microbiota alterations that are associated with NAFLD, which are, at least partly, involved in liver injury [64].

Another study experimented with FMT from human NAFLD patients or healthy individuals into gnotobiotic recipient mice [65]. In mice that received the microbiome of NAFLD patients, this resulted in a 4.6-fold increase in liver triglycerides, liver steatosis and inflammation, increased proinflammatory genes and associated signs of systemic inflammation, and an increase in LPS production [65]. Interestingly, when these mice received an HFD, the alterations showed to be even more pronounced [65]. The increased intrahepatic lipid concentrations, steatohepatitis, dysbiosis of the gut microbiome, proinflammatory profile, and endotoxemia all showed to be reversible when FMT was performed after 8 weeks of HFD of healthy mice into the affected individuals [66].

Another important finding was that the intestinal permeability increased in mice fed 1 week with an HFD, which was also associated with liver steatosis, fibrosis, inflammation, and translocation of bacteria within the liver parenchyma [67]. When FMT was then performed from mice with a 1-week HFD or chow diet into specific pathogen-free mice, increased intestinal permeability was only observed in the mice receiving FMT from the HFD-fed mice [67]. However, the change in intestinal permeability showed to be of short duration and intestinal permeability returned to baseline after 1 week of HFD. These findings suggest a strong link between diet, gut permeability, the gut microbiota, and fat metabolism.

Fecal microbiome transplantation in humans

FMT was firstly introduced in humans by Chinese medical and herbal practitioners in the fourth century in China for the treatment of severe diarrhea and food poisoning [68]. It was over 1200 years later that FMT was rediscovered as a therapeutic option for multiple medical conditions such as vomiting, diarrhea, constipation, and fever [68]. FMT with bacteria of healthy donors into patients is now widely used as a treatment for antibiotic-resistant *Clostridium difficile* infection, with numerous RCTs reporting this treatment to be safe and retain durable cure rates of 90% or even higher, clearly favoring this treatment over antibiotics [54,69–71].

Following the tremendous success of FMT for CDI, this treatment approach has been investigated as a potential treatment for a variety of other gastrointestinal and metabolic diseases, including Crohn's disease, ulcerative colitis [72,73], irritable bowel syndrome (IBS) [74], metabolic syndrome [75], nonalcoholic fatty liver disease [76], and obesity [77]. A randomized controlled double-blinded study in patients with IBS found an improvement in fatigue and quality of life in patients that received FMT, associated with specific significant changes in intestinal bacterial profiles [74]. In patients with metabolic syndrome, FMT increased hepatic and peripheral insulin sensitivity. This improvement appeared associated with increased gut microbiome diversity and specific microbiome changes, with a 2.5-fold increase in butyrate-producing bacteria, but not with any improvement in clinical parameters [75,78]. In line with the murine model studies, discussed previously, FMT of donors with metabolic syndrome into patients with metabolic syndrome further decreased insulin sensitivity, resulted in specific changes in bile acids and microbial taxa, and altered the expression of inflammatory genes, strengthening the link between the gut microbiota and the gut–liver axis even further [79]. In obese patients, also changes in bile acids and acetate levels were found after allogenic FMT, however, without a reduction in body weight [78,80]. Although the therapeutic benefits of FMT for these other indications are less pronounced than the success found in patients with antibiotic-resistant *Clostridioides difficile* infections, the research field surrounding FMT is promising, with special interest in the tailoring of FMT bacterial strains to match the needs of the recipient. However, research within this area is still explorative, with the physiological and pathophysiological mechanisms that play a role within the gut–liver axis and the connection with the gut microbiome still remaining largely unknown. Another factor hampering clinical success of FMT for other diseases is the often limited durability of the effects of FMT. This further indicates that the composition of the gut microbiome is based on a variety of complex processes with environmental and host-related factors superseding FMT modulation in determining the bacterial composition, with a lot of factors remaining unknown until this moment [81]. Multiple FMTs might be necessary in chronic diseases to be of clinical relevance and environmental and host-related factors sich as lifestyle and diet may have to be adjusted to retain therapeutic benefits after FMT. Further studies are required to unravel the mysteries of the gut–liver axis, the role of the gut microbiome, and the potential of gut microbiome modulation by FMT. Given the clinical implications including the considerable burden of Clostridium difficile on global healthcare systems, FMT should be widely available to most centres.Stool banks may guarantee reliable, timely and equitable access to FMT for patients and a traceable workflow that ensures safety and quality of procedures (Fig. 27.3).

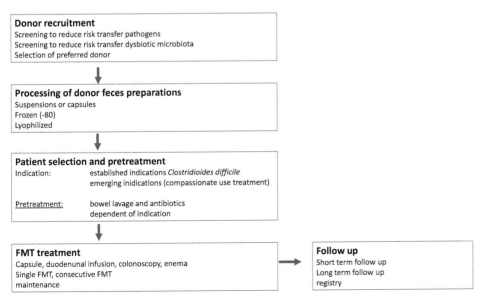

FIGURE 27.3 Workflow for stool banks that ensure safety and quality of FMT procedures.

References

[1] Eckburg PB, Bik EM, Bernstein CN, Purdom E, Dethlefsen L, Sargent M, et al. Diversity of the human intestinal microbial flora. Science (New York, NY) 2005;308(5728):1635–8.

[2] Tripathi A, Debelius J, Brenner DA, Karin M, Loomba R, Schnabl B, et al. The gut-liver axis and the intersection with the microbiome. Nat Rev Gastroenterol Hepatol 2018;15(7):397–411.

[3] Ley RE, Hamady M, Lozupone C, Turnbaugh PJ, Ramey RR, Bircher JS, et al. Evolution of mammals and their gut microbes. Science (New York, NY) 2008;320(5883):1647–51.

[4] Savage DC. Microbial ecology of the gastrointestinal tract. Annu Rev Microbiol 1977;31:107–33.

[5] Kurokawa K, Itoh T, Kuwahara T, Oshima K, Toh H, Toyoda A, et al. Comparative metagenomics revealed commonly enriched gene sets in human gut microbiomes. DNA Res 2007;14(4):169–81.

[6] Bäckhed F, Roswall J, Peng Y, Feng Q, Jia H, Kovatcheva-Datchary P, et al. Dynamics and stabilization of the human gut microbiome during the first year of life. Cell Host Microbe 2015;17(5):690–703.

[7] Faith JJ, Guruge JL, Charbonneau M, Subramanian S, Seedorf H, Goodman AL, et al. The long-term stability of the human gut microbiota. Science (New York, NY) 2013;341(6141):1237439.

[8] LeBlanc JG, Milani C, de Giori GS, Sesma F, van Sinderen D, Ventura M. Bacteria as vitamin suppliers to their host: a gut microbiota perspective. Curr Opin Biotechnol 2013;24(2):160–8.

[9] Kamada N, Seo S-U, Chen GY, Núñez G. Role of the gut microbiota in immunity and inflammatory disease. Nat Rev Immunol 2013;13(5):321–35.

[10] Hooper LV, Littman DR, Macpherson AJ. Interactions between the microbiota and the immune system. Science (New York, NY) 2012;336(6086):1268–73.

[11] Thaiss CA, Zmora N, Levy M, Elinav E. The microbiome and innate immunity. Nature 2016;535(7610):65–74.

[12] Schmidt TSB, Raes J, Bork P. The human gut microbiome: from association to modulation. Cell 2018;172(6):1198–215.

[13] David LA, Maurice CF, Carmody RN, Gootenberg DB, Button JE, Wolfe BE, et al. Diet rapidly and reproducibly alters the human gut microbiome. Nature 2014;505(7484):559–63.

[14] Muegge BD, Kuczynski J, Knights D, Clemente JC, González A, Fontana L, et al. Diet drives convergence in gut microbiome functions across mammalian phylogeny and within humans. Science (New York, NY) 2011;332(6032):970–4.

[15] Barton W, Penney NC, Cronin O, Garcia-Perez I, Molloy MG, Holmes E, et al. The microbiome of professional athletes differs from that of more sedentary subjects in composition and particularly at the functional metabolic level. Gut 2018;67(4):625–33.

[16] Clarke SF, Murphy EF, O'Sullivan O, Lucey AJ, Humphreys M, Hogan A, et al. Exercise and associated dietary extremes impact on gut microbial diversity. Gut 2014;63(12):1913–20.

[17] Le Bastard Q, Al-Ghalith GA, Grégoire M, Chapelet G, Javaudin F, Dailly E, et al. Systematic review: human gut dysbiosis induced by non-antibiotic prescription medications. Alimentary Pharmacol Ther 2018;47(3):332–45.

[18] Bonder MJ, Kurilshikov A, Tigchelaar EF, Mujagic Z, Imhann F, Vila AV, et al. The effect of host genetics on the gut microbiome. Nat Genet 2016;48(11):1407–12.

[19] Goodrich Julia K, Waters Jillian L, Poole Angela C, Sutter Jessica L, Koren O, Blekhman R, et al. Human genetics shape the gut microbiome. Cell 2014;159(4):789–99.

[20] Franzosa EA, Morgan XC, Segata N, Waldron L, Reyes J, Earl AM, et al. Relating the metatranscriptome and metagenome of the human gut. Proc Natl Acad Sci USA 2014;111(22):E2329–38.

[21] Roager HM, Hansen LBS, Bahl MI, Frandsen HL, Carvalho V, Gøbel RJ, et al. Colonic transit time is related to bacterial metabolism and mucosal turnover in the gut. Nat Microbiol 2016;1(9):16093.

[22] Tigchelaar EF, Bonder MJ, Jankipersadsing SA, Fu J, Wijmenga C, Zhernakova A. Gut microbiota composition associated with stool consistency. Gut 2016;65(3):540–2.

[23] Schirmer M, Franzosa EA, Lloyd-Price J, McIver LJ, Schwager R, Poon TW, et al. Dynamics of metatranscription in the inflammatory bowel disease gut microbiome. Nat Microbiol 2018;3(3):337–46.

[24] Turnbaugh PJ, Hamady M, Yatsunenko T, Cantarel BL, Duncan A, Ley RE, et al. A core gut microbiome in obese and lean twins. Nature 2009;457(7228):480–4.

[25] Ley RE, Backhed F, Turnbaugh P, Lozupone CA, Knight RD, Gordon JI. Obesity alters gut microbial ecology. Proc Nat Acad Sci USA 2005;102(31):11070–5.

[26] Larsen N, Vogensen FK, van den Berg FWJ, Nielsen DS, Andreasen AS, Pedersen BK, et al. Gut microbiota in human adults with type 2 diabetes differs from non-diabetic adults. PLoS One 2010;5(2):e9085.

[27] Ott SJ, Musfeldt M, Wenderoth DF, Hampe J, Brant O, Fölsch UR, et al. Reduction in diversity of the colonic mucosa associated bacterial microflora in patients with active inflammatory bowel disease. Gut 2004;53(5):685–93.

[28] Manichanh C, Rigottier-Gois L, Bonnaud E, Gloux K, Pelletier E, Frangeul L, et al. Reduced diversity of faecal microbiota in Crohn's disease revealed by a metagenomic approach. Gut 2006;55(2):205–11.

[29] Zhang X, Zhang D, Jia H, Feng Q, Wang D, Liang D, et al. The oral and gut microbiomes are perturbed in rheumatoid arthritis and partly normalized after treatment. Nat Med 2015;21(8):895–905.

[30] Karlsson FH, Tremaroli V, Nookaew I, Bergström G, Behre CJ, Fagerberg B, et al. Gut metagenome in European women with normal, impaired and diabetic glucose control. Nature 2013;498(7452):99–103.

[31] Le Chatelier E, Nielsen T, Qin J, Prifti E, Hildebrand F, Falony G, et al. Richness of human gut microbiome correlates with metabolic markers. Nature 2013;500(7464):541–6.

[32] Aron-Wisnewsky J, Prifti E, Belda E, Ichou F, Kayser BD, Dao MC, et al. Major microbiota dysbiosis in severe obesity: fate after bariatric surgery. Gut 2019;68(1):70–82.

[33] Vandeputte D, Kathagen G, D'hoe K, Vieira-Silva S, Valles-Colomer M, Sabino J, et al. Quantitative microbiome profiling links gut community variation to microbial load. Nature 2017;551(7681):507–11.

[34] Kayser BD, Prifti E, Lhomme M, Belda E, Dao M-C, Aron-Wisnewsky J, et al. Elevated serum ceramides are linked with obesity-associated gut dysbiosis and impaired glucose metabolism. Metabolomics 2019;15(11):140.

[35] Yuan J, Chen C, Cui J, Lu J, Yan C, Wei X, et al. Fatty liver disease caused by high-alcohol-producing Klebsiella pneumoniae. Cell Metabol 2019;30(4):675–88.

[36] Coppola S, Avagliano C, Calignano A, Berni Canani R. The protective role of butyrate against obesity and obesity-related diseases. Molecules 2021;26(3).

[37] Endesfelder D, Engel M, Davis-Richardson AG, Ardissone AN, Achenbach P, Hummel S, et al. Towards a functional hypothesis relating anti-islet cell autoimmunity to the dietary impact on microbial communities and butyrate production. Microbiome 2016;4(1):17.

[38] Wu X, Wu Y, He L, Wu L, Wang X, Liu Z. Effects of the intestinal microbial metabolite butyrate on the development of colorectal cancer. J Cancer 2018;9(14):2510–7.

[39] Shoaie S, Ghaffari P, Kovatcheva-Datchary P, Mardinoglu A, Sen P, Pujos-Guillot E, et al. Quantifying diet-induced metabolic changes of the human gut microbiome. Cell Metabol 2015;22(2):320–31.

[40] Seganfredo FB, Blume CA, Moehlecke M, Giongo A, Casagrande DS, Spolidoro JVN, et al. Weight-loss interventions and gut microbiota changes in overweight and obese patients: a systematic review. Obes Rev 2017;18(8):832–51.

[41] Kristensen NB, Bryrup T, Allin KH, Nielsen T, Hansen TH, Pedersen O. Alterations in fecal microbiota composition by probiotic supplementation in healthy adults: a systematic review of randomized controlled trials. Genome Med 2016;8(1):52.

[42] Ahn SB, Jun DW, Kang BK, Lim JH, Lim S, Chung MJ. Randomized, double-blind, placebo-controlled study of a multispecies probiotic mixture in nonalcoholic fatty liver disease. Sci Rep 2019;9(1):5688.

[43] Jakobsson HE, Jernberg C, Andersson AF, Sjölund-Karlsson M, Jansson JK, Engstrand L. Short-term antibiotic treatment has differing long-term impacts on the human throat and gut microbiome. PLoS One 2010;5(3):e9836.

[44] Jernberg C, Löfmark S, Edlund C, Jansson JK. Long-term ecological impacts of antibiotic administration on the human intestinal microbiota. ISME J 2007;1(1):56–66.

[45] Maier L, Pruteanu M, Kuhn M, Zeller G, Telzerow A, Anderson EE, et al. Extensive impact of non-antibiotic drugs on human gut bacteria. Nature 2018;555(7698):623–8.

[46] Forslund K, Hildebrand F, Nielsen T, Falony G, Le Chatelier E, Sunagawa S, et al. Disentangling type 2 diabetes and metformin treatment signatures in the human gut microbiota. Nature 2015;528(7581):262–6.

[47] Imhann F, Bonder MJ, Vich Vila A, Fu J, Mujagic Z, Vork L, et al. Proton pump inhibitors affect the gut microbiome. Gut 2016;65(5):740–8.

[48] Rogers MAM, Aronoff DM. The influence of non-steroidal anti-inflammatory drugs on the gut microbiome. Clin Microbiol Infect 2016;22(2):178.e1–9.

[49] Flowers SA, Evans SJ, Ward KM, McInnis MG, Ellingrod VL. Interaction between atypical antipsychotics and the gut microbiome in a bipolar disease cohort. Pharmacotherapy 2017;37(3):261–7.

[50] Jalanka J, Salonen A, Salojärvi J, Ritari J, Immonen O, Marciani L, et al. Effects of bowel cleansing on the intestinal microbiota. Gut 2015;64(10):1562–8.

[51] Tremaroli V, Karlsson F, Werling M, Ståhlman M, Kovatcheva-Datchary P, Olbers T, et al. Roux-en-Y gastric bypass and vertical banded gastroplasty induce long-term changes on the human gut microbiome contributing to fat mass regulation. Cell Metabol 2015;22(2):228–38.

[52] Seekatz AM, Aas J, Gessert CE, Rubin TA, Saman DM, Bakken JS, et al. Recovery of the gut microbiome following fecal microbiota transplantation. mBio 2014;5(3):e00893–14.

[53] van Nood E, Vrieze A, Nieuwdorp M, Fuentes S, Zoetendal EG, de Vos WM, et al. Duodenal infusion of donor feces for recurrent Clostridium difficile. N Engl J Med 2013;368(5):407–15.

[54] Brandt LJ, Aroniadis OC, Mellow M, Kanatzar A, Kelly C, Park T, et al. Long-term follow-up of colonoscopic fecal microbiota transplant for recurrent clostridium difficile infection. Am J Gastroenterol 2012;107(7):1079–87.

[55] Gupta A, Khanna S. Fecal microbiota transplantation. JAMA 2017;318(1):102.

[56] Li SS, Zhu A, Benes V, Costea PI, Hercog R, Hildebrand F, et al. Durable coexistence of donor and recipient strains after fecal microbiota transplantation. Science (New York, NY) 2016;352(6285):586–9.

[57] Vermeire S, Joossens M, Verbeke K, Wang J, Machiels K, Sabino J, et al. Donor species richness determines faecal microbiota transplantation success in inflammatory bowel disease. J Crohn's Colitis 2015;10(4):387–94.

[58] Hugenholtz F, de Vos WM. Mouse models for human intestinal microbiota research: a critical evaluation. Cell Mol Life Sci 2018;75(1):149–60.

[59] Nguyen TLA, Vieira-Silva S, Liston A, Raes J. How informative is the mouse for human gut microbiota research? Dis Models Mechanisms 2015;8(1):1–16.

[60] Chinwalla AT, Cook LL, Delehaunty KD, Fewell GA, Fulton LA, Fulton RS, et al. Initial sequencing and comparative analysis of the mouse genome. Nature 2002;420(6915):520–62.

[61] Treuting PM, Valasek M, Dintzis SM. In: Treuting PM, Dintzis SM, editors. Upper gastrointestinal tract. London: Academic Press; 2012.

[62] Treuting PM, Dintzis SM. In: Treuting PM, Dintzis SM, editors. Lower gastrointestinal tract. London: Academic Press; 2012.

[63] Henao-Mejia J, Elinav E, Jin C, Hao L, Mehal WZ, Strowig T, et al. Inflammasome-mediated dysbiosis regulates progression of NAFLD and obesity. Nature 2012;482(7384):179—85.

[64] Le Roy T, Llopis M, Lepage P, Bruneau A, Rabot S, Bevilacqua C, et al. Intestinal microbiota determines development of non-alcoholic fatty liver disease in mice. Gut 2013;62(12):1787—94.

[65] Chiu CC, Ching YH, Li YP, Liu JY, Huang YT, Huang YW, et al. Nonalcoholic fatty liver disease is exacerbated in high-fat diet-fed gnotobiotic mice by colonization with the gut microbiota from patients with nonalcoholic steatohepatitis. Nutrients 2017;9(11).

[66] Zhou D, Pan Q, Shen F, Cao HX, Ding WJ, Chen YW, et al. Total fecal microbiota transplantation alleviates high-fat diet-induced steatohepatitis in mice via beneficial regulation of gut microbiota. Sci Rep 2017;7(1):1529.

[67] Mouries J, Brescia P, Silvestri A, Spadoni I, Sorribas M, Wiest R, et al. Microbiota-driven gut vascular barrier disruption is a prerequisite for non-alcoholic steatohepatitis development. J Hepatol 2019;71(6):1216—28.

[68] Zhang F, Luo W, Shi Y, Fan Z, Ji G. Should we standardize the 1,700-year-old fecal microbiota transplantation? Am J Gastroenterol 2012;107(11):1755. author reply p.-6.

[69] de Groot PF, Frissen MN, de Clercq NC, Nieuwdorp M. Fecal microbiota transplantation in metabolic syndrome: history, present and future. Gut Microb 2017;8(3):253—67.

[70] Grehan MJ, Borody TJ, Leis SM, Campbell J, Mitchell H, Wettstein A. Durable alteration of the colonic microbiota by the administration of donor fecal flora. J Clin Gastroenterol 2010;44(8):551—61.

[71] Cammarota G, Masucci L, Ianiro G, Bibbò S, Dinoi G, Costamagna G, et al. Randomised clinical trial: faecal microbiota transplantation by co-lonoscopy vs. vancomycin for the treatment of recurrent Clostridium difficile infection. Alimentary Pharmacol Ther 2015;41(9):835—43.

[72] Fuentes S, Rossen NG, van der Spek MJ, Hartman JHA, Huuskonen L, Korpela K, et al. Microbial shifts and signatures of long-term remission in ulcerative colitis after faecal microbiota transplantation. ISME J 2017;11(8):1877—89.

[73] Narula N, Kassam Z, Yuan Y, Colombel J-F, Ponsioen C, Reinisch W, et al. Systematic review and meta-analysis: fecal microbiota transplantation for treatment of active ulcerative colitis. Inflamm Bowel Dis 2017;23(10):1702—9.

[74] El-Salhy M, Hatlebakk JG, Gilja OH, Bråthen Kristoffersen A, Hausken T. Efficacy of faecal microbiota transplantation for patients with irritable bowel syndrome in a randomised, double-blind, placebo-controlled study. Gut 2020;69(5):859—67.

[75] Vrieze A, Van Nood E, Holleman F, Salojärvi J, Kootte RS, Bartelsman JFWM, et al. Transfer of intestinal microbiota from lean donors increases insulin sensitivity in individuals with metabolic syndrome. Gastroenterology 2012;143(4):913—916.e7.

[76] Craven L, Rahman A, Nair Parvathy S, Beaton M, Silverman J, Qumosani K, et al. Allogenic fecal microbiota transplantation in patients with nonalcoholic fatty liver disease improves abnormal small intestinal permeability: a randomized control trial. Off J Am Coll Gastroenterol|CG 2020;115(7):1055—65.

[77] Jung Lee W, Lattimer LD, Stephen S, Borum ML, Doman DB. Fecal microbiota transplantation: a review of emerging indications beyond relapsing Clostridium difficile Toxin colitis. Gastroenterol Hepatol 2015;11(1):24—32.

[78] Kootte RS, Levin E, Salojarvi J, Smits LP, Hartstra AV, Udayappan SD, et al. Improvement of insulin sensitivity after lean donor feces in metabolic syndrome is driven by baseline intestinal microbiota composition. Cell Metabol 2017;26(4):611—619.e6.

[79] de Groot P, Scheithauer T, Bakker GJ, Prodan A, Levin E, Khan MT, et al. Donor metabolic characteristics drive effects of faecal microbiota transplantation on recipient insulin sensitivity, energy expenditure and intestinal transit time. Gut 2020;69(3):502—12.

[80] Allegretti JR, Kassam Z, Mullish BH, Chiang A, Carrellas M, Hurtado J, et al. Effects of fecal microbiota transplantation with oral capsules in obese patients. Clin Gastroenterol Hepatol: Off Clin Pract J Am Gastroenterol Assoc 2020;18(4):855—863.e2.

[81] Moss EL, Falconer SB, Tkachenko E, Wang M, Systrom H, Mahabamunuge J, et al. Long-term taxonomic and functional divergence from donor bacterial strains following fecal microbiota transplantation in immunocompromised patients. PLoS One 2017;12(8):e0182585.

Index

Note: 'Page numbers followed by "f" indicate figures and "t" indicate tables.'

A

Abdominal obesity, 8–9, 8t, 22, 22t
Abnormal lipid metabolism, 270
Adipocytokines, 86
Adipokines, abnormalities in, 272
Adiponectin, 222
Adipose tissue, inflammation of, 66–67, 272
  chronic low-grade inflammation, 205
    weight gain, 206–208, 207f
    weight loss, 208–209, 209f
    weight regain, 209–211, 210f
  determining, 211–212
  global obesity, 205
  immune cell subsets residing, 206t, 207f
  obesity, 211
    atherosclerosis, 211
    insulin resistance, 211
Adipose tissue remodeling, diabetic heart disease
  adiponectin, 222
  cardiovascular disease (CVD), 217, 221–222
  imaging ectopic adiposity, 222–223
  proinflammatory adipocytokines, 222
  sex differences, 221–222, 221f
  signaling pathways, 218–221, 220f
  type 2 diabetes mellitus, 222–223
Adults, 269
  clinical studies, 269
Aerobic training interventions, 323–325, 325f
Aging, 106
Airway hyperresponsiveness, 266
Airway inflammation, 271, 271f
Antiobesity medication, 345
Apoptosis, 90
Artificial intelligence (AI), 125–126
Asthma
  abnormal lipid metabolism, 270
  adipokines, abnormalities in, 272
  adipose tissue, inflammation in, 272
  adult clinical studies, 269
  adults, 269
  airway inflammation, 271, 271f
  children, 267
  disease pathogenesis, 270
  epidemiology, 267–270
  genetic background, 265
  genetic factors in, 266–267
  lung function and genetic factors, 265–267
  obesity-related complications, 270

  oxidative stress, 270–271
  pediatric clinical studies, 267, 268f
  phenotypes, 269, 269f
  physical effects, 265
  pregnant mothers, weight gain in, 268
  racial differences, 266
  respiratory function, 265–266, 265f–266f
  sex differences, 270
    children, 268
  weight change, 267–268
Atherosclerosis, 44–47, 45f, 46t–47t
Athletes, 107
Atrial fibrillation (AF), 47, 237–238, 238f

B

Bariatric surgery, 345, 363
Behavioral determinants, 21–22
Behavioral interventions, 341–345
  behavior therapy principles, 341–342, 342t
  cognitive techniques, 343
  goal setting, 342
  multicomponent behavioral interventions, 343–344
  problem-solving, 343, 343f
  self-monitoring, 342
  treatment structure, 341
Big data, 125–126
Bile acids, 87, 90, 383, 384f
Biopsy, 75, 120–121
  myocardial lipids, 99
Body composition, 373
Body fat distribution
  abdominal obesity, 8–9, 8t
  ectopic fat accumulation, 11
  health consequences, 11–13
  lipid overflow hypothesis, 11
  sex differences, 11–13
  subcutaneous adipose tissue, 9–11
  visceral adipose tissue, 9–11, 9f–10f, 12f
Body mass index, 106–107, 282
Bone marrow adipose tissue (BMAT)
  bone marrow fat origin, 170–171, 171f
  cancer, 181
  computed tomography, 174–176
    dual-energy CT (DECT), 174–176
    single-energy CT (SECT), 174
  endocrine regulation, 178f
  hematopoiesis, 180–181
  magnetic resonance imaging (MRI), 176–177

    proton magnetic resonance spectroscopy (¹H-MRS), 177, 177f
    T1-weighted MRI, 176
    water-fat imaging, 176
  metabolic diseases, 181–182
  physiology, 171–174
    caloric restriction, 173
    characteristics, 171
    exercise, 173
    microscopic aspect, 174
    regional specific differences in, 172–173, 173f
    unloading, 173–174
    variation during growth, 171–172, 172f
    variation with aging, 172
  secretory profile, 178f
  skeletal health, 179–180
  in vivo imaging, 174–177, 175t
Bone marrow fat, 67–68, 303
  origin, 170–171, 171f
Brain
  body mass index, 282
  diffusion tensor imaging, 283, 285f
  fat distribution, 283, 284f
  functional brain imaging, 285–287, 286f
  future directions, 290–291
  genome-wide association studies, 288–289
  hypothalamic function, 284–285, 286f
  mendelian randomization, 290
  pathophysiology, 282f
  polygenic risk scores, 290
  structural imaging, 281–285
  visceral fat, 283–284
Breast, 68
Brown adipose tissue (BAT)
  background on history of, 25–26
  clinical applications, 28f, 32–33, 32f
  human health, 25–26, 26f
  molecular targets, 31–32
  physiology, 25, 26f, 27t
  potential analysis techniques, 26–30
    invasive techniques, 29
    noninvasive techniques, 29–30
  scientific interest, 25–26

C

Calorie restriction, 173, 301–302, 302f
Cancer, 181
Cardiac function
  abnormalities, 250–252
  CKD, 252–253

Cardiac function (*Continued*)
  renal function, abnormalities, 252
Cardiac imaging, 42—43, 43f—44f
Cardiac lipid deposition, 301—302, 302f
Cardiac triggering, 103
Cardiometabolic risk factors, 20
Cardiorenal dysfunction
  atherosclerosis, 244—245
  dyslipidemia, 244—245
  epidemiological and translational studies,
    253—258
  five-part classification system for, 243—244,
    244f
  heart failure, 246
  hyperuricemia, 247
  leptin, 246
  metabolic syndrome, 244, 246f
  microvascular dysfunction, 246
  multiorgan imaging in, 258—259
  obese animal models, 247—250, 248t—249t
  obesity's risk for, 253—254, 254f
  pathophysiology of, 244—247, 245f
  personalized approach, 259
  preclinical studies, 247—253
  preclinical studies, novel developments in,
    258
  renin-angiotensin-aldosterone system
    (RAAS), 247
  sex differences, 253
  sympathetic activation, 246
  systemic inflammation, 246
  Zucker rat and substrains, 250, 251f
Cardiovascular disease (CVD), 87—88, 142,
    217, 221—222
  obesity hypertension, 229—230, 230f
    atrial fibrillation (AF), 237—238, 238f
    coronary artery disease, 234—237,
      236f—237f
    fat deposits in, 230—232, 233f
    function, 232—234, 235f
    heart failure, 238—240, 239f—240f
    magnetic resonance imaging (MRI),
      229—230
    structure, 232—234, 235f
Chronic kidney disease, 142
Chronic low-grade inflammation, 205
  weight gain, 206—208, 207f
  weight loss, 208—209, 209f
  weight regain, 209—211, 210f
Chronic pancreatitis, 120
Chronic stress, 21
Circulating biomarkers, 121
Class 1 obesity, 387, 387t
Combination therapy, 90
Computed tomography (CT), 121, 174—176
  dual-energy CT (DECT), 174—176
  single-energy CT (SECT), 174
Controlled trials, 372
Coronary artery disease, 234—237,
    236f—237f
Cortisol, 198, 199f

D

Data acquisition, 61—64, 61f—63f, 63t, 64f
Diffusion tensor imaging, 283, 285f

Disease pathogenesis, 270
Dissemination, challenge of, 344—345
Dominant water signal, 103—104
Dual-energy CT (DECT), 174—176

E

Ectopic fat, 11, 385
  storage, heart and kidney
    dietary effects on, 255—257, 256f—257f
    glycemic control on, 258
    metabolic imaging studies, 254—255,
      255f
  very-low-calorie diets (VLCDs)
    bone marrow fat, 303
    calorie restriction, 301—302, 302f
    cardiac lipid deposition, 301—302, 302f
    hepatic ectopic fat, 299—300
    skeletal muscle lipid metabolism,
      302—303
    type 2 diabetes, 300—301, 301f
    visceral adipose tissue, 297—298,
      299f—300f
Ectopic lipids
  biopsy, 75
  ^{1}H-magnetic resonance spectroscopy (MRS),
    75, 76f
  negative energy balance, 75—78
    fasting, 78
    single bout of exercise, 75—77, 77f
  positive energy balance, 78
    high fructose/glucose diet, 78, 79t
    long-term high fat diet, 78
    short-term high fat diet, 78
Elipse, 372
Endobariatric interventions, 363, 363t, 365t,
    366f, 366t, 367f, 368t—369t
Endocrine regulation, 178f
Endoscopic sleeve gastroplasty, 364—371
  case series, 367—370
  meta-analyses, 365
  metabolic effects, 370—371, 370f
Epicardial adipose tissue (EAT)
  anatomical characteristics, 40—41
    autopsy, data based on, 40, 43f
    clinical settings, 41
  atherosclerosis, pathomechanism of, 44—47,
    45f, 46t—47t
  atrial fibrillation, 47
  biochemical features, 41—42
  cardiac imaging, 42—43, 43f—44f
  COVID-19 patients with, 49—50
  epicardial fat necrosis, 48
  heart failure, 47—48
  inflammation, 48
  metabolic diseases, 49
  physiological function, 41—42
  terminology, 39—40, 39t, 41f
  treatment options for, 50
Epicardial fat necrosis, 48
Excessive kidney fat, clinical implications of,
    142—143
  after intervention, 143
  cardiovascular diseases, 142
  chronic kidney disease, 142
  implications, 143, 143f

insulin resistance, 142
Exercise, 107, 173
  aerobic training interventions, 323—325, 325f
  definition, 321, 322t
  recommendations, 321—323, 324t
  regular physical activity, 321, 323f
  resistance training interventions, 326—327
    aerobic and resistance training
      interventions, 327
    chronic disease, prevention and
      management of, 328—330
    intensity, 327
    mechanisms, 327—328
    visceral and ectopic adipose tissue,
      327—328

F

Fasting, 78
Fat deposits, 230—232, 233f
Fat distribution, 283, 284f
Fat infiltration imaging, postprocessing and
    assessment of, 157—159
  MRS, 158—159, 159f
Fecal microbiome transplantation, 90, 393,
    394f
Fecal transplant
  fecal microbiome transplantation,
    393, 394f
  gut microbiome, 391—392
    modulation, 392—393, 393f
  humans, 395
  murine models, 394—395, 395f
Fibrosis, 90
  formation, 86
Functional brain imaging, 285—287, 286f

G

Gastric volume reduction interventions
  bariatric surgery, 363
  endobariatric interventions, 363, 363t, 365t,
    366f, 366t, 367f, 368t—369t
  endoscopic sleeve gastroplasty, 364—371
    case series, 367—370
    meta-analyses, 365
    metabolic effects, 370—371, 370f
  intragastric balloon therapy, 372—373
    body composition, 373
    controlled trials, 372
    elipse, 372
    meta-analyses, 372
    metabolic and visceral fat effects of, 373
    metabolism, 373
    NAFLD, 373
    NASH, 373
    obalon, 372
    orbera, 372
    types, 372
  primary obesity surgery endoluminal
    (POSE) procedure, 371
    meta-analysis, 371
    metabolic effects, 371
Gender, 106
Genetic and epigenetic determinants, 84, 84f
Genome-wide association studies, 288—289

GLP1
  analogs, 89
  receptor agonists, 89
Glucagon-like peptide 1 receptor agonists,
    356–357
  action/side effects, mechanisms of, 355f,
    356–357
  clinical efficacy, 357
Growth hormone (GH), 196–197, 197f
Gut microbiome, 391–392
  modulation, 392–393, 393f

H

Healthy human myocardium, 106–108
  aging, 106
  athletes, 107
  body mass index, 106–107
  exercise, 107
  gender, 106
  nutrition, 107–108
Heart, 69
  failure, 47–48, 238–240, 239f–240f
Hematopoiesis, 180–181
Hepatic ectopic fat, 299–300
Hepatic steatosis, causes of, 84t
Hepatocellular carcinoma, 87
High fructose/glucose diet, 78, 79t
^{1}H-magnetic resonance spectroscopy (MRS),
    75, 76f
1H-MR spectra from skeletal muscle,
    159–160, 160f
Hypothalamic function, 284–285, 286f

I

Imaging ectopic adiposity, 222–223
IMAT fatty infiltration, flexibility of,
    151–152
IMCL, flexibility of, 154–155, 154f
Immune cell subsets residing, 206t, 207f
Infiltration, 149–152, 150f–151f, 151t
Inflammation, 48, 86, 90
Insulin, 193–195, 194f
  resistance, 86, 108–109, 142
  sensitivity, 89
Intermittent energy restriction (IER)
  animal models, health parameters in,
    308–311
    metabolic parameters, 310, 311f
    weight and fat, 308–310, 310f
  humans, 311–315, 313f
    continuous energy restriction, 315
    metabolic parameters, 314
    other health parameters, 314–315
    weight and fat, 312–314
  methods, 307
  physiology of, 308, 309f
  potential risks of, 316–317
  sustainability of, 316
Intermittent fasting. *See* Intermittent energy
    restriction (IER)
Intragastric balloon therapy, 372–373
  body composition, 373

controlled trials, 372
elipse, 372
meta-analyses, 372
metabolic and visceral fat effects of, 373
metabolism, 373
NAFLD, 373
NASH, 373
obalon, 372
orbera, 372
types, 372
Intramyocellular lipids, 152–154
In vivo magnetic resonance spectroscopy,
    60–61

L

Lifestyle interventions, 88–89
  antiobesity medication, 345
  bariatric surgery, 345
  behavioral intervention, 345
  behavioral interventions, 341–345
    behavior therapy principles, 341–342,
      342t
    cognitive techniques, 343
    goal setting, 342
    multicomponent behavioral interventions,
      343–344
    problem-solving, 343, 343f
    self-monitoring, 342
    treatment structure, 341
  dissemination, challenge of, 344–345
  medical nutrition therapy, 333–337
    dietary patterns, 333–336, 336t
  physical activity
    adipose tissue, 339
    benefits of, 337–338
    introduction, 337
    recommendations, 338–340, 338f
    type and duration of, 339–340
  sleep, 340–341
    obstructive sleep apnea (OSA), 341
    recommendations, 341
Lipid composition, 60, 60f
Lipid overflow hypothesis, 11
Lipotoxicity, 86, 89
Liver, 68–69, 69f
  cirrhosis, 87
Long-term high fat diet, 78

M

Magnetic resonance imaging (MRI), 66, 121
  automated segmentation, 122
  cardiovascular disease (CVD)
    obesity hypertension, 229–230
  fat fraction, 122–123
  fatty acid composition, 123
  information from, 122–125
  pancreas fibroinflammation, 125, 125f
  pancreas morphology, 123–125
  pancreas volume, 122
  proton magnetic resonance spectroscopy
    (^{1}H-MRS), 177, 177f
  T1-weighted MRI, 176

water-fat imaging, 176
Magnetic resonance spectroscopy (MRS)
  adipose tissue, 66–67
  analysis of, 64–66, 65f
  applications, 66
  bone marrow fat, 67–68
  breast, 68
  data acquisition, 61–64, 61f–63f, 63t, 64f
  heart, 69
  lipid composition, 60, 60f
  liver, 68–69, 69f
  magnetic resonance imaging (MRI), 66
  skeletal muscle, 70
  in vivo magnetic resonance spectroscopy,
    60–61
Medical therapy
  glucagon-like peptide 1 receptor agonists,
    356–357
    action/side effects, mechanisms of, 355f,
      356–357
    clinical efficacy, 357
  metformin, 354–355
    action/side effects, mechanism of, 354,
      355f
    clinical efficacy, 354–355
  nutrition, 333–337
    dietary patterns, 333–336, 336t
  orlistat
    actions/side effects, mechanism of, 355,
      356f
    clinical efficacy, 356
  sodium glucose cotransporter-2 inhibitors
    action/side effects, mechanisms of,
      357–358, 358f
    clinical efficacy, 358
  thiazolidinediones, 353
Mendelian randomization, 290
Meta-analyses, 372
Metabolic diseases, 49, 181–182
Metabolic risk factors, 23
Metformin, 354–355
  action/side effects, mechanism of, 354,
    355f
  clinical efficacy, 354–355
Microbiome, 87
Murine models, 394–395, 395f
Muscle, assess lipids in, 155–157
  Computed tomography (CT), 155–156,
    155f
  MRI, 156–157, 156f
Myocardial lipids
  assessment of, 100f
  biopsy, 99
  cardiac triggering, 103
  disease, 108–110
    insulin resistance, 108–109
    type 2 diabetes, 108–109
  dominant water signal, 103–104
  healthy human myocardium, 106–108
    aging, 106
    athletes, 107
    body mass index, 106–107
    exercise, 107

Myocardial lipids (*Continued*)
 gender, 106
 nutrition, 107–108
 localized proton magnetic resonance
  spectroscopy of the heart, 99–106,
  101f, 103f
 myocardial metabolite content,
  quantification of, 104–106, 105f
 respiratory gating, 103
Myocardial metabolite content, quantification
 of, 104–106, 105f

N

NAFLD, 373
NASH, 373
Necroapoptosis, 86
Negative energy balance, 75–78
 fasting, 78
 single bout of exercise, 75–77, 77f
Non-alcoholic fatty liver disease (NAFLD),
 117
 clinical care paths, development and
  implementation of, 91–92
  primary care, 91
  secondary and tertiary care, 91–92
 clinical consequences
  cardiovascular disease, 87–88
  hepatocellular carcinoma, 87
  liver cirrhosis, 87
 diagnostics, 88
 hepatic steatosis, causes of, 84t
 pathogenesis, 84–87
  adipocytokines, 86
  bile acids, 87
  fibrosis formation, 86
  genetic and epigenetic determinants, 84,
   84f
  inflammation, 86
  insulin resistance, 86
  lipotoxicity, 86
  microbiome, 87
  necroapoptosis, 86
  nutrition, 85–86
  urea cycle dysregulation, 86
 treatment, 88–91
  apoptosis, 90
  bile acids, 90
  combination therapy, 90
  fecal microbiome transplantation, 90–91
  fibrosis, 90
  GLP1 analogs, 89
  GLP1 receptor agonists, 89
  inflammation, 90
  insulin sensitivity, 89
  lifestyle, 88–89
  lipotoxicity, 89
  nutrition, 89
  obesity, 88–89
  oxidative stress, 89–90
  probiotics, 90–91
  SGLT2 inhibitors, 89
Nutrition, 85–86, 89, 107–108

O

Obalon, 372
Obesity, 88–89, 117
 abdominal obesity, 19–20
 adipose tissue, inflammation of, 211
  atherosclerosis, 211
  insulin resistance, 211
 asthma
  abnormal lipid metabolism, 270
  adipokines, abnormalities in, 272
  adipose tissue, inflammation in, 272
  adults, 269
  airway inflammation, 271, 271f
  children, 267
  clinical studies, 269
  disease pathogenesis, 270
  epidemiology, 267–270
  genetic background, 265
  genetic factors in, 266–267
  lung function and genetic factors,
   265–267
  obesity-related complications, 270
  oxidative stress, 270–271
  pediatric clinical studies, 267, 268f
  phenotypes, 269, 269f
  physical effects, 265
  pregnant mothers, weight gain in, 268
  racial differences, 266
  respiratory function, 265–266, 265f–266f
  sex differences, 268, 270
  weight change, 267–268
 brain. *See* Brain
 cardiac function
  abnormalities, 250–252
  CKD, 252–253
  renal function, abnormalities, 252
 cardiorenal dysfunction
  atherosclerosis, 244–245
  dyslipidemia, 244–245
  epidemiological and translational studies,
   253–258
  five-part classification system for,
   243–244, 244f
  heart failure, 246
  hyperuricemia, 247
  leptin, 246
  metabolic syndrome, 244, 246f
  microvascular dysfunction, 246
  multiorgan imaging in, 258–259
  obese animal models, 247–250,
   248t–249t
  obesity's risk for, 253–254, 254f
  pathophysiology of, 244–247, 245f
  personalized approach, 259
  preclinical studies, 247–253
  preclinical studies, novel developments
   in, 258
  renin-angiotensin-aldosterone system
   (RAAS), 247
  sex differences, 253
  sympathetic activation, 246
  systemic inflammation, 246
  Zucker rat and substrains, 250, 251f

 childhood obesity, 19
 definition of, 3–4, 4t
 ectopic fat storage, heart and kidney
  dietary effects on, 255–257, 256f–257f
  glycemic control on, 258
  metabolic imaging studies, 254–255,
   255f
 molecular markers in, 381
 mortality and diseases, 6–8, 6f–7f
 prevalence of, 5, 5f–6f
 visceral fat, children and adolescents,
  21–22
  abdominal obesity, 22, 22t
  behavioral determinants, 21–22
  chronic stress, 21
  ethnicity, 21
  genetics of, 21
  imaging techniques, 22
  metabolic risk factors, 23
  sex, 21
  waist/height ratio, 22, 22t
Obesity hypertension
 cardiovascular disease (CVD), 229–230,
  230f
  atrial fibrillation (AF), 237–238, 238f
  coronary artery disease, 234–237,
   236f–237f
  fat deposits in, 230–232, 233f
  function, 232–234, 235f
  heart failure, 238–240, 239f–240f
  magnetic resonance imaging (MRI),
   229–230
  structure, 232–234, 235f
Obesity-related comorbidities, 380
Obesity-related mortality and diseases, 6–8,
 6f–7f
Obstructive sleep apnea (OSA), 341
Orbera, 372
Orlistat
 actions/side effects, mechanism of, 355,
  356f
 clinical efficacy, 356
Overweight
 definition of, 3–4, 4t
 obesity-related mortality and diseases, 6–8,
  6f–7f
 prevalence of, 5, 5f–6f
Oxidative stress, 89–90, 270–271

P

Pancreas ectopic fat
 anatomically, 118
 artificial intelligence (AI), 125–126
 big data, 125–126
 biopsy, 120–121
 chronic pancreatitis, 120
 circulating biomarkers, 121
 computed tomography (CT), 121
 future directions, 126–127
 magnetic resonance imaging (MRI), 121
  automated segmentation, 122
  fat fraction, 122–123
  fatty acid composition, 123

information from, 122–125
   pancreas fibroinflammation, 125, 125f
   pancreas morphology, 123–125
   pancreas volume, 122
non-alcoholic fatty liver disease (NAFLD), 117
obesity, 117
pancreas state assessment, 120–121
pancreatic cancer, 120
physiologically, 118
proton magnetic resonance spectroscopy (MRS), 121
regional assessment, 120
type 2 diabetes mellitus (T2DM), 117
ultrasound, 121
Pancreas state assessment, 120–121
Pancreatic cancer, 120
Pediatric clinical studies, 267, 268f
Perirenal fat and renal sinus fat
   anatomical characteristics, 131–134, 132f–133f
   histological and pathophysiological characteristics, 134–135
   imaging-based quantification, 135–139, 135t
   quantification of, 135–139, 136f–139f
Physical activity
   adipose tissue, 339
   benefits of, 337–338
   introduction, 337
   recommendations, 338–340, 338f
   type and duration of, 339–340
Physiological function, 41–42
Polygenic risk scores, 290
Positive energy balance, 78
   high fructose/glucose diet, 78, 79t
   long-term high fat diet, 78
   short-term high fat diet, 78
Potential analysis techniques, brown adipose tissue (BAT)
   invasive techniques, 29
   noninvasive techniques, 29–30
Pregnant mothers, weight gain in, 268
Primary care, 91
Primary obesity surgery endoluminal (POSE) procedure, 371
   meta-analysis, 371
   metabolic effects, 371
Probiotics, 90
   fecal microbiome transplantation, 90–91
Proinflammatory adipocytokines, 222
Proton magnetic resonance spectroscopy, 121, 177, 177f

R

Racial differences, 266
Regional assessment, 120
Regular physical activity, 321, 323f
Renal parenchyma triglyceride
   excessive kidney fat, clinical implications of, 142–143
      after intervention, 143
      cardiovascular diseases, 142
      chronic kidney disease, 142

      implications, 143, 143f
      insulin resistance, 142
   histological characteristics, 139–141, 140f
   imaging-based quantification, 141, 141f
Resistance training interventions, 326–327
   aerobic and resistance training interventions, 327
   chronic disease, prevention and management of, 328–330
   intensity, 327
   mechanisms, 327–328
   visceral and ectopic adipose tissue, 327–328
Respiratory function, 265–266, 265f–266f
Respiratory gating, 103
Roux-en-Y gastric bypass
   adipose tissue
      changes in, 382–383, 382f
      obesity through, 381, 382f
   bile acids, 383, 384f
   class 1 obesity, 387, 387t
   ectopic fat, 385
   mechanisms of, 377–380, 379f
   metabolic and bariatric surgery, 383, 384f, 387
   metabolic benefits after, 386, 387t
   obesity, molecular markers in, 381
   obesity-related comorbidities, 380
   procedure description, 377, 378f
   subcutaneous fat, 386
   visceral fat, 383–385, 384f
   weight loss, 380

S

Secondary and tertiary care, 91–92
Secretory profile, 178f
Sex, 21
   differences, 11–13, 270
      children, 268
   hormones, 198–200
SGLT2 inhibitors, 89
Short-term high fat diet, 78
Signaling pathways, 218–221, 220f
Single bout of exercise, 75–77, 77f
Single-energy CT (SECT), 174
Skeletal muscle, 70
   lipid metabolism, 302–303
Skeletal muscle fat
   fat infiltration imaging, postprocessing and assessment of, 157–159
      MRS, 158–159, 159f
   1H-MR spectra from skeletal muscle, 159–160, 160f
   IMAT fatty infiltration, flexibility of, 151–152
   IMCL, flexibility of, 154–155, 154f
   infiltration, 149–152, 150f–151f, 151t
   intramyocellular lipids, 152–154
   muscle, assess lipids in, 155–157
      Computed tomography (CT), 155–156, 155f
      MRI, 156–157, 156f
Skeletal health, 179–180

Sleep, 340–341
   obstructive sleep apnea (OSA), 341
   recommendations, 341
Sodium glucose cotransporter-2 inhibitors
   action/side effects, mechanisms of, 357–358, 358f
   clinical efficacy, 358
Subcutaneous adipose tissue, 9–11
Subcutaneous fat, 386

T

Terminology, 39–40, 39t, 41f
Thiazolidinediones, 353
Thyroid hormone, 195–196, 196f
T1-weighted MRI, 176
Type 2 diabetes mellitus (T2DM), 108–109, 117, 222–223, 300–301, 301f

U

Ultrasound, 121
Urea cycle dysregulation, 86

V

Very-low-calorie diets (VLCDs)
   bone marrow fat, 303
   calorie restriction, 301–302, 302f
   cardiac lipid deposition, 301–302, 302f
   hepatic ectopic fat, 299–300
   skeletal muscle lipid metabolism, 302–303
   type 2 diabetes, 300–301, 301f
   visceral adipose tissue, 297–298, 299f–300f
Visceral adipose tissue (VAT), 9–11, 9f–10f, 12f, 297–298, 299f–300f
Visceral fat, 283–284, 383–385, 384f
   children and adolescents, 21–22
      abdominal obesity, 22, 22t
      behavioral determinants, 21–22
      chronic stress, 21
      ethnicity, 21
      genetics of, 21
      imaging techniques, 22
      metabolic risk factors, 23
      sex, 21
      waist/height ratio, 22, 22t

W

Waist/height ratio, 22, 22t
Water-fat imaging, 176
Weight
   change, 267–268
   gain, 206–208, 207f
   loss, 208–209, 209f, 380
   regain, 209–211, 210f
White adipose tissue (WAT)
   cortisol, 198, 199f
   growth hormone (GH), 196–197, 197f
   insulin, 193–195, 194f
   sex hormones, 198–200
   thyroid hormone, 195–196, 196f